Assessment of the Spine

Contentment is one part love, one part silliness, and one part emotional rescue. Thanks, Meg, for bringing all three into my life and for your warm encouragement to create our dreams through our shared freedom to learn, act, and teach.

For Churchill Livingstone:

Editorial Director, Health Professions: Mary Law
Project Development Manager: Dinah Thom
Project Manager: Morven Dean
Designer: Judith Wright
Illustration Manager: Bruce Hogarth

Assessment of the Spine

Phillip S. Ebrall **BAppSc(Chiropractic), PhD, FICC**
Senior Lecturer in Chiropractic and Program Leader (Chiropractic) (Acting)
School of Health Sciences, RMIT University, Melbourne, Victoria, Australia

Forewords by

Louis Sportelli DC
President of NCMIC Group, Inc, PA, USA

Phillip R. Donato BAppSc(Chiropractic), CCSP
Chairman, Council of Chiropractic Education Australasia, Adelaide, Australia

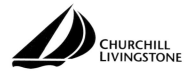
CHURCHILL
LIVINGSTONE

EDINBURGH LONDON NEW YORK OXFORD PHILADELPHIA ST LOUIS SYDNEY TORONTO 2004

CHURCHILL LIVINGSTONE
An imprint of Elsevier Limited

First published 2004

ISBN 0 443 07228 0

British Library Cataloguing in Publication Data
A catalogue record for this book is available from the British Library

Library of Congress Cataloging in Publication Data
A catalog record for this book is available from the Library of Congress

Notice
Medical knowledge is constantly changing. Standard safety precautions must be followed, but as new research and clinical experience broaden our knowledge, changes in treatment and drug therapy may become necessary or appropriate. Readers are advised to check the most current product information provided by the manufacturer of each drug to be administered to verify the recommended dose, the method and duration of administration, and contraindications. It is the responsibility of the practitioner, relying on experience and knowledge of the patient, to determine dosages and the best treatment for each individual patient. Neither the Publisher nor the author will be liable for any loss or damage of any nature occasioned to or suffered by any person acting or refraining from acting as a result of reliance on the material contained in this publication.

The Publisher

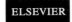 your source for books, journals and multimedia in the health sciences
www.elsevierhealth.com

The publisher's policy is to use **paper manufactured from sustainable forests**

Printed in China

Contents

Foreword

Louis Sportelli

The greater danger for most of us is not
*that our aim is too high and we miss it, but
that our aim is* too low *and we* reach *it!*

Michelangelo

Thankfully, Dr Ebrall has aimed high with his new text,
Assessment of the Spine, and has written a provocative book
which will serve many constituencies seeking to incorporate
any form of manual therapy into their armamentarium.
Chiropractic has now grown in global significance, and today
more educational institutions are located outside the USA, the
birthplace of chiropractic, than in it. This worldwide acceptance
and expansion of chiropractic require a text that is broader in
scope and uniquely specific to provide a global standardization
of approach to spinal assessment.

With the universal expansion of interest in conservative care,
alternative therapeutic applications, and cost-effective approaches
to healthcare, the focus on manual approaches to healthcare
needs requires a text to bring about a comprehensive understanding of the disparate views which exist concerning chiropractic and the universally acknowledged manual approach to
healthcare.

In this text, Dr Ebrall has achieved a level of sophistication,
innovation, insights, observations, and practical, pragmatic, useful approaches to this complex, fascinatingly controversial, and
often misunderstood baseline requirement for the assessment
of the spine.

The author has departed from the traditional teaching of
spinal assessment and may have – by intent, design, or fortu-
itous coincidence – created a minimal set of clinical skills which
must be attained and achieved by every practitioner who desires
to employ a manual approach to patient problems. This universal standard will hopefully be the benchmark against which all
others are measured.

The growing worldwide interest in chiropractic will of
necessity formulate a need for the creation of an evidence-
based benchmark for any practitioner who employs a manual
approach to attain clinical competence in the diagnosis of spinal
dysfunction.

While significant controversy rages within the chiropractic
community and in other professions claiming to employ manual
methods regarding the term "subluxation", this text clearly identifies and demystifies this unique phenomenon. Dr Ebrall has
developed a level of credibility for the term "subluxation complex" and has, with methodical precision, systematically structured the clinical evidence which should be looked for in terms of
components of the model of the vertebral subluxation complex.

Individual chiropractic practitioners, as well as the profession,
have attempted to lay claim to the subluxation complex. In order
to support that claim, it is incumbent upon the profession, and
thus the practitioners, to identify changes in neural function by
spinal levels, as well as changes within the vascular, muscular, and
connective tissues and kinematic changes. Thanks to texts of this
nature, and with a sound foundational basis for the fundamental
understanding of this spinal lesion called a "subluxation complex",
the chiropractic profession will have established its comprehensive protocols and thus rightful claim to develop standards.

While this text may provide a global foundation for chiropractic
skill-sets required to be considered competent, the groundbreaking
concepts will play a pivotal role in chiropractic undergraduate
education. Creating the requirement for evidence-based knowledge to attain the clinical competence determined by the profession, chiropractic will be in a primary position to mandate
educational qualifications.

This book is clearly written by an academic who is truly a
practitioner and who attaches importance to a significant aspect
in any care plan – recognizing that every patient is an individual
with a unique presentation and thus must be provided with the
opportunity for individual management.

There will hopefully be those who disagree with portions of
this text or with conclusions reached by the author. No text
should be without challenge, and undoubtedly this text will
generate spirited discussion, debate, dialogue, and direction for
the chiropractic profession in the prime area of focus.

The profession can be grateful for the incredible effort put into
the development of this text. The aims spoken of by Michelangelo
can be echoed by the words of Ralph Waldo Emerson – "Do not
go where the path may lead; go instead where there is no path
and leave a trail". Dr Ebrall has blazed a new trail.

L.S.

Foreword

Phillip R. Donato

As a student some 20 years ago, although our education and training were thorough and excellent, unfortunately we lacked quality referenced textbooks and resources. Our information was often a conglomerate of lecture manuals and prepared photocopies which students were required to integrate and assimilate. While as students we labored in excitement at this new-found knowledge, nonetheless it took time, organization, and much cross-referencing. From students to professionals, we all know that time, organization, and resource availability are crucial to performance and efficiency.

Thankfully, today's student has greater access to better texts, materials, and resources. Dr Ebrall's *Assessment of the Spine* takes current availability to a further level, providing an encompassing, comprehensive, structured, and integrative approach towards manual assessment of the spine. Rather than students needing to access a variety of resources, much of the information can now be found in one text, which will become a valued and precious commodity for future students.

Ebrall very ably integrates time-honored concepts, principles, and methods with contemporary thinking. There is great input into spinal anatomical information and its applications to both holistic (global) and segmental (detail) considerations. Ebrall has succeeded in extracting and compiling the most current literature and referencing. A pleasing and innovative aspect has been the separation of three spinal regions into smaller regions, allowing a better opportunity for students to grasp and master the various intricacies of the segmental areas.

Once students qualify as practitioners, they will become the portal of entry for patients for the provision of healthcare services. Practitioners must have developed a comprehensive understanding of the human organism, the disease and dysfunction processes that may affect it, examination and assessment, differential diagnosis, and the services that must be rendered with competence.

The education must be both specific and broad so that practitioners not only seek to master their healing art but are also fully cognizant of social and preventive aspects of health, their interrelationship with other members of the health team, and an understanding of their professional limitations.

Public accountability and a demand for safe, competent, and effective practitioners are ever-increasing and become paramount in the delivery of uniform and optimal clinical outcomes. This becomes the ultimate aim for educational institutions in their endeavor to produce practitioners of such ilk who will go forth and serve the community to the best of their abilities. Educational institutions must consider their strategies and provision of resources wisely to enable their students to gain the necessary skills to take on the demands and challenges of practice.

Today's healthcare practitioner faces a great challenge to balance the many aspects of what is considered appropriate and necessary care. This is no easy task – as professionals we need to maintain quality in a cost-conscious way, and yet still need to provide preventive and optimal healthcare solutions.

I am reminded of Stanley J. Bigos MD, Professor of Orthopaedics and Environmental Health, who stated that "traditionally, healthcare practitioners have relied upon assumption-based science providing so-called objective indicators of physiology and function, only to learn that many of these tests and examination findings have selected value, are mostly not reproducible, and at times even fail to accomplish what is expected".

With these thoughts in mind, I implore that we do not become set in our ways and our thinking, that we are receptive and assimilate new information when it arrives. Tradition, passion, experience, intuition, and accumulative observation have a place in our approach to our patients. A solid foundation in our learning is important, but we must be flexible and mature enough to utilize new information when and where applicable.

Furthermore, we must be ready and able to deal with rapidly changing professions, society, and the economy. A useful analogy is a well-founded and solid tree with its roots firmly planted, yet able to adapt to the ever-changing environment; strong and flexible enough to withstand storms, yet able to deliver its outcomes, whether these be fruit, leaves, flowers, oxygen, or simply shade.

On another equally important level, the focus on outcomes directs us to have a patient focus. To this end we need to concentrate on what is important to our patients and their lives rather than the often indirect clinical indicators we have been trained to rely on when making treatment decisions. The public in their quest for the alleviation and prevention of their ailments, and the latest and greatest in healthcare, deserve the best from us.

My congratulations on an insightful and integrative text which challenges all students to do better while reinforcing high and uniform standards of education, competencies, and professional responsibilities.

Although primarily aimed at the chiropractic student, I believe it becomes an ideal text for students of other manual health professions, and equally ideal for existing practitioners to redefine, re-equate, and become aware of current information, applications, and expectations.

P. R. D.

Preface

When you've read this book you'll understand a good many things you don't understand now; but whether it is worth the while going through so much to learn so little, as the charity-boy said when he got to the end of the alphabet, is a matter of taste

(adapted from the words of Sam Weller, written by Charles Dickens).

This book is written for the student who wants to build a comprehensive set of practical skills for the clinical assessment of the spine. All persons claiming to have expertise with the neuromusculoskeletal system must be able to demonstrate the highest level of competency in this field. The intent of this text is to guide the development and attainment of high-order clinical skills to assess the spine for the purpose of better directing therapeutic intervention which restores normal function and health.

The concept of altered spinal function producing negative effects on health seems as old as antiquity. The consideration that this altered function represents spinal subluxation dates from the mid-18th century and was codified as chiropractic in the mid-1890s. The contemporary concept of subluxation implies altered movement within one or more motion units of the spine along with changes in other clinical elements.

The essential premise is that the spinal motion unit (SMU) is the smallest clinical unit of the spine which can be manually assessed. The SMU is defined as two adjacent vertebrae complete with soft tissues. These include the disk, ligaments, and other connective tissues, the neural and vascular structures, and the muscles, which are either intrinsic or extrinsic to the SMU and may either affect its function or indicate dysfunction at a particular spinal level. We therefore have a definable motion unit within the spine with a number of elements which represent clinically identifiable markers or components of the functional spinal lesion or subluxation complex (SC).

This book advances this model of the SC. It describes the essential skills needed to identify and establish the evidence-base required to consider a working diagnosis of SC for each SMU, from occiput–C1 to the sacroiliac joints (SIJs). The reader will learn how to assess each of the elements of the SC in turn and how to consider each from both the subjective and objective perspective in terms of our current understanding of their components.

The process of spinal assessment is the identification and documentation of clinical changes to these various elements. It allows the generation of a diagnosis to guide and direct defendable therapeutic intervention. Further, when changes are identified which are associated with poor health, pain, or other dysfunction, they automatically define the most relevant outcomes measurements for the applied therapy and management.

The chapters of Part 1 describe the components of assessment and the principles which underpin this vital clinical process. The nature of the evidence which must be identified is described – and the preferred clinical methods are presented in order to facilitate the attainment of competency. In turn, competency gives rise to precision, as the ability to obtain similar information of a particular structure or function over time, and to reliability as the ability to return the same finding from the same given set of conditions. This process of assessment includes gathering clinical data from both the subjective and objective perspective.

The chapters within Part 2 build on the basic generic skills presented in Part 1 and apply them to each individual SMU of the human spine and pelvis. The spine is considered as six distinct regions – the upper cervical complex, the mid cervical spine, the cervicothoracic junction, the mid thoracic spine, the thoracolumbar transitional spine, and the lumbosacral spine and pelvis. Each of the six chapters of this part deals with one of these clinically distinct regions, presenting the different critical thinking and clinical decision-making protocols which are unique to the structure and function of each region.

Assessment is incomplete without the documentation of evidence which is supportive of the findings. The reader should appreciate that, while not all clinical evidence can be tested by the scientific method, it must still be recorded. This book attempts to steer a course between the extremes of science and empiricism, and does so with respect for the range of empirical observations gathered and reported from a variety of perspectives. There is also a healthy leaning on the scientific literature, with over 700 individual references, the majority being papers from the contemporary peer-reviewed, indexed literature.

This combined knowledge is essential to help the reader appreciate the rich tapestry of clues available to guide us, as practitioners, in the assessment of our patients. To ignore the accumulated wisdom of over 100 years of documented chiropractic and related practice, and instead rely solely on scientific proof, is to act in a fatally flawed manner. Similarly, to cling to old vitalistic beliefs while ignoring contemporary evidence and society's demand for responsible, accountable practice is to be irrelevant.

There is a happy medium on the continuum between science and empiricism and readers are encouraged to find their own place on it while avoiding the extremes. The clinical skills in this text are intended to form a broad-based foundation and the limitations of restrictive technique constructs or philosophical paradigms are avoided; after all, we are collectively learning to assess the human body, and human anatomy and function remain constant across multiple disciplines, paradigms, and philosophies.

It is essential that spinal assessment is conducted within the context of a comprehensive patient history and a complete physical examination and, where appropriate, diagnostic images of the spine and laboratory reports of the individual patient's physiological and biochemical status. While these skills are learned elsewhere they are reinforced by this text so they may be integrated into the student's total learning package. The components of the clinical record, methods to improve history taking, and the process of diagnosis are presented in Part 3.

Particular attention has been paid to illustrating this text. Every effort has been made to use figures which communicate clearly, and where they do not exist, they have been created. The text is comprehensively illustrated and each spinal segment from C1 to the sacrum is shown. The theories of visual communication have been applied and the illustrations are oriented so they best relate to readers in their role as practitioners. For example, each illustration of a vertebral body in the transverse plane is drawn as if the reader is standing behind the patient, the position from which the spine is assessed.

Assessment is an art, and as such, its skills can be learned. Looking, touching, and listening are also learnable skills, as is the ability to integrate clinical findings and attain an understanding of our patients better to direct their treatment and management. This book is offered as a contribution to assist this learning.

ASSOCIATED READING

This book is but one small part of a practitioner's library. It makes frequent reference to a number of other texts which are, in the writer's opinion, essential works for providing a complete and supportive reference collection for the clinical practice of the disciplines of chiropractic and related manual therapies. Works considered essential associated reading are:

Adams MA, Bogduk N, Burton K, Dolan P 2002 The biomechanics of back pain. Churchill Livingstone, Edinburgh

Cramer GD, Darby SA 1995 Basic and clinical anatomy of the spine, spinal cord, and ANS. Mosby, St Louis, MO

Fuller G 1999 Neurological examination made easy, 2nd edn. Churchill Livingstone, Edinburgh

Herzog W 2000 Clinical biomechanics of spinal manipulation. Churchill Livingstone, New York, NY

Jamison JR 2001 Maintaining health in primary care. Guidelines for wellness in the 21st century. Churchill Livingstone, Edinburgh

Jenkins DB 1998 Hollinshead's functional anatomy of the limbs and back, 7th edn. WB Saunders, Philadelphia, PA

Lumley JSP 2002 Surface anatomy, 3rd edn. Churchill Livingstone, Edinburgh

Taylor JAM, Resnick D 2000 Skeletal imaging atlas of the spine and extremities. WB Saunders, Philadelphia, PA

P. E.
Melbourne, 2004

Editorial advisory board

A text of this nature cannot be written in isolation. I am privileged to enjoy strong support in many ways from my professional colleagues. In particular I wish to acknowledge and appreciate the inspiration, support, advice, and guidance from the following people at various stages of my growth as a teacher and practitioner, and during my journey of preparing and writing this book:

Acknowledgements

Given that this text is written specifically for the student, I am honored to have been guided by a review panel of students from the RMIT Chiropractic program. Their critical and challenging appraisal continues to inspire me as a teacher: Ashley Duffield, Ari Mihailidis, and Simon Brice have all now graduated and are conducting private practice, while Lyndall Daley and Kristin D'Antonio still have a few months to go.

There are some special colleagues who have been generous with their time and whom I also count as friends. Thanks Donald, MAC, Jim, Joe, Meridel, and Annie B. I value your love and your thoughtfulness.

PART 1

Assessment principles and procedures

PART CONTENTS

You only see what your eyes want to see

Madonna & Leonard P 1998 *Frozen*. WB Music Corp.

1

The process of assessment

KEY CONCEPTS

The practitioner does not always see what is there to be seen unless the process of assessment is structured and conducted in a disciplined manner.

There is a specific skills base for the assessor to learn and apply in order to improve the outcomes of clinical assessment.

Touch is an important component of clinical assessment and has its own specific dimensions which must be understood and applied.

The reliability of clinical assessment can be improved by understanding the science of measurement and increasing the critical self-awareness of one's own performance as an assessor.

The process of assessment is influenced by the environment; however, the environment can be managed to improve the assessment outcomes.

The important stages in the clinical assessment process are triage, contextualization, and socioculturalization.

INTRODUCTION

The words of Madonna form an appropriate warning for the practitioner: "You only see what your eyes want to see". Every doctor–patient interaction is preconditioned by past experiences for both the doctor and the patient. The practitioner can be led to see something which is not present, such as a fifth elephant leg (Fig. 1.1), or *not* to see something which *is* present, such as parallel lines (Fig. 1.2). To complicate the situation, there will always be the possibility that the practitioner makes a mistake in his or her own processing of information (Box 1.1).

Similarly, it is easy to ask closed-ended questions which draw simple responses from the patient which support the practitioner's preferred diagnostic hypothesis; it is easy to revert to the mode of "does it hurt when I press here?"; it is easy to adopt

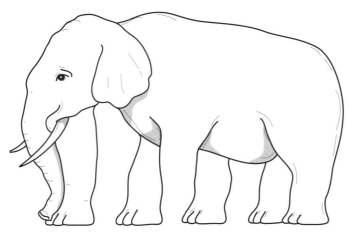

Figure 1.1 How many elephant legs do you see?

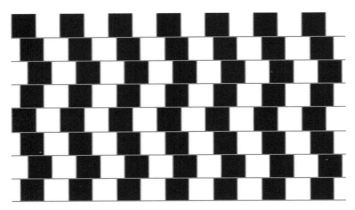

Figure 1.2 Are the horizontal lines sloping or parallel? This image, taken from www.du.edu/~jcalvert/, is a classic optical illusion called "café-wall" believed to have been first published by Hering in *Herman's Handbuch der Physiolog*, vol. 1, p. 372 (1879).

Box 1.1 How reliable are you?

Perform this simple exercise of addition in your mind. Do not use a calculator or pen and paper:

- Take 1000 and add 40 to it.
- Now add another 1000.
- Now add 30.
- Add another 1000.
- Now add 20.
- Now add another 1000.
- Now add 10.
- What is the total?

Your answer is probably 5000. The correct answer is 4100.

---

a commercially marketed technique package in the false belief that it holds all the answers for every patient in every clinical situation – such a panacea clearly does not exist.

The process of assessing the vertebral column is the process of gathering, ordering, interpreting, and managing the clinical status, function, and interaction of the nervous system, muscles,

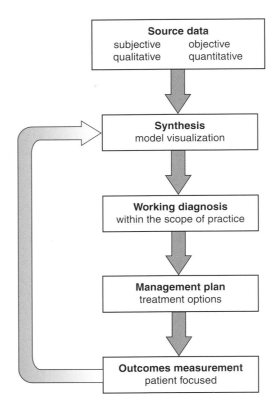

Figure 1.3 Steps in the assessment process.

skeletal components, connective tissues, and vasculature in general and about the spine in particular. It follows five sequential steps (Fig. 1.3), the broadest of which is the collection of the source data. Here the practitioner will elicit information which ranges between subjective and objective, and qualitative and quantitative. It must be noted that subjective is not synonymous with qualitative; neither is objective synonymous with quantitative. The collected data allow a synthesis that reflects the individual practitioner's paradigm of practice. Both the working diagnosis and management plan are a reflection of the practitioner's knowledge and experience.

The management plan is the point at which the patient is presented with the options for care. Any material risk is explained so that the patient may give informed consent. The absence of a management plan and an informed patient represents the most common cause of exposure to litigation for manual healthcare physicians. The identification of relevant patient-focused outcomes measures reflects a blend of outcomes measurements identified in the literature and the personal goals of the individual patient and reflects both the intention of the management plan and the ownership of the patient of his or her own health improvement process. All findings are documented in the common, contemporary language of the clinical professions so they may be understood by all who assess and manage such disorders.

Assessment does not end with the working diagnosis or the management plan. It is ongoing throughout the management of the patient, including the various treatment options, and is used to feed the measured outcomes of intervention back into the active cycle of clinical decision making. The objective is the restoration and maintenance of health.

The concept of altered spinal function producing negative effects on health seems as old as antiquity. The consideration of this altered function being "spinal subluxation" dates from generic medicine of the early 19th century (Harrison 1820). D D Palmer codified the identification and adjustment of spinal subluxation as "chiropractic" in the mid-1890s, and what is believed to be this new profession's first formal text, *Modernized Chiropractic,* published in 1906, described "a subluxated verte-bra" as differing "from normal *only in its field of motion"*, suggest-ing "its various positions of rest are differently located than when it was a normal vertebra and its *field of motion* may be too great in some directions and too small in others" (Smith et al 1906).

THE ASSESSMENT PROCESS

Today, the spinal motion unit (SMU) is widely acknowledged as the location of functional spinal lesions which may be conceptu-alized as a subluxation complex (SC). The stages within the assessment process have now come to reflect clinically identifi-able markers or components of the SC, in particular alterations to posture and kinematics, connective tissue, the nervous sys-tem, musculature, and vasculature.

In the same manner, the steps involved in the assessment process have become more sophisticated and reflect various models of clinical decision making which include *inductive* and *deductive* reasoning. Inductive reasoning is an interpretation based on existing knowledge and is therefore limited by the scope of the knowledge base. Deductive reasoning is based on a hypothesis which, more often than not, is itself derived from inductive thinking. The model of the process of assessment pre-sented in this text (Fig. 1.3) incorporates these modes of think-ing where appropriate and encapsulates them into five defined stages.

Stage 1 – source data

Source data refers to the collection of information gathered in the course of clinical interaction with the patient. It variously includes quantitative and qualitative data which may be gener-ated either within the practitioner's office or externally by other services, such as providers of diagnostic imaging. The source data will also be a mix of objective and subjective data, and cumulatively represent the sum of the clinical knowledge of and about the patient. It must also include knowledge of the indi-vidual diagnostic probabilities which are subsequently associ-ated with the patient.

These data may vary within a short time span as the patient's anxiety decreases or increases during the assessment. It must also be appreciated that these data will vary from one assess-ment to the next, and also that some dimensions will exhibit a diurnal or circadian nature, being cyclically different at various times during a 24-h period. An obvious short-cycle variation is the changing dimension of the thorax with inspiration and expi-ration. Another common example is height, which is typically greater in the morning and lesser in the evening, and there is some evidence that there is also a temporal variation in the size of the sagittal curves of the spine (Ebrall et al 1993).

Stage 2 – synthesis

Synthesis is the process of interpreting and assembling the source data, and is the more active time for inductive and deductive reasoning. The hypothesis draws together existing elements of source data and proposes a resultant which may lie outside the bounds of the practitioner's current knowledge. This is considered to be a hypothetico-deductive process of clin-ical decision making. The more experienced practitioner may also introduce elements of pattern recognition, with the result-ant process of synthesis being an intellectually active interplay of a variety of theoretical decision-making models.

The processes of synthesis is *how the practitioner thinks about and interprets the data,* and this is reliant upon the particular models of visualization used. Regardless of the process of think-ing, the practitioner must have an end-model in mind to work towards. Practitioners typically utilize a model of a spinal lesion or subluxation within the paradigm that structure governs func-tion. The process of visualization within the stage of synthesis is discussed later in this chapter as being an important attribute of the assessment process. The old "bone-out-of-place" model of chiropractic (Forster 1920 pp. 6–39), while grossly inadequate in so many ways, nevertheless remains a useful tool for visualizing the unseen dynamics of the SMU during assessment.

Whilst we have some evidence that C1 and C2 can be imaged in positions of rotation about the *y*-axis (Ebrall & Molyneux 1993), and that lumbar vertebrae will move so as to gap a zygapophy-seal joint (Cramer et al 2000), we don't really *know* that "the spin-ous has moved superior and to the left", or the "right side of the vertebral body has rotated posteriorly". Yet these simplistic con-cepts allow visualization of complex clinical events which we interpret as "findings", to be then constructed into the concept of kinematic change within an SMU. The anecdotal literature (Herbst 1968) argues for the acceptance of this construct as descriptive of any actual kinematic change associated with the SC.

Notwithstanding the questionable nature of the models chosen for synthesis and construction, the practitioner uses this information as evidence for a working diagnosis to explain the clinical condition of the patient. In fact, the purpose of assess-ment is to arrive at a relevant working diagnosis in order to direct intervention and the management plan.

Stage 3 – working diagnosis

The working diagnosis is that considered to be most likely, taken from a list of probable diagnoses constructed during the synthe-sis stage. The list of probable diagnoses is ideally ranked from least to most likely. The practitioner then specifically tests each either to rule it out or rule it in. A working diagnosis should not be a best guess, yet it is difficult for it to be conclusive. The process of testing to allow exclusion or inclusion should be followed until the clinical evidence supports the most likely probability and gives reasons why the others are less likely.

The working diagnosis is best written in a descriptive manner which integrates the key clinical findings into a story which explains what, why, when, and how, and provides a rational series of steps to redress the problem. The processes of con-structing and writing a working diagnosis are discussed in detail in Chapter 17.

Stage 4 – management plan

The management plan is constructed after the working diagnosis to represent the best practice known for the clinical conditions and patient circumstances described in the working diagnosis. It allows for a range of treatment options which may change over time to reflect the nature of the healing process, for example, ice may be used in the early phase of an acute injury, and muscle reconditioning in the later phase of rehabilitation. It is important to appreciate that every intervention is considered a test of the working diagnosis, and consequently the fact that the assessment process is constant and may quite likely require amendments of the management plan to reflect patient response. There is a close relationship between this constant, informal feedback, and that of the final stage, outcomes measurement.

Stage 5 – outcomes measurement

Outcomes measurement is typically conceived as being summative and thus applied at or towards the conclusion of treatment. It is better to view outcomes measurement as a formative indicator of the result of each intervention and the cumulative progress of the patient. The dynamic integration of outcomes measurement precludes formula-driven practice where a cookbook approach is applied to specific presentations. Every patient is an individual with a unique presentation and, while there are broad approaches thought to be better in general cases, the individuality of the patient warrants an individual management plan.

The inclusion of outcomes measures into daily practice is a powerful tool for patient improvement. The information gathered is fed back into the synthesis stage of the assessment process and can thus illuminate the probable diagnoses which were, at an earlier time, excluded as less likely. This feedback loop is a crucial component of a successful assessment process, with the result being a heightened clinical awareness of the patient and the rate of his or her progress towards injury resolution and health.

The art of assessment is to balance data which range from the theoretical to the quantifiable within a context of common descriptive language to arrive at a relevant working diagnosis. The art of treatment is the interpretation of this diagnosis within an appropriate management plan with measurable outcomes. The doctor–patient interaction cycle reflects the standard quality assurance cycle, namely assessment, intervention, measurement, reflection, and reassessment.

It is challenging to learn to coordinate one's senses to assess the patient in a manner which is complete while addressing the broad spectrum of human dysfunction. A staged assessment process, combined with specific attributes of the assessor and applied with a solid skills base, is an important contributor to successful practice.

ATTRIBUTES OF THE ASSESSOR

The underlying concept is that the practitioner must learn to use all senses to see what is *really* there, not just what he or she may *want* to see. This approach broadens the base of clinical interaction in that if one only looked for those findings which

---

Box 1.2 Five attributes of a clinical assessor

These five attributes represent components of a quality improvement process in clinical practice; each may be measured, reflected upon, and improved. The enhancement of individual attributes has a synergistic effect in that the overall improvement of the assessment will be greater than any singular improvement in any one attribute.

- knowing and using appropriate language
- holding a duty of care for the patient
- utilizing subjective and objective data from the qualitative and quantitative perspective
- applying visualization within a constructed paradigm
- recognizing the nature of the constant change of the assessment process.

---

demonstrated high inter- and intraexaminer reliability, one would only see a tiny part of the patient. Similarly, these are those who drift into the esoteric overload themselves with opinions which are peculiar to understand and interpret, and even harder to replicate and justify, again leaving little to work with.

There are five attributes which the practitioner must apply in order to attain competence with patient assessment (Box 1.2). The attributes are expressed as actions and each sits within the specific sociocultural environment of both the doctor and the patient. They represent a triple conjunction of practical skills performance within the biopsychosocial model of pain and disability (Waddell 1998) and the contemporary understanding of practitioners as primary care providers at the leading edge of mind–body medicine (Jamison 1998, 2001).

Appropriate language

The first attribute is an understanding and use of the language of those whom one wishes to become, in this case experts in the assessment, treatment, and management of humans with spine-related disorders. These clinical skills, along with the language which describes and documents the resultant findings, are the skills and the language of chiropractic and related health professions. A Chinese proverb reminds us that *the beginning of wisdom is the ability to call something by its name.*

In this context, language does not refer to the dialect of a particular country or region. Chiropractic's global presence requires that it be practiced in many national and regional languages. The logo of the *European Journal of Chiropractic* is testimony to the profession's multilingual status; the word chiropractic appears in 20 different languages. Similarly, the *Journal of the Canadian Chiropractic Association* carries abstracts in both English and French and the website of the World Federation of Chiropractic offers a choice of three languages (www.wfc.org).

There will always be variation in the shade of clinical language due to socioculturalization; however the core, common professional language is that which students and practitioners alike must come to use for the purpose of standardizing technical terminology. In the case of chiropractic, that which is a "hypertonic splenius capitis muscle" to one practitioner should be a "hypertonic splenius capitis muscle" to another, and so on. The intraprofessional disagreement which exists over the meaning and clinical use of the term "subluxation" is not a language issue; rather it seems to be an attempt by some chiropractic "researchers, academics and others" (Chance & Peters 2001) to appear more understandable to others. The question of where this argument will end was addressed by the editors of the *Chiropractic Journal of Australia*, who ask the question: "if one is exploring uncharted territory, will renaming the landmarks help?" (Chance & Peters 2001).

Duty of care

The second attribute is an understanding and application of the duty of care appropriate for a generalist practitioner who is a primary contact, primary healthcare provider. Primary contact means that any person can seek consultation and treatment at any time by making direct, initial contact without referral from another practitioner or gatekeeper. A primary healthcare provider is one who provides the primary or initial care for a particular presentation. In most of the world's countries practitioners directly accept patients and proceed to provide the majority of them with care.

The duty of care owed by a practitioner to the patient includes the identification of what is most likely ailing the patient and then either referral to a more appropriate provider or acceptance within the paradigm of chiropractic management, and at times both, to comanage the patient. This is the process of triage leading to a working hypothesis and carries the responsibility both to exclude differential problems and to include those most probable. The duty of care continues through the development and application of an appropriate management plan, including treatment, for the most probable problem, in conjunction with the measurement and consideration of the outcomes of the intervention.

The duty of care is broader than the simple identification of spinal lesion or subluxation, which is, in some respects, a technical task performed as one component of patient assessment. The recognition of triage within the duty of care begins to define the contribution of the practitioner and other healthcare providers in public health terms and reflects the societal obligations associated with primary contact status.

Subjective and objective data

The third attribute is an appreciation of the distinctions between subjective and objective findings, and the value of both qualitative and quantitative clinical data. A common characteristic of the healing arts is the need for the practitioner to integrate data from both subjective and objective assessment of the patient. Objective assessment is generally that which can be observed by a third party as well as by the examiner. An example is facet asymmetry at the L5–S1 SMU as seen on the anteroposterior (AP) lumbar plain film.

Subjective assessment derives data from two perspectives: the first is the experience of the patient as reported to the practitioner, and the second is the interpretation of subjective findings by the practitioner. While the raw data which allow objective assessment are more readily defended than that which allows subjective assessment, the individual practitioner's interpretation of these sets of data is similar in both cases. The common element is the internal construction by the practitioner of the findings obtained during specific assessment.

Pain is a good example of a subjective finding, being one which the immediate practitioner and other assessors have to rely on the patient to report and describe. A reliable patient can go a long way towards helping the practitioner construct a chart of the pain experience, but no matter how "objective" this may appear on paper, it remains a document of the patient's subjective perspective. A higher-level example is the nature of end-feel, or the nature of the movement of a spinous process at a particular SMU at the end-range of segmental movement palpation. The statement of findings relies on the internal constructs used by the practitioner to interpret data only the practitioner can feel. The findings are not quantifiable and thus not comparable in the scientific sense with findings from another assessor. This is one reason why the interexaminer reliability of subjective data gained during many clinical assessment procedures may not be strong.

Visualization

The fourth attribute is therefore the development and application of a constructed paradigm within which all findings can be synthesized into a model to direct clinical intervention. The individual nature of data collection suggests that such a paradigm can only be an individualized experience, and while the most common paradigm in contemporary chiropractic is that of the vertebral SC (VSC), it must be appreciated that it may exist in as many forms as there are individual practitioners. Notwithstanding this complexity, the VSC can be considered as a metaphor which includes changed kinematics of or about the spine. There are many testable dimensions associated with the supposition of such changes, and as the metaphor is expanded to include other suppositions, such as changes to connective tissue, the dimensions which can be tested by applying the scientific method from a variety of disciplines increases.

The use of a metaphor in clinical practice is as acceptable as the use of visualization in elite sports. The purpose of visualization is to let the mind of the athlete rehearse specific moves, such as those required for a high dive. The power of the mind is such that, in the few seconds allowed for the actual performance, the diver's body will execute an intricate series of three-dimensional movements, from walk-up to toe-off, rise, half-pike, several twists and turns, and controlled water entry.

Clinical assessment is also a time-limited performance and one in which both participants must feel at ease. Visualization is a powerful tool to drive the performance from the front end, giving a meaning and sense of direction for integrating the many components of the assessment process and the directional changes which may occur as a result of real-time data found during the process. It is also a powerful tool at the back-end of the performance where it is used by the practitioner to construct his or her own belief system for receiving, integrating, and interpreting the found data. Chiropractic is far from unique in being a clinical art driven by belief systems; the history of western medicine and surgery is a story of one belief after another.

Over time the beliefs are tested and, as evidence is gathered, both the belief and the associated clinical behaviors evolve to new beliefs and behaviors. For example, the use of X-radiation essential for clinical radiography has long been considered dangerous (Remier 1957) but it has taken time to understand the cumulative effects (Hall 1994) which suggest the risks to the fetus during pregnancy (Toppenberg et al 1999) and to pediatric orthopedic patients (Bone & Hsieh 2000) are quite small. On the other hand, exposure to radiation and/or magnetic resonance imaging during the period of organogenesis significantly increases malformation in mice (Gu et al 2001) and long-term exposure to ionizing radiation in the environment is both mutagenic and teratogenic (Sviatova et al 2001). Great care must be taken with protective equipment (Zorn 2002).

Health beliefs are also socioculturally dependent. Cigarette smoking remains an acceptable custom in many countries but is legally controlled in others and has become an issue in government-funded health promotion campaigns (Macklin 1993). Others consider smoking to be substance abuse and a risky health behavior (Jamison 2001, pp. 191–192). It was also once believed that extensive bed-rest was the treatment of choice for low-back pain and leg pain; now we know the opposite is true (Waddell 1998).

The role of science is to test belief in a search for that which is repeatable under set conditions, a state humans consider as a truth. The more adept science becomes in understanding biomechanics (Panjabi & White 2001), psychoneuroimmunology (Jamison 1996, Morgan 1998), four-dimensional negentropic energy fields (Freeman et al 2001), and consciousness research and quantum physics (Peters 2001), the closer it will come to revealing the more subtle components and complex effects of the belief that less-than-optimal spinal kinematics have a negative effect on body function, expressed as less-than-optimal health.

Assessment as a constant process

The fifth attribute of assessment is the constant nature of the process. This includes a loop to feedback from the outcomes assessment into the synthesis, thus allowing a constant cycling of monitored data and activities which is, in fact, a quality improvement cycle. Such processes are vital to maintain and improve the quality of patient care. On the more immediate level, the source data are identified and the statement of findings is synthesized in as much of a uniform manner as possible, to allow greater agreement on the subsequent clinical decisions of intervention and management plan. The steps in this process are summarized in Figure 1.4.

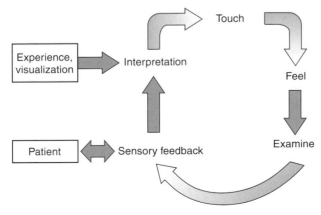

Figure 1.4 The palpation cycle. After Field (2001), with permission.

THE SKILLS BASE

When all is said and done, the science of manual healthcare is essentially the science of applied anatomy and clinical biomechanics, set within the broader context of basic sciences such as biochemistry and physiology. There is no substitute for a deep knowledge of anatomy and a thorough understanding of biomechanics. The anatomy of the human may be learned at five levels relevant to clinical practice: (1) surface anatomy; (2) internal anatomy; (3) neuroanatomy; (4) functional anatomy; and (5) clinical anatomy (Box 1.3).

The practitioner draws from these levels during interaction with the patient to utilize the skill set which best reflects the particular presentation of the patient during the assessment process. At times the skills will focus on surface anatomy, especially during palpation, while at times the practitioner will draw on neuroanatomy to explain altered function, or internal anatomy to create links for further assessment, or functional anatomy to understand a mechanism of injury, or clinical anatomy to develop a suitable rehabilitation exercise. It is therefore evident that a knowledge of anatomy is one thing, while its application to the body so it may be read and interpreted is another.

All senses are used within the process of assessment, the prime being the sense of touch. Palpation is the art of clinical touch and is the mechanism by which the practitioner comes to see deep into the body as the hands and fingers become the eyes. The nature of touch is governed by strong sociocultural influences (Bowers 2000). In western societies there are four levels of touch, as described below.

Box 1.3 A schema of anatomy for practitioners

A high level of competence with surface and internal anatomy is just the starting point for a satisfactory clinical encounter; the fields of neuroanatomy and functional anatomy are the essential elements which must be integrated within the context of the patient to direct intervention and determine the measurable outcomes. The field of clinical anatomy takes the practitioner to the next level to underpin the attainment of effective rehabilitation and patient health.

- Surface anatomy – the road map of the body, for identifying bony landmarks, joint spaces, soft tissues, including muscles and their attachments, and the characteristics of the skin, hair, and nails
- Internal anatomy – visualization of the unseen internal structures, including bones and joints, as well as viscera and vessels, for the purpose of understanding structural and physiological relationships and pathoanatomy
- Neuroanatomy – knowledge of the afferent neural pathways and mechanisms essential for human function, including nociception, pain interpretation, and proprioception; of the efferent pathways for posture, locomotion, and all functioning; and of the reflex pathways between the two and among the autonomic and conscious systems
- Functional anatomy – an understanding of how the parts function as a whole to appreciate mechanisms of injury and strategies for prevention
- Clinical anatomy – an understanding of the clinical interactions among body parts and the principles of treatment, rehabilitation, and recovery.

THE NATURE OF TOUCH

- therapeutic touch
- friendly touch
- familial touch
- sensuous (erotic) touch.

Therapeutic touch, which is the only form of touch appropriate for use in clinical practice, is touch which is deliberate yet gentle, purposeful yet non-invasive. Therapeutic touch is driven by both a knowledge of the structures being palpated and an appreciation of the nature of information being elicited.

The application of therapeutic touch is preceded by an explanation to the patient of the reasons for procedure and the expected outcomes in order for the patient to provide an informed consent to be touched. Touching without informing the patient and gaining consent may be considered as battery, even when the practitioner has the best interests of the patient in mind (Forrester & Griffiths 2001).

Friendly touch, which ranges from the formal handshake to a pat on the back or, in some close friendship groups, a modest hug, is also strongly dependent on the sociocultural environment. In western countries friendly touch is evident in most daily activity but in practice should be limited to a handshake upon greeting a patient. Friendly touch in the Asian context is a very different matter: in Japan touch may be excluded and the greeting in the waiting room is more likely to be a reverential bow; in Indonesia the head of a child is never touched by an adult outside an approved clinical interaction; in South Korea the handshake between males is attended by specific gestures drawn from historical and cultural events.

Familial touch is that which is evident between family members and ranges from the Italian tradition of a kiss on both cheeks to longer and loving hugs, as between parent and child. Familial touch is not demonstrated by the practitioner at any time, even when treating a member of his or her own family. The nature of touch is the mechanism by which a professional boundary is established, and as unwise as it is to manage a family member as a patient, there are times when careful intervention after basic diagnosis may be warranted; on these occasions the practitioner must be careful to exhibit only therapeutic touch.

Sensuous or erotic touch is reserved for persons in an intimate relationship and has no place within clinical practice. At no time should either the doctor or the patient imagine themselves to be in any situation where sensuous touch could be considered. Sensuous touch may occur inadvertently during the assessment or treatment phases and may be initiated, perhaps unknowingly, by the patient. At times the practitioner may feel sexual arousal when with a particular patient. Bowers (1994) describes these feelings as normal and warns that they are the beginning of the "slippery slope" to professional oblivion. The practitioner must be aware of the potential for therapeutic touch to be misunderstood, and always act to maintain the clear professional boundary which is imperative for the successful application of therapeutic touch.

PALPATION

- superficial
- light
- deep.

There are three levels of palpation used for assessment and the art is to move seamlessly back and forth through the levels while maintaining constant communication through touch with the patient. These levels of palpation are applied within a cycle (Fig. 1.4) which includes the actions of feeling and examination, which are acts of touch. The palpation cycle is a positive-feedback loop within the practitioner which is impacted by both the endogenous level of experience and the practitioner's skills of visualization and the exogenous input of the patient. The former reflects the training and competence of the practitioner while the latter reflects the biopsychosocialization of the patient.

A crucial component is sensory feedback and it must be remembered that this is bidirectional; the patient will sense the fear or confidence of the examiner through his or her interpretation of the nature of the touch equally as well as the examiner will receive clinical information. A nervous or insecure examiner will have sweaty, moist hands which do not inspire confidence. The feedback given by the patient will be dependent on his or her tolerance and understanding of their clinical condition and perception of pain. These factors result in the palpation cycle being dominated by both subjective and qualitative elements. It is thus much more of an art than a science. The final component of the cycle is the interpretation of the findings by the examiner, and again this is reliant on both the past experience and the examiner's process of visualization.

Superficial palpation is the introductory touch between the practitioner and patient, and is used to determine the characteristics of the skin, including temperature. The feel of skin changes with age and health status. It may be wet or dry; resilient and able to spring back when pressed, or stodgy and edematous to retain the finger mark characteristic of pitting edema; it may be loose and pliable or taut, like a drum skin. These characteristics are to be noted and explored to determine if they are local effects or a generalized status.

Light palpation is the level of touch appropriate for identifying structures within the skin, such as scar tissue, and in some subcutaneous tissues. Bony landmarks are identified by lightly palpating the tissues around them, and then the landmark itself. This level of touch may move areas of skin and subcutaneous tissue around and over the underlying body structures, and is used for gaining a sense of tissue compliance, preference, and direction. Deep palpation is used to sense and visualize muscle and other structures which lie beneath the subcutaneous tissues. Care must be used with deep palpation to respect the patient's pain and comfort levels.

Exercises to develop touch

Appropriate exercises can be created to develop skill with each level of palpation. The better exercises are those which accompany everyday activities, such as shopping. Superficial palpation can be developed by exploring the textures of labels and various consumer products. The temperature of items throughout the supermarket can be assessed to distinguish those items just taken from a storeroom and placed in a chiller from those which have been chilled for an acceptable period. Light palpation is appropriate in the produce section, especially to select the perfect avocado. Deep palpation is better with a model spine, where increasing layers of cloth or foam rubber can be placed over the spinal segments to replicate skin and muscle, and one's skills can be developed by palpating known structures through such barriers.

Another excellent exercise to develop general palpation skills is to use a disarticulated spine and, with one's eyes closed, arrange the vertebrae in correct sequence purely by palpating each for its shape and structural characteristics. Atlas and the sacrum are easy, but the desired level of achievement is attained when it is possible to palpate the differences between segments such as T9 and T10, and C6 and C7.

RELIABILITY OF ASSESSMENT

The assessment process flows from source data obtained by measurement, and measurement may include the use of an instrument, as with measuring height or blood pressure. The use of an instrument introduces a further suite of questions regarding the level of measurement error, subsuming reliability, accuracy, precision, drift, bias, and hysteresis. It is not the intent of this chapter to explore the intricacies of instrumentation in clinical practice; however, in order to understand the sources of variation in practitioner–patient assessment, several basic concepts must be appreciated.

First, the very act of making a measurement will introduce a change, loosely based on both the Hawthorn effect (Stewart 1972), in which any change in the environment seems to result in a positive change in performance, and the Pavlov's dog effect (Keating 1992b) which conditions the patient for a certain response. The patient's personal environment is invaded by the practitioner and thus it is changed during the process of assessment. Care must be taken to avoid the process creating a positive-feedback loop to the patient regarding his or her clinical behavior.

Second, the basic rule of thumb is that the greater source of error in any measurement arises more from the human interface than from most instruments themselves. The ongoing emphasis in this text is for the practitioner to work toward achieving a higher consistency and thus lower level of error at this interface.

The key dimensions of instrumentation and their relevance to the practitioner–patient interface are:

- level of measurement error
- reliability
- accuracy
- precision
- drift
- positional drift
- temporal change.

Level of measurement error

The level of measurement error is a mathematical expression of the comparative size of the compound error in relation to the quantity being measured, expressed scientifically as coefficient of variation ($V\%$) (Dunn 1989, Ebrall 1992b, He & Oyadiji 2001), and clinically as $\pm$ a unit value. $V\%$ is the size of the error expressed as a percentage of the overall dimension and thus is a value of uncertainty.

For example, a certain method of measuring a patient's height may be tested and found to have $V\% = 0.26\%$. Assuming the many variables associated with height measurement are controlled, this value means a typical human height measurement of 180.55 cm has a level of measurement error of ±4.7 mm, meaning the actual height is somewhere between 180.08 and 181.02 cm. The variables include whether the patient is measured in bare feet or shoes, head position, the landmarks used by the practitioner, the practitioner's ability to locate the same landmark, repeatedly, and so on. When these are taken into the equation it becomes clear that it is better to express clinical values as a range instead of as absolute values.

Further, in clinical terms the size of the error of measurement is often larger than the differences one tries to measure. An example is line drawing on radiographs, where a left/right difference of 1 or 2 mm may be held by some to be significant. Leaving alone the questions of variation due to patient positioning, a dimension as small as 1 or 2 mm may be less than the acceptable level of error of measurement between lines drawn with a soft lead pencil, where the line itself may be 1 or 2 mm wide. Further examples arise from movement palpation where the amount of movement, for example rotation in the lumbar spine, may be as small as 1° or 2° in either direction.

Reliability

Reliability is the characteristic of returning the same measurement of a stable dimension upon repeated use. Given that repeated measurements will provide data with a normal spread about the actual value, the term "reliability" becomes a misnomer in that it will more likely be by chance that two exact values are returned. It is the actual spread of the data obtained on multiple readings which produces the coefficient of variation ($V\%$) as an indicator of the level of error.

In clinical terms, the dimensions are rarely stable, reflecting the dynamic nature of the living human body. The question of intraexaminer reliability may be addressed by standardizing as much of one's technique and processes as possible in order to minimize the variance of the practitioner. The patient will continue to be the greater source of variance and this can be controlled for by careful selection of tests and procedures which provide the greatest isolation of the area of interest from the global patient presentation.

Accuracy

Accuracy is the property that the resultant measurement will bear some semblance to a known scale of values. To be accurate, an instrument used to measure a dimension, for example 30 cm, would be expected to return a group of values around 30 cm. If it returned values around 20 or 40 cm for this dimension it would not be viewed as being accurate. As a quantity, accuracy can be estimated from one reading by an instrument if the value of the dimension is known to some degree.

Precision

Precision is the ability to obtain similar measured values of a stable dimension over time. As such, it is inversely proportional to the level of error. The smaller the level of error, or the more tightly the data from multiple measures of a constant dimension are grouped, the higher the precision of the instrument. The property of precision can only be estimated from a series of readings.

The need for accuracy and precision in clinical assessment is essentially limited to quantifiable dimensions such as those associated with the patient demographics (height, weight) and those vital signs recorded by instrument (blood pressure, pulse, temperature). Fortunately, while the variation in these dimensions may be considerable over time, good-quality instruments, used carefully, are sufficient to obtain a clinically relevant estimate. The questions of accuracy and precision with manual skills become quite complex because the data remain inherently subjective. The quality of accuracy is perhaps the most challenging, as the descriptive measurement scales themselves are subjective.

Instrumentation allows practitioners to quantify dimensions of the patient and thus achieve a degree of accuracy in some findings. These findings should remain similar among different practitioners with common training and using common instruments, allowing good interexaminer reliability.

However, the nature of many patient variables, such as the end-feel of a spinous process, may only be quantified by touch, and the emphasis shifts to intraexaminer reliability. It is important for the practitioner to label successively matching clinical findings, such as end-feel, with the same descriptor, and thus achieve a level of clinical precision. The effective use of palpation to examine the patient requires the highest level of anatomical knowledge.

For example, not only does the examiner need to know that "this is the posterior superior iliac spine (PSIS)", he or she must know the surface texture and shape of the bony structure labeled as the PSIS, the ligaments and fascia which attach to and about it and which may confound palpation, the typical surface area of the landmark and how this may vary with the different types of pelves, and how this landmark may vary in persons of differing somatotypes. The acquired level of qualitative clinical precision reflects the examiner's knowledge of the schema of anatomy (Box 1.3) and supports the observation that the clinical encounter is, in reality, considerably more than applied anatomy and biomechanics and the ability to palpate and label landmarks; it is about understanding and interpreting the compilation of all anatomical, physiological, and biomechanical data relevant to the landmark.

Drift

Drift is the attribute of any group of measured values slowly moving away from the real value. It represents a slow change in accuracy over time and is usually so subtle that it is not noticed until the data are reviewed and it is then realized that the measured value no longer approximates the actual dimension. Drift is controlled by calibration, the act of regularly determining the error level and precision of the instrument. Hysteresis is a parallel characteristic with drift and is the effect of the instrument lagging behind any change in the value being measured. Most clinical instruments marketed today are quite stable with little, if any, drift or hysteresis.

The practitioner is human and also exhibits diurnal variation in the ability to perform clinical skills at a consistent level. The most obvious cause of human drift is a lapse in concentration, perhaps secondary to low blood sugar or breathed-oxygen levels. Less obvious is the drift associated with tiredness or boredom. The wise practitioner will become aware of the manner in which these parameters affect his or her own clinical performance and will learn to control for them, for example, by working for shorter periods between breaks and maintaining a clean-air environment.

Positional drift

Positional drift is an aberration which occurs when the object being measured is placed in different positions within the instrument's envelope of acquisition. The resultant variance in measurements of a known constant dimension demonstrates bias, and this is representative of a systematic error, albeit variable in direction (negative or positive bias).

Systematic errors within manual assessment arise from the natural and often unrecognized bias of the practitioner, including the fundamental characteristic of the dominant hand and eye. Little is known about relationships between the frequency of a particular clinical finding and parameters such as the handedness of the practitioner and his or her philosophical paradigm. It has been said that when one's only clinical instrument is a hammer, then every finding can only be a nail. Handedness is poorly understood and it is only recently that suspicions have been raised that modern interventions, such as diagnostic ultrasound during pregnancy, may be implicated in an increased incidence of sinistrality or left-handedness (Kieler et al 2001). The question of handedness and any relationship between a bias in findings, such as a determination that a spinal segment is found to be "left posterior", has yet to be explored, however, this is a potential element of positional drift.

Temporal change

No matter how experienced the practitioner becomes, he or she will at times be thwarted by the inherent variance among human subjects, particularly those which arise from the patient being in pain. These endogenous effects of living include temporal changes which are emphasized with longitudinal or time-series measurement, and the physiological changes attendant to a living human. For example, if "chest diameter" is the dimension of interest then the physiological variation of the subject may be as subtle as the changes in rib angle which accompany inspiration and expiration. In all cases the practitioner must ensure the patient is consistently prepared on each occasion such measurement is taken, preferably in full expiration. Such variance may be controlled for by consistency in both patient and doctor positioning, which requires a number of steps in the assessment process.

The first step is *awareness*. The second is the application of this awareness during the learning process. All learning exercises should be constructed to challenge the natural comfort zone of students to ensure they are challenged in such a manner that all senses and biases are tested. The third step is a level of critical self-awareness of the practitioner during the performance of these tasks. This can be illustrated by student practitioners realizing that if they were fashion models, or had received basic training in deportment, they would forever more always step out from a standing position by moving the right foot first. The question of *why* does not matter; the reality remains that a model has sufficient self-awareness always to commence ambulation with right-leg toe-off.

Surely the practitioner should have sufficient self-awareness to create a structured performance which accounts for details like handedness, dominant eye, the preferred side of the patient from which to assess, and so on. This level of awareness is crucial for raising intraexaminer reliability, and while a highly systematized and rigid approach to the patient may on the one hand improve reliability, it may on the other hand narrow the clinical options rather than enhance individual performance. Such a narrowing is akin to wearing blinkers and the general rule of thumb for the various technique approaches is that they should challenge the practitioner by increasing the range of options available as opposed to creating a comfort zone by automating responses. The wise practitioner will study many different techniques and build the broadest selection of clinical options better to match treatment with individual patients.

THE PREFERRED ENVIRONMENT

- present-time consciousness (PTC)
- sound
- lighting
- color.

Successful assessment of a patient may only be achieved within an environment conducive to appropriate clinical behaviors and patient compliance. Bowers (1994) emphasizes the contribution a professional environment makes to the minimization of boundary issues for the chiropractic physician. Her work focuses on the maintenance of protective behaviors which are, in essence, microcomponents of the environment in which the doctor–patient interaction occurs. These components include physician and patient clothing and the matters of confidentiality as well as the "place and space" of the interaction.

Present-time consciousness

The greatest asset a practitioner can bring to patient interaction is PTC. This is the aggregation of the practitioner's senses in the absence of external influences or thoughts while working with a patient. PTC has become a buzz-phrase for those who peddle practice-building tips but it simply boils down to the principle of giving the doctor–patient interaction the respect it deserves.

Astute readers will know from their experiences that the art of patient assessment requires a stream of consciousness to be established between the two parties. This relationship is fragile and easily disrupted. The practitioner should arrange for an assistant to intercept phone calls, messages, and other demands during the period of assessment, especially in the initial and establishment phases. The practitioners must also bring self-control to the interaction and ensure their mind is clear of mundane matters. It may appear as a paradox; however, the more successful the practitioner is in relegating non-clinical matters to non-clinical time, the greater the PTC during the clinical action and the more easily the mundane matters will be resolved.

An important factor for maintaining an appropriate level of PTC throughout the practice day is the quality and nature of the air in the clinic environment. Both the practitioner and the patient benefit from breathing clean air of reasonable humidity and at about 21°C. Warmer temperatures induce drowsiness and cooler temperatures challenge the body's automatic regulation of its temperature. Efficient ventilation is required as deoxygenated air induces drowsiness and decreases human performance.

Sound

Background music is appropriate, especially if there is a low level of street noise or the chance of cross-talk between rooms. Much has been written on the psychology of music; however the choice really belongs to the practitioner and must be sensitive to both the sociocultural environment of the practice and the broad characteristics of the patient base. Whenever patients are conscious of the music it could be either that they identify with it in a positive manner or that it is an inappropriate choice, too loud or intrusive. Patient input is valuable and the question of background music can be explored in feedback questionnaires.

Lighting

Lighting is second only to sound for establishing a healing environment. There are many chiropractic treatment maneuvers which require the patient to lie in the supine position, yet how many clinics pay attention to the lighting fixtures? It is quite inappropriate for migraine sufferers to lie on their back and stare at bright fluorescent tubes. The preferred lighting is indirect, and if fluorescent tubes are used they can be hidden in side recesses along each wall, resulting in a diffuse, soft light in the room. There are times during the assessment when control of light is needed, such as when assessing intercostal muscle activity during respiration, and a movable, incandescent light source is a valuable inclusion in each room.

Color

The color of the clinic in general and of the practitioner's rooms in particular is also important. There are various theories on the preferred colors for healing but the basic rule is to avoid strong, primary colors and move toward pastels at the green end of the spectrum. Color coordination is important to convey the psychological image of the clinic to the patient through appointment cards, report stationery, and other documents. The underlying theory is that a peaceful color scheme will assist patients to relax, and a relaxed patient is more cooperative and participatory in the assessment process. If this achievement is able to be conveyed to patients when they are away from the clinic environment, through such devices as an appointment card or patient information sheet, then better in-clinic doctor–patient interaction is more likely to be achieved.

THE ASSESSMENT CONTINUUM

The assessment of a patient should not be considered to be an isolated event; rather it is seen as a point on a continuum which commences when the patient experiences the cause which then drives the appointment for the consultation. There are many opportunities along this continuum, prior to the actual assessment, to gain the confidence and cooperation of the patient. These opportunities include the dialogue of the receptionist who establishes the appointment and the circumstances, including time and payment, under which it will occur. The receptionist also has a vital role to play upon the arrival of the patient to ensure that the patient's mind is free of concerns about cost and other matters.

These hidden dimensions of assessment can be summarized as the process of ensuring the comfort of the patient. Apart from the physical factors such as supportive chairs and current reading material in the waiting room, patient comfort is largely influenced by the processes involved in attaining the initial appointment. If these processes are obstructive, confusing, or poorly organized, the patient can only come to the assessment in a confused and uncooperative frame of mind. It is difficult to assess a patient successfully in such conditions.

The other hidden issues affecting the assessment interaction include matters of the clinic location. In some societies it could be seen as imperative that patients have convenient access to the clinic and its services. In other situations, such as outreach clinics conducted in developing communities, the patients may attend regardless of the degree of personal effort required to travel. Convenience is therefore a sociocultural dimension; in a western city it includes matters such as reliable elevator access in a multistory building, closeness to public transport, and parking spaces without threat of time limits. Patient cooperation during assessment could quickly be tested when the time frame approaches the limits of the parking meter.

Another environmental consideration is the matter of privacy, both for the performance of the assessment, and for the information so obtained. Typically the assessment interaction will be between one practitioner and one patient. It may not be unusual for the practitioner to be assisted by an associate or intern; however, this should be explained to the patient and specific consent obtained. There are some assessment protocols which require a chaperone and, again, these should be explained. The circumstances under which a second party may be present with the patient are those where the patient is a child or adolescent, an older person with unreliable faculties, or one with impaired faculties who is under guardianship. The agreement for privacy of information derived during the assessment must be made and understood by all parties who become involved in the process.

The information derived from patient assessment should remain confidential and private to the patient, although again this is a socioculturally dependent issue. In some communities it is now a legal matter and patient privacy in Australia is mandated under the federal Privacy Act. In other communities the patient's privacy may not be of great importance given the power imbalance granted by the society towards the practitioner.

In general terms and from a broad humanistic perspective, there is benefit in the question of patient privacy being an aspirational issue in order to raise the standard of the clinical interaction. The practitioner should be explicit in informing the patient as to the privacy policy of the clinic and ensure that all staff respect and adhere to this. The ethics of the doctor–patient interaction require confidentiality for matters which are antecedent to the assessment, such as the fact a particular patient has an appointment, and expressly for all matters which are subsequent to the assessment. The patient has the right to be informed of these matters and this can be seen as an act appropriate to facilitating a competent patient assessment.

PRINCIPLES OF ASSESSMENT

- triage
- contextualization
- socioculturalization.

A safety model of practice requires practitioners to have a reasonable idea of what problems they may be facing in conjunction with a knowledge and understanding of the humanistic dimensions of the patient. While the rule of thumb is to expect the unexpected, a more consistent clinical performance can be attained through the application of three basic principles: triage, contextualization, and socioculturalization. Figure 1.5 depicts the commonality of responsibility of all practitioners practicing as primary contact, primary care health providers, and the point at which divergence to various modalities of care is appropriate and defensible.

All practitioners who are registered for primary contact are held under law to be responsible to triage each and every patient to determine the most timely and appropriate provider of care for them. Only when the elements of emergent (such as cauda equina syndrome) and inappropriate (such as meningococcal infection) presentations are ruled out or identified and referred in a timely manner can the manual healthcare physician accept the patient for a program of care. All primary care practitioners share a common responsibility to the point of triage; after this there is a wide variety of both disciplines and subdisciplines which the patient may elect to follow. There are prescribed procedures to achieve effective triage; however, once a patient elects a particular paradigm of care, he or she is subject to the variability of that paradigm. It is therefore difficult – if not impossible – to standardize the processes of contextualization and socioculturalization.

Triage

Triage is the act of receiving and screening the patient better to direct the subsequent intervention. The typical musculoskeletal example is the patient who presents complaining of low-back and leg pain with saddle paresthesia and perhaps loss of control of excretory functions. This is the classic presentation of cauda equina syndrome where surgical intervention may be preferred over manipulation, and where the desired action could be appropriate and timely referral for surgical opinion.

Triage is conducted as a face-to-face interaction with the patient on presentation and is most important given the primary contact status of manual healthcare practitioners, where patients may not preselect themselves as an appropriate musculoskeletal case. Patients reserve the right to present with any ailment of their choosing, and often present with a combination of other complaints which may or may not be better managed with referral to the appropriate specialist, such as a dermatologist for suspicious skin lesions. In some cases patients who are new to a particular practice may complete a questionnaire eliciting details

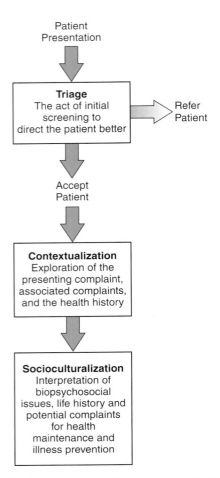

Figure 1.5 The three basic principles of assessment are triage, contextualization, and socioculturalization.

of their present and previous health status. Such instruments may provide some useful information to guide the interaction with the patient but can never be considered as a replacement for the triage process.

The first principle of assessment is therefore the selection and acceptance of patients who may be considered appropriate for clinical intervention in accord with the training of the practitioner, and adequate referral of those who are more appropriate for assessment and intervention by those with more relevant expertise. Triage is an act at the source data level of the assessment process (Fig. 1.5). The second and third principles of contextualization and socioculturalization are ongoing acts at all levels of the assessment process, from source data to outcomes measures.

Contextualization

Contextualization is the exploration by the practitioner of the patient's presenting complaint and seeks to place the complaint within a context which includes temporal and physical dimensions. The temporal dimension includes characteristics such as

acute, subacute, and chronic, as well as the broader life-cycle status of the patient, be it child, adolescent, young adult, adult, or aging. The physical dimensions include those factors which may be causative of the complaint, and these may be exogenous or endogenous to the patient. Endogenous factors are those within the patient and include physical qualities such as osteopenia, while exogenous factors lie outside the patient and may represent the mechanism of injury in cases where the complaint is of traumatic origin.

The required instruments include the history of the presenting complaint, sometimes called an eight-point history, a specific pain history, the health status history, sometimes called a review of systems, and the record of examination, either directed or full physical. These are explored in later chapters.

Socioculturalization

Socioculturalization requires the practitioner to identify and interpret the biopsychosocial issues associated with the patient and his or her specific presentation. These factors include the life history of the patient and allow a judgment of the patient's health locus of control (Härkäpää et al 1991). It has been determined that chiropractors have traditionally practiced in a patient-centered, humanistic manner (Ebrall 2001c) but it is only recently that the importance of this approach has been recognized (Coulter 1991, Gatterman 1995b, 1997). Other complementary disciplines have also been described as also demonstrating patient-centered, humanistic skills (Coulter 2000) and this may be seen as one reason for the increasing use by western health consumers (Micozzi 2001).

The biopsychosocial model of pain identified by Waddell (1998) is a powerful tool for interpreting and understanding where patients have come from in respect to their pain experience. With a little imagination it also becomes a tool to predict where the patient may progress to, and in this manner it becomes enveloped with a higher level of value as a tool to aid wellness and preventive care. Jamison (1996, 1998, 2001) has addressed this issue in detail. If manipulative medicine in general, and chiropractic in particular, are the more relevant forms of the developing mind–body medicine paradigm, then issues of socioculturalization and biopsychosocialism must become a commonplace component of the assessment process.

Socioculturalization can be politicized (Ebrall 2001a) but such ploys are a negative influence at the level of the doctor–patient interaction. Socioculturalization in the clinical sense must be paramount in practice, and sadly, in today's society, it includes issues such as previous exposure of the patient to torture and abuse. It is a covert component of the curriculum in those educational institutions which conduct outreach clinics and activities to expose their students to the realities of the broadest possible patient base. Healing interactions can only occur to their fullest potential in an environment which recognizes and incorporates the patient's social and cultural dimensions. The topic is explored further in Chapter 16.

A final thought on the principles of assessment is for the practitioner to look to find what is *not* there. Often it is the unspoken or the concealed which conveys the more significant information. In this regard the characteristics of eastern philosophy and social behavior hold a salutary lesson for the budding practitioner. It must always be remembered that greater meaning may be conveyed by silence and lack of action, as opposed to words and actions.

SEQUENCING THE ASSESSMENT TASKS

The reality of the primary learning process is that individual tasks must be individually addressed, allowing for task deconstruction and then reconstruction by students to facilitate their progress towards task competence. The individual steps and tasks are typically learned as discrete units, such as "examination of the heart" and "examination of the pulses"; however, they are rarely applied to the patient in such an individual manner.

The secondary learning process is integrative and takes many individual mini-performances and assembles them into the total performance which becomes the doctor–patient interaction. An analogy is the motion picture; a complete story is told through the successful compilation of 24 or so individual frames per second; the movie represents secondary learning while each individual frame represents a primary learning process.

The integration of the essential elements within the secondary learning process is guided by a few basic concepts which may collectively result in a smooth and effective performance package. These concepts demonstrate an awareness of the imbalance of power which exists between the doctor and the patient, and work towards building a cooperative compliance within the patient by strategically applying the psychology of human interaction. For example, no human is comfortable standing with the back to a stranger in a close environment. Second, while variations in cultural background result in variations of the size of the personal space envelope, the basic principle remains that confidence and trust are established during face-to-face contact.

The tertiary level of learning occurs in both real time and reflection during practical application in practice. Primary learning is quite straightforward; a muscle test can be taught for a particular muscle and the subtleties of the task can be deconstructed into components such as patient position, doctor position, contact hand, indifferent hand, and so on. These can then be practiced and reassembled into a performance of the singular task. The tertiary process gives meaning to the story. It is continuous learning and represents the combination of theoretical knowledge with the experience of practical application so typical of clinical practice. The essential element at this level is an awareness by the practitioner that every interaction is indeed a learning process.

The outcome is the many assessment tasks are integrated into an "assessment performance" where multiple tasks are conducted to obtain the required clinical findings. The sequencing of tasks given in Table 1.1 is based on minimizing the impact on the patient, who is often in pain and discomfort. The tasks are thus sequenced so as to maximize the patient comfort by grouping tasks which can be performed in a common patient position. The sequence starts in a comfortable face-to-face seated mode which allows the gathering of vital signs and the various oral histories. The preferred seating arrangement is across the corner of a desk, where the practitioner can easily reach around and

Table 1.1 Sequencing of assessment

Position	Some possible assessments
The patient is seated	Vital signs Oral histories
The patient is standing	Posture, gait analysis, range of motion Lower-limb orthopedic Central nervous system testing Spinal assessment (scoliosis)
The patient is seated	Physical assessment of heart and lungs Head and neck Ear, nose, and throat Upper-limb orthopedic and neurological Lower-limb orthopedic and neurological Spinal assessment (cervical and thoracic)
The patient is prone	Segmental spinal assessment Pelvic and lower-limb orthopedic Upper-limb orthopedic Various extensor muscle tests about the neck, upper limbs, trunk, and lower limb
The patient is supine	Physical examination of the chest and abdomen Cardiovascular assessment, including jugular venous pulse pressure Lower-limb orthopedic and neurological Various flexor muscle tests about the neck, upper limbs, trunk, and lower limb

touch the patient to reinforce a question, or the patient can readily stand or move to demonstrate a particular point to the examiner. The process then moves through the application of relevant tests with the patient standing, then sitting, lying prone, and finishing with the patient lying supine and then returning to the seated position for the report of findings.

The challenge with this sequencing is the need to categorize all relevant tests into delivery modes based on patient position. This is compounded by the need for the practitioner's mind to be sufficiently flexible so it may freely range over a variety of activities as opposed to following a strict algorithmic pathway. The student must come to develop mental relationships between those tests which may, for example, be performed seated, and the different clinical information they may reveal. For example, intellectual connections need to be constructed to relate a seated patellar reflex test to the taking of blood pressure in a seated patient. The disparity of some of these connections emphasizes the benefits of lateral thinking and a free-flowing mental process, again in contrast to the rigidity of a list of tests or a cause-and-effect algorithm.

CONCLUSION

Patient assessment is a dynamic process which has multiple layers of interaction and responsibility. The assessment of the patient, particularly for change in parameters such as kinematics, is an act which is fully integrated and sits on both sides of the eventual intervention. Not only should assessment be based on as much evidence as possible, where thorough and accurate documentation is obtained within a context of high intraexaminer reliability, but its close integration in turn creates more evidence of each individual clinical encounter. This is notwithstanding the range of the evidence from subjective to objective, and qualitative to quantitative.

There should be no suggestion of weakness in the inclusion and utilization of such evidence by the practitioner. To the contrary, these skills should be practiced and refined to strengthen interexaminer reliability. The use of defined skills in a controlled clinical environment and the expression of findings in a common language will contribute to this goal. It should be the objective of the practitioner to increase the reliability of the assessment of the human patient through providing a comprehensive, structured approach to gathering evidence and describing it in a consistent manner.

2

The spinal motion unit

KEY CONCEPTS

The functional spinal unit of the biomechanists is a component of the clinician's spinal motion unit (SMU).

Variations in the biomechanical characteristics of the SMU affect its function. The art of clinical assessment is to identify and describe these changes in quantitative and qualitative terms.

Movement within the SMU is in six degrees of freedom and is typically a complex coupled movement with a variable center of rotation.

The SMU is a complex unit of the spine which has an inbuilt intelligence such that it generates a continuous stream of data which manages the position of the spine, protects the spine by sequencing the timely recruitment of supportive musculature, and informs the central nervous system of such developments.

Extremely small displacements of the SMU can dramatically alter the distribution of axial load and other forces, leading to altered function, structural change, and clinical signs and symptoms.

The nervous system is the paramount system of the body; it is responsible for posture and movement through muscle, for proprioception and balance through ligaments as connective tissues, for the senses and visceral function, and the balance between arterial inflow, venous outflow and lymphatic drainage.

There are five dimensions of the SMU which can be clinically assessed; kinematic change, connective tissue change, muscle change, neural change, and vascular change. Any assessment of the spine is incomplete without data for each of these dimensions.

The spinal adjustment is a high-velocity, low-amplitude thrust delivered within the end-zone of the elastic barrier of joint movement.

INTRODUCTION

The functional spinal unit (FSU) was defined in 1978 (White & Panjabi) as the term of choice for a spinal motion segment. It consists of two adjacent vertebrae and the connecting ligamentous tissues. Significantly, it is the smallest segment of the spine that exhibits biomechanical characteristics similar to those of the entire spine. This definition was clarified in White & Panjabi's second edition (1990) by naming the connecting disk as a ligamentous component.

This definition is appropriate for any discussion of spinal biomechanics; however, it is limited in the clinical context by both the specific exclusion of muscle and its restriction to the typical intervertebral complex. Any assessment of the spine beyond its pure biomechanical performance must include the associated musculature and soft tissues, including vasculature. The operational definition must also allow the inclusion of the atypical articulations of the spine and pelvis, particularly the upper cervical and sacroiliac joints, and the symphysis pubis.

An early definition was derived from the German *Bewegungssegment* (literally *movement segment*) used by Junghanns to describe the three-joint spinal motion segment, but it suffered in translation and modification (Gatterman 1995c). A previous operational definition by Schafer (1983) was confined to vertebral segments and was thus termed *intervertebral motion unit*. Gatterman & Hansen's consensus process in the 1990s agreed on the term *spinal motion segment* (Gatterman & Hansen 1994) and this was endorsed by the *Chiropractic Research Journal* Editor's Council (Chance & Peters 2001).

The biomechanical term FSU correctly describes the smallest segment of the spine in which motion may occur as a *unit* consisting of two typical vertebral segments. This term and that derived from consensus within the chiropractic community can be brought together by substituting *unit* for *segment* in the latter. This establishes the contemporary clinical term of choice as *spinal motion unit* (SMU) and it is used in this text to incorporate all relevant articulations of and about the spine.

THE SPINAL MOTION UNIT

The SMU is therefore the smallest *unit* of the entire *spinal* complex in which movement or *motion* can occur in response to action of the associated musculature. Given that the SMU allows movement within the context of normal spinal function, it follows that restrictions in movement may affect spinal function and that such effect may in turn be reversed by removal or correction of the cause of restriction. Triano describes such changes in function as representing an evidence-based manipulable lesion, functional spinal lesion, or subluxation (Triano 2001a, 2001b). He consequently describes spinal manipulation as an act applied to such a lesion with the intention to direct specific forces and biomechanical moments in such a way that the internal mechanical stresses which generate symptoms are reduced (Triano 2001b).

The SMU is thus the target of the spinal adjustment and a thorough knowledge of its components, structure, and function is essential for its assessment. It is not the intent of this text to present the detailed anatomy, neuroanatomy, or biomechanics of the SMU; it is assumed the reader has or is gaining this knowledge at an appropriate level. The following will merely revisit aspects of that knowledge to provide a clinical context relevant to assessment of the spine with the intention to stimulate a greater excitement for and interest in the key sciences which underpin clinical assessment.

As the smallest unit of the complete spinal complex in which motion can occur, the SMU includes both the typical vertebra–vertebra articulations and the atypical atlanto-occipital articulation, the atlantoaxial articulation, the lumbosacral junction of L5 on S1, each sacroiliac joint, and the symphysis pubis. Clinical assessment must also include the articulations of the ribs, both posteriorly about the vertebral segments, and anteriorly about the sternum, manubrium, and clavicles, as these joints may reflect spinal dysfunction, particularly through the upper and mid thoracic regions. The following discussion is a general introduction to a generic SMU in order to establish key concepts. The unique characteristics of each SMU will be presented in the relevant regional chapter.

THE SPINAL COMPLEX

The human spinal complex provides the axis of the body and through its mechanical qualities of rigidity and plasticity provides support and structure while allowing movement. As the central structural axis arising from the foundation of the pelvis, the spinal complex provides attachments for the viscera and extremities, and carries the rib cage which supports and protects the vital organs of the thorax. It houses and protects the brain and spinal cord, allows distribution of spinal and peripheral nerves, and supports the ganglia of the autonomic nervous system. As such the spinal complex can be considered the neural axis of the body.

The rigidity of the spinal complex derives from both form and function. *Form rigidity* is the result of structural design, such as the keystone manner in which the sacrum sits within the pelvis, while *functional rigidity* arises from the ligaments and muscles which provide both intrinsic and extrinsic support. *Intrinsic structures* are those within and about the spinal complex itself, such as the multifidi muscles, while *extrinsic structures* are those away from the complex yet essential for its maintenance of balance, such as the gastrocnemius muscle.

There is little question that altered function within the spinal complex is associated with altered function of the body in a basic manner, such as radiating posterior leg pain arising from nerve root compression and irritation by a posterolateral disk protrusion in the low lumbar spine. The unknown questions, in the scientific sense, revolve around the extent to which minor functional change in the form of the subluxation complex (SC) may affect whole-body function. The chiropractic paradigm as adopted by the World Federation of Chiropractic (WFC) links the SC with compromised neural function which may in turn influence organ system function and general health (Association of Chiropractic Colleges 1996).

The clinical viewpoint is unequivocal: any assessment of the spine is only complete when it is undertaken in the global context

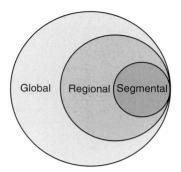

Figure 2.1 Assessment progression. The assessment of the spine commences with a global perspective and moves through a regional assessment to arrive at the segmental level. Examples: (1) whole spine ⇒ lumbosacral spine ⇒ L4–5; (2) whole spine ⇒ thoracic spine ⇒ posterior aspect of left rib 1; (3) whole spine ⇒ upper cervical spine ⇒ right atlanto-occipital articulation.

of the patient. On the one hand the process of assessment is designed to provide information about a particular set of functional dimensions about one or more specific segmental levels of the spine as they interplay within the SMU, while on the other it places this in the context of regional and global spinal function. The rule of thumb for approaching assessment is to think globally, then regionally, then segmentally (Fig. 2.1).

THE TYPICAL SMU

The *typical* SMU consists of two contiguous vertebrae (Figs 2.2–2.4). These vertebrae are bound together by the intervertebral disk and a largely interconnected network of ligaments (Ch. 5). The supportive soft tissues, muscles (Ch. 6), neural components (Ch. 7), and vasculature (Ch. 8) are added to this foundation to form the clinical entity. Similarly, the architecture and relationships of each SMU vary greatly from spinal level to spinal level and these details are specifically described in the regional chapters.

The movement which occurs within each SMU can only occur within the three-joint complex comprising the disk and the bilateral facet joints (Fig. 2.5). Experimental data show that between 60 and 86% of axial compressive load is carried by the disk as forming an anterior column with the vertebral bodies (Giles 1992). The remaining 14–40% of load is shared bilaterally by the articular processes and their facet joints which form paired posterior columns. In the cervical spine the lateral and posterior margins of the disk are supported by uncinate processes arising from the vertebral body which may form synovial joints (of Luschka) with the inferior surface of the body above (Cramer & Darby 1995), thus expanding the single anterior joint to a multiple anterior joint complex in this region. The distribution of the compressive load in the lumbar spine is associated with the lordosis of this region, and as the lordosis increases, the load is distributed more to the posterior annulus and posterior columns (Dolan & Adams 2001).

The response of the SMU to compressive loads is best known for the lumbar region. An increase in the axial compression load substantially increases the intradiscal pressure, facet loads, and disk fiber strains (Shirazi-Adl & Parnianpour 1999). The axial

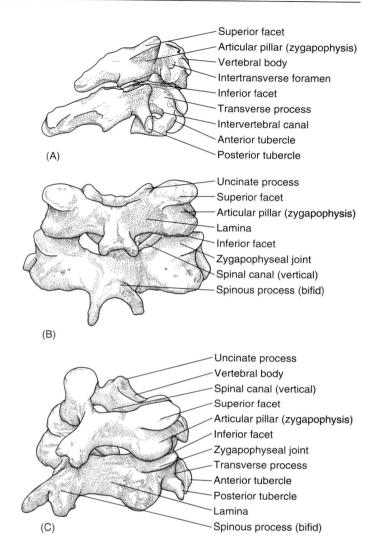

(A)

- Superior facet
- Articular pillar (zygapophysis)
- Vertebral body
- Intertransverse foramen
- Inferior facet
- Transverse process
- Intervertebral canal
- Anterior tubercle
- Posterior tubercle

(B)

- Uncinate process
- Superior facet
- Articular pillar (zygapophysis)
- Lamina
- Inferior facet
- Zygapophyseal joint
- Spinal canal (vertical)
- Spinous process (bifid)

(C)

- Uncinate process
- Vertebral body
- Spinal canal (vertical)
- Superior facet
- Articular pillar (zygapophysis)
- Inferior facet
- Zygapophyseal joint
- Transverse process
- Anterior tubercle
- Posterior tubercle
- Lamina
- Spinous process (bifid)

Figure 2.2 Views of a typical cervical spinal motion unit. (A) Right lateral; (B) posterior; (C) right posterolateral superior.

compression vector is considered to act perpendicular to the plane midway through the disk. Generally it is only the plane of the L3–4 disk which is horizontal, allowing a vertical compression vector, as the other disks are angled to allow the lumbar lordosis (Dolan & Adams 2001).

A resultant shear force is associated with the axial load and angled disk (Fig. 2.6). As the axial load increases, the tensile and compressive strains at the base of the pedicle increase (Hongo et al 1999). This shear force, secondary to compressive load, also produces sagittal rotation of the vertebra, resulting in further stresses in the pedicles and pars interarticularis (Arai et al 1985, Shirazi-Adl & Parnianpour 1999). The shear forces are resisted primarily by a combination of intervertebral disk shear and facet compression or tension (Miller et al 1983).

The clinical relevance is that the anterior shear load in the lumbar spine has been shown to be highly related to the risk of reporting a back injury (Norman et al 1998). The shear stress may lead to injury in the form of small stress fractures within the posterior elements of the SMU (Jayson 1983). The pars has

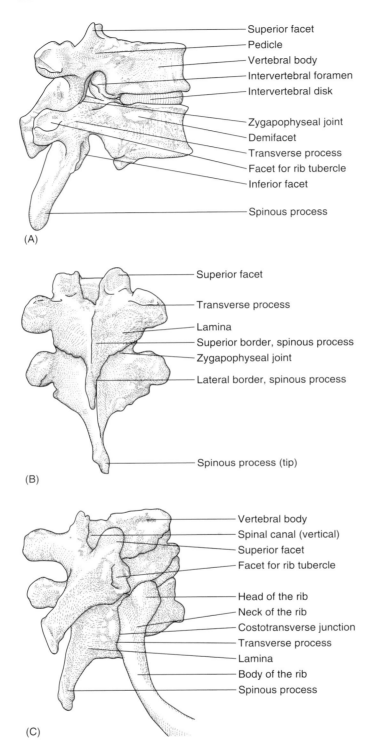

Figure 2.3 Views of a typical thoracic spinal motion unit. (A) Right lateral; (B) posterior; (C) right posterolateral superior.

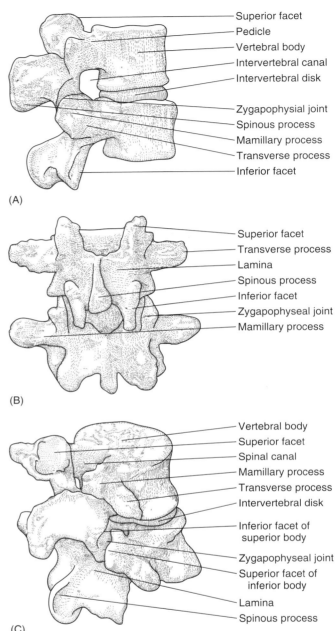

Figure 2.4 Views of a typical lumbar spinal motion unit. (A) Right lateral; (B) posterior; (C) right posterolateral superior.

been shown to be the primary site of failure with increased anterior shear (Yingling & McGill 1999) leading to the clinical entity of a pars defect with *spondylolisthesis*. Within the disk the peak stresses have been observed in the posterior lateral annulus, corresponding to the common clinical finding of posterolateral disk protrusion where herniation has occurred in this region of the disk (Edwards et al 2001).

The zygapophyseal facet joints

The zygapophyseal joints form two of the three joints of the typical SMU. They lie posterior to the column formed by the disk and body combination and can be thought of as a two-part (left and right) posterior column of the spine. The articular processes project superiorly and inferiorly from the junction of the pedicles

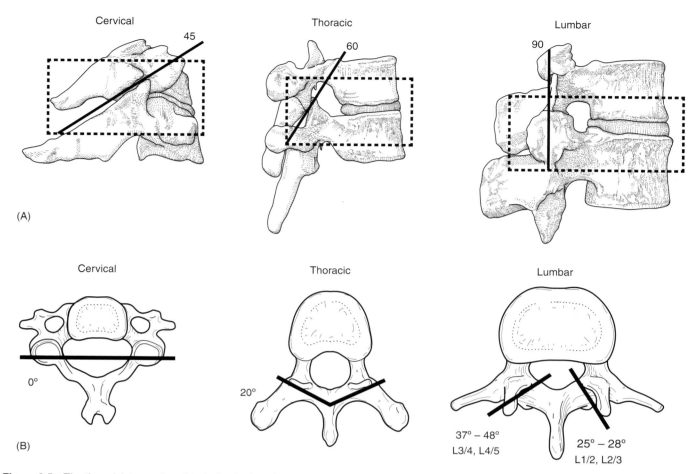

(A)

(B)

Figure 2.5 The three-joint complex of typical spinal motion units, including facet orientation. (A) Sagittal plane; (B) transverse plane – superior surface. Data from White & Panjabi (1990).

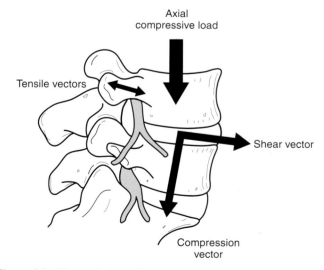

Figure 2.6 Vectors in the spinal motion unit (SMU). The axial compressive load within the SMU creates a shear vector parallel with the disk, leaving a lesser vector of compression. The tensile vectors result from the shear force and are mainly concentrated in the posterior elements. After Sandoz (1976), with permission.

and laminae in the vertebral arch. The superior facet essentially faces posteriorly and the inferior anteriorly; however, their angulation in both the sagittal and transverse planes varies considerably throughout the spine (Fig. 2.5). Their position in the cervical region facilitates great mobility, especially in rotation and lateral flexion, while those in the thoracic region better facilitate flexion and extension. The facet joints in the lumbar spine allow less movement but provide increasing support in the lower levels, especially the control and stabilization of torsional forces (Bough et al 1990). Their angulation is more vertical and sagittal in the upper lumbar spine, moving towards more oblique and less sagittal at the lower levels. This helps to explain why the proportion of compressive load resisted by the lower lumbar facets (around 20%) is about double that of the facets at the higher levels (Adams et al 2002).

The facets in the lumbar spine also exhibit a degree of asymmetry, most notably about the lumbosacral junction, but multiple-level asymmetries are not unknown. Two studies looking for any correlation between facet joint asymmetry and protrusion of the intervertebral disk found there was no significant relationship (Hagg & Wallner 1990, Yu et al 1998); however, it is thought that asymmetry will influence the direction of protrusion from and below L4 as disk protrusion did occur more frequently on the side of a sagittally oriented facet (Yu et al 1998). On the other hand a significant relationship has been found between the degree of facet tropism and far lateral lumbar disk herniation, where the protrusion of the disk is within or lateral to the intervertebral foramen or tunnel (Park et al 2001a).

The zygapophyseal joints are true diarthrodial joints complete with capsule and synovial lining (Giles & Singer 1997) and are richly innervated with both *nociceptors* and *proprioceptors* (Yamashita et al 1990). Parts of the synovial folds project into the joints (Giles & Singer 1997) and intra-articular structures have been identified, including adipose tissue pads, fibroadipose meniscoids, and connective tissue (Bogduk & Twomey 1987, Giles & Singer 1997). The connective tissue is thought to assist in load distribution, and the adipose tissue pads and meniscoids are thought to provide some protection to the articular cartilages as they separate during flexion (Bogduk & Twomey 1987).

The diarthrodial nature of the joint renders it susceptible to degeneration and its mechanosensitive afferent innervation suggests an involvement in pain generation. The biomechanical importance of the facet joints and their capsules is well established, and while they have been considered to be involved in low-back pain for almost a century, it is probably simplistic to consider "facet syndrome" as a reliable clinical diagnosis (Jackson 1992).

The intervertebral canal

The intervertebral canal (IVC) is an integral component of the SMU and is best thought of as a dynamic tunnel or canal as opposed to the traditional foramen. It is bounded by the pedicles superiorly and inferiorly. The anterior boundary is formed by the posteroinferior margin of the superior vertebral body, the intervertebral disk, and the posterosuperior margin of the inferior body. The ligamentum flavum and the superior and inferior facets form the posterior boundary. The canal has sufficient depth for there to be three clearly identifiable zones: the entrance or lateral recess zone, the midzone, and the exit zone defined as the area surrounding the IVC without specific definition of the area itself (Jenis & An 2000). The IVC is angled anterolaterally in the cervical region and obliquely inferiorly in the lumbar region.

The contents of the IVC include the mixed spinal nerve root and the *dorsal root ganglion* (DRG) surrounded by the dural root sleeve and which, in the lumbar region, account for about 30% of the area. They are accompanied by fat, radicular vessels, lymphatic channels, and two to four recurrent meningeal (sinuvertebral) nerves (Cramer & Darby 1995). The canal also contains a variable number of accessory or transforaminal ligaments which form a lattice about the neural and vascular contents and which may be implicated in clinical disorders (Cramer & Darby 1995).

The canal is susceptible to stenosis, typically secondary to degenerative hypertrophy of the zygapophyses and facet joints, loss of disk height, and posterolateral osteophytes from vertebral endplates (Jenis & An 2000). There is also the phenomenon of dynamic stenosis where, in the lumbar region, extension has been shown to reduce the cross-sectional area of the canal by 15% (Inufusa et al 1996). This increased the incidence of nerve root compression within the canal from 21% in neutral to 33.3% in extension (Inufusa et al 1996). The clinical relevance is that dynamic stenosis may result in an intermittent nerve root compression related to positional change during physical activity (Jenis & An 2000).

The spinal canal

The purpose of the spine is to provide osseous protection for the soft neural axis of the body while maintaining structural strength and allowing movement and flexibility. The spinal canal is the vertical space within the spinal column which contains the spinal cord, its protective covering, blood and nerve supply, lymphatic vessels, and adipose tissue. The spinal canal follows the normal contour of the spinal column, and is relatively large and triangular in the cervical and lumbar regions and smaller and more circular in the thoracic regions (Cramer & Darby 1995).

The anterior border is formed by the posterior longitudinal ligament (PLL) adhering to the posterior surfaces of the vertebral bodies and the disk. The PLL commences as a broad band attached to the occiput and remains fairly broad as it descends. It narrows over the centers of the bodies in the thoracic and lumbar spines, and broadens more at the level of the disk. It is firmly attached to the disks and the adjacent portions of the bodies but is fairly loose about the middle of the body to allow small arteries and veins to enter and leave the body (Jenkins 1998).

The lateral borders of the spinal canal are the combination of the pedicles of the vertebra and the opening of the IVC. The pedicles extend to form the lamina which represents the posterior arch which, together with the ligamenta flava, forms the posterior border of the spinal canal. The ligamenta flava consist of the paired ligamentum flavum which runs between the laminae of adjacent vertebrae throughout the spine. They are thinnest in the cervical region and become thickest in the lumbar region. Even though they are paired, they often blend with each other and with the interspinous ligament (Cramer & Darby 1995). The ligament is unique in that is contains yellow-colored elastin which gives it elastic properties and allows it to constrict naturally. Cramer & Darby (1995) note that it may actually do work and assist in extension of the spine. While it is also an elastic barrier to slow the last few degrees of flexion, the most important function of the elastin may be to prevent buckling of the ligament into the spinal canal during extension (Cramer & Darby 1995).

There is a natural variability in the canal/body ratio which, in the cervical spine, is significantly larger in women than in men (Hukuda & Kojima 2002). This may implicate the male prevalence of cervical myelopathy. It remains unclear whether congenital anomalies in the form of transitional vertebrae are associated with a congenitally narrowed canal. Oguz et al (2002) found no relationship while Santiago et al (2001) report that patients with lumbarization showed smaller diameters of the spinal canal. The transitional vertebrae may be a risk factor for lumbar disk herniation (Otani et al 2001); however, a 7-year follow-up study of findings about the spinal canal from magnetic resonance imaging (MRI) were not predictive of the development or duration of low-back pain (Borenstein et al 2001).

The space within the spinal canal may be compromised through a number of mechanisms including trauma, neoplastic processes, infection, prior surgery, or degenerative changes (Daffner & Vaccaro 2002) which result in an intrusion into the space of the spinal canal and thus compromise the contents, including the cord itself, the rootlets or spinal nerve roots. Stenosis is typically symptomatic only in a single spinal region, although it may rarely involve both cervical and lumbar spines (Naderi & Mertol 2002). There are rare causes such as atlanto-axial anomalies consisting of posterior arch hypoplasia in a bipartite atlas with an os odontoideum (Atasoy et al 2002) and the presence of an autologous loose body termed a spinolith (Tambe et al 2002); however, the most common causes are disorders of the ligamenta flava.

The ligamentum flavum may ossify with calcific deposits. While this is a common finding in Japan (Akhaddar et al 2002), it has been reported in Caucasians, being first reported in Australia (Hankey & Khangure 1988) and subsequently in the UK (Arafat et al 1993, Parekh et al 1993), the Netherlands (van Oostenbrugge et al 1999), France (Debiais et al 2000), and Spain (Ugarriza et al 2001). It is rarely found in Blacks (Rivierez & Vally 2001), although the incidence in Blacks is probably under-recognized (Cabre et al 2001). The ossification of the ligament may result in nodules on the ligament and these may also be found on the outer surface of the ligament as well as on the surface within the spinal canal (Mak et al 2002). The ossification may be unilateral or bilateral and the lower thoracic spine is commonly involved (Xiong et al 2001), more frequently in middle-aged men (Shiokawa et al 2001). Ossification of the ligamentum flavum may be associated with osteoblastoma (Okuda et al 2001). It may develop a ganglion cyst (Yamamoto et al 2001), a hematoma (Maezawa et al 2001), or exhibit myxomatous degeneration (Yoshii et al 2001).

A nerve supply, including sensory fibers, has been demonstrated reaching into the ligamentum flavum (Bucknill et al 2002) which suggests it may be a pain generator. The abnormal sensations which occur in the lower extremities of patients with lumbar spinal canal stenosis are thought to result from the failure of coordination between the sympathetic nerve function and somatosensory nerve function (Banzai & Aoki 2001). Stenosis of the spinal canal may require surgical intervention, although spontaneous remissions are thought to occur in some 60% of cases (Mayer 2001) and, while the traditional approach is decompression by open laminectomy, minimally invasive microsurgical techniques have been shown to be safe and as effective as open decompression (Nystrom et al 2001, Guiot et al 2002).

The intervertebral disk

The integrity of the disk is clearly significant to the integrity of the SMU. The maximum value of disk height is found at the L3–4 level in younger adults and at L5–S1 in older adults (Al-Hadidi et al 2001). A database of age-related normative disk and vertebral height values in males and females has been established (Frobin et al 1997). The mean disk height in the lower lumbar spine has been reported at $11.6 \pm 1.8\,mm$ for the L3–4 disk, $11.3 \pm 2.1\,mm$ for the L4–5 disk, and $10.7 \pm 2.1\,mm$ for the L5–S1 disk (Zhou et al 2000). It can readily be appreciated that any decrease in disk height will result in an approximation of the facet surfaces with a concomitant increase in the load carried by each facet joint (Dunlop et al 1984, Dai et al 1992, Luo et al 1996).

A loss of disk height of just 1 mm causes the peak compressive stresses on the articular surfaces of the (lumbar) facet joints to

move from the middle to the upper region in flexed postures, and to the inferior margins in extension or lordotic postures (Dolan & Adams 2001). Under laboratory conditions it has been found that these changes in stress distribution occur with very small movements; just 2° of extension can significantly shift the load to the facets, while just 2° of flexion is sufficient to unload the posterior columns completely (Adams & Hutton 1980).

Similarly, the increase in lumbar lordosis increases the total loading of both the facet joints and the posterior annulus of the disk (Dolan & Adams 2001). It is also known that lateral bending (lateral flexion) will increase the ipsilateral facet load (Buttermann et al 1991). It is little wonder that the greatest risk of back injury seems to be associated with the asymmetrical loading occurring in tasks which combine lifting, causing an increase in compression load, and twisting, which concentrates the load to one side (Cheng et al 1998).

The force and moment changes associated with load redistribution will be accompanied by changes in movement about those joints; however, such change is also mediated by the degree of hydration within the disk (Dolan & Adams 2001). The disk loses water during the day, leading to a mild diurnal decrease in disk height. Dolan & Adams found that a loss of disk height of just 2 mm reduced tension in all collagenous tissues which hold the SMU together and that this slacking was proportionately greater in the short collagen fibers of the annulus than in the longer fibers of most intervertebral ligaments. The result is the annulus is most resistive to bending in the early morning when the disk is fully hydrated (Dolan & Adams 2001).

The findings that disk tissue becomes more elastic as its water content falls suggests that disk prolapse becomes more difficult later in the day. These diurnal changes in the disk also vary the distribution of load among the neural arch, posterior elements, and associated ligaments. The clinical relevance is the need to explore the time of onset of signs and symptoms with the patient, and to explore any diurnal variation in their severity (Adams et al 1990).

A decrease in disk height does not only alter load distribution. Narrowing of the lumbosacral disk space has been shown to result in compression of the fifth lumbar spinal nerve (Briggs & Chandraraj 1995). The mechanism is not "bone on nerve", as historically considered by practitioners; rather it is compression of the neural structures, including the DRG, by additional fibrous bands within the lumbosacral ligament; these appear to develop as a mechanical response to anatomical variation in the region as well as instability (Briggs & Chandraraj 1995). This instability leads to a chain of degenerative changes.

Functional integration

The elements of the SMU should be considered clinically as being integrated, not only in a structural manner but also in a functional manner. Recent evidence demonstrates that stimulation of the nerves within the posterolateral annulus of the disk will elicit reactions in the multifidus and longissimus muscles of the pig (Indahl et al 1997). The ligaments about the SMU are innervated by spinal and autonomic nerves and a direct relationship has been established in humans between the receptors in the supraspinous ligament and the multifidus muscles (Solomonow et al 1998). The multifidii are important stabilizers of the spine, especially in the lumbar region when coactive with their antagonist, the psoas major (Quint et al 1998).

It is also known that the multifidus muscles play an important role in position sense of the lumbosacral spine. When the proprioceptive sensors in the muscle have been distorted by the manual application of vibration to the muscles for 5 s, the repositioning accuracy of human subjects in the sitting position was significantly altered (Brumagne et al 1999). Brumagne et al (2000) also found that multifidus muscle vibration induced a significant muscle-lengthening illusion that resulted in healthy subjects undershooting the target position while subjects with low-back pain actually improved their positioning ability. This suggests an active role for paraspinal muscle spindle afference in controlling spinal position.

The sensitivity of the lumbar spine to sense a change in position has been reported to decrease with fatigue (Taimela et al 1999) and more work needs to be undertaken to explore whether there is a significant difference in trunk repositioning errors in subjects with low-back pain (Newcomer et al 2000a), notwithstanding the findings of Brumagne et al (2000). The manner in which proprioception about the thoracolumbar spine alters in subjects with pain is also being studied (Koumantakis et al 2002). The size and direction of the repositioning error are variable and seem dependent on whether the spine is in flexion or extension (Newcomer et al 2000b).

It is quite evident that there is a bidirectional flow of proprioceptive and other information among the elements of the SMU, including its supportive musculature. Afferents capable of monitoring proprioceptive and kinesthetic information are abundant in the disk, capsule, and ligaments (Holm et al 2002). The muscular excitation is most pronounced at the level of stimulation and has weaker radiation one to two levels above and below (Holm et al 2002). The structures of the SMU are well suited to monitor sensory information and control spinal muscles at each particular level. Holm et al (2002) suggest they probably also provide kinesthetic perception to the sensory cortex. Afferents from the ligaments of the SMU allow direct polysynaptic reflex effects on to ascending pathways and skeletomotoneurones (Sjolander et al 2002). The outcome is the provision of information on movements and posture to the central nervous system (CNS) through ensemble coding mechanisms (rather than via modality-specific neural pathways). This is interpreted by Sjolander et al (2002) as continuous control of muscle activity through feedforward, or preprogramming, mechanisms, as opposed to the concept that there is a threshold beyond which the ligamentomuscular protective reflexes occur in response to potentially harmful load.

This continuous flow of proprioceptive information from the structures of the SMU may explain why human spinal position sense is independent of the magnitude of movement (Swinkels et al 2000). Healthy subjects were able to reposition their spine with considerable accuracy as measured in the laboratory and this ability does not change significantly on a day-to-day basis (Swinkels & Dolan 1998). Even though proprioceptive information flows continuously, there are mechanical neutral zones in the spine where there is an absence of activity in the supporting muscles. Experiments on the cat show that the low lumbar multifidii displacement and tension thresholds are lower for flexion than extension and are triggered earlier in flexion and terminated earlier in extension as the frequency cycle of movement increased (Solomonow et al 2001). This means that the lumbar spine is unprotected by the multifidii for a substantial part of the extension movement and that this zone of weakness increases as the speed of extension increases (Solomonow et al 2001).

The collective understanding of how the spine and its components integrate and function has accelerated over the past decade, yet there is still so much to learn. Practitioners must also continue to read and apply the research findings which are increasingly emerging from labs around the world in an effort to develop and refine clinical models to understand better the SMU and its role in human health and function. Solomonow et al's (2001) model of the neutral zone and the variable decrease in muscular protection of the spine in extension suggests that injury to the SMU has a greater likelihood as the spine is being extended. On the other hand, his team has also demonstrated that prolonged lumbar flexion will elicit spasm in the multifidus muscles (Williams et al 2000) which may also decrease muscular protection of the SMU and allow injury.

There are also new data which do not support the long-held hypothesis that stimulation of the group III and IV muscle afferents sensitive to algesic or inflammatory metabolites increases the stretch sensitivity of muscle spindles via a reflex pathway involving γ-motoneurons (in the cat) (Kang et al 2001). It has been thought that the reflex increase in muscle spindle activity in turn reflexively increased the excitability of α-motoneurons leading to enhanced muscle tone and further accumulation of muscle metabolites and subsequent pain.

What is clear is that the SMU is a complex unit of the spine which has an inbuilt intelligence such that it generates a continuous stream of data which manages the position of the spine, protects the spine by sequencing the timely recruitment of supportive musculature, and informs the CNS of such developments. The premise of spine-centric disciplines such as chiropractic which maintain that normal spinal function is an important element of whole-body function is starting to be seen in a new light.

Degenerative change

Degeneration associated with altered biomechanics has been explored in the clinical context by Kirkaldy-Willis, who developed a schema of the phases of degenerative change. He ordered these as dysfunction, the unstable phase, and the stabilization phase (Kirkaldy-Willis 1992b). It appears this degenerative cycle may commence with minor damage to a vertebral body endplate resulting in inhibited cell metabolism within the disk with subsequent internal disk disruption (Adams et al 2000). Adams et al (2002) have formalized a four-point grading system for the lumbar disk (Box 2.1). The stress profiles found by Adams et al suggest the unstable phase of degeneration is at grade 3, while their grade 4, although particularly variable in its stress response, does become more stable.

The classic paper by Adams & Hutton (1982) associated endplate failure with degenerative change of the disk. They considered it could be sufficiently large to allow nuclear material to enter within the vertebral body (Adams & Hutton 1982). It is now known that the disk can only function normally if the

Box 2.1   A scale of aging and degenerative changes for lumbar disk

Grade 1
Normal disk with defined annular fibers and distinct, intact nucleus pulposus.

Grade 2
Mild degeneration. The nucleus has become fibrous with some brown pigmentation typical of aging; however, the disk structure is intact. While the degeneration is more biochemical than biomechanical, these disks do not distribute loading evenly on to the vertebral body. The stress is usually concentrated posterior to the nucleus.

Grade 3
Moderate degenerative change is seen. Commonly, but not invariably, this takes the form of the annulus bulging into the nucleus, typically associated with damage to the inferior endplate. Structural disruption may also take the form of radial fissures, rim tears, and disk protrusion/extrusion. The distribution of the brown pigmentation is inconsistent.

Grade 4
Severe degeneration with a reduction in disk height secondary to the internal collapse of the annulus, with disruption to one or both endplates. Brown pigmentation is widespread. The narrow disk allows less movement.

From Adams et al (2002), with permission. The personal communication of Dr. Adams, Senior Research Fellow in the Department of Anatomy at the University of Bristol, is acknowledged and appreciated.

endplate is intact (Chandraraj et al 1998). The endplate weaknesses have been attributed to vascular scars (Harris & MacNab 1954) and regression of the notochord (Schmorl & Junghans 1971). Chandraraj et al (1998) traced the fate of vascular canals in the endplate and consider that regression of the canals while the nucleus of the disk was still turgescent could be a cause of vertical herniation and endplate failure in patients up to about the fourth or fifth decade.

It is quite clear that degenerative change is a complex physiological process which occurs at microlevels below simple increases in total compressive load and it is now apparent that the origin of pain is multifactorial and that inflammation probably predominates over merely mechanical mechanisms (Leonardi et al 2002). Factors such as regression of the vascular structures in the vertebral endplates (Chandraraj et al 1998), biochemical changes about the endplates, small redistribution of compressive load among the three columns, and the tensile forces which arise as vectors associated with compressive load may all play a role. It must also be remembered that these events occur within the unique biopsychosocial context of the individual patient.

The process of assessment must attempt to identify and evaluate these hidden dimensions. This is not so easy clinically; however, it is known that degenerative annular change is significantly correlated with decreased disk height in the lumbosacral spine (Vanharanta et al 1988). More recently, an association has been reported between decreased disk height and abnormal (high) signal intensity from MRI and with disk disruptions extending into or beyond the outer annulus (Milette et al 1999, Lam et al 2000, Luoma et al 2001); however, others feel the association may not be reliable (Carragee et al 2000) or has low

predictive value (Smith et al 1998) with respect to discogenic pain. If the MRI findings are indeed representative of painful degenerative changes within the disk, then such changes may be inferred from a finding of decreased disk height as measured from plain radiography.

It is quite clear that changes in the anatomical dimensions of any component of the typical SMU will result in changes to the load distribution among the three-joint complex, in turn altering the biomechanics of motion within the unit. The physical changes, demonstrable on diagnostic imaging, and the resultant biomechanical changes are thought to produce kinematic change which is associated with and predictive of a dysfunctional SMU.

If such kinematic change is real, and science is yet to show that it is not, and if it reflects alterations to the functional characteristics of the SMU, as it is reasonable to predict, then it is entirely plausible that a trained practitioner would be able to form an opinion of the nature of such changes during a controlled assessment of a particular SMU. This proposition is the essence of chiropractic and other disciplines which manually assess the spine. It also underscores the purpose of this text.

BIOMECHANICAL BEHAVIOR

In order to understand the kinematic changes within an SMU which lead to the clinical suspicion of SC one must first understand and appreciate the normal range of expectations. This text will provide a general overview of the generic behavior of a typical SMU and will happily leave the detail to the specialist biomechanists, most notably White & Panjabi (1990), Herzog (2000), Panjabi & White (2001), and Triano (2001a). The behavior of the sacroiliac joints and the other atypical articulations will be discussed in the relevant regional chapters.

Axes and planes

Movement in the body is commonly described in accord with the right-handed Cartesian coordinate system (also known as the orthogonal, international or rectangular coordinate systems), consisting of three straight lines mutually perpendicular and intersecting one another (Panjabi & White 2001). Each line represents an axis about or along which movement may occur. Their point of common intersection is termed the origin and in the human this is typically about the cornua of the sacrum, as shown in Figure 2.7. Any two axes define one of the three planes of the body. The frontal (coronal) plane is defined by the x- and y-axes, the sagittal by the y- and z-axes, and the transverse (horizontal) by the x- and z-axes (Fig. 2.7).

The axes as they apply to the typical SMU are depicted in Figure 2.8. In simple terms, movement is either a rotation about an axis, or a translation along an axis. Each movement, either rotation or translation, around or along an axis is considered a degree of freedom, regardless of its direction. Given that a vertebra can rotate around any of the three axes as well as translate along any of the three, it is said to have six degrees of freedom. The actual movement within an SMU is typically a *coupled* movement about or along one or more axes requiring the generation of an instantaneous axis of rotation or center of rotation (Panjabi & White 2001).

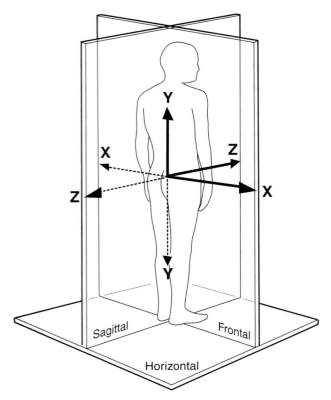

Figure 2.7 Axes and planes of the body. Each plane of three planes of the body is defined by two axes. For example, the frontal plane is formed within the x- and y-axes.

The direction of translation may be positive or negative with reference to the origin. Positive translation is up the *y*-axis, to the left on the *x*-axis, and frontwards on the *z*-axis. Similarly, negative translation is down the *y*-axis, right on the *x*-axis, and backwards on the *z*-axis. Rotation about an axis may also be positive or negative. The convention is to consider oneself at the origin, looking along an axis. Positive rotation is clockwise and negative is counterclockwise (Panjabi & White 2001).

Descriptions of movement

Lateral translation does not commonly occur within an SMU except in the upper cervical spine, where it may be either a left or a right translation, usually of C1 but occasionally of occiput or of C2. In such cases it is termed either *left lateral* or *right lateral*. Forward translation along the *z*-axis is a frontward slippage and is thus termed *anterolisthesis*. A common clinical finding is an anterolisthesis of the body of L5, usually secondary to *spondylolysis* or separation of the pars interarticularis. Posterior translation is *retrolisthesis*. Translation in the *y*-axis results in either an increase in disk height or, more commonly, a decrease in disk height. Chiropractors have long considered such change indicative of disk degeneration (Herbst 1968) and current clinical research confirms this (Vanharanta et al 1988, Milette et al 1999, Lam et al 2000).

Rotation about an axis may be described in many ways, from the formal terminology of the Cartesian system as used by Plaugher (1993), to the clinical terminology used in this text. Movement about the *y*-axis is either *left* or *right rotation* where

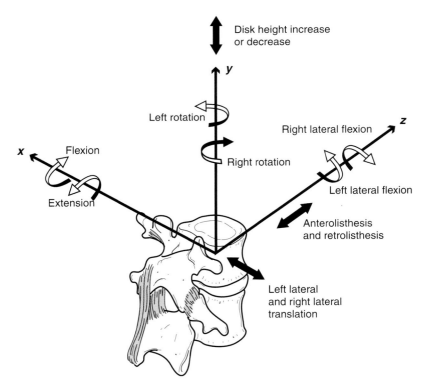

Figure 2.8 Axes and movements of the spinal motion unit (SMU). Movement within the SMU is typically a coupled movement. The components are the pure movements of translation along an axis, and rotation about an axis. After Herzog (2000), with permission.

the front of the patient's body is the reference point. When patients turn to their left they induce left rotation about the y-axis within the SMU.

Forward bending is *flexion* about the x-axis, and backward bending is *extension*. This represents the traditional language of anatomy in which the approximation of surfaces is a movement into flexion. In biomechanical terms some authors differentiate between forward flexion and backward flexion of the spine, where the latter is the return to neutral from a flexed starting point, and extension is backward movement beyond the neutral position to open or separate the anterior surfaces. Forward extension is thus the return to neutral from an extended position.

Movement about the z-axis is commonly considered *lateral flexion,* although some prefer lateral bending. Left lateral flexion is therefore lateral bending to the patient's left, and right lateral flexion is lateral bending to the right, from a neutral starting point.

A simple mnemonic to aid the understanding of the axes is *Why, what's up, Zorro?* "Why" represents the y-axis, which runs "up" (positive) and down, and "Zorro" is the fictional horse-riding swordsman who cut a "z" into the front of his enemies (think of his sword from the front, forming the z-axis into the victim). Naturally, a sword thrust into a victim has a negative outcome (for the victim), thus movement into the body is negative z translation. The unfortunate victim will then fall down, which represents a negative y translation. The remaining axis is, of course, the x-axis.

Sagittal spinal curves

The spinal complex exhibits three clinically relevant curvatures in the sagittal plane. The cervical and lumbar curvatures are *lordotic* and the thoracic curvature is *kyphotic* (Fig. 2.9). Some consider the sacral kyphosis as a fourth curve. The curves are formed by a combination of the shape of the vertebral body and the structure of the disk. These in turn respond to the stress of muscle forces and it is considered that their development coincides with the progression of muscle use in childhood.

Panzer et al (1990) associate the development of the cervical lordosis with the increasing use and strength of the cervical extensor muscles as the child begins to sit and then crawl. A trend has been shown for the bending angles of the cervical lordosis of the fetus in utero to be directly proportional to the overall motility of the fetus (Panattoni & Todros 1989); however, this does not suggest that the lordosis is present at birth. It is known that the occipitocervical lordosis increases at a rate of about 1° per year per level fused until skeletal maturity in children who have undergone arthrodesis about the occipitocervical junction (Rodgers et al 1997). It is also known that in mature humans the cervical lordosis tends to flatten with increasing age, particularly in males, and that this may reflect an increase in the thoracic kyphosis (Boyle et al 2002). The mechanism is thought to be a cranial migration of the cervicothoracic inflexion point (the point where the lordosis meets the kyphosis) from T3 to C7–T1 (Boyle et al 2002).

The lumbar curve is kyphotic at birth and progresses to neutral by about 13 months (Kapandji 1974). The development of the lordosis is associated with the gaining of erect posture (Panzer et al 1990) and becomes identifiable around age 3 or 4

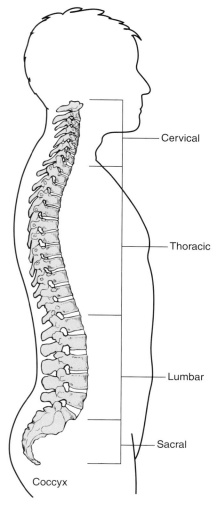

Figure 2.9 The sagittal spinal curvatures. There are four notional curves of the spine in the sagittal plane. Anatomically each is defined by named vertebral segments. Typically there are seven cervical, 12 thoracic, five lumbar, and a collection of sacral and coccygeal segments which form the sacral kyphosis. Clinically, the transition point between the curves is less defined and may vary over several segments. After Adams et al (2002), with permission.

years, reaching the definitive adult state by about 10 years (Kapandji 1974, Keats & Smith 1988). There is little clinical use in attempting to assign typical values to each curve as these values vary widely, as reported in the literature (White & Panjabi 1990, p. 155). It is also thought they vary on a temporal basis (Ebrall et al 1993).

The purpose of the sagittal curves is to provide resistance to axial forces while allowing mobility and flexibility. Harrison et al (2000) have modeled the curvatures of a theoretical ideal spine and demonstrated how such curves allow optimal distribution of axial load. The sagittal curves are dynamic and responsive to intrinsic factors such as pelvic tilt, and extrinsic factors, such as the work-place interface. The cervical lordosis is particularly related to a person's posture and gender (Visscher et al 1998).

Panzer et al (1990) liken the spine to a flexible rod balancing on the sacrum. An anterior tilt of the pelvis, accompanied by an increase in the sacral angle, will increase the lumbar lordosis. This change is compensated for by increases in both the thoracic and cervical curves, and conversely, a decrease in sacral angle will allow a decrease of all curves in the spine. These changes are accompanied by variations in posture and any assessment of the spine is incomplete without an analysis of posture, both static while standing, and dynamic while walking.

Coronal spinal balance

The ideal balance of the spine in the coronal plane is for the skull and vertebrae to be centered over the pelvis, with the scapulae and iliac crests level. This has led to the simplistic depiction of the spine as two coaxial triangles with the sacrum forming an inverted foundation triangle within the pelvis, and the vertebral column forming an elongated triangle balanced on the first. Pragmatically this "ideal balance" is rare and the clinical presentations of posture in the coronal plane are many and diverse, ranging from the mild variances characteristic of the handedness posture (Petty & Moore 2001, p. 42) through a range of postures thought to be associated with muscle imbalance and/or spinal lesion, as described in Chapter 4.

Typically there is a small physiological curve in the coronal plane concave to the left in the upper thoracic region, thought to accommodate the aorta (Panzer et al 1990). All curves are either *structural* and secondary to altered anatomy, such as the presence of a hemivertebra, or *functional* and secondary to either a functional or structural imbalance. As examples, a functional imbalance may arise from hypertonicity of the paraspinal musculature along one side of the spine, causing an ipsilateral concave curve. On the other hand, this same curve may be secondary to hypotonicity along the side contralateral to the concavity. Structural imbalance may arise secondary to an anatomical leg-length inequality resulting in a tilt of the pelvis towards the side of the shorter leg. In this case compensatory curves will develop in the spine to bring the center of mass back to the central gravity line.

Curves which become pronounced are regarded as forming a *scoliosis*, either structural or functional, and this necessitates specific clinical protocols for assessment and management. While these curves are seen and measured in the coronal plane, it is a mistake to consider them as two-dimensional. All curvatures of the spine should be considered as three-dimensional and it is of value to imagine an axial view of the spine in order to appreciate the interplay of curves along the full length of the spine. Investigators are now specifically exploring the mechanical properties of the spine by generating three-dimensional load-displacement curves (Panjabi et al 2001).

Much is made of the role of the sacrum as the structural base of the spine; however, Kapandji (1974, p. 92) considers L3 significant in that it acts as a functional relay station for forces transmitted along fibers of the latissimus dorsi and of the spinalis (Fig. 2.10A). This role is appreciated further in the lateral view (Fig. 2.10B), which places L3 at the apex of the lumbar lordosis. Kapandji argues that the ascending iliolumbar fibers of the latissimus (and the thoracolumbar fascia) provide a firm anchor of the lower lumbar segments on to the sacrum, while the ascending fibers of the spinalis muscles arise from L3 and stabilize the column above. Kapandji thus sees L3 acting as a relay station for the stabilization forces, a principle explored clinically by others (Dvořák & Dvořák 1990).

Adams et al (2002) have explored the distribution, direction, and attachments of muscle fibers in this region and hold that L2 is the pivotal stabilizing segment receiving individual fascicles of the multifidus, iliocostalis lumborum, and longissimus thoracis. The major stabilizer of the region is the quadratus lumborum, being always active in flexion, extension, and lateral flexion (Herzog 2000). Its superficial and deep fibers form a diagonal lattice about each side of the lumbar spine involving the 12th rib, iliac crest, and all lumbar bodies (Dvořák & Dvořák 1990). Adams et al (2002) propose a diagonal transmission of force across the lumbar spine from the latissimus dorsi on one side into the gluteus maximus on the other (Fig. 2.10C). These concepts are supported by Barker & Briggs (1999) who propose that the posterior layer of the fascia acts as an intermediary in the transfer of forces in three directions: between the upper and lower limbs, between the left and right sides of the body, and between the abdominal walls and the spine. It is clearly simplistic to reduce such complex arrangements to a left–right balance within a single plane.

The role of muscles in balance and movement about the spine is best considered in three dimensions. Triano's (2001a) description of the spine as a "viscoelastic system of linkages that are mechanically coupled" is highly appropriate. The interplay of forces about the spine results in complex and related displacements along the length of the spine (Triano 2001a). It is incomplete to think that a low right shoulder may be secondary to either an ipsilateral hypotonic upper trapezius muscle or an ipsilateral hypertonic lower trapezius. If considered solely in the coronal plane, the practitioner may see a left head tilt and possibly a mild scoliosis concave to the left by way of compensation. However, assessment in the sagittal plane may reveal that the right shoulder has moved anteriorly and this may be accompanied by anterior head carriage and a straightening of the cervical lordosis. The practitioner must learn to synthesize a three-dimensional interpretation of the patient from data gathered in each of the two-dimensional planes.

In general terms, three-dimensional spinal balance is maintained by the muscles of the trunk and, with reference to the spine, these are considered as lying anterior (spinal flexors), lateral (spinal rotators and lateral flexors), or posterior (spinal extensors). It must also be remembered that, for any muscle to act on a joint or a collection of joints, as in the spine, the corresponding antagonist muscle or muscles must relax. The larger muscles which cross several or many segments are best thought of in the broad regional context and they will be described in this manner in the regional chapters.

The small, intrinsic muscles of the SMU, the rotatores and intertransversarii, have been described as fulfilling the role of creating axial twisting torque within the SMU; however, this role is questioned by Herzog (2000). He argues these muscles are of such small physiologic cross-section and have such a small moment arm that they may not generate forces sufficient to effect movement. The muscles are reported to be highly rich in muscle spindles and Herzog suggests their role is more as length transducers or vertebral position sensors, thus proposing a likely role as proprioceptors for vertebral joint

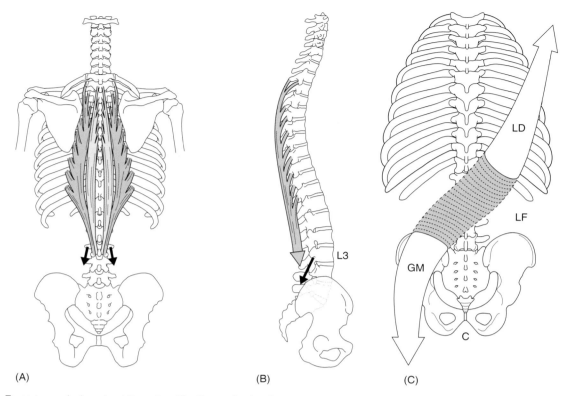

(A) (B) (C)

Figure 2.10 Force transmission about the spine. The thoracolumbar fascia plays a key role in mediating the transfer of loads about the spine. Load can transfer from the upper to the lower limbs, between the left and right sides of the body, and between the abdominal walls and the spine. The mid lumbar spine (L3) and the lumbar fascia (LF) act as relay mechanisms. There is a crossover of forces between the latissimus dorsi (LD) of one side and the gluteus maximus (GM) of the other. (A, B) from Kapandji (1974), with permission; (C) from Adams et al (2002), with permission.

position (Herzog 2000) and contributing to the inbuilt intelligence of the SMU.

Movement within the typical SMU

Three views of a typical SMU from each of the traditional regions of the spine are given in Figures 2.2–2.4. All movement occurs within the three-joint complex of the disk and the two zygapophyseal joints (Fig. 2.5). By convention the superior vertebra is considered the descriptive vertebra with reference to the vertebra below. The two types of pure movement within the SMU are either rotation about an axis or translation along an axis. The major purpose of the facets is essentially to guide movement and this is specifically reflected in their variable design and orientation (Fig. 2.5). The tensile and compressive characteristics of the disk both permit and limit movement.

The six degrees of freedom are given as left or right rotation about each of the three axes, and positive or negative translation along each of the three axes (Fig. 2.8). In the clinical situation, the movement within any SMU is typically a *coupled movement* of rotation and translation which results in a three-dimensional pattern of movement. Understanding the pattern of movement in just one degree of freedom is the start to understanding these complexities in the clinical context.

The Sandoz model of joint movement (Fig. 2.11) is a two-dimensional representation of one degree of freedom within a diarthrodial joint. In that figure, movement is possible to either the left or right of the neutral position. This movement may be left or right rotation about any one axis, or positive and negative translation along any one axis.

The first phase is active movement. This is movement initiated by the patient under either conscious or subconscious neural control. This is the normal movement which occurs tens of thousands of times every day in joints throughout the body and is essential for life. Active movement is limited by the muscles, tendons, and ligaments. There is a degree of resilience in these tissues and they collectively form an *elastic end-zone* or *barrier* which provides a gentle, protective restriction to normal, active movement.

Passive movement is that movement induced by an external force. In the clinical situation the force is provided by the examining practitioner in a controlled manner. Passive movement may commence from either the neutral position or from within the zone of active movement and ends within the region of the elastic barrier. The end-point of the elastic zone represents the summation of the individual elastic characteristics of each soft tissue and will vary to reflect the temporal changes in these tissues. Movement beyond the end-point will damage various tissues, producing a strain/sprain injury. Movement which exceeds the integrity of the soft tissues is traumatic as it moves the joint into its anatomical limits and may result in fracture of the bony components of and about the joint.

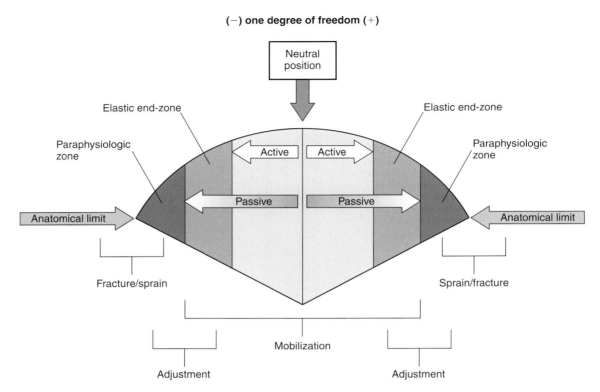

Figure 2.11   The Sandoz model of joint movement. Pure movement is either translation along an axis or rotation about an axis. The movement on one axis, as either translation or rotation, is one degree of freedom. As there are two types of movement and three axes, there is a total of six degrees of freedom within a joint. The nature of the movement within one degree of freedom is either positive or negative from the neutral starting position. There is a quantity of active movement which is restricted by the elastic barrier of connective tissue. Passive movement intrudes into this elastic zone, beyond which is a paraphysiologic space within the anatomical limits of the joint. Joint mobilization is movement into the elastic end-zone, and joint adjustment is rapid movement from deep within the elastic zone into the paraphysiologic zone. Modified from Sandoz (1976), with permission.

Coupled movement

In clinical terms the movement within an SMU is a coupled movement, combining rotation and translation in two or more degrees of freedom and being reflective of the contributions of the disk and facets to the end-result. An example is the end-result of left rotation within the cervical spine. As a cervical vertebra rotates to the left on the vertebra below, the angulation and orientation of the facets are such that the vertebra will rise on the right and move lower on the left. The pure movements are left rotation about the *y*-axis and left rotation about the *z*-axis. The first movement causes the second, and both movements are coupled.

The clinical result is that pure movements are rare and the practitioner is typically required to assess a coupled movement within which the point of reference may describe three-dimensional arcs as opposed to a simple vector. Coupled movement occurs about a constantly changing axis of rotation which is termed the *instantaneous axis of rotation* or the *center of rotation* (Panjabi & White 2001). These findings are evident at all spinal levels, and vary depending on the structure of the particular SMU. White & Panjabi (1990) have reported approximate locations for the instantaneous axis of rotation/center of rotation for the typical SMU in each spinal region. While these data

are useful for researchers, the practitioner simply needs to appreciate that all movement within any SMU is movement within a living system and, as such, has a high level of complexity and variability. For this reason it is as important for the practitioner to assess the *quality of movement* as it is to assesses the *quantity of movement*. The quality is dependent on the integrity of all structures which generate the center of rotation and includes the condition of the disk and its nucleus as well as the articular surfaces of the facet joints.

The center of rotations

The center of rotation for flexion and extension lies to the anterior of the disk and lower body in the cervical spine. This allows maximal opening and closing of the spinous processes which can be observed by palpation. It moves towards the center of the lower body in the thoracic spine and allows a consistent palpatory feeling in both flexion and extension. In the lumbar spine the center of rotation for extension is located towards the posterior disk, closer to the facets, while that for flexion remains at the anterior of the SMU. This finding helps to explain why small movements in flexion and extension can greatly vary the load on the facets in the lumbar spine.

The center of rotation for lateral flexion in the cervical spine is unclear; however, in both the thoracic and lumbar regions it lies to the contralateral side. The elongated nature of the thoracic articular pillars places the center of rotation into the lower vertebra of each SMU, while in the lumbar region it remains in and about the disk and endplates for the reason that, as the upper vertebral body is laterally flexed to the left, the right side of the disk space is opened, allowing the nucleus to move to the right assisted by compression of the left side of the disk. The healthy nucleus is considered to be the pivot point for lateral flexion within the lumbar SMU (Kapandji 1974). An important biomechanical finding with clinical significance is the resultant direction of movement of the spinous process during lateral flexion and the nature of the movement which may be suggestive of the pliability or otherwise of the nucleus within the disk complex.

Movement of the spinous process

In the cervical and upper thoracic spines the spinous process moves contralateral to the side of lateral flexion, namely with left lateral flexion the spinous process moves to the right or away from the regional concavity created by lateral bending. In the lower thoracic and upper lumbar spines the movement of the spinous process may be in either direction, while in the lower lumbar spine it is thought to be ipsilateral: with left lateral flexion the spinous should move to the left and into the concavity of the regional curve (White & Panjabi 1990). In reflecting on their findings, White & Panjabi (1990) considered the variability in the direction of movement to be a result of differences in the specimens used. Panjabi et al (1989) noted that, in the laboratory, the specimens exhibited variations in coupling as the posture changed between full flexion and full extension.

In clinical practice it is observed that the direction of spinous movement in lateral flexion is dependent on the degree of lordosis or kyphosis in the lumbar spine (Pletain 1997). Pletain agrees that in the normal lordotic lumbar spine the spinous process should move into the concavity created by lateral flexion (to the left with left lateral flexion) but states that, when the patient is seated with a slight degree of kyphosis in the lumbar spine, the direction of movement will reverse and move towards the convexity (to the right in left lateral flexion).

Grice (1979) categorized the motion patterns during lumbar lateral flexion as:

- Type I – movement of the spinous *into* the concavity (the spinous moves to the left with left lateral flexion). This is considered by many to be the normal clinical finding in the lumbar spine, notwithstanding the caveat of Pletain.
- Type II – movement of the spinous away from the concavity and into the convexity (the spinous moves to the right with left lateral flexion). This is considered to be the normal clinical finding in the cervical and upper thoracic spines.

Grice (1979) included two further types which essentially describe an individual vertebra breaking the regional pattern by either not laterally flexing (type III) or by moving its spinous in the reverse direction to those above and below it (type IV). Haas et al (1992) report that around half of symptomatic and asymptomatic patients demonstrate type II movement at various levels of the lumbar spine during lateral flexion. What is not known is whether or not the spines used for these studies were normal or if levels of segmental fixation were present in vivo, which could account for such variability of spinous movement secondary to coupled movement within the SMU.

The clinical relevance is that close attention must be paid to the positioning of the patient for assessment of kinematic change in the spine, particularly during lateral flexion. The examiner must maintain control of the patient as he or she is taken though each passive range of movement. It is also worth realizing that the concept of "average" may have little relevance in the clinical context. What is more relevant is the ability to establish what is normal for an individual patient within anatomical, physiological, and biopsychosocial contexts.

Mobilization and adjustment

The clinical act of joint *mobilization* is considered to be movement induced by an external party, the practitioner, which remains within the zone of normal or active joint movement. Mobilization is typically a repetitive movement aimed at rehabilitating the normal ranges of movement for the joint.

The clinical act of joint adjustment is a *high-velocity, low-amplitude* thrust applied by the practitioner within the elastic end-zone of joint movement, as depicted in the Sandoz model (Fig. 2.11). The forces of the adjustment must be finely controlled. They commence deep within the end-zone where the joint surfaces are *open-packed* and maximally separated but still approximated by the elastic resistance of the soft tissues. The adjustive thrust takes the joint beyond the elastic barrier and into the *paraphysiologic zone*. This is the fine region between the passive end of the elastic zone and the commencement of the anatomical limits.

Any force, no matter how small, applied to a muscle will cause the muscle spindles to fire. In the case of the adjustment, there will be low-level firing in the muscles surrounding the SMU during the set-up, and the faster the thrust is applied, the stronger they will fire. The clinical relevance is the need to achieve the force application of the adjustment before the muscle spindle reflex response can loop back. If this reflex response is strong enough there will be a twitch response and if the twitch response happens while the practitioner is still applying the load of the adjustment, it will alter the intended load vectors, perhaps adding or subtracting, depending on which muscles fire.

The safety of the adjustment is derived from its elements of high velocity and low amplitude and these skills represent the essential psychomotor skills of the chiropractic physician. Chiropractic is unique among the numerous health disciplines which assess and treat the spine in that it can be said that the profession is defined by its focus on the adjustment being the treatment of choice for the vertebral subluxation complex.

The characteristics of the adjustive thrust

The duration of the adjustive thrust must be shorter than the twitch response time of the surrounding muscles. A thrust which is longer will cause the muscle to contract during the application of the adjustive load, resulting in a thrust into active, contracting muscle. This decreases the clinical effectiveness of the adjustment and may result in injury to the muscle.

A thrust which is faster than the response time allows maximal separation of the joint surfaces, which is typically accompanied by cavitation of the joint's synovial fluid. Triano (2001a) reports the typical time to peak force application in a series of adjustments throughout the spine as ranging from 32 to 140 ms. If the twitch response arrives after the adjustive force has been applied it may provide a second impulse to the joint, and again this may promote or interfere with the desired treatment effect. Should the neuronal pool activity be inhibited when the muscle spindle activation reaches it, there may be no muscle response at all.

It is also essential for the patient to relax. If the patient is tense and actively contracting muscles about the SMU there will be a splinting effect and that region of the spine will be stiffer, which in turn will attenuate the effective treatment loads as they pass to the spine.

The second safety dimension arises from the control of the magnitude of the thrust. The magnitude is the amplitude of the total force, moment, velocity, or displacement. It is obvious that this must remain well within the anatomical limits of the joint; however, there are numerous other factors which must be considered with regard to the desired vectors. These include the amount of preload applied within the elastic zone, the status of the tissues in the elastic zone as to whether they are normal and healthy or traumatized with inflammation or other disorders including contracture, and the status of those tissues such as the disk which may affect the neural elements. Finally, the practitioner must control the peak force and moment which occur during the thrust phase of the adjustment.

The clinical relevance is the need for the practitioner to develop and maintain a high level of psychomotor skill to ensure the many variables of the adjustment are controlled in order to achieve the intended end-result while maintaining patient safety by limiting potential risk. It is only by a complete assessment of the spine that sufficient clinical information can be obtained or inferred to guide the clinical application of the spinal adjustment safely.

ASSESSABLE DIMENSIONS OF THE SPINAL MOTION UNIT

The purpose of assessing the spine is to determine levels of clinically relevant dysfunction with a view to optimizing therapeutic intervention and management. The concept that dysfunctional levels may be described as an SC allows for the development of a model (Fig. 3.1) which in turn facilitates the identification of those dimensions of the SMU which may be assessed, either in a quantitative or qualitative manner. This model incorporates five clinical dimensions: kinematic change, connective tissue change, muscle change, neurologic change, and vascular change. These dimensions are addressed in holistic terms in the remaining chapters of this part to provide a broad context for each as it relates to the typical SMU and the SC. The chapters in Part 2, which examine each of the six regions of the spine, explore the dimensions in depth as they relate to the individual SMUs described in those chapters.

CONCLUSION

The SMU is the clinical term of choice for the smallest individual unit of the spinal complex. It is highly sensitive to variations in its biomechanical behavior and extremely small displacements of the SMU can dramatically alter the distribution of axial load and other forces, leading to altered function, structural change, and clinical signs and symptoms.

The art of clinical assessment is to identify these changes in quantitative and qualitative terms with the realization that the nervous system is the paramount system of the body and is responsible for posture, proprioception, and balance. It also allows for sensation and visceral function, and balances the arterial inflow with the venous outflow. Recent studies also show lymphatic drainage to be under neural mediation.

Movement within the SMU has six degrees of freedom and is typically a complex, coupled movement with a variable center of rotation. This places greater responsibility on the practitioner to ensure that his or her skills are sufficiently advanced reliably to generate qualitative and quantitative data for this dimension.

The spinal adjustment is a high-velocity, low-amplitude thrust delivered within the end-zone of the elastic barrier of joint movement. It requires a high level of training to achieve the physical characteristics of velocity and magnitude to ensure its safe application in typical presentations. There are well-defined reasons and protocols for assessing the dimensions of the SMU and these are specifically expounded in this volume.

3

The functional spinal lesion

KEY CONCEPTS

The functional spinal lesion (FSL) is any lesion in the spine associated with altered function. The term is commonly used in biomechanics where the altered function is described in terms of altered biomechanical performance.

The subluxation complex (SC) is the preferred clinical term for FSL as it incorporates a number of clinical dimensions beyond simple biomechanical change along with a number of subclinical dimensions.

The most accepted contemporary model of the SC is one which incorporates the clinical dimensions of kinematic change, connective tissue change, muscle change, neural change, and vascular change within a context which acknowledges the subclinical dimensions of biochemical change, inflammatory response, pathological anatomical change, and biopsychosocial considerations.

The term "subluxation" has appeared in the clinical literature since the mid 18th century and was originally used by medical practitioners with an interest in orthopedics. The term became codified into the chiropractic discipline at the start of the 20th century and it has been chiropractors alone who have furthered its understanding and developed the contemporary models.

The SC is an abstract object. It may be understood through the process of visualization and described in the clinical sense by the development of a series of diagnostic statements. Each statement should document both the subjective and objective dimensions believed to be associated with a particular SC as they are manifested in the patient.

The diagnostic statements are gathered in a structure which represents the clinical dimensions within the contemporary model of subluxation. These multiple statements should address the dimensions of kinematic change, connective tissue change, muscle change, neural change, and vascular change. Where technically possible, the statements may also address the subclinical dimensions.

Diagnostic imaging, mainly in the form of plain radiographs, has a role to inform the practitioner of the spinal anatomy as it exists in a particular patient, and to identify functional and pathological change. Given that the SC exists as a functional and physiological entity, it is not evident on radiographs which depict only structure.

There are conventions and protocols for describing the SC as it may be found to exist in a particular patient. These act to "list" the perceived effect of kinematic change in order to direct the preferred therapeutic intervention which is the spinal adjustment, a high-velocity, low-amplitude mechanical input into the SMU.

THE BEGINNING

The concept of altered spinal function producing negative effects on health is as old as antiquity; however, there is little agreement among manual healthcare physicians today as to how to name this phenomenon. In biomechanical terms, a lesion associated with altered function is a "functional lesion" and when it occurs in the spine, the preferred technical term becomes functional spinal lesion (FSL), hence the title of this chapter.

The consideration that this altered function represents spinal subluxation is found in western medical literature from the mid 18th century (Terrett 1987). A discussion of its relationship to the function of the nervous system is found in generic medicine of the early 19th century (Harrison 1820). Harrison was a former president of the Royal Medical and Royal Physical Societies of Edinburgh, and in 1827 published an illustrated text of his observations on spinal diseases. He described subluxation as a "small irregularity in the height, distance, and lineal direction of particular vertebrae in respect to others" (Box 3.1) and considered this type of spinal dysfunction was of "great consequence to future health". He even developed an instrument of brass and leather to assist him manipulate the spine to correct subluxation (Harrison 1827).

Chiropractic's founder, Daniel David Palmer, codified the identification and adjustment of spinal subluxation as chiropractic from the mid-1890s. Any discussion about the spinal subluxation and its role in health and disease should therefore be within the context of the profession which grew from Palmer's efforts. Although Harrison (1827 p. 53) had associated

---

Box 3.1 A discussion of subluxation – 1827

A small irregularity in the height, distance, and lineal direction of particular vertebrae in respect to others is perceptible, on examination, in most delicate females. This disorderly arrangement and disposition of the component parts of the vertebral column, though hitherto overlooking and wholly neglected, are, I am persuaded, of great consequence to future health. The effects of this subluxation, not being distinguishable by the symptoms, have never been traced to their origin in the spine. A very slight and partial compression of the cord, or some of its nerves at their origin, will disturb the organs to which they run … When we take into account the number, the size, and the distribution of the spinal nerves among the viscera and muscles, we are led to conclude that scarcely a complaint can arise in which they do not participate [from p. 11].

As far as relates to my own opinions, it is really of no importance whether it be said that the vertebrae are luxated or displaced. All that I contend for is that the articular ligaments elongate before the vertebrae change their position [Harrison defines the effect of the ligaments, p. 133].

The first takes place when one of the bones is wholly removed from its fellow. The dislocation is then said to be complete, perfect, or entire. In the second, the bones still remain more or less intact with each other. This latter example is denominated and in perfect dislocation, a subluxation, or partial disjunction. Most joints admit of both dislocation and in every degree [Harrison divides luxations into two stages or species].

Paraphrased from Harrison (1827), pp. 11, 133, with thanks to Dr. Donald McDowall.

Box 3.2 A discussion of subluxation – 1906

In case of a simple vertebral subluxation, the vertebra is not lodged in a fixed and permanent abnormal position like the displaced brick in the wall; to consider it so is preposterous for it is a movable bone in a flexible and movable column. A simple subluxated vertebra differs from a normal vertebra only in its field of motion and the center of its field of motion, but because of its being subluxated, its various positions of rest are differently located than when it was a normal vertebra.

A vertebra, because of its peculiar shape, because of its articular cartilages, the intervertebral cartilage above and below it and the muscles and ligaments attached to it, is capable of certain circumscribed movements, and it must, therefore, have a certain definite center of movement just as a wheel has a hub. It is therefore obvious that when a change takes place in the bone itself or when any of the attached muscles, ligaments, or cartilages are changed from normal tonicity, consistency, or tension, the center and also the field of motion of the bone are changed. Like a wheel with its hub off-center, its field of motion may be too great in some directions and too small in others.

By *position of rest* we mean the positions assumed by bones while the body maintains certain poses. If, by subluxation, the center of motion and field of motion are changed it follows that the positions of rest will also be changed from the normal in case of subluxations.

Paraphrased from Smith et al (1906), pp. 24–26, with thanks to Dr. Donald McDowall.

---

altered tone of the body with subluxation, Palmer (1910) specifically related it to altered nerve supply. He became assertive of the concept of tone, so much so that the title page of his seminal collection of writings stated that chiropractic is "Founded on

Tone". Palmer himself said: "I founded the science of chiropractic upon the basic principle of tone" (Palmer 1910 p. 878). His writings emphasized the importance of appropriate tone for optimal human function and the principle of "too much or too little tone" can be accepted as the extension of the founding principle of chiropractic (Ebrall 2001b).

Palmer considered tone to be the neurally mediated health of individual cells and body parts (Keating 1992a). His notion of tone provided a theoretical bridge between vitalism and subluxation, and allowed the dual concepts of either an increase or a decrease in functional tension within the nerve (Keating 1992a). Either would alter the vibration rate of impulse transmission, reflecting a variation of the flow of life force or innate intelligence. Palmer vigorously recommended the spinous process of a subluxated vertebra be used to restore its position and correct the hypothetical cause of presumed nerve interference, thus normalizing neural tone.

The first formal text of the new chiropractic profession, *Modernized Chiropractic,* described "a subluxated vertebra" as differing "from normal only in its field of motion", suggesting "its various positions of rest are differently located than when it was a normal vertebra and its field of motion may be too great in some directions and too small in others" (Box 3.2, Smith et al 1906). The essential concepts up to this time were understood as including small changes in vertebral position, small changes in movement of a vertebra, and an impact on the proper functioning of the nervous system.

BEYOND NERVE IMPINGEMENT

Arthur L Forster MD, DC published the first edition of *Principles and Practice of Chiropractic* in 1915 and an enlarged, second edition in 1920 (Forster 1920). He was a graduate of the Medical Department of the University of Illinois and became Professor of Symptomatology and Diagnosis at the National School of Chiropractic and Editor-in-Chief of the *National Journal of Chiropractic.* He specifically addressed the theoretical basis, anatomical basis, and physiological basis of chiropractic (Forster 1920 pp. 6–46) and wrote in detail on the physiology and functioning of the nervous system and the manners in which it may be compromised, resulting in various clinical presentations.

The depth of Forster's writing was greater than the simplistic subluxation-causes-nerve-pressure concept. He considered the importance of both arterial and venous blood, as well as lymph, to maintain balanced neural nutrition and function, and included a chapter in his book dealing with the internal causes of vertebral malalignment (Forster 1920 pp. 188–198), in which the various reflex arcs were discussed. In essence he introduced the concept that subluxation had associated dimensions other than altered movement causing nerve impingement.

In 1927 the Palmer School of Chiropractic published the *Chiropractic Textbook* written by Ralph W Stephenson, with a second edition some 20 years later (Stephenson 1948). He defined subluxation as "the condition of a vertebra that has lost its proper juxtaposition with the one above, or the one below, or both; to an extent less than a luxation; and which impinges nerves and interferes with the transmission of mental impulses" (Stephenson 1948 p. 320).

Significantly, Stephenson identified a causative role for ligaments and muscles. He suggested an abnormal disk offered "considerable resistance to adjustment" and tended to "misplace the vertebra again"; that abnormal ligaments about the spinal motion unit (SMU) "do not assist much in keeping the vertebrae in normal position, when they are adjusted, until enough time is allowed for them to regain their normal form and texture"; and that "the muscles are the means of subluxations occurring" (Stephenson 1948 pp. 314–315).

DIVERGENT THOUGHT

The prevailing concept at the mid-point of the 20th century was that vertebral subluxation was a disrelationship between two adjacent vertebrae; however, it was considered that the nature of the altered relationship ranged from "minute" (Firth 1948) to "extreme" (Janse 1948a). The need for organized research into the putative clinical entity was clear.

The National (American) Chiropractic Association (NCA) established the Chiropractic Research Foundation (CRF) to "receive money from the sincere and enthusiastic practitioners and also from the friends and patients" (Editorial 1945). The officers of the CRF determined that research would be a funding priority and a National Chiropractic Research Council was formed. Its long-range research program, first presented at the 1944 NCA convention, had a largely biomechanical focus.

The research agenda was set to improve knowledge of postural distortions; the degree to which distortions seen in a particular X-ray exposure were fixed; the nature of any corrective effects produced by various adjustive procedures, using before and after radiographs; and the correlation of individual and multiple distortions with change in function. Contact was re-established with European practitioners, who had been entirely cut off from the USA during World War II.

These developments occurred in the times when Palmer's charismatic son, Bartlett Joshua (BJ) Palmer, had established himself as the chiropractic profession's most vocal spokesperson in the 1920s and 1930s. While advancements were made in understanding and developing the original concepts of Palmer, Firth, and others as the profession spread around the globe, BJ remained insistent there was only one constant of chiropractic philosophy principle. In his final volume, *Our Masterpiece,* published after his death in 1961, he maintained that "disease is only two kinds", either a decrease in the quantity of nerve flow or the inability of the body to function adequately with a decreased flow (Palmer 1966 p. 29).

While acknowledging that his father "discovered" the vertebral subluxation, he effectively halved its potential influence on the body by insisting on the model of occlusion producing impingement causing reduced carrying capacity in neural structures resulting in reduced organ function (Palmer 1966 p. 35). This claim captures the essence of the debate regarding subluxation, which is not so much about whether or not subluxation exists, but quite clearly about its supposed effects and influence on health and disease. Palmer (BJ) maintained a reductionistic constant he called the chiropractic philosophy principle, namely that a vertebral subluxation occluded an opening, producing pressure on the spinal cord or spinal nerves. In turn this interfered with the quantity of transmission of mental impulses between the brain and the body which reduced the energy flow and slowed down tissue cell actions (Palmer 1966 p. 58).

These ideas are not uniquely chiropractic; the medical physician Harrison wrote the following over a century earlier, in 1827:

Distortion of the spine produces an alteration in the canal, and the vertebral holes are necessarily forced into unnatural directions. In consequence of these changes, the tender substance of the cord gets pressed against the hard sides of its sheath. The nervous filaments which issue from it have to travel over a longer course, become unduly stretched, and encounter angles and projections in their way through the bony holes of the vertebra, by which their energies are impaired, interrupted and morbidly affected (Harrison 1827).

THE BROADER VIEW

Other writers took a much broader view of the cause and effect of subluxation. The cause was seen as trauma or muscle contraction (Firth 1948, Stephenson 1948) and other tissues were thought to be involved, including the disk and ligaments (Stephenson 1948) and blood vessels and lymph (Forster 1920). Altered tone was the result of impingement of nerves by the vertebrae, although the neural reflex arc was also implicated (Forster 1920).

Joseph Janse, President of the National College of Chiropractic from 1945 to 1983, argued that the subluxation could be seen as introducing the construct of being a complex of altered components, including neural (impingement), vascular (congestions), and connective tissue (adhesions). His concept of altered movement being an extreme ignored the subtleties inherent in Smith et al's description of 1906. Today's understanding of changes in movement is much broader and will be discussed in Chapter 4.

A contemporary of DD Palmer, Andrew Taylor Still formalized a system of manual medicine he termed *osteopathy*, a discipline with strong parallels to chiropractic in that it emphasizes the importance of homeostasis and balance within the body. Still placed specific emphasis on the unimpeded arterial flow and venous and lymphatic drainage to and from the organs (Coughlin 2001). After Still's death in 1917, osteopathy sought to gain legal, if not philosophic, equality with the allopathic medical profession which had, by then, established itself as the gold standard of medical practice (Coughlin 2001).

While primarily a manipulative profession, osteopaths found manipulation was not cost-effective in a medical system driven by insurance company reimbursements and it is considered that manipulation will become the lost art of osteopathic practice. Coughlin (2001) considers that the current imbalance between the number of osteopaths (40 000) and the number of medical doctors (more than 600 000) in the USA indicates that osteopathic medicine's days as a distinct profession are numbered. Notwithstanding this situation in North America, osteopathy remains a manipulative profession (Gibbons & Tehan 2000) separate and distinct from drug-based medicine in the UK and Australia. The FSL is osteopathy's "local disturbances or lesions of the musculoskeletal system" (Gibbons & Tehan 2000) or its "somatic dysfunction" (Coughlin 2001).

During the latter half of the 20th century a number of medical practitioners explored and published in the field of manual medicine. Most notable are Dvořák & Dvořák (1990) of Europe. They

---

Box 3.3 Components of subluxation – 1995

1 Biomechanical
1.1 Vertebral malposition
1.2 Fixation caused by adhesion
1.3 Fixation caused by meniscoid entrapment
1.4 Fixation caused by nuclear fragmentation
1.5 Disk deformation caused by tissue creep
1.6 Hypermobility and ligamentous laxity
1.7 Mechanical joint locking

2 Neurologic
2.1 Nerve, root, dorsal root ganglion compression or traction
2.2 Spinal cord compression or traction
2.3 Somatosomatic reflexes
2.4 Somatovisceral and viscerosomatic reflexes
2.5 Motor system degeneration
2.6 Psychoneuroimmunology

3 Trophic
3.1 Aberrant axoplasmic transport
3.2 Intraneural microcirculation ischemias
3.3 Macrocirculation ischemias
3.4 Altered cerebrospinal fluid flow

4 Psychosocial
4.1 Placebo effect
4.2 Stress reduction
4.3 Lifestyle modification

Modified from Mootz (1995), with permission.

---

interpret the FSL or SC as a spondylogenic reflex syndrome and have amassed reasonable clinical evidence to support their diagnostic and treatment approaches (Dvořák & Dvořák 1990). Other medical writers (Cyriax & Cyriax 1996, Maigne 1996, Murtagh & Kenna 1997) advocate manual treatment to levels of the spine which are restricted in movement and painful on palpation. These writings, along with those of the noted manipulative therapist Maitland (et al 2001), are devoid of any philosophical construct for the FSL. By way of contrast, the orthopedic surgeon Kirkaldy-Willis writes with chiropractors (Cassidy et al 1992) and osteopaths in the broad field of low-back pain, and has identified dimensions beyond the mechanical which are integral to the successful clinical intervention (Kirkaldy-Willis 1992a).

Palmer (DD) considered the FSL in the form of subluxation to be a physical reality yet, over a century later, science has yet either to demonstrate or disprove its existence. Unless the subluxation concept is discussed in terms of testable dimensions, it can only be considered a metaphor (Keating 1992a, O'Malley 1997). This has value, particularly when the metaphor is expanded to be considered as a complex involving a number of dimensions. Gatterman (1995a) and her contributors summarized the many types of subluxation (Box 3.3) and effectively entrenched the SC as the most accepted model of the subluxation today (Chance & Peters 2001). The further development of our understanding is essentially a refinement of these dimensions and an exploration of each in greater depth.

THE SUBLUXATION COMPLEX

When the SC is thought to exist within the spine and between two or more contiguous vertebrae, it is termed the vertebral

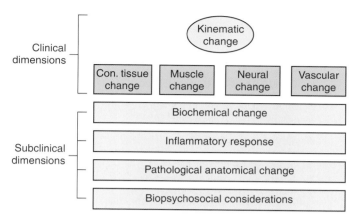

Figure 3.1 A contemporary model of the vertebral subluxation complex. After models developed by Lantz and Gatterman.

subluxation complex (VSC), and when it is thought to exist in the atypical articulations of the spinal complex, such as the sacroiliac joint, it may be considered as a sacroiliac joint SC. The concept of "complex" brings the key dimension of altered movement within the SMU (kinematic change) together with the clinical dimensions of change in the connective tissue about the SMU, change in the musculature which is both intrinsic and extrinsic to the SMU, change in the suite of neurological considerations ranging from pain to reflex effects, and change in the associated vasculature. These clinical dimensions are accompanied by various subclinical changes (Fig. 3.1).

The concept of the subluxation complex grew out of the work of noted European chiropractic researchers Fred Illi and Henri Gillet. Illi was a graduate of the Universal Chiropractic College in Pittsburgh (Gillet 1972) and studied with Janse at the National College until 1943, when he returned to Europe and continued his research and practice in Geneva (Wardwell 1992). Gillet also gained his chiropractic education in the USA but generated his significant contribution to chiropractic research in Europe.

They and their colleagues represented the productive "European school" of chiropractic science and in the 1950s their research focus was guided by the desire to understand the fundamental chiropractic principles. Illi was a prolific investigator of orthopedic mechanisms associated with the subluxation which he felt was an effect more than a cause (Gillet 1972), while Gillet made strong gains towards understanding the association between the fundamental principles and the vertebral subluxation (Wardwell 1992).

In some respects this could be seen as a very mechanical approach, in contrast to both the vitalism of BJ Palmer and others in North America, and the neurophysiological understanding of Janse (1948a,b,c) and Homewood (1981), to name but two. However, it is unwise to attempt to dichotomize the history of subluxation in this manner.

A cornerstone of the European investigative approach was analysis of segmental movement which became formalized as motion palpation, first presented in the USA in New York by Gillet in June 1951 (Gillet & Gaucher-Peslherbe 1996). John L Faye, an American, observed their work in Europe and, on returning to the USA, commercialized it in the 1970s as Motion Palpation (Faye 1986). It is reported that Faye considered the term

"subluxation" historically had a static connotation and that it had outlived its usefulness (Sandoz 1989).

While it seems Faye was the first formally to adopt the term "subluxation complex" to take into account his perception that this clinical entity was characterized by the variable interplay of articular, neurological, muscular, physiological, and possibly even visceral phenomena (Sandoz 1989), it is clear his work was abstracted from Janse (1948a, b, c) and the developments of Illi and Gillet (Lantz 1995b).

In the 1990s Gatterman and other participants in the Consortium for Chiropractic Research drove a consensus process designed to attain an acceptable level of agreement on subluxation terminology and usage (Gatterman 1992, 1995a, Gatterman & Hansen 1994). The outcomes encapsulated Lantz's earlier work with the construct of the VSC (Lantz 1989) and led to the publication in 1995 of what is now accepted as the most articulate understanding of the functional spinal lesion, the VSC (Lantz 1995a).

It has been suggested (Bolton 2002) that the terms "subluxation" and "subluxation complex" are jargon terms, unique to chiropractic. Bolton continues by arguing that these terms, together with other terms unique to chiropractic, including the words "chiropractic" and "chiropractor" themselves, have become weapons in the politics of power as played out in the western world by political medicine against the developing profession of chiropractic. It is not the intent of this text to discuss political matters; the contemporary facts are that chiropractic has been established and practiced as a discrete profession for more than a century, which is far longer than many medical specialties. It is also fact that the term "subluxation complex" is in daily use around the globe. The purpose of this text is to increase the collective clinical understanding of the SC for the ultimate benefit of the patient.

The model depicted in Figure 3.1 has its genesis in the models of Lantz, Gatterman, and others and integrates the contemporary appreciation of the role played by the various biopsychosocial dimensions (Waddell 1998). It is difficult to give specific credit for this model on the basis of the rich historical developments which have stimulated a number of writers and practitioners to reflect and comment. Similarly, no credit is taken by this writer for this current iteration. The SC must be considered as now being a firmly established clinical entity, and, while many have contributed over time to the contemporary model shown in Figure 3.1, tomorrow it must be redrawn to reflect an ever-expanding knowledge and understanding.

The complexities of subluxation

The interplay of the dimensions of the SC represents a complexity which is beyond the capacity of any single list to capture. It is only recently that researchers have begun to consider that there may be various categories of subluxation (Triano 2001b). It may well be that the diversity in practice seen among practitioners of manual healthcare in general and among chiropractors in particular is a reflection of a diverse range of subluxation presentations. This is compounded by the clinical fact that definitive diagnosis is quite rare in neuromusculoskeletal health problems and, rather than being seen as a weakness, Coulter (1999) suggests this lack of clarity regarding the central focus of the chiropractic clinical encounter is a strength of that profession.

This chapter presents a range of concepts, both historic and contemporary, regarding the SC and takes the broad view that, while the SC is a clinical entity which exists in a wide variety of forms, there are sufficient common elements which allow the practitioner to reach a working diagnosis and develop an appropriate plan of treatment. For example, one form of SC may exhibit significant loss of motion at a particular SMU but present no other findings, while another form may exhibit signs such as nerve root pain to the ankle of one leg (neural change) with a mild component of edema (vascular change) and unilateral hypertonic iliocostalis musculature (muscular change), with barely discernible restrictions to movement. Clearly both scenarios are descriptions of findings commonly encountered in clinical practice and, equally as clearly, both are distinctly different.

The high degree of variation in the SC challenges its identification and scientific validation and explains the mediocre interexaminer reliability reported in the literature in studies which typically do not offer any control for the different types of subluxation (Hestback & Leboeuf-Yde 2000). It may also be that this variation in the type of lesion has contributed to the development of the broad spectrum of interventions and technique systems now characteristic of the practice of manipulative medicine in general and of chiropractic in particular. As Triano went on to suggest, these subcategories of lesions may well be better treated by one form of manipulation over others (Triano 2001b). Notwithstanding the matrix of testable dimensions which may be drawn to represent this complex variety of subluxations, it is one thing to obtain credible evidence of the SC and another to associate any such SC with altered health. However, once the former is clearly established, the latter question may be more effectively addressed.

CATEGORIES OF SUBLUXATION

The construct of a subluxation matrix goes beyond the types of subluxations described previously by writers and practitioners such as Forster (1920), Gonstead (Herbst 1968), Howe (1975), Hildebrandt (1977), Schafer (1983), Sandoz (1989), and Gatterman (1995c).

The various forms of subluxations which are believed to occur have been described in detail from the very early days of chiropractic (Forster 1920). In some respects Forster's work can be considered as the beginnings of a system of listing the subluxated vertebrae in order better to direct the intervention. The requirement of the US government in 1972 that payment for chiropractic services under the Medicare scheme would only be made where subluxations were demonstrated to exist on X-ray led to the formalization of a scheme to classify subluxations formally. The classifications adopted by the profession were based on work in the 1960s by Howe and Winterstein of the National College of Chiropractic (J Winterstein, personal communication, 2002) and subsequently presented by Howe at the 1975 national workshop on the research status of spinal manipulative therapy conducted at the National Institutes of Health (USA) (Box 3.4, Howe 1975).

Notwithstanding the objection of the profession to enforced radiation of all patients regardless of clinical indicators, this scheme entrenched the notion that dynamic and physiological processes could be reliably demonstrated on a radiograph. The point has been well made that the identification of altered structure on a radiograph does not in itself imply clinical significance.

Box 3.4   Radiographic classification of subluxation – 1970s

A Static intersegmental subluxations
1. Flexion malposition
2. Extension malposition
3. Lateral flexion malposition – right or left
4. Rotational malposition – right or left
5. Anterolisthesis and/or spondylolisthesis
6. Retrolisthesis
7. Lateralisthesis – right or left
8. Altered interosseous spacing – decreased or increased
9. Osseous foraminal encroachment

B Kinetic intersegmental subluxations
1. Hypomobility – fixation subluxation
2. Hypermobility – loosened vertebral motor unit
3. Aberrant motion

C Sectional subluxations
1. Scoliosis and/or alteration of curves secondary to structural asymmetries
2. Scoliosis and/or alteration of curves secondary to muscular imbalance
3. Decompensation of adaptational curvatures
4. Abnormalities of motion

D Paravertebral subluxations
1. Costovertebral/costotransverse disrelationships – primary or secondary
2. Sacroiliac subluxation – primary or secondary

After Hildebrandt (1977).

It is emphasized that such findings must be correlated with other clinical findings for confirmation, while on the other hand it must be appreciated that a symptomatic patient may not demonstrate any findings at all on imaging. Further, clinical findings such as disk protrusion may appear to have worsened on subsequent imaging while the patient has actually improved and become symptom-free (Ebrall 1993).

Radiographic classification

Notwithstanding the above, there is a valuable role for X-ray findings in structural diagnosis. This was given by Howe (1975) as being: (1) anatomical depiction; (2) functional assessment; and (3) pathological assessment. Safe clinical practice does not happen until it is made to happen, and the use of diagnostic images in specific circumstances is one way to create safe practice.

The most common imaging modality used by practitioners is plain film radiography and the guidelines for its use are given in Box 3.5 (Phillips 1992). It is currently acknowledged that there are some circumstances where imaging may be useful for suspecting subluxation; however, the use of radiographs as a routine screening tool for this purpose is questioned (Schultz & Bassano 1997). Howe's observations (1975) remain valid; the clinical purpose of radiographs is to allow visualization of anomaly and anatomical variation, and to depict spinal pathology. Such pathology may be causative of the clinical presentation or may inform the practitioner regarding relative or absolute contraindications to adjustment and manipulation.

The third purpose is functional assessment, which includes full biomechanical analysis, both in standard orthopedic terms

---

Box 3.5 Guidelines for requesting plain film images

1. Age more than 50 years
2. Presentation with significant trauma
3. Presentation with neuromotor deficits
4. History of recent unexplained weight loss
5. Suspicion of ankylosing spondylitis
6. History of drug or alcohol abuse
7. History of cancer
8. Use of corticosteroids
9. Adult with increased temperature (>37.8°C, 100°F)
10. Recent visit for same problem with a lack of improvement
11. Patients seeking compensation for back pain

From Phillips (1992), with permission.

---

and in the terms of the structural changes which may be indicative of subluxation (Box 3.4). A further level of analysis is that used within the Gonstead technique system (Herbst 1968). The clinical value of radiographs is enhanced when they are requested in accord with the guidelines given by Phillips (1992) (Box 3.5).

Radiographic evidence

Radiographs of the spine, when taken with the patient erect and weight-bearing, allow detailed biomechanical analysis which includes identification of signs which may infer degrees of either structural or functional change thought to be associated with the SC. Such films also allow the application of inclusion and exclusion criteria for spinal manipulation and adjustment. Gillet (1973) commented on the radiographic definitions of subluxation as decided upon in the early 1970s by a group of practitioners representative of the American Chiropractic Association's Governor's Council, the Council of Chiropractic Roentgenologists, and the (American) Council of Chiropractic Orthopedists, and considered it was the first real attempt to define the entity around which the whole basis of chiropractic revolved.

Perhaps it was the intent to provide definitions which could link perceived vertebral malpositions with descriptive terminology which led to subsequent attempts to define the subluxation in the language of mathematics (Dulhunty 1987, 1996, 1997) and engineering (Troyanovich 1997). A brief consideration of these and other papers is relevant in assisting the reader to appreciate that there is actually very little common understanding of normal spinal dynamics, let alone the lesion on which the various fields within manipulative medicine are built.

Dulhunty described the "Basic mechanics of the vertebral subluxation" in terms of displacement, resistance, load, and time (1987) and published "A mathematical basis for defining vertebral subluxations and their correction" in (1996). He also applied these concepts in a review of the literature to determine the normal parameters for the sagittal lumbar spine (1997) but was dismissed by Troyanovich (1997) who, in association with Harrison, had instead defined normal spinal parameters in engineering terms (Harrision et al 1996a). One could be forgiven for thinking that the considered application of the pure sciences to describe the subluxation would be without controversy, but this is not so and Harrison's work has received critical review (Jutkowitz 1997, 1998, Morgan 1997, Owens 1997).

In addition to the fundamental work of Dulhunty, there are interesting suggestions that practitioners should apply linear algebra to understand posture better (Harrison et al 1996c); use a "flopping doctor" model to understand the biomechanics of spinal manipulation (Solinger 1996a); or use the theory of small oscillations to describe manipulation as a therapeutic intervention (Solinger 1996c, 2000). It has been claimed (Harrison et al 1996b) that practitioners misuse the term "torque" in their literature and that this misuse is perpetuated by chiropractic colleges; that claim was rebutted (Herzog 1998). Finally, the physics of spinal manipulation were carefully explained in a four-paper series by Haas (1990a, b, c, d), only to be labeled later by Solinger (1996b) as erroneous with invalid conclusions.

Rather than being discouraging, this level of disagreement among scientists such as biomechanists, engineers, mathematicians, physicists, and statisticians may be seen as highlighting the challenges associated with the objective application of science to describe the subluxation and its correction by spinal adjustment. The real concern is the observation that it is only a handful of chiropractors who are writing on these issues (Lawrence 2000), and perhaps even fewer practitioners from the related disciplines.

Even more destabilizing is the use of the pseudoscientific descriptor "biomechanical joint dysfunction" which some prefer over the term SC. Those who use terms like this, along with others who use the term "posterior joint dysfunction" to describe all spinal dysfunction, clearly limit their description of the spinal lesion to only its kinematic dimension. This is not to suggest that posterior joint dysfunction may not be a component of the SC; indeed, the practitioner must attempt to identify the most likely structures causing movement restriction, including the specific components of the posterior joint complex, such as capsule, meniscus, articular cartilage, osseous degenerative change, ligamentous creep, muscle hypertonicity, and so on.

The SC has come to represent the heritage of the chiropractic profession and there is no credible reason why practitioners the world over cannot fully embrace the term in daily practice, no matter what their discipline. There is a rich body of scientific evidence emerging about the function of the body which makes greater sense when understood within the SC paradigm of human function and health.

Clinical classifications

In addition to radiographic findings, seven commonly recognized clinical types of subluxation were described by Schafer (1983) and are given in Box 3.6. He also included Howe's classification. Schafer's list of clinical types seems to draw from work published by Janse in 1948 (a, b, c), particularly with its emphasis on off-centering, which is included in the definition given by Janse:

A vertebral subluxation may be interpreted as an off centring of a vertebral segment, in relation to the one above and below and usually at the extreme or slightly beyond the normal range of movement. As a result the vertebra is no longer capable of the physiological demands of normal movement, resulting in a variable degree of fixation, vertebral joint strain, a pathological altering of the diameters of the intervertebral foramina, with possible consequent nerve trunk

---

Box 3.6 Seven clinical types of subluxation described in the 1980s

1. Functional subluxation – a functional and slight off-centering with partial fixation in an otherwise normal articular bed
2. Pathologic subluxation – an off-centering derangement in an articular bed that has become deformed as the result of degenerative changes
3. Traumatic subluxation – in consequence to an extraneous or intrinsic force and the associated muscle spasm
4. Reflex subluxation – off-centering induced by asymmetrical muscle contraction from aberrant visceral or somatic reflexes
5. Defect subluxation – of an anomalous or developmentally defective spinal or pelvic segment
6. Fixation subluxation – hypomobile fixation wherein a spinal or pelvis segment that is in a neutral position of mobility fails to participate fully in that movement
7. Hypermobile subluxation – pathologic segmental increase in movement consequent to the loss of integrity of the retaining mechanism caused by trauma or degenerative pathology

From Schafer (1983), with permission.

---

impingement, paraforaminal congestions, and eventual development of adhesions (Janse 1948a).

The American Chiropractic Association's Council on Technic published a report of chiropractic terminology in 1988 (ACA Council on Technic 1988a, b) which identified dynamic listing nomenclature for the purpose of designating the abnormal movement of one vertebra in relation to its subjacent segment. This scheme formalized the term "restriction" as meaning the limitation of movement and being descriptive of the direction of such limitation in a dysfunctional joint. The nomenclature included the descriptive terms flexion restriction, extension restriction, lateral flexion restriction (left or right), and rotational restriction (left or right) (Bergmann et al 1993).

Gatterman & Hansen have conducted an extensive consensus process to clarify the terminology of subluxation (Gatterman & Hansen 1994) and Gatterman has monitored advances in terminology and usage (Gatterman 1995a). The contemporary understanding is that there may be up to four major components of subluxation as understood from the chiropractic perspective, and that each component has a number of subcomponents. These are given in Box 3.3 and are seen to draw together the long-standing historical considerations with the more recent developments in neurology and mind–body medicine.

Compensations

Various systems of spinal analysis and treatment have developed nomenclature specific to their understanding of the FSL and the nature of the resultant entity within the spine as inferred by clinical findings. Gonstead technique is one such system and it is quite proscribed in its description of the perceived directions of misalignment which may be found in various components of the spinal complex. Typically this terminology includes descriptors like posterior misalignment, body rotation, and lateral wedging (Herbst 1968). The Gonstead system makes two specific points about spinal misalignment: the first is that, while there may be many misalignments in a spine, there are only few subluxations.

The point is that when a vertebra is misaligned due to subluxation, the architecture of the spine is affected to some degree. At some time in the spine, one or more vertebrae must compensate for the loss of balance and equilibrium by misaligning in a direction opposite to the subluxation. This form of misalignment secondary to the misalignment of subluxation is considered to be a compensation. This concept reinforces the notion that a subluxation cannot be determined solely from X-ray; it can only be hypothesized when there is sufficient clinical evidence, perhaps including X-ray findings (Herbst 1968).

Gillet described spinal compensation in terms of primary and secondary fixation (Pletain 2001). A primary fixation is a major fixation in both quantitative and qualitative terms. An articular fixation is characterized by joint movement restriction accompanied by loss of joint play, as opposed to a ligamentous fixation which is typically of a chronic nature. The compensating fixations are secondary and usually of a muscular type (Pletain 2001). Clinical observation shows that the secondary fixations appear to be complementary to each other and typically resolve when the primary fixation is corrected (Pletain 2001).

Anterior subluxation

The second belief of Gonstead is that the typical vertebra cannot subluxate anteriorly (Herbst 1968). The clinical finding of thoracic segments appearing to be anterior or somewhat dished, with an edematous feel and tenderness on palpation, has been interpreted as a compensation for a subjacent flexion fixation (Plaugher 1993 pp. 248–249).

Others consider such findings are indicative of segmental anterior subluxation and Bergmann provides a spectrum of both supine and standing adjustive techniques for this clinical finding (Bergmann et al 1993 pp. 375–383; 385–390). Gatterman acknowledges both the flexion fixation and the related supine adjustment, as well as the prone adjustment with a superior (S) to interior (I) vector (Gatterman 1990 pp. 189–190).

On the other hand, Walther describes the concept of the anterior thoracic subluxation in detail, and provides empirical clinical assessment procedures (Walther 1981 pp. 60–62). These include specific palpation for exquisite tenderness at the tip of the spinous process, thought to be reflective of interspinalis muscle weakness. It is thought that the tip of the spinous process of the inferior segment in the anterior SMU will also be tender (Walther 1981).

The finding of anterior thoracic segments has also been considered to represent a sectional subluxation in an attempt to understand the signs and symptoms which accompany a flattening of the thoracic kyphosis over several segments (Zachman et al 1989). The mechanism is that which Plaugher describes, namely a flexion fixation with multiple extension fixations above, and it is considered that the supine adjustive approach is more sensible. Zachman also related this sectional subluxation to many of the patient's symptoms, a clinical approach expanded by Patriquin who suggested that diminished minor motion between two or three adjacent segments is indicative of viscerosomatic reflex activity, secondary to visceral disease (Patriquin 1992 p. 7). He added that a finding of thinned, atrophic, fibrous deep paraspinal musculature in one area represented a long-standing problem, while vigorous edema, swelling, and tenderness, perhaps with increased local muscle tone, was more suggestive of acute visceral disease (Patriquin 1992).

DIAGNOSTIC CRITERIA

The beauty of the model of the SC given in Figure 3.1 is that it identifies both clinical and subclinical dimensions, each of which becomes a criterion within the diagnostic process. Further, when the elements are separated out in this manner they have a use which reaches beyond the clinical application and into the research environment. The greatest strength, however, may come from the model facilitating the practitioner to visualize an abstract clinical entity.

The theory of abstract objects

The theory of abstract objects is a method which allows the SC to retain its clinical abstractedness while its presupposed properties, which individually have validity within our scientific conceptual framework, become the stories which the practitioner is able to document. Such sentences allow logical analysis about the abstract object. The following discussion of diagnostic criteria represents a sequence of stories which, while each complying with the various laws governing our current understanding of reality, can still only be seen as descriptive of an abstract object, the SC.

The SC cannot be excised and put on display in a bottle. It is believed to exist as a functional and physiological entity and thus may only have a presence in the living mammal. In order to describe this abstract entity, a series of statements about it can be developed. Each statement in itself should hold true to the fundamental laws as we know them, so then each statement itself is testable and repeatable. However it must be remembered that the SC only remains abstract because science does not yet have the skill or expertise to observe and measure the parameters of each statement at this time. This does not render the statements invalid; rather it gives one a greater appreciation of the "art" of clinical practice where the art is the understanding of the empirical evidence.

The statements which are generated can be structured to reflect the model depicted in Figure 3.1. The next step in the clinical sequence is that a specific act is generated in order to execute each diagnostic statement. If, for example, one diagnostic statement is that a particular vertebra is rotated to the right relative to the vertebra below it, such that the practitioner thinks of it as being "right posterior", the sequential clinical act is an intervention designed to remove the element of right posteriority and restore normal position and movement. Thus the truth of the statement of treatment is built on the truth of the diagnostic statement. The diagnostic statement is derived from the practitioner's perception of the SC as an abstract object and the intervention statement is then applied to the SC, again as an abstract object.

The diagnostic procedures

A survey of the variety of methods commonly used by practitioners to detect spinal subluxation (Walker 1998) identified the

---

Box 3.7 Sources of diagnostic statements about the subluxation complex

Assessment of kinematic change
Postural assessment
Static palpation
Radiographic analysis
Objective structural change of spinal motion unit (SMU) mechanics
Other diagnostic imaging assessment
Subjective nature of movement
Objective nature of movement
Assessment of the individual joints

Assessment of connective tissue change
Ligaments of the SMU
Other ligaments of the region
The intervertebral disk
Fascia and other connective tissues

Assessment of muscle change
The small intrinsic muscles of the SMU
Muscles affecting the SMU
Muscles affected by the SMU

Assessment of neural change
Local pain
Referred pain
Sensory change
Motor function
Autonomic effects
Central neural change
Muscle stretch (deep tendon) reflex change

Assessment of vascular change
Palpable vascular dimensions
Vertebrobasilar insufficiency
The inflammation cycle
Subclinical vascular change
Lymphatic change

---

following which were regarded by the respondents as reliable (in the clinical, not scientific sense):

- visual posture analysis
- pain description of the patient
- plain static erect X-rays
- leg-length discrepancy
- neurological tests
- motion palpation
- static palpation
- orthopedic tests.

These procedures can be grouped according to the SC model, namely:

- assessment of kinematic change: visual postural analysis, plain, static erect X-rays, leg-length discrepancy, static palpation, motion palpation, orthopedic tests
- assessment of muscle change: orthopedic tests
- assessment of neural change: pain description of the patient, neurological tests.

There are many more clinical procedures available to the practitioner than those which are identified as being commonly used. One possible scheme is given in Box 3.7. The structure of the chapters in Part 2 loosely follows this scheme and attempts to step the reader through specific clinical changes which may be observed and quantified, and perhaps associated with the SC at a particular spinal level.

Palpation

The act of palpation is crucial to developing most of the diagnostic statements. Palpation occurs whenever the practitioner touches the patient with diagnostic intent, which is frequently indistinguishable from touching with therapeutic intent. Traditional palpation has been considered as being either static or dynamic. The reality is that any diagnostic touch of the patient is dynamic as it involves both an action by the practitioner and a response (usually subconscious) from the patient sufficient to generate a tactile response from the tissues as data input to the practitioner.

Dynamic palpation has been extended to become movement or motion palpation and, while the concept of altered vertebral movement has long been entrenched in chiropractic practice, the use of movement palpation to detect such change is a relatively recent development, being first presented in the USA in New York by Gillet in 1951 (Gillet & Gaucher-Peslherbe 1996). The clinical skills needed for the analysis of SMU movement became systematized as Motion Palpation and were commercially marketed by the Motion Palpation Institute (Faye 1986). This text refers to dynamic or movement palpation in its generic sense as opposed to the systematized Motion Palpation.

Diagnostic statements

There is a twofold purpose for generating clinical data in response to the diagnostic statements which flow from the categories given in Box 3.7:

- to determine the presence of the SC by generating a series of statements which document both the subjective and objective dimensions believed to be associated with a particular SC as they are manifested in the patient
- to visualize the SC as a physical entity to which a physical intervention can be directed. In this sense, the listing becomes the directions for specific intervention which is believed to have a therapeutic and corrective effect.

The visualization of the SC is mostly drawn from the assessment of kinematic change and the specific clinical protocols for determining the presence and nature of such change are presented in Chapter 4. An understanding of its effects on the patient is drawn mostly from the assessment of changes in the connective tissues, muscles, nervous system, and vascular system. Protocols relevant to these dimensions are presented in Chapters 5–8.

The data gathered during the assessment of the spine allow the practitioner to apply some mode of predication to help imagine the SC in order to understand it and the forces which may have formed it, the dimensions which may now describe it, the clinical effects which may be associated with it, and the therapeutic forces which may correct it.

The process of visualizing the SC as an abstract object raises the possibility that the SC exists more in the mind of the practitioner than in the patient's spine. Visualization should not be confused with fantasy. The latter allows one to imagine something which does not exist, while visualization allows one to imagine substance which may not be able to be seen, or action

which has not yet happened. Examples of visualization for a future event are widely apparent among athletes, especially high divers. The processes of visualization allow them to create the appropriate neural pathways in their mind for the intricate positioning of their body in three-dimensional space and these pathways then provide a pattern to control their body during the performance over time.

Visualization allows the practitioner to gather an array of subjective and objective clinical data and then integrate, correlate, and extrapolate it to generate a valid entity as the focus of subsequent clinical intervention.

DESCRIPTIVE TERMINOLOGY

Some conventions have developed for the descriptive terminology applicable to the SC in a typical SMU. The first is that the superior vertebra is taken as the segment to describe the perceived kinematic change, with reference to the inferior segment. It must be remembered that the SC is not a displaced vertebra; it is the collection of signs and symptoms arising from a variety of small changes within a specific SMU. The superior vertebral segment is simply used to describe one dimension of those changes, namely altered position or movement of that vertebra, in the understanding that the effects of the SC arise from the effects of change within the entire SMU.

Diversified listings

Different methods of describing the FSL are used by each manual discipline. The most commonly used system within chiropractic is that codified by the National College of Chiropractic and broadly considered a "diversified" system. This system simplifies the second convention that a specific structure or location on a vertebra is used to identify its perceived position. Diversified listings describe the perceived position of the vertebral body in terms of its most posterior aspect secondary to rotation about any of the three axes (Fig. 3.2). Exceptions are translation along the z-axis which is termed anterior, and flexion about the x-axis, which is termed anterior inferior, with reference to the anterior margin of the body.

When the trunk of the patient rotates to the left so the patient faces to the left, the vertebral body follows. In the manner in which the patient's left shoulder has become more posterior than the right, the left side of the vertebral body is considered to have rotated more posteriorly than the right.

There is a congruency between movement and the listing, which makes clinical sense given that the general treatment approach is to take an adjustive contact on the most posterior aspect of the vertebral body. The intent is to deliver a therapeutic adjustive thrust to correct the posteriority by driving that part of the vertebral body towards the anterior. If the posteriority represents kinematic change then correction with an anterior thrust represents the therapeutic intervention.

Gonstead listings

A second listing system is used by practitioners who practice the Gonstead system where the spinous process of the typical vertebra is the reference point, causing the congruency between

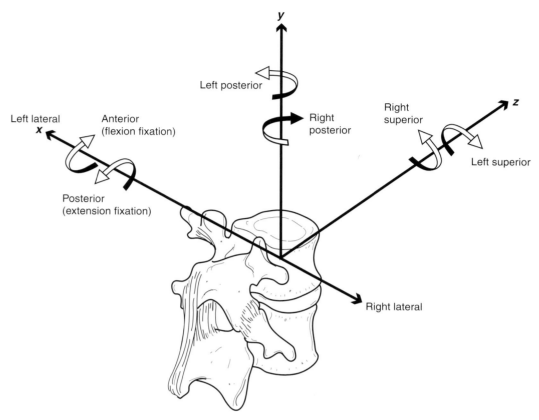

Figure 3.2 Possible movements for listing within a typical spinal motion unit (SMU). The possible movements within the SMU have been given in Figure 2.8. This is the same diagram, labeled to identify the listing associated with those movements. The listing for a typical SMU describes the supposed fixation of the superior segment relative to the inferior segment. For example, RPS would mean the superior segment has both rotated to the right about the y-axis (RP = right posterior) and to the left about the z-axis, so that the posterior side (right) has become superior (S). This listing suggests the practitioner would contact the right posterior-superior side of the body to correct the perceived malposition with an anterior-inferior thrust.

movement and listing to be lost. As before, when the trunk of the patient rotates to the left so the patient faces to the left, the vertebral body follows but the spinous process moves to the right. Regardless that the left side of the vertebral body is considered to have rotated more posteriorly than the right, the segment is listed as spinous right.

An essential additional component of the Gonstead listing system is the belief that a typical vertebra can only subluxate into extension. The corollary is that extension equates to a posteriority of the spinous, therefore the initial component in every spinous listing is the letter P to represent this perceived mandatory movement. The "spinous right" listing thus becomes simply PR. It is assumed that the spinous is the reference point, therefore it does not need to be named in the listing. PR thus means posterior right (spinous).

Rotation about the z-axis is similarly listed with reference to the perceived movement of the spinous process. Left lateral flexion of a segment, which is left rotation about the z-axis, will raise both the right side of the vertebral body and the spinous process. This is emphasized if lateral flexion is accompanied by left rotation, which would move the spinous to the right. The letter "S" is then added to the simple PR listing to indicate the spinous, which has rotated to the right, has also moved superior

or to the side of the perceived open disk wedge. The full listing is PRS, the reverse of the diversified equivalent, LPI.

Fluency in listing

Regardless of it being initially quite confusing, the student is strongly encouraged to become fluent in both systems and to select the most appropriate listing to describe best the perceived findings of kinematic change. This flexibility accommodates the third convention of listing a vertebra, which is the principle that the adjustive thrust is always directed into the convex side of the spine when any scoliosis is present.

Many adjustments of the lumbar spine are delivered with the patient in a side-lying position. The convention is that the concave side of any scoliosis is "down" and the convex side is "up". In the typical instance the convex side of the scoliosis is also the side of any open wedge of the disk within the involved SMU. The vertebral rotation about the y-axis is such that in some cases the spinous process will be on the upside, the side of the open wedge (Fig. 3.3A), and in other cases it will be on the downside, the side of the closed wedge (Fig. 3.3B).

In order to remain compliant with the convention that the adjustive force is delivered on the convex side of scoliosis, which

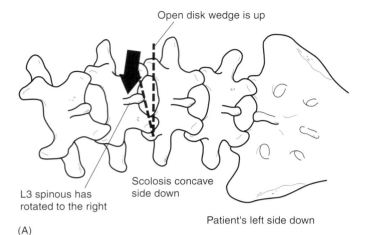

Open disk wedge is up

L3 spinous has rotated to the right

Scolosis concave side down

Patient's left side down

(A)

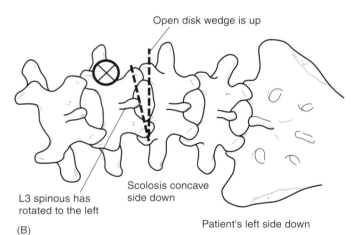

Open disk wedge is up

L3 spinous has rotated to the left

Scolosis concave side down

Patient's left side down

(B)

Figure 3.3 Selection of the most appropriate listing. (A) The L3 spinous process is perceived to have rotated to the right, which is the side of the open wedge of the disk and also the side of convexity of the lumbar scoliosis. All conventions are met when the L3–4 SMU is listed as L3 PRS to indicate the adjustive contact will be on the upside of the L3 spinous process (filled arrow). (B) The L3 spinous process is perceived to have rotated to the left, which is towards the side of the closed wedge of the disk. In order to comply with convention, the correct contact point is the up-side mamillary process of L3, which is on the side of the open wedge of the disk and on the side of convexity of the lumbar scoliosis. The most appropriate listing in this case is L3 RPS to indicate the adjustive contact will be on the upside mamillary process (crossed circle).

conveniently ensures the side of the open wedge of the disk is on the upside, the practitioner will need to switch between listing systems. In cases where the spinous process has rotated to the upside, the Gonstead listing system is appropriate (Fig. 3.3A) as it identifies the preferred adjustive contact as being on the upside of the spinous process (filled arrow). In cases where the spinous process has rotated to the downside, the diversified listing system is appropriate (Fig. 3.3B), as it identifies the posterior side of the body, or the mamillary process, as being the appropriate adjustive contact (crossed circle). Gonstead accounts for this second situation by adding an additional identifier to the listing, which in this case would become PLI-M to indicate the spinous has rotated to the inferior side of the disk wedge and

Table 3.1 Simple listings for specific vertebral positions

Perceived body position	Listing
Flexion about the x-axis	Anterior inferior
Extension about the x-axis	Posterior inferior
Right rotation about the y-axis	Right posterior
Left rotation about the y-axis	Left posterior
Right lateral flexion about the z-axis	Right inferior
Left lateral flexion about the z-axis	Left inferior
Right lateral listhesis as right translation along the x-axis	Right lateral
Left lateral listhesis as left translation along the x-axis	Left lateral
Superior translation along the y-axis	Increased disk height
Inferior translation along the y-axis	Decreased disk height
Anterior translation along the z-axis	Anterolisthesis
Posterior translation along the z-axis	Retrolisthesis

that the contact should be on the opposite mamillary (M). This is an unnecessary level of complication, and, given that Gonstead listings at times conflict with other concepts, it is preferable for the practitioner to be fluent between systems to allow the greatest level of choice.

Simple and compound listings

It is generally accepted (Peterson & Bergmann 2002 pp. 52, 53) that the simple vertebral positions which may result from kinematic change, and their associated listing, are as given in Table 3.1. These movements simply reflect the "movement within a typical SMU" as discussed in the preceding chapter.

It will also be recalled that it is quite unusual for there to be any pure movement within the SMU and that movement is typically coupled. Therefore any rotation about the y-axis is likely to be accompanied by rotation about the z-axis. In this case the more posterior side is then described as being either superior or inferior in the frontal plane. The resultant listing becomes compound to reflect two or three movements (Table 3.2).

For example, a left rotation about the y-axis with a left lateral flexion (rotation to the left about the z-axis) will result in the left posterior aspect of the body being more posterior than the right (hence listed as LP) and more inferior in the frontal plane (hence listed as I), to give a compound listing of LPI. Given the convention that the upside of the SMU should be listed to identify the adjustive contact, the preferred listing relates to the spinous process and would be PRS. The converse compound listing (RPS) is described in the caption of Figure 3.2. The four most common compound listings for the typical SMU are described in Table 3.2.

Given that chiropractors can't come to a common consensus to use one system it is extremely unlikely that all manual disciplines would ever agree on a universal listing system. The principles given in this section should help the practitioner determine the best listing to use for any given set of clinical findings. The listings given here are universally portable and reflect the reasonable application of visualization to dysfunction within the SMU.

Atypical spinal regions

The possible listings described above are just for the typical SMU. Matters become more complex when the atypical regions

Table 3.2 Compound listings for specific vertebral positions (lumbar spine)

Perceived vertebral body position	Listing
Right rotation about the y-axis with right lateral flexion about the z-axis. This places the spinous on the high side of the disk wedge (left) and the preferred reference point is the spinous, which will have rotated to the left and become superior to reflect the right lateral flexion	The preferred listing is posterior left superior (spinous) or PLS
Right rotation about the y-axis with left lateral flexion about the z-axis. This places the spinous on the low side of the disk wedge (left) and the preferred reference point is the body or mamillary process, which will have rotated to the right and become superior to reflect the left lateral flexion	The preferred listing is right posterior superior (with reference to the mamillary) or RPS
Left rotation about the y-axis with left lateral flexion about the z-axis. This places the spinous on the high side of the disk wedge (right) and the preferred reference point is the spinous, which will have rotated to the right and become superior to reflect the left lateral flexion	The preferred listing is posterior right superior (spinous) or PRS
Left rotation about the y-axis with right lateral flexion about the z-axis. This places the spinous on the low side of the disk wedge (right) and the preferred reference point is the body or mamillary process, which will have rotated to the left and become superior to reflect the right lateral flexion	The preferred listing is left posterior superior (with reference to the mamillary) or LPS

of the spine are considered, particularly the upper cervical complex and the lumbosacral spine and pelvis. The occiput, atlas, and C2 are described in Chapter 9.

The listings for the ilia and sacrum are quite complex and are described in Chapter 14. It is empirically observed that the L5–S1 SMU may exhibit more complex patterns of kinematic change than those typical segments above. In particular, the side of the open disk wedge may not always appear on the convex side of any lumbar scoliosis. These alternatives are more readily discernible from radiograph than from palpation and they dictate the need for two more listing options. These are described in Chapter 14.

CONCLUSION

The fact that a listing is applied to the superior segment of a SMU does not imply that the vertebra has necessarily "moved out of place". Rather, it is a means to standardize the description of clinically identifiable changes in movement. At times the radiograph will clearly demonstrate an altered position of a vertebra which is subsequently shown to have been returned to its normal position after adjustment, but this model of thinking depicts only a few categories of SC and should not be considered as the dominant model.

The challenge for the practitioner is to learn to respond to the evidence as found in the patient and not to succumb to identifying only those findings in the patient which support a preconceived expectation. In essence, this is the weakness of adopting only one paradigm or system of practice, complete with its blinkers. When the practitioner's only tool is a hammer, every patient problem has to be a nail and the practitioner adds little value.

Wise practitioners will realize they need competency with a reasonable range of tools so they can efficiently manage the screw, the bolt, and the nut, as they are identified, along with the occasional nail. This necessitates competency in a variety of paradigms and technique systems and a high degree of fluency among them.

In essence, the SC or FSL must exist as a visualization in the practitioner's mind before it can be successfully identified and treated in the patient. The listings which are proposed as appropriate to describe the typical visualized entity combine the best of two established systems within the discipline of chiropractic on the basis that they fit the models which can be visualized and reflect the preferred treatment options. This alone may be considered heresy by some but the bottom line is that today's practitioner must move beyond the traditional, insular approaches while respectfully drawing from them, to arrive at a destination which best integrates time-honoured methods with contemporary thinking. The purpose is simply to be able to do the best for every individual patient.

4

Assessment of kinematic change

KEY CONCEPTS

Kinematic change is perhaps the most commonly recognized dimension of the subluxation complex (SC), with static malpositions being described over 200 years ago and dynamic changes a century ago.

There are a number of elements of kinematic change which can be identified. Some are subjective and others are objective. The found data represent the source data of the assessment process and will include both qualitative and quantitative dimensions for various elements.

Postural alignment is the end-result of multiple microprocesses designed to maintain the body's position in space. Deviations may be gross and indicative of significant structural or functional disorder, or subtle and suggestive of minor changes in muscle balance, neural organization, and spinal function. While certain patterns are typically associated with muscle dysfunction and subluxation, the practitioner should not jump to conclusions.

Gait is an essential component of movement and can be considered as the most fundamental form of dynamic posture. It is the basis of holistic biomechanical analysis of the patient. Once neurological gait has been excluded the practitioner must assess for mechanical gait changes. Weakness or other dysfunction of certain muscles, and some subluxations, particularly about the pelvis, may be reflected in altered gait patterns.

All palpation is dynamic in the sense that it evokes a reactive response from the patient; however, static palpation refers to the identification of landmarks and structures of the body while dynamic or movement palpation refers to the process of assessing the quantity and quality of movement and the quality of end-feel for particular joints and spinal motion units (SMUs).

Movement palpation as a form of assessment of the SMU is a high-level clinical art and its success begins with careful positioning of the practitioner and the patient. This is to ensure an interaction most conducive to detecting reliably very small changes in the quantity and quality of movement as well as changes in the quality of end-feel in a particular SMU.

INTRODUCTION

Kinematic change is perhaps the one dimension of the five represented in the contemporary model of the vertebral subluxation complex (VSC: Fig. 3.1) which has the longest recognition by practitioners. In 1827 Harrison described subluxation as including static kinematic change described as a "small irregularity in the height, distance, and lineal direction of a particular vertebra in respect to others" (Harrison 1827). A century ago dynamic kinematic change was described in chiropractic's first formal textbook as a vertebra differing from normal only in its field of motion, with the observation that its various positions of rest were differently located than when it was a normal vertebra (Smith et al 1906). During the first half of the 20th century, BJ Palmer viewed subluxation from a more vitalistic perspective and it was essentially the European school of Illi and Gillet from the mid 20th century which kept the focus on its biomechanical dimensions and kinematics (Gillet 1972).

The model of the VSC generated by Gatterman and other participants in the Consortium for Chiropractic Research (Gatterman 1992, 1995a, Gatterman & Hansen 1994) first utilized the term "kinesiopathology" to describe the dimension of movement within the SMU. The term evolved to "kinesiology". The more appropriate term for describing altered movement is "kinematic change", on the basis that altered movement may or may not be associated with pathology, and the accepted use of the term "kinesiology" to describe a specific clinical science in its own right (the study of human muscular movement). The word "kinematic" is familiar within the broad context of manual medicine (Biedermann 1992) as well as chiropractic (McCarthy 2001).

Kinematic change, in itself, is not necessarily a pathological finding. It may simply identify a pattern of movement altered by anatomical asymmetry. The term becomes clinically useful as a dimension of the SC when it is associated with findings indicative of clinical change. Asymmetrical joint geometry is common (Ross et al 1999) and difficult to detect by static palpation (Jende & Peterson 1997). Radiographs of the spine are useful to establish the existence of joint asymmetry as well as for biomechanical analysis (Howe 1975); however, these changes alone do not infer the presence of SC.

As with all of the assessable dimensions of the SMU, kinematic change must be placed within the global then regional and then segmental context (Fig. 2.1). The approach to the assessment of kinematic change in the patient as presented in this chapter follows that scheme. The global context includes posture, gait, and range of motion while the regional assessment is focused on determining the dynamics of a specific spinal region within the global context. Finally, the segmental assessment looks at the smallest unit of the spine in which movement can occur. This is the SMU in the typical regions of the spine, and specific joint complexes in the atypical regions, such as the atlanto-occipital joint in the upper cervical spine and the sacroiliac joint in the lumbosacral spine and pelvis.

BIOPSYCHOSOCIAL CONTEXT

All clinical assessment should be conducted with recognition of and respect for the individual patient's biopsychosocial environment. Waddell (1998) recognized common elements found in patients suffering chronic low-back pain and identified their interrelationships. This led to the publication of a biopsychosocial model of low-back pain and disability (Fig. 4.1), yet the wisdom of this model lies in its ready applicability to most, if not all, doctor–patient relationships.

The general debilitating nature of spine-related pain, such as mechanical low-back pain which so frequently becomes chronic, and headache which can be cyclic-disabling, renders Waddell's model particularly useful in the context of spinal dysfunction. Pain remains the dominant driver of the patient to the practitioner and pain lies at the core of the biopsychosocial model. Pain is modified by the patient's attitudes and beliefs and, when unresolved, leads to psychologic distress and illness behavior. These patient behaviors sit within their particular social environment where they are modified, nullified, or reinforced, depending on the interactions of the patient with others in that environment. The social environment also represents the sociocultural dimension of patients, particularly their individual response to the pain experience.

The assessment of the patient, particularly for the presence of and effects associated with kinematic change, must recognize the biopsychosocial context. The specific importance of this stems from the simple fact that many of the tests used within the

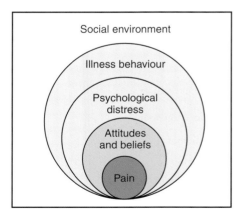

Figure 4.1 The biopsychosocial context. Pain lies at the core of the biopsychosocial model and is modified by the patient's attitudes and beliefs. When unresolved, it leads to psychologic distress and illness behavior, which are modified, nullified, or reinforced by the patient's environment and sociocultural dimension. From Waddell (1998), with permission.

assessment of the spine will reproduce pain. Further, the assessment of kinematic change requires patients to demonstrate their capabilities, however limited or painful these may be.

Patients must be prepared physically and mentally for this experience and their understanding and cooperation enlisted to maximize the reliability of the examination. If patients report they "can't walk" then the practitioner must determine whether there is a physical disability preventing them from walking, or whether it is a self-imposed limitation based on fear that it they do move they may worsen their pain and further damage themselves.

The practitioner must therefore be very clear in communicating with the patient and remain compassionate yet firm during the assessment.

THE ELEMENTS OF KINEMATIC CHANGE

There are a number of elements of kinematic change which are able to be identified and subsequently assessed in the patient. Some elements are subjective, such as postural findings, while others are objective, such as the presence of degenerative change in an SMU as seen on radiograph. A listing of the assessable elements is given in Box 4.1.

The found data represent the source data of the assessment process and will include both qualitative and quantitative

---

Box 4.1   Assessable elements of kinematic change

Subjective position at rest assessed in terms of
Postural alignment
Antalgia
Symmetry of structures
Static palpation

Objective position at rest by means of diagnostic imaging assessment
The plain radiograph
  Orthopedic line drawing and analysis
  Chiropractic line drawing and analysis
The computed tomography (CT) scan
The magnetic resonance image (MRI)

Objective structural change of spinal motion unit mechanics
Fracture
Dislocation
Avulsion
Lysis
Apophysitis
Reactive osseous hypertrophy
Pathological hypertrophy

Subjective nature of movement
Gait analysis
Active global range of motion
Active regional range of motion
Passive regional range of motion

Objective range of movement in each of the six degrees of freedom
Active global range of motion
Active regional range of motion

Subjective segmental movement in each of the six degrees of freedom
Quantity of movement in each plane
Quality of movement in each plane
Quality of end-feel at each elastic barrier

---

dimensions for various elements. The starting point for assessment of the SMU for kinematic change is an awareness of those factors which can potentially affect its movement. This is followed by a discovery of the nature of its movement.

Assessment therefore commences with observation of the patient to form a clinical opinion about the underlying mechanics of the SMU, and progresses through an objective assessment of information from radiographs or quantified measurements, and then both objective and subjective assessments of the quantity and quality of movement. These assessment steps are performed for the global spine, then the particular regions of interest, and finally at a segmental level for each relevant SMU.

Subjective position at rest

The subjective response of the patient to palpatory touch usually varies with increasing familiarity. This means that a patient in pain will initially overreact to touch in an effort to protect against the unknown. Anxiety can prompt a false response at the initial touch, in which case the careful continuation of assessment and the revisiting of each area usually provides more reliable information. As the doctor–patient bond develops, the patient becomes more trusting, less generally reactive, and more specifically reactive to the touch of assessment which causes pain.

The same principle applies to postural assessment. The patient may initially respond by attempting to stand as correctly as possible, thus masking the subtle changes the practitioner is looking for. On the other hand, some patients may have such anxiety that they exaggerate the postural change associated with their condition. Examples are the patient with acute torticollis and the patient with lower-quadrant nerve root pain secondary to disk protrusion. These conditions are quite frightening to patients and they become afraid to move in case they worsen the problem or increase their pain.

Perhaps the most important role of the practitioner is patient reassurance and the skills of communication are an integral part of the assessment process. The verbal instructions to patients should be in a language which they understand, and should be spoken gently but authoritatively to guide the patient clearly to stand and move where and how the practitioner requires.

Requests of patients should be preceded by a simple face-to-face explanation of what it is the practitioner requires them to do, and perhaps why it needs to be done. This is especially important if the particular procedure is likely to reproduce the patient's pain. It must also be remembered that at all times the practitioner's "touch" of patients may be considered as an invasion into their personal space. The extent to which this occurs will reflect the sociocultural environment of the individual practice. For example, it is offensive to touch an Indonesian child on the head, and it may be offensive to touch any part of a female Muslim patient without her husband being present and giving approval.

Postural alignment about the frontal plane

The maintenance of whole-body balance is a complex task, involving the interaction of three major sensory input systems (visual, vestibular, and somatosensory) and the precisely coordinated motor output at many joints (Radebold et al 2001). Postural assessment may be thought of as a simple task, yet it is able to reveal many subtle indicators of changes in the complex interplay between the input and the output systems. Inappropriate muscle responses may reflect spinal reflex, brainstem balance, or cognitive programming changes, or local change within the muscle. Patients with low-back pain demonstrate impaired postural control of the lumbar spine with poorer balance performance than healthy patients (Radebold et al 2001) and this is indicated by greater postural sway.

The patient should be gowned and wearing only underwear so the back can be exposed to view. Ask the patient to "stand comfortably still for a couple of moments while I look at you closely to see how the various parts of your body relate to each other". If the instruction specifically tells the patient the practitioner is inspecting posture the results are likely to be biased through the patient attempting to stand correctly.

Patients are instructed where to stand and it is useful to ask them to fix their gaze on a marker in front of them. A peaceful framed print hanging on the wall is useful for this, as the patient can be asked to "stand comfortably here and look at the boy in the boat in that picture" or whatever the preferred landmark is. It should be at eye level for patients so their head is level in the sagittal plane.

As the patient moves into position the practitioner comes to stand behind him or her and places a hand on each shoulder to support the patient while he or she shuffles the feet to about shoulder width, and looks at the marker. This action will assist the patient to relax and be compliant.

The following bilateral landmarks are assessed in the order given, from behind the patient (Fig. 4.2):

- mastoid processes
- acromioclavicular joints
- inferior angles of the scapulae
- flank angles
- iliac crests
- ischial tuberosities
- gluteal creases
- popliteal fossae
- Achilles tendons
- medial foot arches.

The level of the mastoid processes can be assessed by using the pad of the thumbs or the lateral border of the index finger, flexed at the proximal interphalangeal joint. The mastoids are gently palpated from inferior to superior to ensure the head is in its natural resting position. The same technique can identify the inferior angles of the scapulae.

The pad of the straightened index finger can palpate the acromioclavicular joints and the iliac crests with a superior to inferior touch. The "flank angle" is the angle of the lateral border of the body between the lower ribs and the iliac crests and should be symmetrical. Left/right asymmetry may suggest a high iliac crest or perhaps a scoliosis altering the lower margins of the rib cage.

The ischial tuberosities are palpated with the thumbs and with the fingers, taking a broad but gentle contact over the greater trochanters. If the gluteal crease is assessed, then it is convenient to use the lateral border of the first finger when it is held horizontally. The lateral contour of the gluteal bulk is also assessed for symmetry. Changes may suggest sacroiliac joint fixation, particularly about the y-axis. Altered ischial tuberosity

height suggests structural change in a leg or about the pelvis, while altered gluteal crease heights suggest soft-tissue or muscle change about the pelvis.

The popliteal fossae are palpated with the posterior aspect of the flexed index finger, in a posterior to anterior manner to assess for differences in tension or tone of the soft tissues about the knee. A unilaterally increased tone is secondary to increased activity of associated postural muscles, which in turn is suggestive of altered pelvic or lower-limb biomechanics. A decreased tone suggests the knee is being held in slight flexion.

Similarly, the tonicity of the Achilles tendons is assessed by palpating either with the finger as for the popliteal fossae, or

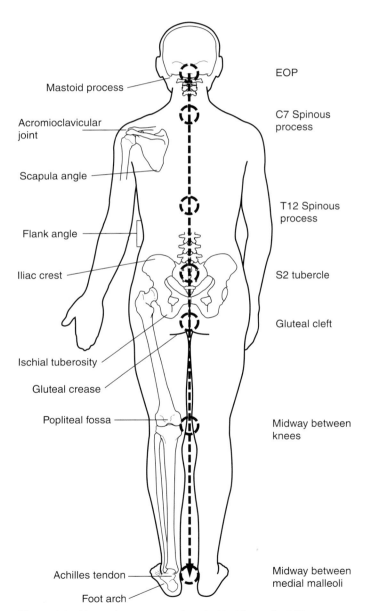

Figure 4.2 Postural assessment from behind the patient. The landmarks are palpated bilaterally in sequence, starting with the mastoid processes. The gravity line falls from the external occipital protuberance.

with the pad of the thumb. The patient is specifically asked about tenderness when palpating this structure, as it is thought that a tender Achilles tendon in the absence of significant sciatic nerve root pain may indicate sciatic entrapment by the piriformis muscle, rather than irritation by a lumbar disk. This finding may only be considered when local pathology about the tendon has been excluded.

The integrity of the medial arch of the foot is assessed by slipping the fingers of the contralateral hand under the medial side of each foot in turn, looking for the presence of an arch and its left–right symmetry. An increased arch is pes cavus and a decreased arch or flat foot is pes planus.

Any unleveling of these bony landmarks suggests rotation about the z-axis; however, in addition to these findings, the fall of the gravity line is assessed to determine any translation (lateral shift) or rotation of body segments away from a symmetrical, balanced standing posture.

The gravity line (Fig. 4.2) should fall from the external occipital protuberance (EOP), and pass through the following:

- the spinous process of C7
- the spinous process of T12
- the S2 spinous tubercle
- the gluteal cleft
- midway between the knees (medial femoral condyles).

It should fall midway between the medial malleoli. It is particularly important to document a visual impression of the spine and to note whether there are obvious curves or deviations away from the "normal" idealized straight alignment.

A final observation is made from in front of the patient to review the effects of any posterior findings and to assess the angle of carriage of the arms. This is the angle of the surface of the antecubital fossa to the frontal plane of the body when the arms are held in neutral with the palms facing towards the thighs. It will vary considerably from patient to patient but should be a symmetrical finding. It is distinctly different to the carrying angle, which is the angle of the forearm as it angles away from the body at the elbow. Observation of the carrying angle requires the arms to be held in the anatomical position, with the palms of the hands facing anteriorly. This angle is typically greater in the female than in the male.

A number of chiropractic authors have described patterns of postural change with scoliosis, ranging from a single C-type curve representing a broad scoliosis of the thoracic and lumbar spines with a low shoulder and high iliac crest on the concave side, to more complex patterns of muscular distortion (Schafer 1983). Common patterns of postural distortion associated with subluxation are given in Part 2 for the upper cervical region (Fig. 9.7 A–D), the thoracolumbar region (Fig 13.6 A–D), and the lumbopelvic region (Fig. 14.5 A–F).

The findings of the posterior postural assessment can be recorded on an outline of the posterior body similar to that used in Figure 4.2; however, it must be appreciated that this method of recording is a two-dimensional representation of three-dimensional clinical findings. The better practice is to proceed to assess the posture in the lateral view of the patient, and then revisit the posterior assessment in terms of integrating the findings about the x-axis and the gravity line as seen from the side, with those findings about the z-axis and the gravity line as seen from behind. The result will be an understanding of postural change to include rotations about the y-axis, such as head rotation, within the context of possible head tilt (as seen from behind), and forward head carriage (as seen from the side).

Postural alignment about the sagittal plane

The gravity line is assessed from the side of the patient (Fig. 4.3). With ideal posture, the gravity line will pass through the following structures:

- the external auditory meatus (EAM)
- the acromioclavicular joint

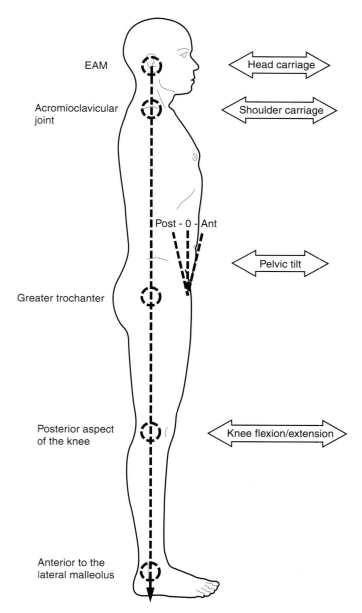

Figure 4.3 Postural assessment from beside the patient. The landmarks and relationships are observed in sequence, starting with head carriage. The gravity line falls from the external auditory meatus (EAM).

- the greater trochanter
- about the posterior aspect of the knee
- just anterior to the medial malleolus.

The relationships of the following body parts are then assessed:

- Head carriage: is the head held forward or backwards? Is the neck curved or straight?
- Shoulder carriage: are the shoulders relaxed and neutral, or are they hunched, or drooping? How does this affect the upper thoracic spine? Does it increase the kyphosis?
- Thoracic kyphosis: is it within normal limits, reduced and flattened, or exaggerated and hunched?
- Abdominal carriage and pelvic tilt: does the patient have a large abdomen? Is the pelvis rotated about the x-axis? The neutral pelvis will have the anterior superior iliac spine (ASIS) vertically above the pubic symphysis. An anterior pelvic tilt is recorded when the ASIS rotates anteriorly over the pubis, and a posterior tilt is when the ASIS is posterior and the pelvis appears to be thrusting.
- Knee flexion: are the knees held in slight flexion or are they hyperextended? Is one knee held markedly different (usually into flexion) than the other?

The findings from lateral observation can be recorded on a lateral body outline similar to that used in the figure; however, as noted above, the findings are not simply recorded on to a two-dimensional sheet; they must be interpreted. Further, it must be appreciated that the spine undergoes changes during the day which are sufficient to reduce the patient's height and alter the values of the sagittal curvatures (Ebrall et al 1993). When sequential findings are sought over time, probably as outcome measures for a particular patient, they should be gathered as far as possible at about the same time each day.

The interpretation and integration of findings are done within the context of the history obtained from the patient, but should not be focused on any preconceived pattern. The practitioner should "look to see" to identify what is found in each individual patient. These findings represent a component of the impression on the subjective position at rest and must be considered with other findings in this category, and then with findings from movement, and particularly findings from muscle assessment.

Some practitioners include the context of the patient's somatotype, as being endomorphic, mesomorphic, or ectomorphic. In the middle of the last century, attempts were made to associate behavioral profiles with body type; however, these dated concepts have been replaced by more evidence-based approaches which allow the determination of a body profile through the application of surface anthropometry in general and girth measurement in particular (McArdle et al 1999). These are advanced techniques, more suited to specialist practice, particularly sports chiropractic.

Antalgia

Postural change which reduces pain is called antalgia and represents movement of the patient to the postural position of least pain. Perhaps the most common antalgic finding is with a patient who has a protruding lumbar disk causing unilateral nerve root pain. The patient will tend to lean forward to create flexion about the injured disk, thus reducing compression on the posterior aspect about the damaged, protruding fibers.

The patient may also lean to one side, again in an attempt to lessen the pain; however, the side to which the patient leans is not consistently away from the side of leg pain. It is thought possible to differentiate clinically between a posterolateral and a posteromedial disk protrusion on the basis of the antalgic lean of the patient (Schafer 1983, Gatterman 1990, Plaugher 1993).

The theoretical mechanism is simple; however, the clinical application and interpretation are somewhat complex. The disk protrusion is considered as a mechanical extension of disk material either lateral to the involved nerve root or medial to it. If the protrusion is medial to the nerve root, the patient would want to lean toward the involved side in order to lessen the mechanical tension of the involved nerve medially over the protruded material (Fig. 14.5A, B). On the other hand, if the protrusion is lateral to the nerve root, the patient would want to lean away from the involved side in order to draw the spinal cord and the involved nerve root medially, to lessen mechanical contact with the laterally protruded material (Fig. 14.15C, D).

The association between antalgic posture and anatomical pain generators is explored dynamically by guiding the movements of the patient. It is important to include any observation of antalgia at this stage of assessment because it will be an important guide to following actions.

SYMMETRY OF STRUCTURES

Humans may like to think they are symmetrical; however, symmetry usually exists only at the gross level of the existence of paired structures. Quantified assessment clearly demonstrates the body is quite asymmetrical; for example, the arm and shoulder of the dominant hand usually have more developed musculature; one breast of the female is usually larger; and one testicle of the male is lower in the scrotum than the other.

The subjective assessment of symmetry is firstly to ensure the gross pairing of structures, and then to look for the subtle differences within the context of expected changes which may provide clues to the presenting problem of the patient. An example is the more developed musculature of the dominant-hand side of the patient. Is the greater muscle bulk becoming hypertonic and causing an imbalance in head carriage which may, in turn, be reported as a headache by the patient? Or is the lesser developed musculature being overworked and developing trigger points which refer pain, possible about the head?

Asymmetry may represent agenesis, as found with the pectoralis muscles. One side may be congenitally absent, significantly altering the expected dynamics of the shoulder girdle. Such findings must be noted and, in the case where the pectoralis major is absent, the area should be palpated to determine whether there is hypertrophy of associated musculature as compensation.

STATIC PALPATION

Having looked, observed and "seen" the patient, it is appropriate to proceed to palpate areas or structures which require clarification. Strictly speaking, static palpation elicits clinical

---

Box 4.2 Essential clinical landmarks identified by static palpation

Each landmark may be used within more than one assessment. The list below avoids needless repetition.

For spinal assessment
Superior nuchal line
Inferior nuchal line
Posterior tubercle of C1
Each spinous process
Each transverse process
Articular pillars of the typical cervical segments
Scapulae, including the spine, superior angle, medial border
Supra- and infraspinous fossae
Neck and angle of each typical rib
Mamillary process of each lumbar segment
Sacral tubercles
Posterior superior iliac spines (PSIS)
Ischial tuberosities

For postural assessment in the frontal plane
Mastoid process
External occipital protuberance (EOP)
C7 spinous process
Acromioclavicular joint
Inferior angle of the scapula
Flank
Iliac crest
Ischial tuberosity
Gluteal crease
Popliteal fossa
Achilles tendon
Medial arch of the foot

For postural assessment in the sagittal plane
External auditory meatus (EAM)
Anterior superior iliac spine (ASIS)
Symphysis pubis
Greater trochanter
Lateral malleolus

For assessment of the head and neck
Vertex
Styloid process
Glabella

Nasion
Zygomatic bone
Angle of the mandible
Temporomandibular joint
Lateral canthus
Cricoid
Laryngeal cartilage
Carotid artery

For assessment of the upper quadrant
Manubrium and the jugular notch
Sternum and the sternal notch
Clavicle
Coracoid process
Anterior borders of ribs 2, 3, 4, and 5
Intercostal spaces #2, 3, 4 and 5, left and right
Nipple
Bicipital groove
Medial epicondyle
Lateral epicondyle
Radial head
Olecranon
Radial styloid

For assessment of the lower quadrant
Umbilicus
Quadrants of the abdomen
Inguinal ligament
Femoral triangle
Iliotibial tract
Medial and lateral condyles of the femur
Patella
Margins of the tibial plateau
Tibial tuberosity
Fibula
Medial malleolus
Calcaneus
Great toe

---

information by inducing micromovement which, of course, is not a true static finding. The skills of this type of assessment are most valuable at the specific, segmental SMU level; however they are used in the first instance to identify clinical landmarks.

Box 4.2 lists the basic clinical landmarks which can be identified by static palpation. These form the essential framework within which all palpation is conducted. The process of learning to identify these landmarks must include the development of verbal descriptors of how each landmark feels. In addition to whether the landmark is palpated superficially or deep, each has a certain typical palpatory feel.

Readers can quickly learn these different types of palpatory feel by palpating their own nose (Fig. 4.4): the nasal bone of the bridge of the nose will give a hard, non-resilient bony feel on palpation; the junction between the nasal bone and the lateral nasal cartilage has a springy end-feel, quickly regaining its shape after deformation; the end of the nose, over the alar cartilage, is more elastic. It can deform more than the lateral nasal cartilage and is a little slower in regaining its shape. Palpation over the cheek produces a spongy, edematous feel, especially

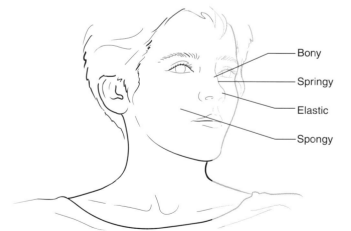

Figure 4.4 Types of tissue feel on palpation. The bridge of the nose has a bony feel on palpation. The junction between the bony bridge and the nasal cartilage has a springy end-feel, while the end of the nose is more elastic. Palpation over the cheek produces a spongy, edematous feel, especially when the tongue is pressed against the cheek.

when the tongue is pressed against the cheek. These terms are also applicable in the assessment of the quality of movement of joint components at the elastic barrier to normal range of motion, or end-feel.

OBJECTIVE POSITION AT REST

The inherent nature of patient assessment by practitioners of manual healthcare is that the data are largely subjective and qualitative. Diagnostic images provide one form of objective and quantitative data and should be included wherever possible given the importance of a risk–benefit analysis for the patient. Plain radiographs remain the most common form of diagnostic images for manual assessment, with both axial and sagittal images from computed tomography and magnetic resonance imaging usually being supplementary. Diagnostic ultrasound is also a useful supplementary image in certain presentations, such as tendinopathies.

The plain radiograph is a snapshot of structure-in-time. Function may be inferred if certain stress views, such as flexion and extension, are taken, but active physiological processes are not captured. Pathological changes may be identified and these include fracture, dislocation, avulsion, lysis, apophysitis, reactive osseous hypertrophy, and pathological hypertrophy. Physical changes to the bony structures caused by these mechanisms will result in altered SMU mechanics and represent a means of quantifying objective structural change.

A fundamental principle with obtaining plain radiographs is that two views, perpendicular to each other, are the minimum views needed of any spinal region. The two views most relevant to imaging the spine are the anterior to posterior (AP) projection and the lateral projection. Supplementary views may be taken in an oblique plane in the cervical and lumbar regions to visualize the intervertebral foramina. Some practitioners prefer a full-spine radiograph, while others are content with the sectional or regional views which are traditionally provided by radiology services. There is some debate as to which method provides the least projectional distortion and the least radiation to the patient. The view of this writer is that, all things considered, the sectional views are preferable.

The mandatory requirement is that the plain radiographic images are obtained with the patient erect and weight-bearing. The seven views which constitute a standard postural series are:

1. lateral cervical neutral: to visualize occiput through to C7 or T1
2. AP lower cervical: to visualize C3 or C4 to T1 or T2
3. AP open-mouth (APOM): to visualize occiput, C1, and C2
4. lateral thoracic: to visualize C7–L1
5. AP thoracic: to visualize C7–L1 and the posterior rib articulations
6. lateral lumbar neutral: to visualize T12 to sacrum and coccyx
7. AP lumbar: to visualize T12 to sacrum and coccyx, and the ischial tuberosities.

The lateral cervical and lumbar views are termed "neutral" to distinguish them from flexion and extension views in the sagittal plane, which may also be taken of these regions. Gonad shielding should be used for the pelvic views and care is taken to ensure bony structures are not obscured.

There is a range of orthopedic lines which may be drawn on each view to assist with the analysis of relationships. There are several standard lines which are considered essential in the cervical and lumbar regions and these are discussed in the relevant chapters. The remaining lines are drawn as indicated by the clinical presentation and the reader is referred to Yochum & Rowe (1996 pp. 139–196) for detailed descriptions of these.

There is also a collection of lines which may be drawn to reflect particular paradigms of practice, such as the Gonstead approach in chiropractic; however, the validity and reliability of these may not be as acceptable as for the standard orthopedic lines. These lines should not be dismissed, however, as they represent a broad empirical experience which at times can provide useful data to assist clinical decision making.

SUBJECTIVE AND OBJECTIVE NATURE OF MOVEMENT

Once the static parameters of the patient are identified, assessed, and recorded, the practitioner may progress to the dynamic parameters which include the objective and subjective nature of movement in each of the six degrees of freedom.

The global range of motion is an active procedure. Values are given in Figure 4.5 but it must be remembered that these are approximations and there are many factors which will cause them to vary, including the somatotype and age of the patient. The important finding is any left/right asymmetry within the context of what can be considered normal for a particular individual.

Flexion is assessed by asking the standing patient to "bend forward and see how far you can reach towards the floor". This is an open-ended command, as opposed to the closed-ended command "touch the floor". The latter is an instruction for a specific task and does not encourage the patient to reach further than the nominated end-point of touching the floor. The former is open-ended in the sense that it encourages the patient to reach as far as possible which, in some cases may mean they place their palms flat on the floor.

Extension is assessed by showing standing patients how to extend and internally rotate their arms so they can lock their fingers and hold their arms out as ballast. The patient is asked to "lean backwards gently and look up to the ceiling". The practitioner must be in a position to support and stabilize patients as this procedure requires neck extension which may destabilize patients and cause them to fall.

Lateral flexion is assessed in standing patients by asking them to "run the fingers of one hand down your leg, as far as possible without bending your waist or knees". The practitioner may stand behind and to the side of patients to ensure they are stable and to check they do not crib by bending forward. The practitioner should mark the point of furthest reach with the finger against the patient's leg. If this is reduced on one side then the distance between the maximal reach point at the patient's fingertips and the floor can be measured and recorded in the file. This value is an easy quantification of any restriction or increase in lateral flexion. Clinically, patients will laterally flex further on the side opposite hypotonic erector spinae as they provide less resistance to the contralateral movement.

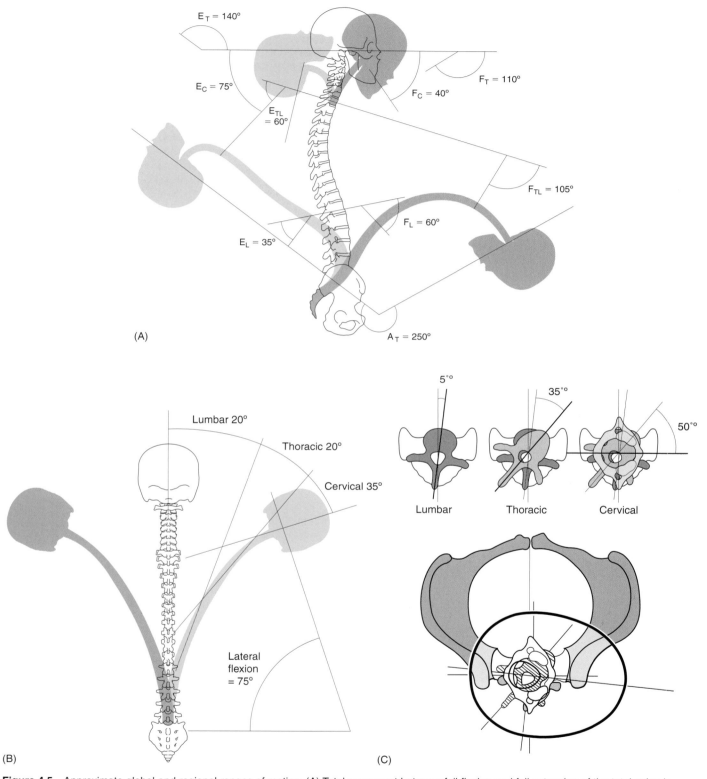

Figure 4.5 Approximate global and regional ranges of motion. (A) Total movement between full flexion and full extension of the total spine is 250°. This consists of 110° of flexion and 140° of extension. The regional values are given in the figure, where E = extension, F = flexion, $_C$ = cervical, and $_{TL}$ = thoracolumbar. (B) Total lateral flexion is 75° to either side. The regional values are given in the figure. (C) Total axial rotation from pelvis to cranium exceeds 90° to either side. The regional values are given in the figure. From Kapandji (1974), with permission.

Rotation in reasonably mobile patients may be assessed with them standing while the practitioner supports the pelvis and asks them to "turn and look as far as possible over each shoulder". Patients in pain or with a reasonable level of dysfunction will be more compliant if they are sitting on a bench for this procedure. The practitioner will stand behind the patient and observe any restriction in axial rotation.

There is little point is attempting to quantify these active, global movements of the spine in terms of absolute measurement in degrees. All patients have a maximum range which is normal for them and which may fall outside any perceived "average". In such cases there will be reasons why this occurs and these must be identified and documented. The remaining patients will typically demonstrate a marked restriction on one side, usually limited by pain. Once the pain-free maximal range is established, the restricted range can be expressed in comparison, usually in the form "left rotation is limited to about 50% (or whatever) of right rotation by pain (if true) in the ... region".

Active range of motion by region is subsumed within the global movements and this requires close observation by the practitioner to ensure that, as far as possible, things remain equal for reciprocal movements. In other words, a keen eye must be kept open for recruitment or other subtle changes in body position which can occur in order to assist a dysfunctional movement in one direction to approximate a normal movement in the opposite direction.

The quality of the movement during global and regional range of motion assessment is particularly important in this regard. The practitioner must observe to ensure the movement is smooth and fluid, and, in cases where it isn't, attempt to identify and describe the causative factors. It is important to appreciate that the assessment of movement involves a judgment of both the quantity and the quality, where the former is more objective and the latter much more subjective. These movements are active, and passive range of motion is not really assessed in the global sense except in the cervical spine.

Passive regional range of motion

While there is little value in attempting to assess passive range of motion in the lumbar and thoracic spines, it is extremely valuable in the cervical spine. The patient is seated and the practitioner stands behind with a hand on each shoulder.

The basic movements of flexion, extension, and left/right lateral flexion may be assessed actively, with the cervical spine of the patient in the neutral position. A good level of clinically relevant information is elicited with these procedures, especially as the patient with neck pain and/or headache attempts to verbalize the nature, location, and extent of any restriction. Chapters 9–11 emphasize the extensive soft-tissue relationships throughout this region. Painful restriction to cervical spine movement may arise from dysfunction as low as the mid thoracic spine.

The movements of axial rotation provide the most pointed clinical information, for the simple reason that, when rotation is conducted in full flexion and then full extension, different regions of the cervical spine are emphasized. Flexion of the cervical spine opens the facet joints of the typical segments, which lessens their participation in rotation, which is therefore concentrated into the upper cervical complex. Conversely, extension

close-packs the facets and locks the upper cervical segments, thus concentrating rotation into the lower cervical spine.

Active range of rotation of the cervical spine must therefore be assessed in neutral, flexion, and extension, and passive range of motion is highly informative in flexion and extension. The practitioner's hands guide the passive movement. In flexion the ipsilateral hand (of patient head rotation) may cup the mandible while the contralateral hand supports the ipsilateral parietal region. The hand on the mandible gently draws the head into the elastic end-zone. In extension both hands cup the parietal region and assist rotation into the elastic end-zone. A restriction, with or without pain, to axial rotation while the neck is in flexion is strongly suggestive of upper cervical involvement, while restriction with the neck in extension points to subluxation within the lower cervical spine.

The next assessment of movement is at the segmental level and, while specific guidance is given in the regional chapters of Part 2, especially for the atypical spinal levels, a generic discussion of typical segmental assessment by movement palpation is given in this chapter. First, however, the patient should be assessed for gait. It is equally as reasonable to assess gait as a component of postural assessment and before any range of motion assessment as it is to assess gait after knowing how the patient can perform during the range of motion assessment. The actual sequencing as applied in the clinical situation is the practitioner's choice.

Gait analysis

Gait is an essential component of movement and can be considered as the most fundamental form of dynamic posture. It is the basis of holistic biomechanical analysis of the patient (Schafer 1983 p. 107) and it is sometimes said that the observation of gait starts in the waiting room as the patient is observed getting out of the chair. While this may provide important early clues to the practitioner, a more structured approach is required.

The patient should be seated in a firm chair and be wearing minimal clothing. The first observation remains that of the way the patient rises from the chair. The patient is asked to stand and the practitioner is looking for signs of the patient shifting the body weight to a pain-free, uninvolved side of the body. This is Minor's sign (Evans 2001 pp. 576–577) and is positive when the patient is seen to support the body while sitting by balancing on the uninvolved leg and then using the hands to raise the body from the chair. A positive finding suggests sacroiliac involvement, lumbosacral sprains and strains, disk protrusion with nerve root pain into a leg, and other more worrisome conditions such as lumbopelvic fractures, muscular dystrophy, and dystonia (Evans 2001).

A patient with a positive Minor's sign will obviously demonstrate a significantly altered gait, restrictions to range of motion, and possibly an antalgic lean, especially with non-central disk protrusion (Fig. 14.15). There is little point in forcing such patients through a series of provocative intermediate tests and it is more appropriate to proceed with a directed examination which focuses on the process of ruling in and ruling out the relevant differential diagnoses.

Once patients are standing they are asked to walk a short distance, turn, and walk back to the chair. They may need to repeat this process a number of times, pain permitting.

Observations are made by the practitioner from the side, front, and back. The essential premise is that the body should progress smoothly and fluidly through space with symmetry of movement and elegance of balance.

The manual physician is primarily concerned with mechanical gait but must first consider and rule out neurologic gait. The key observation is whether the gait is symmetrical or asymmetrical. Mechanical problems usually produce asymmetrical gait, such as an antalgic lean due to pain or a limp due to bony deformity; however, an asymmetrical gait with one leg swinging out to the side suggests a hemiplegic gait while one knee lifting higher suggests foot drop (Fuller 1999). The hemiplegic gait is clearly a neurologic gait; however, the causes of foot drop range from a pyramidal lesion to a lumbopelvic SC causing L5 nerve root compromise. Mechanical gait changes range from those which are subtle and secondary to SC and associated changes, through restricted motion gaits due to soft-tissue contractures, to antalgic gaits which include the painful limp.

A quick guide to identifying neurologic problems is to associate a waddling gait with muscle disease, a wobbling gait with cerebellar disorders, a shuffling gait with Parkinson's disease, and a jerking gait with chorea (Wilkinson 1993). The following discussion of gait is most relevant for patients with subtle kinematic change, most likely secondary to subluxation, as opposed to those who demonstrate gross change secondary to a more severe clinical presentation.

Normal gait is a smooth progression through consecutive walking cycles, where one cycle is two steps, one with each lower limb (Fig. 4.6A). Some 60% of the walking cycle is the stance phase, where the foot is in contact with the ground, progressing through heel strike, foot-flat and toe-off. The remainder of the cycle is the swing phase where the limb progresses through toe-off (acceleration), midswing, and heel strike (deceleration). The following clinical notes are summarized from Schafer (1983 pp. 103–120) and Fuller (1999 pp. 35–40):

The following are specifically assessed in the side view:

- Symmetry of the stance phase: it should be equal left and right.
- Stride length: it should be even left and right.
- Vertical excursion: the body should smoothly rise and fall several centimeters during each cycle.
- Carriage of the head and trunk: it should be vertical and maintain balance. A ramrod back suggests thoracic subluxation or erector spinae hypertonicity.
- Arm swing: it should be free, equal, and alternate to leg swing.
- Heel strike: an altered pattern suggests bursitis, a heel spur, or a blister. A harsh heel strike suggests weak hamstrings.
- Knee extension: failure to extend fully during heel strike suggests weak quadriceps, as does excessive flexion in midstance.
- Lateral gravity line: paraspinal muscle hypertonicity is suggested in a patient who leans backwards during the cycle. Problems of the posterior mechanical spinal columns, such as facet irritation, tend to cause the patient to lean forward during the cycle.
- Toe-walking: a patient with painful lumbosacral or cervical lesions may try to walk gently, more on the toes, in an attempt to reduce jarring the spine.

The following are specifically assessed from in front of and behind the patient:

- The pelvis: it should remain centered over the line of progression; however, it will shift laterally a couple of centimeters to each weight-bearing side during the cycle. Accentuated lateral shifting suggests gluteus medius weakness. It should also rotate and tilt smoothly in the manner described by Greenman (1990, Fig. 4.6B) and restrictions in these movements may indicate sacroiliac joint fixation. A forward lurch of the hip suggests a weak gluteus maximus. Significant anterior rotation of the pelvis to provide thrust for the leg suggests weak quadriceps. A pelvis which "waddles" indicates weak or ineffective proximal muscles caused by proximal myopathies. It may also suggest bilateral congenital dislocation of the hip.
- Base width: the distance between the heels is normally 5–10 cm. A wider-based gait is assessed for whether it is high-stepping or not. A high-stepping wide-based gait suggests sensory ataxia as a loss of joint position sense (with a positive Rhomberg's test) and is commonly caused by peripheral neuropathy or posterior neural column loss. A wide-based gait without high stepping suggests cerebellar ataxia and the patient will veer towards the side of the lesion. Common causes include cerebrovascular disease and multiple sclerosis. This gait is also caused by alcohol and drugs (phenytoin). A decreased base with a "scissor" crossover action of the legs suggests spastic paraparesis. Common causes include cerebral palsy, multiple sclerosis, and cord compression.
- Leg swing: weak adductors may allow the leg to swing outwards from the hip, while weak medial hamstrings may allow the foot to rotate externally and flare during the swing phase. The foot may appear to turn outwards with a normal piriformis if the contralateral piriformis is weak. An inturned foot may suggest a weak psoas on the same side.
- Shoulder rotation and arm swing: these should be even and in opposite direction to the advancing leg. The level of greatest rotation within the spine should lie about T6–7. Restrictions to shoulder rotation suggest thoracic subluxation or shoulder and arm disorders.
- AP gravity line: the gravity line is distorted with a lean to one side in cases of lumbar disk lesions and the patient's hand may be used to support the pelvis on the painful side. The gravity line may deviate to the side away from weak erector spinae and may also lean away from the side of a weak gluteus medius during the stance phase on that side.

The findings from the gait analysis must be considered with the postural findings in an attempt to direct the regional and segmental examinations better.

SEGMENTAL ASSESSMENT

The specific purpose of segmental assessment of a specific SMU is to determine:

- the quantity of movement in each degree of freedom
- the quality of movement through each degree of freedom
- the quality of end-feel, within that SMU.

These findings are placed within the context of all other findings discovered and recorded during the process of assessing the patient for kinematic change through posture analysis, range of motion, gait, radiographic findings, and so on. These data are

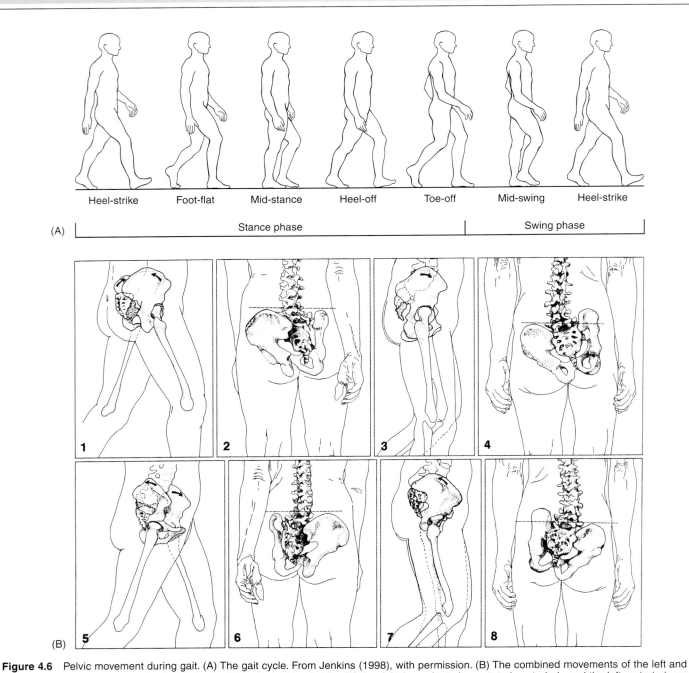

Figure 4.6 Pelvic movement during gait. (A) The gait cycle. From Jenkins (1998), with permission. (B) The combined movements of the left and right innominates, sacrum, and spine during walking. At right heel strike (1) the right innominate has rotated posteriorly and the left, anteriorly and (2) the anterior surface of the sacrum has rotated to the left and the superior surface is level, while the spine is straight but rotated to the left.

At right midstance (3) the right leg is straight and the right innominate is rotating anteriorly and (4) the sacrum has rotated right and tilted to the left while the lumbar spine has laterally flexed to the right and rotated to the left.

At left heel strike (5) the left innominate begins to rotate anteriorly after toe-off and the right innominate beings to rotate posteriorly and (6) the sacrum is level but with the anterior surface rotated to the right. The spine is straight but rotated to the right, along with the lower trunk.

At left leg stance (7) the left innominate is high and left leg straight and (8) the sacrum has rotated to the left and tilted to the right, while the lumbar spine has laterally flexed to the left and rotated to the right. From Greenman (1990), with permission.

integrated within the clinical decision-making process in order to demonstrate some relationship with any SMU which may demonstrate altered movement.

The whole idea is to integrate any segmental change with change in the whole being and at this point those other changes

are also kinematic in nature. The subsequent chapters address changes which may occur in connective tissue, muscle structure and function, the nervous system and the vascular system, and will demonstrate how those changes may also be related to segmental change within a specific SMU.

Movement palpation

Segmental kinematics are assessed by dynamic or movement palpation, a process by which the practitioner induces specific movements into an SMU for the purpose of aiding an assessment of its function in terms of the quantity and quality of movement in each of the six degrees of freedom, and the nature of the end-feel, again in each degree of freedom.

The six degrees of freedom in correct terms are rotation about each of the x-, y-, and z-axes, and translation along each of the x-, y-, and z-axes. Given that pure movement of this nature is unlikely within the SMU, a little license is taken and the six degrees of freedom, in the clinical sense, become flexion, extension, left rotation, right rotation, left lateral flexion, and right lateral flexion.

Movement within each of these degrees must be assessed first for its quantity. This finding is a cross between an objective and a subjective measure because the amount of movement is typically so small within any SMU that it is less than the level of error of any instrument which could measure it. Therefore it becomes a judgment of the practitioner (subjective) based on that which is visualized as an objective dimension.

On the other hand, the quality of movement during the normal range of motion, no matter how small it might be, of a particular SMU can only be a subjective measure. The practitioner must use every skill available to observe and palpate the movement of one spinal segment on another to make a judgment of the quality of movement within the context of its quantity. The quality of movement may be continuous or intermittent, smooth or jerky, or slow-starting or late-starting. The subjective finding of the practitioner leads to a diagnostic statement which can be accepted as a truth and become subject to reassessment on a subsequent occasion.

The final information is a subjective judgment of the quality of the end-feel of the segment in each degree of freedom. In practical terms this translates to a judgment of how the spinous process moves under provocation at the end of rotation, lateral flexion, and flexion/extension. End-feel has palpatory qualities similar to those of tissue palpation (Fig. 4.4). A bony end-feel suggests the segment has a major degree of fixation, such that almost no movement is possible. A springy end-feel is normal as the ligaments about the SMU do their duty and gently limit the degree of movement. An elastic end-feel suggests ligamentous involvement, perhaps a weakening on one side which allows a little more movement on the other side such that the segment moves beyond normal and is restrained by the elastic qualities of the ligaments. A spongy, edematous feel is suggestive of inflammation and segmental pathology.

Practitioner position

All manual assessment and therapeutic procedures require careful consideration of the placement of both the practitioner and patient. The benefits are manifold and include a relaxed, cooperative patient amenable to control by the practitioner, with the result being a greater level of reliability and reproducibility. Given that the movement of the patient is passive, the practitioner position must be optimized to ensure the examiner is able to exert and maintain full control as the full range of passive movement is induced in each of the six planes of the SMU.

The essential element of the practitioner position is the stance. As with a trained dancer, all control and the subsequent beauty

of movement flow from correct foot placement. The different types of practitioner stance are shown in Figure 4.7. It may be square behind the patient for seated assessment of the cervical spine (Fig. 4.7A) or as a fencer stance (Fig. 4.7D) at a posterolateral position to the patient for the assessment of the thoracic spine. The offset square (Fig. 4.7B) stance is used for assessment of the atlanto-occipital joints and the square to the side stance (Fig. 4.7C) is used for assessing components of cervical spine movement, and other movements in the sagittal plane. A combination of square to the side and posterolateral fencer stance is also used for assessment of the thoracic spine (Fig. 4.7E).

The patient position must be carefully managed to achieve maximal comfort, relaxation, and compliance while meshing

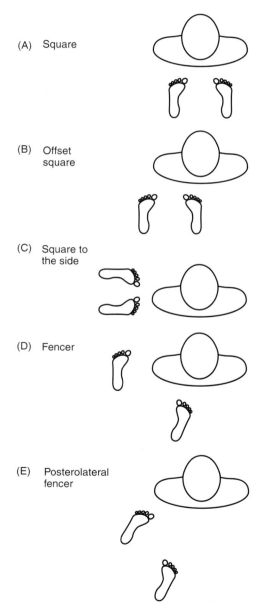

(A) Square

(B) Offset square

(C) Square to the side

(D) Fencer

(E) Posterolateral fencer

Figure 4.7 Types of stance with reference to a seated patient. Displacement of the practitioner may be either to the left, as shown, or to the right.

with the practitioner's height and build. For example, assessment of the upper cervical spine is optimized when the seated patient is placed so the atlanto-occipital complex is level with the practitioner's hypogastrium. This allows the practitioner to assess the region with the elbows flexed to 90° and stabilized against his or her own body in order to afford optimal control of the particular joint being assessed.

Most movement palpation is conducted with the patient seated; however, the cervical spine and upper thoracic spine and upper ribs may be assessed with the patient supine, and many spinal articulations can be assessed with micromovement palpation in the prone patient.

It is important to use the appropriate contact point of the doctor's hand. The basic contact points have evolved over time as the chiropractic profession developed and were codified in 1988 (ACA Council on Technic 1988b) (Fig. 4.8). The palpating hand is a bidirectional instrument which both receives information from patients and conveys sensation to them. The hands must be kept clean and dry as they can communicate fear and nervousness to the patient if dirty or sweaty.

The role of the hands is to control movement while receiving the delicate tactile data required of the patient for assessment. A non-greasy hand cream may help keep the skin soft and supple and this in turn will improve the ability to sense by touch. The nails are to be kept trimmed so as not to scratch the patient. Heavy jewelry and finger rings set with stone are a distraction and should not be worn in the clinical context. Above all, the touch must at all times be therapeutic, which is asexual, gentle yet firm, and controlled.

The detailed anatomy of each SMU must be understood and applied to ensure contact is made on the relevant landmarks. For example, the variable relationships of the transverse processes to the spinous process, and indeed, the length and shape of the spinous process itself in the thoracic region can significantly confound contact. A logical pattern of thought must be applied to ensure the optimal contact is held during a specific movement. For example, if the nature of the end-feel of the spinous process of a typical SMU is being assessed in right body rotation, then the palpating finger will firstly contact the right side of the spinous process and press it further into its end-zone, to the left. The finger will then contact the left side of the spinous process and apply a testing force to the right to assess resilient movement away from the end-zone.

Care is taken with all contacts to optimize the control of the patient's passive movement. In this respect the indifferent or non-contact hand is both a stabilizing hand and a movement hand as opposed to being largely only a stabilizing hand for spinal adjustment. A high level of present-time consciousness is required to ensure the best placement of the indifferent hand at all times. The touch of this hand must also be gentle yet firm to guide the movements of the patient through each degree of freedom. It is advantageous first to explain the process to patients and verbally to reinforce the fact they are to remain relaxed while the doctor leads, directs, and controls each movement.

Underlying principles

The underlying principle is that the subluxated segment will move better into subluxation than it will move out of subluxation.

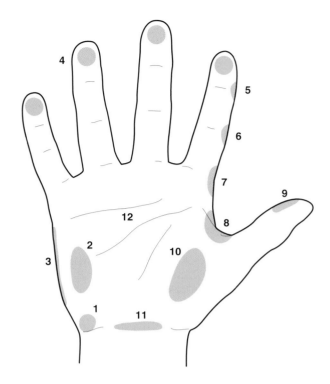

1 Pisiform

2 Hypothenar

3 Metacarpal (knife-edge)

4 Digital

5 Distal interphalangeal (DIP)

6 Proximal interphalangeal (PIP)

7 Metacarpophalangeal (MP)

8 Web

9 Thumb

10 Thenar

11 Calcaneal

12 Palmar

Figure 4.8 Contact points on the hand.

This illustrates the belief that subluxation involves movement into a position from which return movement is restricted. Therefore the segment is thought of as being fixated in the position into which it has moved. Given that movement is largely a continuum and the degree of fixation is variable, the subluxated segment usually retains the ability to demonstrate movement in the direction of fixation. The converse movement, away from the position of fixation, is significantly reduced.

In the situation where muscle contraction has contributed to the SC it can be readily understood that a segment will retain movement in the direction of contraction along the axis of the contracted muscle but will be less able to demonstrate movement away from the contracted muscle. In other words, the muscle will contract and prevent movement in the opposite direction. A simple clinical demonstration of this principle is to have a companion flex the elbow to 90° using the biceps. The reader can support the elbow and will find it is relatively easy to move the forearm into further flexion yet quite difficult to move it out of flexion or into extension.

The practitioner is conducting movement palpation for the purposes of making an informed observation of the quantity and quality of movement in each of the six degrees of freedom of the SMU. The third assessment is of the quality of the end-feel at the end of each passive movement. Given the belief that subluxation occurs as a segment moves into a position from which it is restricted in moving out of, end-feel must be assessed in a bidirectional manner. This means, for example, that with right rotation of the vertebral body which is accompanied by movement to the left of the spinous process, the spinous must be assessed for end-feel both further to the left as well as out of that direction, namely to the right.

The variety of causes of the SC mean it is impossible to identify and explain every conceivable combination of end-feel. Pragmatically, the practitioner must aim to identify a sense of what may be happening and this is where a solid knowledge of anatomy is essential. An end-feel with an elastic quality in one direction and a bony quality in the other suggests fixation in the direction of bony end-feel. An end-feel which has a springy quality, perhaps in both directions, suggests acute strain/sprain of the SMU. It is very difficult to link scientifically the quality of end-feel with a particular clinical condition. This places an emphasis on the practitioner to "look to feel" and to record what is felt, and then to correlate these findings with others to synthesize a working diagnosis which best integrates all findings.

A final principle is to sequence the assessment of movement in an order which recognizes the dominant movement at a particular spinal level over the lesser movements. For example, flexion and extension is a much more significant movement than rotation in the lumbar and thoracic spines, hence the first movement to be assessed should be flexion and extension. Restriction is more likely to be evident in flexion and extension than in rotation, so rotation can be the last movement to be assessed. Lateral flexion may or may not be a component of the SC in this region so it can be assessed after flexion and extension and before rotation.

Lateral flexion and rotation are the pre-eminent clinical movements in the cervical spine and restriction is typically found more easily in lateral flexion and rotation. Given the nature of the lordosis and the involvement of the articular pillars, the movements of flexion and extension are less important. It is for this reason that the assessment of regional rotation with the neck in full flexion and then full extension is a valuable clinical pointer to levels of fixation.

These principles have been stated in an extraordinarily simple manner and the clinical reality is naturally much more complex. The aim of movement palpation is first to assess the left/right symmetry of movement, noting the quantity in terms of any increase or decrease in the absence of known causes such as mechanical change in various elements of the SMU. Second, it is to develop a description of the change in order to direct the therapeutic intervention. The description is the "listing" and its relationship to the movement findings is given below.

An example

The notion of a right rotation fixation of the vertebral body of L1 will be used as the first example. This could be described as either a right posterior mamillary process (**RP**) or a (posterior) left spinous process (**PL**).

In the prone patient a blocking sensation may be palpated over the right mamillary process with posterior to anterior springing, which would suggest posteriority. This may also be reported as tender by the patient. When the spinous process is provoked for end-feel, tenderness may be palpated about the left lateral distal area and this may be emphasized with palpation from the left to right, which will feel blocked. The spinous may feel springy with palpation from the right to the left against the right side and this movement may be painful in the SMU, as opposed to tender at the contact point.

In the seated patient the spinal region is scanned in repetitive flexion and extension movements to identify any levels of restricted or blocked movement. In this case (L1–2) the practitioner will support the patient's folded arms and use this indifferent hand to rock the patient's arms and shoulders up and down to induce flexion and extension in the spine. The contact hand will palpate each SMU during each flexion/extension cycle to identify any particular SMU which may have a restricted or blocked feel.

The practitioner's indifferent hand and arm then control the patient into full flexion and then extension at any suspected SMU (in this case L1–2). The contact hand will provoke the spinous process into further flexion when the patient is in full flexion at this SMU and this should feel blocked and be reported as tender. This finding is suggestive of an extension fixation at this level which limits movement of the L1 segment into flexion. The spinous process of L1 should appear to close normally on that of L2 in extension, representing movement into the extension fixation.

If there is a suggestion (or a belief within the practitioner's paradigm) that there is a component of lateral flexion associated with this SC, then the SMU is assessed for movement in lateral flexion. The practitioner is in a square stance to the side (Fig. 4.7C) and the indifferent forearm lies over the patient's shoulders so that lateral flexion can be induced in the spine at the level of the L1–2 SMU. This current example of PL spinous or RP body will now be visualized with L1 being laterally flexed to the right. This will generate an open wedge of the L1–2 disk on the left and the listing will be PLS (with reference to the spinous) or RPI (with reference to the mamillary).

When right lateral flexion is induced into the SMU, there should be little or no restriction of movement, either in lateral flexion or of the spinous process. The principle here is that a lesion with some lateral flexion to the right of the superior segment will appear to flex laterally more to the right when that passive movement is induced in the SMU. This movement is coupled with rotation and the body is expected to rotate to the right, which will move the spinous process to the left. When right lateral flexion is passively induced into the SMU the spinous will palpate as moving better to the left than to the right.

On the other hand, left lateral flexion will produce blocked findings. First, the SMU is less likely to close down on the side of open wedge and left lateral flexion into the SMU will be limited. Second, given left lateral flexion is limited, the spinous process will similarly have limited movement and may palpate in both directions as blocked.

Restrictions in lateral flexion may also be inferred from the AP radiograph; however, any such finding must be placed in the clinical context of the patient. It may also be possible to visualize more of a regional loss of lateral flexion through close observation of standing patients as they actively laterally flex left and right. This is likely to appear as a kink in the spine at the L1–2 level, particularly with left lateral flexion.

Rotation is the final movement to assess in the seated patient. The practitioner's indifferent hand and forearm induce axial rotation of the spine by again using the shoulders as a lever. With all movements induced from the shoulders, care must be taken to ensure the vectors actually induce the desired movement in the target SMU. Rotation is not a simple turning of the patient's torso to the left and right; it must be controlled to ensure that the movements of rotation occur within the SMU.

Given that the vertebral body has rotated right (with the spinous to the left), the movement of right rotation will palpate without restriction, although there may be some tenderness about the spinous processes, as described above for prone palpation. Rotation to the left will palpate with restrictions in the movement of the spinous process; in particular, it will palpate as blocked and tender when pressed on the left side, from left to right.

The key steps in the performance of movement palpation are summarized in Box 4.3. As with the application of adjustive

---

Box 4.3 Steps in the performance of movement palpation

- Optimize the doctor position.
- Optimize the patient position.
- Use the appropriate contact point.
- Contact relevant landmarks.
- Control the passive movement.
- Assess quantity of movement in each degree of freedom.
- Assess quality of movement through each degree of freedom.
- Assess quality of end-feel.

---

technique, the success of the process begins with the crucial element of the relative positions of the doctor and the patient.

CONCLUSION

The assessment of kinematic change is perhaps the most commonly identified dimension of the SC in clinical practice. This does not infer that the assessment of such change is straightforward; the practitioner must be aware of structural asymmetries, functional changes which are normal to a particular patient, and the concept of compensation versus subluxation.

From postural analysis, through gait analysis and segmental movement palpation, the practitioner is seeking evidence, both subjective and objective, of kinematic change which must inform the ongoing process of assessment for associated dimensions.

5

Assessment of connective tissue change

KEY CONCEPTS

In clinical terms, connective tissue can be thought of as having three distinctly different forms: broad and flat, as with the skin, subcutaneous tissues, and fascial planes; band-like ribbons and cords, as ligaments which are tensile structures; and the intervertebral disk, perhaps the most important form of ligamentous connective tissue in the spine.

The identification of a high-intensity zone in the magnetic resonance imaging (MRI) of the disk is a useful indicator of disk disruption but is not necessarily associated with pain. MRI must be interpreted with consideration of full clinical signs, symptoms, and other relevant background.

The height of the disk space increases with age up to age 69 years, therefore the finding of a loss of disk height on a plain radiograph is a pathologic finding. MRI associates loss of disk height with internal disk disruption.

Fibromyalgia syndrome (FMS) is commonly thought to be a connective tissue disorder which affects the patient in a global manner; however, it is frequently misdiagnosed. Classic FMS is a state of global lowered pain threshold caused by abnormal brain processing of sensory stimuli and is not responsive to manual intervention. Pseudo-FMS is a subset of regional musculoskeletal disorders which do respond to mechanical and other interventions.

Trigger points (TrPs) are hyperirritable spots, usually within a taut band of skeletal muscle or its fascia, and are painful on compression. They give rise to characteristic referred pain, tenderness and autonomic phenomena. An active TrP is tender and prevents full lengthening of the muscle, thus weakening it.

A neurolymphatic point is a circumscribed zone in a predictable location on the body which acts in both a diagnostic and therapeutic manner for a certain muscle or group of muscles. The clinical relevance is that the finding of tenderness about a particular spinal motion unit (SMU) may not necessarily represent local tissue response to kinematic change. Rather, it may represent a reflex finding secondary to remote muscle dysfunction.

The predominant connective tissues at the segmental level are the intervertebral disk and the ligaments about the SMU. Ligaments are specialized for tensile strength and energy absorption and contain nerve endings capable of monitoring tissue stress, strain, and pain. The ligaments of the SMU have only a minor mechanical role in maintaining spinal stability but are important contributors to proprioception and joint position sense, including vertebral position.

The intervertebral disk is perhaps the most important connective tissue of the spine and, in addition to generating pain through mechanical interference with surrounding structures, most notably the spinal nerve roots, the disk itself may generate pain from damage to its own structure, typically as internal disk disruption.

INTRODUCTION

In the absence of connective tissue the body would simply be a pile of bones, muscles, and organs, incapable of function and movement. The body exists in its familiar form because connective tissue invests every component and brings order to chaos. The term "connective tissue" encompasses a broad range of structures, from the largest organ of the body, the skin, to the finest filaments attaching the dural sleeve within the spinal canal and intervertebral canal. The individual and cumulative effects of connective tissues are important to consider in the assessment of the spine.

Given the category of connective tissue is so broad and its involvement in health and disease is so diverse, an ordered approach is needed. The sequence of global, regional, then segmental provides a convenient structure for the assessment. This chapter will consider disorders such as fibromyalgia as global and myofascial pain syndromes as regional. The ligaments about the SMU, including the intervertebral disk, are considered to be segmental.

In clinical terms, connective tissue can be thought of as having three distinctly different forms. The first is broad and flat, as with skin and its underlying connective tissue and the fascial planes which are palpated through the skin. Its assessment is more by compressive palpation and is described in terms of tone, although some fascial sheets have been shown to transfer tensile loads (Vleeming et al 1996, Barker & Briggs 1999). Collectively these tissues can be thought of as skin and fascia. The second form is ligament and can be thought of as defined,

tensile structures. Ligaments vary in their capacity for clinical assessment. Some, such as the cruciate ligaments of the knee, are clearly able to be isolated and assessed for dysfunction, while others, notably the ligaments of the SMU, are implicated more by clinical guesswork than specific testing. MRI, when available, is able to provide quantitative evidence of ligament damage about the SMU.

The third is the intervertebral disk, perhaps the most important form of ligamentous connective tissue in the spine. As with the other ligaments of the SMU, any involvement of the disk as a pain generator is more of a clinical inference than a definitive statement. Even when diagnostic imaging provides quantitative evidence of disk involvement in some way, it is not necessarily a conclusive diagnostic statement that the disk is the cause of the patient's pain.

FASCIA

Fascia may be viewed as a complex, continuous series of interconnected tubes and sheets extending throughout the body, within which muscles, joints, nerves, vessels, and the viscera are enclosed (Bilkey 1992). Superficial fascia lies under the skin and is a moderately loose weave of irregularly arranged fibrous and elastic tissue. This type of loose areolar connective tissue also lies deep to invest the abdominal and thoracic viscera and is termed "subserous fascia". The deep fascia is tough, compacted but still irregularly woven fibroelastic tissue which envelopes tissues, including muscles (Bilkey 1992). The deep fascia has superficial and deep laminae which in turn surround muscles and have multiple fibrous attachments (Barker & Briggs 1999).

The thoracolumbar fascia has been shown to be innervated by free nerve endings as well as two types of encapsulated mechanoreceptors (Ruffini's and Vater–Pacini corpuscles), which suggests it may play a neurosensory role in the lumbar spine mechanism (Yahia et al 1992). A subsequent study failed to identify any specific neural end-organs in samples of thoracolumbar fascia harvested during surgery from patients with back pain who had not undergone previous lumbar surgery. These findings suggest that the thoracolumbar fascia may be deficiently innervated in problem-back-pain patients (Bednar et al 1995).

While the above comments relate specifically to the thoracolumbar fascia, it must be appreciated that fascia forms one integrated and totally connected network through the body (Chaitow & DeLany 2000 p. 2). Fascia is formed of collagen and acts as a colloid in that it tightens against rapidly applied forces but remains plastic and pliant under a slowly applied load. Clinically this requires a gentle touch applied relatively slowly in order to palpate and assess the resting state of the fascia. A hard, rapid touch will induce rigid responses as a reaction and mask the underlying state.

Continuous connective lines have been identified in the fascia of the body (Chaitow & DeLany 2000 pp. 7–8) and, while these may have some clinical application, the more important realization is the high degree of connectivity which does exist. This is more sophisticated than the simple understanding that the plantar fascia links through the gastrocnemius to the hamstrings which link to the thoracolumbar fascia through the sacrotuberous ligament, and so on. As discussed below, the connective tissue systems do more than link together all of the mechanical elements of the body; they also attach to and affect the dura of the central nervous system, within the cranium, spinal canal, and sacrum.

Tissue preference

A second important clinical consideration is the manner in which the asymmetry in the fascia affects body movement at certain levels. It is thought that fascia has an inherent asymmetry which favors tissue movement in one rotary direction over another. Zink & Lawson (1979) described four levels at which this preference could be identified:

1. the upper cervical spine at the atlanto-occipital junction
2. the cervicothoracic junction
3. the thoracolumbar junction
4. the lumbosacral area.

Chaitow & DeLany (2000 p. 12) demonstrate how tissue preference may be assessed at the cervicothoracic junction (Fig. 5.1).

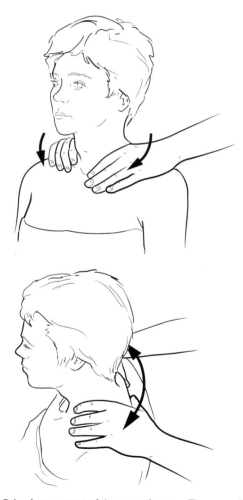

Figure 5.1 Assessment of tissue preference. Tissue preference in rotation is assessed at the cervicothoracic junction in the seated patient. The practitioner's hands rest lightly about the base of the neck and move the tissues slightly left and right, in a rotary manner about the neck. The tissue on one side will have a sense of feeling looser than the other. From Chaitow & DeLany (2000), with permission.

The same principle applies at each of the four sites which are considered crossover sites for the fascia. The tissues at each level are lightly palpated and moved in a rotary manner about the y-axis. It is thought that the tissue on one side will have a sense of feeling looser than the other and that this is the side of "tissue preference". Zink & Lawson (1979) suggest the typical finding is for an alternating left–right preference from the atlanto-occipital junction downwards. They reported that patients who did not demonstrate an alternating pattern had poor health histories.

The clinical implication is that the natural tendency of the body to demonstrate tissue preference at these levels introduces a general level of noise into the overall assessment of connective tissue and fascial tone, and a specific level of noise which acts as a confounder for the assessment of kinematic change at the key transitional areas of the spine.

The patient should be assessed for tissue preference before being assessed with movement palpation. Two things should be noted: the presence or absence of left–right symmetry and the side of looseness, particularly at the atlanto-occipital, cervicothoracic, and thoracolumbar junctions, and whether this demonstrates a left–right–left pattern. The subsequent assessment of kinematic change at these levels must take account of the tissue preference and not automatically consider that any restriction of tissues represents the presence of spinal dysfunction.

GLOBAL CONSIDERATIONS

The interconnectivity of the fascia and ligamentous networks obviously implies that a global effect may arise from any regional dysfunction and this is to be particularly considered in the assessment of posture and gait. Such imbalances however are typically pain-free and represent a chronic adaptation to segmental dysfunction elsewhere in the body. On the other hand, the connective tissues may become associated with pain and tenderness at multiple sites throughout the body. The complaint of multiple sites of soft-tissue pain, often described as "pain all over" and usually presenting with fatigue, is commonly termed the fibromyalgia syndrome (FMS) (Bennett 1999).

Fibromyalgia syndrome

The peak patient group for FMS is females between the ages of 55 and 64 years. The female prevalence is typically about 3%, while for males it is less than 1% (Yunus & Inanici 2001). FMS has a relatively complex multifactorial origin and is not a diagnosis by exclusion. Pain is the predominant symptom and is experienced in widespread locations. The basic classification criteria for FMS rely on the identification of quantified pain in specific predetermined sites about the body (Fig. 5.2). Quantification is by use of an algometer and the applied force is $4\,kg/cm^2$.

The criteria for classifying a patient as having FMS as introduced in 1990 by the American College of Rheumatology (Wolfe et al 1990) are:

- chronic, widespread pain (pain that is present on both sides of the body, above and below the waist, and in the axial skeleton) that has been present for more than 3 months
- pain elicited by the palpation of tender points (TePs) at a minimum of 11 of 18 predetermined sites (Fig. 5.2).

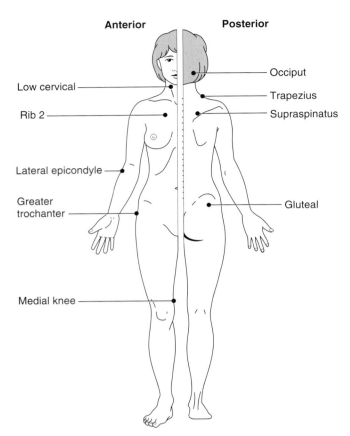

Figure 5.2 Assessment of FMS. The locations of nine bilateral tender point sites introduced in 1990 by the American College of Rheumatology as the criteria for classification of fibromyalgia syndrome patients. From Baldry (2001), with permission.

The Copenhagen Declaration of 1992 (Jacobsen et al 1993) associated the basic physical findings with persistent fatigue, non-refreshing sleep, and generalized stiffness. FMS may present as part of a wider syndrome encompassing headache, irritable bowel syndrome, irritable bladder, dysmenorrhea, cold sensitivity, Raynaud's phenomenon, restless legs, atypical patterns of numbness and tingling, exercise intolerance, and complaints of weakness (Schneider & Brady 2001).

Schneider & Brady (2001) consider there is a falsely high rate of diagnosis of FMS in the absence of adequate laboratory tests to rule out differentials such as anemia, Lyme disease, hypothyroidism, inflammatory arthritides, autoimmune disorders, multiple sclerosis, and occult malignancy. They also found some patients experienced substantial and long-term relief with manual treatment while others derived little or no benefit from the same therapy. Further, it seems the response of patients with FMS remains quite variable to a range of interventions, including low-dose antidepressants, dietary manipulation, vitamin supplementation, herbal remedies, and thyroid or estrogen replacement therapy.

Patients with fibromyalgia report seeing a variety of complementary and alternative medicine (CAM) practitioners; however, empirical research data exist to support only mind–body techniques, acupuncture, and manipulative techniques

(Berman & Swyers 1999). The data are strongest from biofeedback, hypnosis, and cognitive behavioral therapy, and weakest for manipulative techniques such as chiropractic and massage; however, these findings may reflect the falsely high rate of diagnosis.

Manipulative treatment combined with standard medical care has been shown to be more efficacious in treating FMS than standard care alone (Gamber et al 2002). The outcomes for standard care are more favorable in patients of a younger age (46 vs 51 years) and with less sleep disturbance (Fitzcharles et al 2003). Fibromyalgia patients are typically more anxious and somatically aware than patients with rheumatoid arthritis or musculoskeletal pain, although all patients studied in these three classifications of chronic pain had impaired cognitive functioning on an ecologically sensitive neuropsychological test of everyday attention (Dick et al 2002).

Schneider & Brady (2001) also consider that the traditional view of FMS can be improved by a new classification which first separates classic from pseudo-FMS and then further explores pseudo-FMS for other diagnostic possibilities (Fig. 5.3). Patients with classic FMS do not respond well to standard manual treatments such as chiropractic, physical therapy, or massage, because their condition is not primarily caused by any abnormality of the muscles and joints; it is a state of qualitatively altered nociception (Bendtsen et al 1997) and global lowered pain threshold caused by abnormal brain processing of sensory stimuli (Bennett 1999, Gracely et al 2002). The subset of pseudo-FMS patients with musculoskeletal disorders are those who should respond favorably to manual treatment.

This would appear to be a reasonable approach which allows a more consistent grouping of symptoms within the classic FMS diagnosis and which should result in better diagnosis and treatment of patients with incomplete or confusing symptoms (Schneider & Brady 2001). The practitioner will note the subcategories of pseudo-FMS include a variety of disorders which have a similar global impact on the body's fascia and connective tissue systems.

The underlying principle identified by Schneider & Brady (2001) is that, whenever a practitioner can successfully reproduce a regional pain pattern on physical examination, the patient should not be diagnosed with FMS.

REGIONAL CONSIDERATIONS

Fascial pain is a diagnosis largely reached by the exclusion of other causes and then ruled in by a simple test. First, the pain experience of the patient is one characterized by being relatively diffuse about a spinal region, with or without some radiation into a limb. The complaints are usually either low-back and unilateral buttock pain with radiation into the posterior leg, or upper-back and low-neck pain with unilateral shoulder pain which may radiate into the arm and forearm (Bilkey 1992). There may be dull or sharp aching with some tingling, burning, or numbness but no pins and needles or loss of sensation (Bilkey 1992).

The SMU must be ruled out as a pain generator by establishing there is no kinematic change in, or other changes attributable to, the particular SMUs in a spinal region. Muscle and tendon are then excluded by demonstrating normal muscle function in the absence of pain or tenderness. The major joints

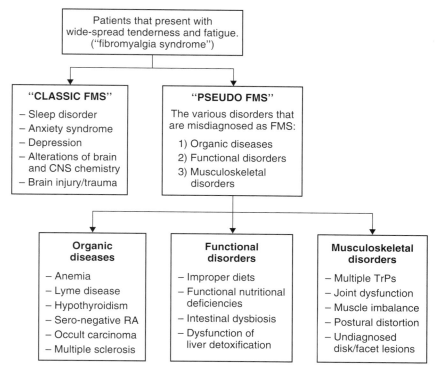

Figure 5.3 A diagnostic approach to fibromyalgia. The diagnostic approach to patients with suspected fibromyalgia should take account of the disorders which may have similar global effects but which are not the classic fibromyalgia syndrome. CNS, central nervous system; RA, rheumatoid arthritis; TrPs, trigger points. From Schneider & Brady (2001), with permission.

(hip, shoulder) are excluded as discrete pain generators by demonstrating normal pain-free range of motion of the joint itself in the absence of tenderness to palpation and any signs of joint inflammation (Bilkey 1992).

When these sources of pain are ruled out, the major joints are reassessed. In the case of low-back pain, the fascia is implicated when the back pain itself is worsened in the supine patient with hip rotation in neutral, and hip distraction. In the case of cervicothoracic pain, the fascia is implicated when horizontal abduction of the shoulder, with the elbow extended, is painful and restricted (Bilkey 1992).

Myofascial pain syndrome

A myofascial pain syndrome is one which involves a muscle or muscles as well as the fascia in one region of the body, in the absence of profound fatigue in the patient (Bennett 1999). Typically there will be a palpable trigger point in the muscle or its myotendinous junction which refers pain in a distinctive pattern when stimulated. TrPs tend to occur in predictable, known locations, and a number of authors have described the pain distribution for TrPs in specific muscles.

Trigger points

A TrP is a hyperirritable spot, usually within a taut band of skeletal muscle or in the muscle's fascia. The spot is painful on compression and can give rise to characteristic referred pain, tenderness, and autonomic phenomena. TrPs may be latent, in which case they exist but do not create pain, or active, in which case they do create pain which refers in a characteristic pattern.

An active TrP is tender and prevents full lengthening of the muscle, thus weakening it. The TrP is distinctly different to a TeP in that it usually refers pain on direct compression, mediates a local twitch response of its taut muscle fibers when adequately stimulated, causes tenderness in the pain reference zone, and often produces specific referred autonomic phenomena, generally in its pain reference zone. An active TrP can cause referred pain and tenderness at rest, or with motion that stretches or loads that muscle.

The twitch response is characteristic of a TrP and is a transient contraction of a group of muscle fibers (usually a palpable band), that contains a TrP. The contraction of the fibers is in response to stimulation (usually by snapping palpation) of the TrP or sometimes of a nearby TrP. The TrP is palpated as a pea-sized nodule in a taut band of muscle fibers.

The TrP typically refers pain unilaterally and, depending on its location, it may refer distally or proximally. As such, the TrP is a regional phenomenon usually associated with muscle dysfunction. The assessment of TrPs is an integral component of the assessment for muscle change. They are discussed here because they may exist in fascia and are frequently encountered while palpating the paraspinal tissues.

Myofascial pain may also arise within the sclerotomal distribution of a dysfunctional spinal segment. This is suspected when the patient reports a vague, deep aching pain which bears little, if any, relationship to known nerve root or dermatomal distributions. Myofascial pain about the thorax is confounded by the pain which arises from irritated spinal structures and which has been mapped by Kellgren (1977; Fig. 12.18). The clinical diagnostic approach to diffuse pain is straightforward: first, determine if there is a local cause and, if not, assume there is a remote pain generator. The task then becomes one of identifying, testing, and ruling out known pain generators until one remains which reproduces the patient's pain. This is the same approach given above for determining the presence of fascial pain and requires the practitioner to have a healthy respect for and knowledge of the soft-tissue pain generators.

Connective tissue systems

The two major regional connective tissue systems are the ligamentum nuchae and the thoracolumbar fascia. The spinal dura about the suboccipital region is linked by connective tissue to muscles about the spine and the ligamentum nuchae (Hack et al 1995, Mitchell et al 1998, Krakenes et al 2001, Dean & Mitchell 2002). Further, it has now been shown that the superficial lamina of the lumbar fascia is continuous with the rhomboid muscles and that the deep layer continues superiorly with the inferior tendinous border of the splenius cervicis and the lower fibers of the splenius capitis (Barker & Brigs 1999). It is quite clear that any assessment of the upper cervical complex is incomplete without assessment of the muscles which contribute to the ligamentum nuchae.

Vleeming et al (1995) have demonstrated that the deep lamina of the thoracolumbar fascia continues inferiorly with the sacrotuberous ligament. Further, they have demonstrated that there is sufficient tensile strength in the fascia to transfer loads about the spine. Barker & Briggs (1999) report that the lumbar fascia which extends to invest the rhomboids and splenii is also capable of transmitting a variable amount of tension.

This new evidence of a virtually continuous connective tissue sheath between the low pelvis (sacrotuberous ligament) and the occiput (splenius capitis), complete with superior contractile elements (the muscles which contribute to the ligamentum nuchae), and the findings that this sheath communicates with the dura of the spine at the suboccipital level place a greater responsibility on practitioners to broaden their assessment processes well beyond the segmental or regional complaint.

The implications are straightforward: assessment of the connective tissues of the upper cervical complex should reasonably include an assessment of the thoracolumbar fascia, and, given that the thoracolumbar fascia plays a key role in load transfer between the upper and lower limbs, it must be considered in the assessment of the upper spine, including the cervicothoracic junction.

Pragmatically, when the interconnectivity between the two is understood and appreciated, the better approach to spinal assessment is one which considers the spine as a single, integrated, functioning unit. It is no longer acceptable to omit cervical spine assessment in patients with low-back pain, nor lumbosacral spine and pelvic assessment in patients with headache.

Neurolymphatic points

A neurolymphatic point is theorized to be a circumscribed zone in a predictable location on the body which acts in both a diagnostic

and therapeutic manner for a certain muscle or group of muscles. The points were developed in the early part of the 20th century by Chapman, an osteopath, and are eponymously termed Chapman's reflexes. The points are also empirically associated with various organs and glands (Walther 1981 pp. 220–223).

The mechanism is discussed in Chapter 8 as the lymphatic system is an important manager of body fluids within the vascular system. The underlying theory is that the lymphatic system about a certain structure may be remotely influenced by sympathetic pathways running to the target from an SMU. If these pathways do exist, then it is conceivable for there to be an interaction between a dysfunctional structure and an SMU, and vice versa. As with much of manual healthcare, the empirical constructs run well ahead of any scientific evidence and it is wise to consider the possibility of such clinical relationships.

There is scientific evidence for an interaction between the ligaments and muscles of the spine to provide a stabilizing system (Solomonow et al 1998). There is also acceptable electrophysiologic evidence for an intersegmental reflex pathway between lumbar paraspinal tissues (Kang et al 2002) and evidence that the viscoelastic structures of the spine are well suited to monitor sensory information as well as to control spinal muscles and probably provide kinesthetic information to the sensory cortex (Holm et al 2002). Further, it has been demonstrated that the optimal control of the innate immune response is dependent on the rate of change of system variables and that the immune system can do its job better when innately enhanced (Stengel et al 2002). Chapter 7 further discusses a number of theories and their contemporary evidence.

The relevance of neurolymphatic points in the assessment of connective tissue change is that the finding of tenderness about a specific SMU secondary to muscle dysfunction may be explained by the somatosomatic reflex. The inference of a therapeutic relationship through these reflex pathways, and any association with particular organs or glands, is a matter for further investigation. In the meantime it is really quite acceptable to relate a specific spinal level with particular muscle dysfunction.

The points have been mapped on both the anterior and the posterior aspects of the body. Some are found on a daily basis by the observant practitioner and do seem both diagnostic and therapeutic for specific muscles. As with most empirical constructs, other points seem somewhat elusive and any indication or effect is dubious. The points have particular currency within the paradigm of Applied Kinesiology; however, the astute practitioner will be aware of the more common locations and will integrate any clinical findings into the overall assessment of the patient.

The most important clinical implication is quite simply the message that tenderness about a particular SMU may not necessarily represent local tissue response to kinematic change. As with the concept of tissue preference, the putative neurolymphatic points may act as confounders to manual palpation and assessment of the spine by providing a background of tenderness which, while meaningful to some, may be considered as noise by others.

Assessment

The patient is positioned to exhibit the region of complaint best. Assessment for head and neck pain may be performed with the patient seated; for posterior pain about the cervicothoracic, mid thoracic, thoracolumbar, and lumbosacral regions the patient may be placed prone. If the upper limb is involved it is better for the patient to be seated, and if the lower limb is of interest, then the patient may be seated, supine, or prone, depending on the structures which need to be palpated.

A flat, digital palpation is applied with mild pressure initially, moving to moderate then deep pressure to vary the depth at which tissues are palpated. At times both hands will work side-by-side or with one covering the other, but generally both will explore the patient bilaterally, level by level. In the prone patient the practitioner takes a fencer stance, facing cephalad, and palpates through the paraspinal zones given in Figure 12.10. A square stance may be taken when a specific level of interest needs to be explored further.

The practitioner is attempting to determine whether the palpated tissue is normal or demonstrates altered tone, where tone is the resilient response to palpatory touch. A simple scheme for differentiating tone is to categorize any increase as mild, moderate, or severe. A circle can indicate normal tone and a vertical line can be added for each degree of increased tone (Fig. 5.4). The symbols are drawn on an outline of the patient in the area where the finding is identified.

It is common to identify a ropy band within the paraspinal tissues, particularly the iliocostalis. These bands may extend over some distance and, while it is possible to palpate an insertion into the inferior margin of a rib, the band often disappears distally into the thoracolumbar fascia. The band is commonly found unilaterally and is often painful, representing hypertonic dysfunction of some fascicles within the muscle. These bands may possibly arise secondary to dysfunction at a nearby SMU and may also represent the spondylogenic reflex syndromes explored by Dvořák & Dvořák (1984).

The information from the assessment is recorded in the clinical file and should also include comment on the nature of the skin if it varies from a normal, warm feeling. Variations include excessive moisture, perhaps secondary to autonomic dysfunction or pain and fear; excessive dryness, perhaps associated with aging; or excessive focal hypersensitivity, which may reflect a dysfunctional SMU which in turn is affecting the cutaneous nerve distribution. When an area of focal tenderness is found in a location considered to be a site for a neurolymphatic point, the practitioner should specifically record the finding and explore the associated muscles.

SEGMENTAL CONSIDERATIONS

The predominant connective tissues at the segmental level are the intervertebral disk and the ligaments about the SMU (Fig. 5.5). They are intrinsic to the SMU while the fascial bands of the paraspinal muscles which span multiple spinal levels, such as the iliocostalis, are extrinsic to the SMU. The fascial planes such as the thoracolumbar fascia, which also span multiple segments, are also considered to be extrinsic to the SMU.

The ligaments are specialized for tensile strength and energy absorption and consist of fibroblasts (in growing tissue) and fibrocytes (in mature, less active tissue) embedded in a fibrous matrix which has some blood supply and a number of nerve endings capable of monitoring tissue stress, strain, and pain (Adams et al 2002). The matrix is composed of collagen type I (80%), proteoglycans, and a variable amount of elastin. The collagen fibers exhibit a zig-zag planar waveform called "crimp" which gradually straightens out with tensile forces and allows the typical ligament to be stretched by about 15% before damage (Adams et al 2002).

The ligamentous structures are considered to have only a small mechanical role in maintaining spinal stability. Solomonow et al (1998) argue that the spinal ligaments are conveniently situated in key locations sensitive to relative motion of the vertebrae in various planes, such that receptors within them can monitor their movement and activate the musculature via spinal neurons and maintain or restore stability. Afferent nerves capable of carrying proprioceptive information have been located in the interspinous, supraspinous, and flaval ligaments as well as in the disk (Swinkels & Dolan 1998) and the small muscles of the SMU (Herzog 2000), conferring a role in joint position sense. Further, the paraspinal muscle spindles may provide the central nervous system with different information regarding vertebral position dependent upon the previous length history of the paraspinal muscle (Pickar & Kang 2001).

Ligament injury

Herzog is of the opinion that damage to the ligaments of the SMU does not occur during lifting or other normal occupational activities. Rather, he sees damage occurring primarily during traumatic events which then leads to joint laxity and acceleration of arthritic changes (Herzog 2000 p. 40). The slow strain rates during occupational tasks seem to produce more avulsion injuries while fast strain rates, as in traumatic accidents, are more likely to produce mid ligamentous failure.

The damage which arises from the application of excessive strain forces to a ligament is termed a sprain and, in the joints of the extremities may be graded as 1, 2, or 3. Grade 1 sprains do not typically affect joint stability; however, the fibers of the ligament are stretched or torn to a small extent. The pain is usually mild and there may be a little swelling with stiffness. A grade 2 sprain tears and separates ligamentous fibers and is associated with joint instability and moderate to severe pain. A grade 3

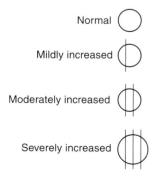

Figure 5.4 Symbols for recording tissue tone. Tissue tone or compliance can be indicated by a circle superimposed with a vertical strike to indicate the severity of the increasing tone. The gradings are normal, mildly increased, moderately increased, and severely increased.

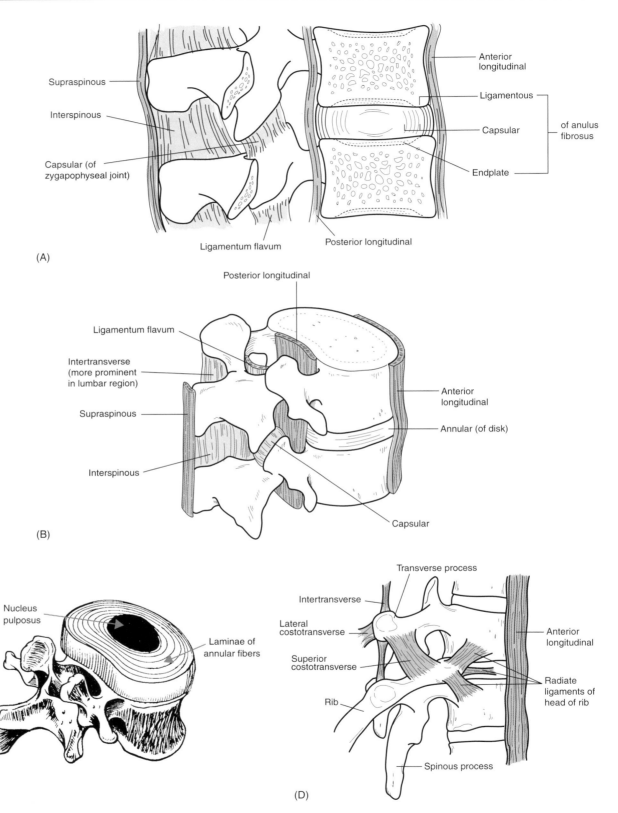

Figure 5.5 The ligaments of a typical spinal motion unit. (A) Sagittal view within the lumbar region; (B) oblique view of the right posterior aspect within the lumbar region; (C) oblique view showing the lumbar disk; (D) lateral view within the thoracic region. (A) After Kapandji (1974), with permission; (B) after Jenkins (1998), with permission; (C) after Schafer (1983), with permission; (D) after Peterson & Bergmann (2002), with permission.

sprain totally ruptures the ligament, resulting in gross instability of the joint. These grades may not be readily transferable to the SMU; however, the principle remains that the ligaments of the SMU may commonly suffer mild or moderate sprain. Severe (grade 3) sprains are typically of such traumatic magnitude that they require hospitalization and intervention beyond the scope of a manual healthcare provider.

Immediately after injury and for about 72 h, there is bleeding from damaged vessels and a migration of inflammatory cells into the injured area. A statistically significant increase in the production of the proinflammatory mediators interleukin-6 and interleukin-8 by damaged disk tissue has been demonstrated in patients with discogenic low-back pain (Burke et al 2002). It is thought the proinflammatory mediators within the nucleus may be a major factor in the genesis of a painful lumbar disk. While the origin of pain is multifactorial, inflammation probably predominates over merely mechanical mechanisms (Leonardi et al 2002).

Mast cells are involved in tissue repair and the induction of angiogenesis. It is now known that the neovascularization of a damaged disk is accompanied by innervation and it is thought the mast cells may be involved in the production of and response to neurotrophic stimuli such as nerve growth factor (Freemont et al 2002b). These findings suggest a role for mast cells in low-back pain, but whether it is causative or therapeutic remains open to investigation.

Healing occurs over the next 6 weeks or so, with new capillary growth and fibroblastic activity. When fibers are torn the ends are reconnected by a fibrin clot which serves as a matrix for the formation of scar tissue by collagen and proteoglycans. These tissues are laid randomly; however, active exercise during this period seems to result in a stronger repair as the collagen tends to realign in response to progressive stresses and strains. Scar maturation may take up to 12 months in extremity joints.

When a disk is damaged by herniation the cells may undergo apoptosis (programmed cell death). A protein related to apoptosis, Fas receptor, has been found on disk cells collected during surgery to repair herniation (Park et al 2001b). The percentage of Fas-positive disk cells correlated significantly with the patient's age but not the degree of disk degeneration seen on MRI. More research is needed to explore the clinical implications of these findings; however it is clear the disk is capable of self-maintenance and has considerable regenerative properties for repair after injury (Humzah & Soames 1988). It is known that the hydrostatic pressure within the disk directly affects the synthesis of collagen and proteoglycans by the intervertebral disk cells. Increased pressure seems to inhibit proteoglycan synthesis but stimulates collagen synthesis by the nucleus cells while inhibiting annulus cells (Hutton et al 2001).

The problem with a strain injury to the fibers of the disk or the ligaments of the SMU is that these processes occur unseen (except by advanced imaging). A patient with a strain injury must be encouraged to remain mobile and restrained from any overexertion which may cause further sprain damage, albeit mild, which perpetuates the injury loop. Poor management during this period allows the psychosocial overlay to become evident and the patient is likely to progress towards chronicity.

Ligaments of the SMU

A number of ligaments about the SMU are relatively consistent at each spinal level. They are mentioned below to provide a broad-based introduction to the general nature and characteristics of these main ligaments with a view to establishing their role as pain generators in spinal dysfunction and the subluxation complex. Given that their main role is to provide strength, support, and stability, it will be appreciated that ligamentous change will also be reflected in kinematic change.

All ligaments are described in detail appropriate to their spinal level in each chapter of Part 2. The ligaments about the upper cervical complex are unique and are discussed in Chapter 9 (Fig. 9.5). The rib attachments throughout the thoracic spine are also unique and are discussed in Chapter 12 (Fig. 12.7). The transforaminal ligaments are a feature of the lumbar spine and the iliolumbar ligament is an important ligament of the lumbosacral junction. These, together with the ligaments of the pelvis, are discussed in Chapters 13 (Fig. 13.7) and 14 (Fig. 14.17).

The regional chapters also contain a discussion about the intervertebral disk relevant to each particular spinal region. The information presented in this chapter serves as a broad introduction, particularly to the clinical concept of the disk being perhaps the most important connective tissue within the spine.

Anterior longitudinal ligament

This is a long band enveloping the anterior and anterolateral margins of the spinal column. It arises from the basilar part of the occiput, attaches about the anterior tubercle of the atlas, then descends to the sacrum. It narrows a little at each disk level and lightly attaches to the anterior disk margin. It firmly attaches to the anterolateral surfaces of the vertebral periosteum and is innervated by gray communicating rami from the sympathetic trunk.

The anterior longitudinal ligament imparts a springy end-feel to the SMU at the end-range of extension as the anterior margins of the vertebral bodies separate.

Posterior longitudinal ligament

This ligament forms the anterior border of the spinal canal and arises from the body of C2 to descend from the transverse ligament complex about C1–2 and attach to the sacrum. It is continuous superiorly with the tectorial membrane. It firmly attaches to the posterior margins of each disk and lightly about the posterior margins of the vertebral bodies to allow the exit of the basivertebral veins from the body.

The ligament is innervated by the meningeal branch of the spinal nerve which enters the spinal canal and divides into ascending and descending branches which fuse with those from adjacent vertebrae. These in turn give off transverse branches which spread to the vertebral segment of the ligament (Kojima et al 1990). Nerve fibers also enter the ligament through the posterolateral portion of the annulus. There are abundant free nerve endings in the peripheral zones of the ligament and it is thought these may have a role in the regulation of movement and posture (Kojima et al 1990).

There is no clear delineation between the deep layer of the ligament and the fibrous layer of the periosteum of the vertebral body. It appears that the periosteum becomes less conspicuous with age after the second decade and that the peridural membrane is its homolog, as there is no periosteum on the vertebral body where this membrane is found (Honda 1983, Wiltse 2000). The presence of this membrane and its relationship with the posterior longitudinal ligament raise the question as to whether there is periosteum on the posterior aspect of the vertebral body within the spinal canal (Wiltse et al 1993).

The loading of pig and human specimens at slow rates in bending and shear suggests that excessive tension in the longitudinal ligaments results most frequently in avulsion or bony failure near the ligament attachment site (Herzog 2000).

Capsular ligaments and zygapophyseal menisci

The capsular ligaments provide the greatest resistance at the end-point of flexion of the SMU. They are most susceptible to damage in flexion with rotation to one side as this movement includes a component of lateral flexion which affects the capsular ligaments contralateral to the side of rotation or bending.

The outer layer of the fibrous capsule is a dense regular connective tissue that is composed of parallel bundles of collagenous fibers. The inner layer of the fibrous capsule consists of bundles of elastic fibers, similar to the ligamentum flavum. In the superior and middle part of the joint the fibers run in the medial to lateral direction, crossing over the joint gap. In the inferior part they are relatively long and run in a superomedial to inferolateral direction, covering the inferior articular recess (Yamashita et al 1996). Substance P, a putative neuromodulator of pain, has been shown to have an excitatory effect on both nociceptive and proprioceptive units in the tissues around and in the lumbar facet joint (Yamashita et al 1993).

The relationship between the zygapophyseal joint capsule and the fibrous intra-articular folds or menisci varies at different levels of the spine. An entrapped meniscus is considered to be an important form of acute spinal pain, usually with joint locking. These variations are discussed in each regional chapter.

Ligamentum flavum

The ligamenta flava are short, yellow ligaments which cover the spaces between the lamina at each SMU. Laterally they extend to the articular capsules where fibers may intermingle. The ligament matrix contains elastin, a fibrous protein which is quite stretchable to impart a high degree of extensibility, perhaps up to 40%, to these ligaments. They form part of the posterior boundary of the spinal canal and stretch with flexion while contracting about 10% in extension to reduce buckling into the canal (Schafer 1983).

Ossification of the ligamenta flava is not an unusual finding in the Japanese (Arafat et al 1993, Xiong et al 2001) and it has been described in Caucasians (Arafat et al 1993, Parekh et al 1993) and reported to compress the spinal cord (van Oostenbrugge et al 1999) and cause femoral neuropathy (Debiais et al 2000). Ossification has also been found associated with osteoblastoma (Okuda et al 2001).

Intertransverse ligaments

These are small, thin ligamentous slips which attach between the horizontal surfaces of each transverse process. They are best developed as strong, cord-like structures in the thoracic region while in the cervical region they may be replaced by slips of muscle fibers. In the lumbar spine they have been described variously as thin and membranous and as a well-developed band (Behrsin & Briggs 1988).

As the ligament extends medially to the outer margin of the ligamentum flavum in the lumbar region, it divides into ventral and dorsal leaves. The ventral leaf passes lateral to the IVF where it is pierced by the ventral ramus of the spinal nerve and the nerve to the psoas muscles. It then passes ventrally to lie over the vertebral body ultimately to blend with the anterior longitudinal ligament. The dorsal leaf passes medially to attach to the arch of the vertebra and blends with the capsule of the zygapophyseal joint. It is pierced by the dorsal ramus of the spinal nerve and related blood vessels (Behrsin & Briggs 1988).

Interspinous ligaments

These thin, almost membranous ligaments run between the inferior margin of the superior spinous process to the superior margin of the spinous process below throughout the spine. They are most developed in the lumbar region and least in the cervical spine. The ventral fibers are said to arise from the ligamentum flavum and pass superiorly and posteriorly to attach to the anterior part of the inferior margin of the spinous process above (Behrsin & Briggs 1988). The midline fibers arise, pass, and insert in a similar manner, while the posterior fibers pass superiorly and posteriorly from the posterior part of the superior surface of the lower spinous process and attach to the supraspinous ligament (Behrsin & Briggs 1988). This description is quite different to most textbook descriptions and is confirmed by Herzog (2000 pp. 37–41).

It is commonly thought that the interspinous ligaments limit flexion; however, the oblique direction of their fibers suggests they play a much more important role in controlling shear forces. Herzog (2000) considers a very likely scenario of interspinous ligament damage is falling and landing on one's behind. This would drive the pelvis forward on impact, creating a posterior shearing of the lumbar joints when the spine is fully flexed. The interspinous ligament is a major load-bearing tissue for anterior shear displacement under high-energy loads (Herzog 2000 p. 38).

Supraspinous ligament or restraint

Cramer & Darby (1995) consider this more of a fibrous restraint than a ligament in the lumbar region. It runs from the spinous process of C7 to the L5 spinous. Superiorly from C7 the midline of the spine is bound by the ligamentum nuchae. It is not unusual for small bursae to form between the restraint and the underlying interspinous ligaments. The structure is the major delimiter of flexion.

Trolard's ligament

This is a sacrodural ligament first described in 1888 (Barbaix et al 1996). It is a strong, medially and sagittally oriented septum in the lumbosacral region (L3 to sacrum) and attaches the lower spinal dura to the posterior longitudinal ligament in many cases. Its actual form is quite variable; however, it is felt that its presence acts as a damper to the spinal cord so that traction forces have less impact on the peridural blood vessels and nerve roots.

The presence of these attachments lends weight to the premise that movements in sacral nutation and counternutation have an effect on dural tension. The variability of the attachments may also explain the variability in the clinical response of patients with similar indications to the same therapeutic techniques (Barbaix et al 1996). Even though they were first described over a century ago, they remain very much a hidden ligament.

Assessment

The intrinsic ligaments of the SMU are very difficult to assess individually and their involvement in various presentations is largely an inference synthesized from the application of skilful palpation, a strong knowledge of anatomy, and an awareness of any mechanism of injury and the likely responses. There are well-known protocols to identify and describe conditions of the intervertebral disk; however, these do not isolate the capsular ligaments in particular or the other intrinsic ligaments in general. The clinical signs and symptoms must be carefully observed and documented.

The behavior of ligaments is hard to classify in a simple manner. While it is accepted that flexion will open the facet joints and stretch the capsular ligaments, it has also been shown that extreme extension of the lumbar spine will cause extensive stretch of the facet joint capsule (Cavanaugh et al 1996). Extension also increases the compressive load on the facets and causes low- and high-threshold mechanoreceptors to fire (Yamashita et al 1990). There is no doubt the lumbar facet capsule is a pain generator as there is an extensive distribution of small nerve fibers and free and encapsulated nerve endings in the capsular fibers and these are sensitive to chemicals released during injury and inflammation (Cavanaugh et al 1997).

Similarly, it is not appropriate simply to conclude that nerve root pain is always secondary to irritation from a bulging disk. In the lumbar region the spinal nerves exit the spine along the intervertebral canal which has been described as an osteoligamentous tunnel (Amonoo-Kuofi & El-Badawi 1997). Here, transforaminal ligaments form a criss-crossing network about the spinal nerve and dorsal root ganglion and cannot be clinically assessed. Amonoo-Kuofi & El-Badawi (1997) suggest they may have a role as pain generators and that they may also create direct mechanical pressure on the neural components giving rise to severe pain and paresthesia along the distribution of the nerve. These ligaments may be implicated in clinical presentations of this nature where there is insufficient evidence to support a discogenic cause.

It is also known that extension of the lumbar spine decreases the area within the intervertebral canal by 15% (Inufusa et al 1996), resulting in dynamic stenosis which may compress neural structures. This must be borne in mind when performing the Kemp's test to differentiate between meniscoid entrapment (local pain) and dynamic stenosis (nerve root pain) (Evans 2001 pp. 534–537).

The clinical relevance of connective tissue assessment must reflect its dual role as pain generators and proprioceptors. It may be that aberrant kinematics within an SMU result in an altered proprioceptive feedback loop which may perpetuate kinematic change, leading to the early stages of degeneration and its sequelae.

Conversely, the high-velocity, low-amplitude spinal adjustment may generate an intense but transient proprioceptive load which allows the SMU to reset and again function normally (Lehman & McGill 2001). Any such feedback loop would also include the lumbar paraspinal musculature (Pickar & Kang 2001), which makes the pragmatic point that, in clinical reality, the distinctions between that which is connective tissue, muscular, neurological, or vascular are somewhat blurred.

The intervertebral disk

The disk is a complex structure composed of several different tissues, including a highly hydrated gel in the center of the nucleus and a tough, ligamentous fibrocartilage in the outer annulus. There is a small amount (less than 20% dry weight) of collagen in the nucleus which increases to about 70% dry weight towards the outer annulus. The endplates resemble an amorphous hyaline cartilage (Adams et al 2002). The basic forms of disk protrusion are discussed in Chapter 14 (Figs 14.12–14.14).

The precursor to disk protrusion and herniation is considered to be internal disk disruption (Bogduk 1991) and it is thought that such disruption may follow a compression injury. While Adams et al (2002) and others have been able to categorize the stages of disk disruption, there is no real knowledge of the role or sequencing of the range of events. It is suggested that disruption to the endplate will transfer load from the nucleus to the posterior annulus, which may in turn cause pain (Adams et al 1996).

Disruption of the endplate typically requires trauma; however, it has been shown that regression of the vascular canals in the endplate during growth may allow a spontaneous mechanism (Chandraraj et al 1998). It appears that the regression of these canals commences during the first decade and leaves "scars" as nodular areas. By the beginning of the third decade, herniation of disk material into these weak spots can be observed, identifying a route for the early formation of intranuclear herniations (Chandraraj et al 1998). These weak spots may also render the endplate more susceptible to damage with mild trauma. It is also reported that the shape of the vertebral body margin at the endplate is an important factor contributing to the development of disk disruption, especially at L4–5 and L5–S1 (Harrington et al 2001).

It is important for the practitioner to appreciate that, in addition to the disk generating pain through mechanical interference with surrounding structures, most notably the spinal nerve roots, the disk itself may generate pain from damage to its own structure. This represents internal disk disruption and is diagnosed by provocative discography with diagnostic imaging evidence of internal disk disruption, provided that, as a control, stimulation of at least one other disk fails to reproduce pain (Schwarzer et al 1995). An increased risk of low-back pain has been found in relation to all signs of disk degeneration, as seen on MRI (Luoma et al 2000).

There are no conventional clinical tests which can discriminate patients with internal disk disruption from patients with other discogenic conditions (Schwarzer et al 1995). The finding of decreased disk space height on MRI is significantly associated with internal disruption of the disk (Milette et al 1999). There is no reason why the finding of decreased disk height as seen on the plain, lateral radiograph should not equally be an indicator of internal disk disruption at that level. The diagnosis is either made as described above, or is accepted as a working hypothesis by exclusion of other possibilities in the presence of decreased disk space height on radiograph.

The stages of disk degeneration are discussed in Chapter 2 (Box 2.1). The key points to bear in mind are:

- The cervical and lumbar disks are morphologically very different and, while our greatest knowledge is of the lumbar disk, this is not automatically applicable to the cervical disk.
- Lumbar disk degeneration appears to begin with biochemical change, followed by biomechanical changes (Adams et al 2002).
- The degenerating disk develops nerve growth into the damaged area and these include nociceptors (Freemont et al 1997). The nerve growth is linked to the production of nerve growth factor by blood vessels growing into the disk from adjacent vertebral bodies (Freemont et al 2002a).

What is not yet known is whether there is any correlation between altered signal intensity on MRI and the grade 2 state of mild degeneration where the nucleus has become fibrous with some brown pigmentation. It is also not yet known whether altered MRI signals only reflect the mechanical changes associated with grade 3 moderate degenerative change. It is known that minor damage to a vertebral body endplate leads to progressive structural changes in the adjacent intervertebral disks

(Adams et al 2000). Clearly this is an area for cooperative research between radiologists and practitioners in an attempt to determine the earliest state of internal disk degeneration or disruption which may be conclusively imaged.

A common misconception is that the disk height decreases with age. Current data clearly demonstrate that the height of the lumbar disks of males and females within the age 20–69 years increases linearly with increasing age. The data show that disk height starts to decrease after the age of 69 years (Shao et al 2002). Any shortening of the spine before that age is more likely due to loss of vertebral body height. Decreased disk height in patients under the age of 69 can therefore be considered an indicator of disk disruption and damage (Yoshimura et al 2000).

The role of MRI

MRI is recognized as the modality of choice for evaluating the spine (Fukuda & Kawakami 2001); however, it is yet to become universally available to manual practitioners. The preferred images are T2-weighted and the finding of a high-intensity zone (HIZ) within the disk is significantly correlated with disruption of the disk tissues (Lam et al 2000). The intraobserver reliability for detecting an HIZ in a given disk has been reported as fair to good (kappa = 0.57; 95% confidence interval = 0.44, 0.70) but while the sensitivity for detecting grade 4 annular disruption and exact pain was poor (31%), its specificity was relatively high (90%) (Smith et al 1998).

Loss of disk height or abnormal signal intensity is highly predictive of symptomatic tears extending into or beyond the outer

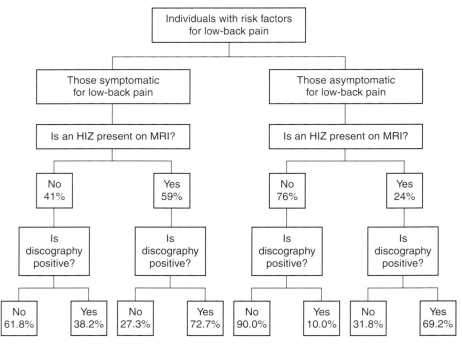

Figure 5.6 The relationship between magnetic resonance imaging (MRI) findings, discography, and back pain. The presence of a high-intensity zone within the disk on MRI does not reliably indicate the presence of symptomatic internal disk disruption. HIZ, high-intensity zone. Data from Carragee et al (2000).

annulus (Milette et al 1999). When the patient is symptomatic for low-back pain, the HIZ is considered to be a reliable marker of painful outer annular disruption (Schellhas et al 1996). The sensitivity of the HIZ as a sign of either annular disruption or pain was found to be modest in a study of 500 symptomatic patients but its specificity was high (Aprill & Bogduk 1992). These findings are similar to those of Smith et al (1998, described above); however, while Smith et al reported a low (40%) positive predictor value of an HIZ for a severely disrupted disk, Aprill & Bogduk (1992) found it to be a more respectable 86%.

The finding of an HIZ is therefore a useful indicator of disk disruption but is not necessarily associated with pain (Ricketson et al 1996, Ito et al 1998). The HIZ is thus not useful as a predictor of pain (Buirski & Silberstein 1993). Some consider that discography may be useful in patients with an equivocal MRI (Brightbill et al 1994) while others consider discography has no proven efficacy in improving patient outcomes and may lead to inappropriate surgery (Bogduk & Modic 1996). Still others consider the non-invasive methods of intradiscal ultrasound and a vibration provocation test of the spinous process to be preferable, and report a sensitivity of 0.90 and a specificity of 0.75 for the vibration test compared to the discographic pain provocation test (Yrjama et al 1996).

The work of Carragee et al (2000) won the Volvo award in clinical studies that year and concludes that the presence of an HIZ does not reliably indicate the presence of symptomatic internal disk disruption. The prevalence of an HIZ in asymptomatic individuals with degenerative disk disease (25%) is too high for meaningful clinical use. When injected during discography, the same percentage of asymptomatic and symptomatic disks with an HIZ were shown to be painful (Carragee et al 2000). The findings from this report are presented diagrammatically in Figure 5.6.

MRI must be interpreted with consideration of full clinical signs, symptoms, and other relevant background (Fukuda & Kawakami 2001).

CONCLUSION

The skills-set required for the assessment of connective tissue change ranges from the basic palpation of skin and fascia about an SMU to high-order inferential analysis required to implicate tissues which are typically not accessible for manual assessment. A thorough knowledge of anatomy is essential to underpin the meaningful interpretation of findings from the history and mechanism of injury, the physical and spinal examinations, and diagnostic imaging interpretation.

6

Assessment of muscle change

KEY CONCEPTS

Skeletal muscle is responsible for function, movement, and grace, and is traditionally categorized as consisting largely of dense red slow-oxidative fibers with slow contraction associated primarily with aerobic-type activities such as postural control, or of predominantly white anaerobic fibers which produce quick, forceful contractions but fatigue more readily.

A contemporary scheme for designating skeletal muscles is to consider them as either stabilizers which tend to weaken and lengthen, or mobilizers which tend to shorten and tighten.

Skeletal muscle progressively declines in strength, beginning in middle age, and the absolute strength of the muscle groups in the upper and lower extremities and the back decreases by as much as 60% between the ages of 30 and 80 years. The ability of some muscles to provide sustained power during repeated contraction may also decline with age.

Feed-forward control mechanisms exist for spinal protection and seem to take the form of a spinal reflex mediated by a direct afferent pathway from the upper limbs or the upper spinal segment to preprogram stiffness in muscles which protect the lumbar spine through reflex modulation of the gamma-muscle system.

The ligamentomuscular stabilizing system of the lumbosacral spine produces a proprioceptive effect at both the local level and projected to the sensory cortex. This ability for kinesthetic perception assists with the control of spinal muscles and is independent of the magnitude of movement.

Tenderness is an early sign of pathologic change in muscle and is generated when the threshold of nociceptors within the muscle is reset to a lower level by endogenous substances released when it is damaged.

Muscle pain arising within the erector spinae modulates the descending voluntary motor commands which significantly alter the motor patterns of the trunk in persons with chronic low-back pain. The reduction in trunk motion is consistent with theories of guarding and models of pain adaptation.

Abnormal posture, movement, and gait arises from muscle weakness and may impair normal functional movement. All muscles have a normal level of power which allows normal healthy living. The ability of a muscle to generate force against resistance is strength and is closely associated with endurance, the ability to perform repetitive muscular contractions against some resistance for an extended period of time.

INTRODUCTION

If it is connective tissue which gives the body form and substance then it is muscle which gives it function, movement, and grace. These three characteristics are controlled by the nervous system, so in many respects the assessment of muscle change can only be performed in conjunction with the assessment of neural change. This truism reflects the overall nature of clinical assessment, namely that all dimensions of the patient are assessed, contextualized, then interpreted within the patient's sociocultural context (Fig. 1.5).

Many texts have been published on muscle testing, muscle assessment, neurologic assessment, exercise and strength training, and rehabilitation, and it is not the intent of this chapter to replicate these in whole or in part. The reader is assumed to have or be developing a comprehensive knowledge of muscle structure and physiology. This discussion is ordered from global through regional to segmental considerations, and is intended to be applied in conjunction with the assessment of changes in kinematics, connective tissue, and the nervous and vascular systems.

The concepts of changes in skeletal muscle presented here are those which may suggest the presence of spinal dysfunction in the form of a subluxation complex (SC) or other spinal lesion treatable in typical chiropractic, osteopathic, and like practices of manual care. This reflects the theory of interneuron dysfunction which says that joint dysfunction or misalignment causes secondary reflex changes in the segmentally related muscles (Schneider 1999). The barrage of nociceptive and mechanoreceptive impulses which are generated by irritated or inflamed joints is received within the spinal cord and spills over to the anterior motor neurons by way of spinal interneurons. This may affect both excitatory and inhibitory interneurons and thus have a variable effect on the segmentally related muscles (Schneider 1999).

Correction of the joint dysfunction reduces the intensity of inputs into the spinal cord and reduces, if not ends, the secondary reflex muscle changes. One effect of spinal manipulation is strong stimulation of the mechanoreceptors about the spinal motion unit (SMU) and this is also thought to lead to interneuron inhibition of motor neurons, again decreasing reflex muscle activity.

Normal, healthy skeletal muscle is responsive to a variety of inputs ranging from subconscious proprioceptive data from the disk and ligaments of the SMU (Indahl et al 1997) to conscious neural data which direct movement. The global overview demonstrates symmetry and balance in the normal subject. Dysfunctional muscles alter symmetry and balance which may lead to compensation in static posture and recruitment in functional activities. Muscle may become dysfunctional through overuse, misuse, abuse, disuse, disease, trauma, and/or disturbances in the neurological or vascular systems (Chaitow & DeLany 2000 p. 16).

The roles of the practitioner are first to identify dysfunctional muscle, second to propose a causal mechanism which reflects the clinical findings, then third to design and implement an appropriate therapeutic intervention to rectify the perceived cause and diminish or correct the dysfunction. Causes of global dysfunction are relatively identifiable; however, as the dysfunction becomes more regional then segmental, while concurrently becoming less quantitative and more qualitative, the cause becomes less identifiable and more speculative. This is not meant to diminish the therapeutic encounter, rather it places a greater importance on concise documentation of both the clinical findings and the therapeutic intervention. As with much of clinical practice, a diagnosis is rarely proven; it typically becomes presumed when there is a positive outcome to a specific intervention.

The practitioner must bear this in mind to ensure a high and consistent level of intraexaminer reliability when assessing muscle. Great care must be taken with patient positioning, doctor positioning, stabilization, and the actual test procedures.

MUSCLE DESIGNATION

Muscle fibers are either dense red fibers classified as slow oxidative (SO) type I, or white fast twitch fibers classified as fast glycolytic (FG) type II. The latter may be subdivided on the basis of their resistance to fatigue (Prentice 2001).

The slow-twitch type I fibers have a slow rate of contraction (100 ms) and take greater time to generate force. Their high concentrations of myoglobulin and mitochondria make them resistant to fatigue and they are typically associated with long-duration, aerobic-type tonic activities such as postural control. The major postural muscles are shown in Figure 6.1. In contrast, the type II fibers act in a phasic manner to produce quick, forceful contractions (30 ms) which are useful in short-term, high-intensity applications. They are anaerobic and fatigue more readily.

All skeletal muscle has a mix of fibers to adapt them best to the role they are required to perform. Muscles which predominantly consist of type I fibers are naturally considered to be type I muscles, and those predominantly consisting of type II fibers are type II muscles. However, things are not this simple in the clinical environment. For example, the paraspinal muscles are essentially phasic, apart from the erector spinae which are generally considered as tonic postural muscles, which also have a variable mix of type I and II fibers depending on their spinal region.

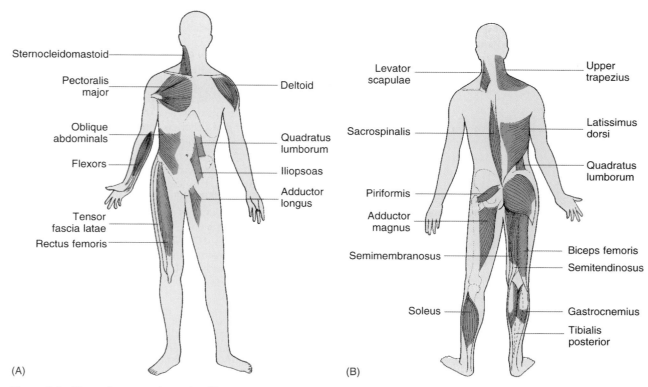

Figure 6.1 The major postural muscles. The postural muscles largely consist of type I slow-twitch fibers which shorten in response to long-term stress. The balance and symmetry of these muscles must be noted during postural assessment. (A) As seen from the anterior; (B) as seen from the posterior. (A, B) From Chaitow & DeLany (2000), with permission.

The behaviors which muscles are thought to exhibit do not, in some cases, match the expectation. Most clinical texts and papers have considered that type I muscles shorten in response to long-term stress and become hypertonic, testing as either strong or weak. Type II muscles have been considered to weaken in response to dysfunction, that is, they become inhibited, test as weak, and may lengthen. These simple categories do not address the inconsistencies which have been observed in the manner in which muscles function, nor do they necessarily reflect the actual proportions of fiber distribution within a muscle.

More relevance has been placed on the proper activation of muscles at the right moment and in harmony with other muscles involved in an activity as being a better indicator of function and the concept of weakness is becoming less relevant. A recent effort has been made to standardize the designation of muscles (Chaitow 2000) and the contemporary opinion of clinical experts is that it is more appropriate to designate muscle as stabilizers or mobilizers, allowing the following designations:

- primary stabilizer – a muscle unable to provide significant joint movement
- secondary stabilizer – a muscle which is able to stabilize and move joints
- tertiary stabilizer – a muscle which can at times provide defensive rigidity
- mobilizer – a muscle which acts to move or mobilize joints.

Stabilizers are usually slow-twitch muscles and have a propensity to weaken and lengthen while mobilizers tend to shorten and show a tendency to tightness through increased resting tone. Mobilizers may be thought of as mostly similar to postural muscles. They tend to dominate movements and may alter posture by restricting movement and preventing optimal segmental alignment (Murphy 2000).

Brief comment is made in the chapters of Part 2 of this text as to the perceived nature of a particular muscle. The terminology used is that of Janda as interpreted by Chaitow and reflects what has been the common view among practicing practitioners of type I vs type II muscles. The "stabilizer/mobilizer" concept is new and still subject to debate. One expert proposes a further scheme which appears quite logical. Richardson (2000) suggests skeletal muscle falls into one of two groups:

1. Group A – more linked with stabilization, more likely to undergo reflex inhibition with injury to the associated joint, more likely to atrophy quickly due to lack of use or lack of gravitational load, and more likely to decrease activity and change function when exposed to ballistic repetitive exercise. These are mainly monoarticular muscles or muscles capable of controlling one joint or one area of the spine.
2. Group B – more linked with efficient movement of joints, more likely to undergo reflex excitation with injury to the associated joint, not prone to atrophy quickly due to lack of use or lack of gravitational load, and more likely to become more active (and tighten) with exposure to ballistic repetitive exercise. These are multijoint muscles capable of moving several joints at the same time.

Both the stabilizer/mobilizer concept and Richardson's groups allow useful conceptualization of muscle which is relevant in the clinical content. However it will take some time for this topic to develop further and achieve common nomenclature across disciplines.

Changes with aging

Skeletal muscle starts to exhibit a progressive decline in strength, beginning in middle age. Decreases in the number and size of muscle cells lead to a loss of muscle mass from about the age of 35 years onward. It is thought that muscle mass declines at an average rate of 4% per decade until the age of 50 years, and at 10% per decade thereafter (Buckwalter et al 1993). This age-related loss of skeletal muscle mass contributes significantly to decreasing strength. The absolute strength of the muscle groups in the upper and lower extremities and the back decreases by as much as 60% between the ages of 30 and 80 years.

In addition to the decrease in strength, the ability of some muscles to provide sustained power during repeated contraction may also decline with age (Buckwalter et al 1993). Age-related changes increase the probability of injury, particularly by their own contractions, especially when lengthened at the time of the contraction, and thus decrease the ability of muscle to heal. The factors which contribute to this decline include decreased exercise, especially fewer contractions against high loads, decreases in hormone levels, including those of growth hormone, testosterone, and thyroxine, and neuromuscular changes, including structural and functional changes in the spinal motor neurons and neuromuscular junction (Buckwalter et al 1993).

Degenerative changes also occur in the fibrous tissues associated with muscles, particularly the tendons, which may result in spontaneous or low-energy level ruptures and strains and sprains of the joint capsules and ligaments, including those of the spine. Normative data of age-related changes in tendons do not seem to have been reported in the literature (Buckwalter et al 1993).

Structural change is evident when a muscle has atrophied, has been torn or previously damaged, or indeed may be absent. Functional changes represent the manner in which the muscle undertakes its intended tasks of stabilization and movement and may be clinically assessed two ways: the myoelectric activity may be measured by electromyography (EMG) and the strength of voluntary contraction may be manually assessed. Age-related changes will be evident in these parameters.

EMG

The use of EMG to assess an individual muscle accurately requires the insertion of needle electrodes into a patient and this is not within the scope of typical manual practice. An opening is therefore created for surface EMG where electrodes may be carefully placed on the skin overlying a specific muscle or muscle group, or placed in a hand-held device which is scanned over the paraspinal muscle groups.

Under controlled conditions *static* surface EMG has been shown to differentiate between subjects with chronic low-back pain and controls by analysis of the flexion relaxation ratio which is calculated from measurements taken during forward flexion and re-extension while standing (Watson et al 1997). A recent development is the application of a new mathematical technique known as wavelet transformation (WT) to analyze the complex, non-stationary signal obtained from surface EMG. It is reported that the use of WT methods improved the analysis of EMG signals in the time domain by facilitating the determination of the time of muscle activity (Pope et al 2000).

On the other hand there is little or no evidence supportive of a diagnostic role for *scanning* surface EMG. The proponents of scanning surface EMG argue that asymmetrical findings from paraspinal musculature may be caused by, or be causative of, spinal subluxation. It is also argued that such information has relevance to clinical decision making and patient management. The arguments in favor of surface EMG confound data supportive of *static* surface EMG with the lack of data supportive of *scanning* surface EMG. At this time the use of the scanning instrument remains investigational.

Age, gender, and body type also vary the proportional distribution of muscle fibers (Mannion 1999), and the clinical implication is twofold:

1. the practitioner must be aware of the likely changes which may be occurring in patients of particular ages and modify the process of assessment to reflect this within the context of the patient's body type and gender
2. there is difficulty in interpreting clinical data from surface EMG, not only between patients of different age, gender, and body type, but also between the thoracic and lumbar levels within the same patient.

CLINICAL APPROACH

Normal posture and movement are predicated on effective and coordinated interaction between opposing muscle groups and the clinical assessment of muscle function is conducted at multiple levels. The first part of any assessment of muscle change is the subjective determination of position at rest. This is in the global, regional, and segmental sense and includes observation of the symmetry of paired muscles. Individual muscles are then palpated for tonicity, flaccidity, atrophy, tender points, trigger points, and myotendinoses.

The global/regional/segmental approach also helps distinguish muscles which are extrinsic to the SMU from those which are intrinsic. The larger, extrinsic muscles are much more accessible than the small intrinsic muscles which are very difficult to assess. The extrinsic muscles are typically included in the global and segmental assessment and the practitioner is looking to see what changes may be identified in these muscles and then whether any such change can be attributable to a dysfunctional SMU.

This process requires the practitioner to have a thorough working knowledge of the segmental levels from which the spinal nerves arise to innervate each particular muscle. This is not to suggest that all muscle dysfunction arises from SMU dysfunction; rather, the spinal level of innervation becomes a piece of evidence in the clinical investigation. Muscle dysfunction may be secondary to peripheral nerve entrapment as well as multiple central causes.

Muscle tenderness

Tenderness is an early sign of pathologic change in muscle. The nociceptors within muscle usually have a high mechanical threshold; after all, they are present within a dynamic microenvironment which is constantly active. It is thought their threshold is reset to a lower level by endogenous substances released from the muscle when it is damaged. They then report normal movements and contractions within their dynamic environment as tenderness and then pain (Mense 1991).

The concept is that the excitability of the nociceptors within muscle is not fixed but is modulated by endogenous sensitizing agents such as bradykinin, serotonin, and E-type prostaglandins (Mense 1991). Investigations of inflamed muscle suggest there are two types of nerve endings to report either pain or tenderness, and that each is affected in a different manner by the biochemical changes which accompany inflammation. Tenderness is probably caused by a lowering of the threshold of group IV nerve endings as a sensitization to the inflammatory metabolites, while pain is probably caused by an increase in the resting activity of group III endings (Mense 1991).

The motor patterns of the trunk are significantly altered in persons with chronic low-back pain (Lund et al 2002). Muscle pain arising within the erector spinae modulates the descending voluntary motor commands but has surprisingly little effect on segmental stretch reflexes (Zedka et al 1999). The reduction in trunk motion is consistent with theories of guarding and models of pain adaptation. The altered motion pattern exposes the non-painful muscles in the area, particularly the contralateral erector spinae, to mechanical overload which could be a mechanism for the spread of pain from an injured muscle to neighboring muscles (Zedka et al 1999).

The diffuse nature of muscle pain may be due to the fact that the afferent fibers from a given muscle are distributed to many spinal segments, terminating mostly in laminae I and V of the spinal cord. The multiplicity of these receptors could form the basis of the referral of deep pain to other deep tissues (Mense 1991). Little is known about the links between the nociceptor afferents and the α-motoneurons in the ventral horns. The γ-motoneurons (fusimotor neurons) receive a complex input from the skin, joints, and muscles and synapse on to the α-motoneurons and this may be the link between pain input and altered motor output (Zedka et al 1999).

The practitioner must distinguish between tenderness on palpation, a mild clinical concern, and pain on resisted movement, a more significant clinical concern. Pain with movement must be localized as either about the tendon, including its bony and muscle junctions, or within the muscle fibers themselves. An attempt should also be made to identify the particular muscle which worsens any diffuse or referred pain, and these findings need to be interpreted within the concepts of Kellgren (1977) (Fig. 12.18), and pain distributions according to sclerotome, myotome, and dermatome.

Assessment of function

The final step is the subjective assessment of function. This includes an assessment of muscle tone and observation during dynamic movements, including gait, and the assessment of individual muscles by manual muscle testing. Function may be quantified where necessary by specifically grading muscle power using a common scale, by quantifying strength through the use of a dynamometer, and by the careful and selective use of surface EMG.

Manual assessment of muscle response to an external force applied by the practitioner's hand has been found to be a method capable of reliably and objectively discriminating the state of conditional facilitation or inhibition of a muscle (Caruso & Leisman 2001) and is a common and useful method in clinical practice. It is noted that, while manual muscle testing has been shown to be an excellent outcome tool when used by a limited number of highly trained clinical evaluators working together, it has the disadvantage of being subjective and requiring extensive experience to score muscle strength reliably (Escolar et al 2001).

GLOBAL CONSIDERATIONS

Global muscle change occurs secondary to a central cause which may be transient, as with emotionally activated limbic system dysfunction, or permanent, as with myasthenia gravis. Chiropractors and osteopaths recognize that upper cervical subluxation or dysfunction may affect many different neural pathways throughout the body (Burns 1937, Cole 1947, Herbst 1968). Palmer (BJ), the chiropractic profession's most vocal spokesperson in the 1920s and 1930s, considered upper cervical subluxation as the "one major element in all disease as it either decreased the quantity of nerve flow or the inability of the body to adequately function with a decreased flow" (Palmer 1966 p. 29).

The above considerations are empirical and dated; however, it is now known in the scientific sense that cervical dysfunction has distant neurological effects (Budgell & Hirano 2001). It remains unclear whether the global function of muscle can be affected by subtle spinal dysfunction, although of course it is accepted that frank trauma such as fracture within the cervical spine has the cataclysmic effect of quadriplegia. Muscle tone is an important indicator of any global change and may indicate central neurologic dysfunction.

Resting tone

A resting muscle has tone secondary to biomechanical elements and not neurological input. Hence the tone in a resting muscle is not measurable by EMG as the muscle is required to perform an active movement in order to generate an electrical signal representative of motor tone.

Resting tone is therefore assessed manually. The patient must be relaxed and the practitioner moves the upper then the lower limb through a range of movements, looking for any change from what is considered normal. The movements include passive supination and pronation of the forearm, rolling the hand around the wrist, and flexing/extending the elbow. Legs are assessed in the supine patient by rolling the knee from side to side, lifting the knee rapidly to see how the heel follows, flexing and extending the knee, and moving the ankle through dorsi- and plantar flexion (Fuller 1999).

According to Fuller (1999 p. 109), the resting tone will be:

- normal and provide slight resistance through the full range of movements and the heel will lift minimally from the bed when the knee is quickly lifted
- decreased with a loss of resistance and the heel will not lift off the bed when the knee is quickly lifted. A marked loss of tone is flaccidity which may be caused by a lower motor neuron disorder or a cerebellar lesion, and, rarely, a myopathy
- increased, where the resistance may catch and increase suddenly, which is spasticity. In this case the heel lifts easily when the knee is quickly lifted. Spasticity indicates an upper motor lesion. The resistance may also be increased through the whole range which is lead pipe rigidity. If there are intermittent breaks in this type of tone then it is cog-wheel rigidity. These patterns indicate an extrapyramidal syndrome such as Parkinson's disease. There may also be the appearance that the patient is attempting to oppose limb movement and this may suggest paratonia secondary to cerebrovascular disease.

Increased muscle tone may also be found in the absence of spasticity and extrapyramidal dysfunction. Janda (1991) identifies the following causes:

- dysfunction of the limbic system
- impaired function at the segmental (interneuronal) level
- impaired coordination of muscle contraction, perhaps secondary to trigger points
- response to pain irritation
- overuse, generally combined with changed elasticity of the muscle and usually described as muscle tightness.

The limbic system activates the excitatory portion of the reticular activating system (RAS) which may, in response to stress in the patient, increase its output, resulting in multiple muscle groups becoming hypertonic and taut (Schneider 1999 p. 20). Intervention in these cases must address the underlying emotional distress.

If marked muscular weakness is observed as 3 or less on the common power scale (Box 6.1), the practitioner must search for a pattern which may suggest a cause:

- weakness of arm extensors with weak leg flexors (a pyramidal pattern), with increased resting tone and increased reflexes, suggests an upper motor neuron lesion
- decreased tone with wasting, fasciculation and absent reflexes suggests a lower motor neuron lesion
- decreased tone with wasting and impaired or absent reflexes suggests muscle disease
- normal or decreased tone with normal reflexes and fatigable weakness suggests a lesion at the neuromuscular junction
- normal tone with normal reflexes without wasting but with erratic power suggests a functional weakness (Fuller 1999).

Postural change

Global postural change is the sum of a number of regional, and perhaps even segmental, changes. The assessment of posture has been discussed in Chapter 4 and, while there are many

---

Box 6.1 Power rating of skeletal muscle

5	Normal power
4+	Submaximal movement against resistance
4	Moderate movement against resistance
4−	Slight movement against resistance
3	Movement against gravity but not against resistance
2	Movement is possible with gravity eliminated
1	A flicker within the muscle
0	No movement

Power should be graded according to the maximum power attained, no matter how briefly this is maintained. The test muscle is isolated as best as possible and is positioned halfway through its normal range of motion. The patient is asked to contract and resist against the static force of the practitioner for no more than 6 s. The practitioner should not overpower the test muscle.

After Fuller (1999), with permission.

---

causes of change, muscle dysfunction is nearly always involved. The process of identifying muscle involvement depends heavily on an accurate knowledge and understanding of a particular muscle's basic function. For example, the sign of unilateral quadratus lumborum weakness can only be a raised rib 12 and not a lowered iliac crest. The ilium is not suspended by the quadratus lumborum, whereas the rib is stabilized by it.

The actions of the muscle must also be considered as to whether it is acting as an agonist which may either be facilitated (strong) or inhibited (weak), or as an antagonist, again either facilitated or inhibited. An example is drawn from the upper trapezius, where head tilt to the right with left rotation of the face may be secondary to a facilitated upper trapezius on the right which overpowers the normal strength of the muscle on the left, or an inhibited upper trapezius on the left which allows a normal upper trapezius on the right to dominate.

The muscle is then considered within the context of the surrounding muscles, which either act as agonists or antagonists. The better examples are within the "crossed syndromes" of Janda, as described by Chaitow. The lower crossed syndrome is described in Chapter 14 (Fig. 14.6) and the upper crossed syndrome is presented here to establish the principles (Fig. 6.2).

Janda considers that a crossed syndrome occurs when postural muscles shorten and phasic muscles weaken. The clinical implication is that muscle activity must be considered beyond the simple concept of a left/right relationship between a muscle pair, such as the upper trapezii, to include the anterior/posterior contributions of muscles which normally act in harmony to maintain normal balance, in this case the muscles of the upper anterior thorax, the pectorals. As these tighten, the deep neck flexors and rhomboids weaken, allowing significant postural distortion of the head, neck, and shoulders.

While a crossed syndrome is usually either about the head and neck (upper) or the pelvis (lower), and is therefore a regional consideration, its effects are not isolated. Any alteration to the carriage of the head and neck will be reflected in postural changes about the arms, pelvis, and lower limbs. This is particularly so because of the principle of quadrupedal coordination (Dietz 2002).

This principle hypothesizes that, during locomotion, corticospinal excitation of the upper limb motorneurons is mediated

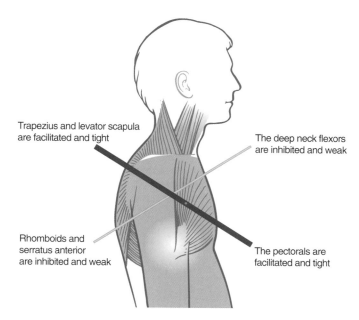

Trapezius and levator scapula
are facilitated and tight

The deep neck flexors
are inhibited and weak

Rhomboids and
serratus anterior
are inhibited and weak

The pectorals are
facilitated and tight

Figure 6.2 Upper crossed syndrome. The upper crossed syndrome is observed in postural assessment from the side and is an imbalance which alters the normal positions of the head, neck, and shoulders. From Chaitow & DeLany (2000), with permission.

indirectly via propriospinal neurons in the cervical spinal cord. This allows a task-dependent neuronal linkage of cervical and thoracolumbar propriospinal circuits controlling leg and arm movements during human locomotion activities (Dietz 2002).

It is known that there is an increased EMG activity in the left erector spinae with right arm abduction (Davey et al 2002). This must involve the latissimus dorsi, a muscle designed to move the upper limb or to raise the trunk in brachiation (Bogduk et al 1998). The clinical application is that the mechanical transfer of forces reported by Vleeming et al (1995) (Figs 2.10 and 13.8) is underpinned by neurologic mechanisms and that dysfunction in these mechanisms may be reflected in postural change.

While these findings have significant application in spinal rehabilitation, they also broaden the scope of spinal assessment. Spinal stability is influenced by posture and, specifically, the control of spinal stability is reduced in asymmetric postures associated with low-back disorders (Granata & Wilson 2001). Postural assessment is a crucial tool for identifying levels of asymmetry and then relating them, both neurologically and mechanically, to global change which may be indicative of segmental dysfunction.

REGIONAL CONSIDERATIONS

A broad range of conditions affect muscle in a regional context. These include changes in muscle tone, muscle strength or power, functional symmetry, myofascial pain syndrome, neurolymphatic points, feed-forward control, and spine position sense. Regional assessment follows global assessment and the same principles apply: observation, palpation, passive range of motion (ROM) and active ROM. An important finding is the nature of motor tone in a particular muscle, set of muscles (an agonist with its antagonist), or group of muscles.

Motor tone

Motor tone is detectable by EMG and is present in a resting muscle only under abnormal circumstances, for example when psychological stress or protective activity is involved. Motor tone is either phasic to move something, or tonic to stabilize something. Motor tone is absent when there is no demand from activity or gravity (Chaitow & DeLany 2000).

Muscle contraction occurs in response to a motor nerve impulse acting on muscle fibers, and such a nerve will always activate a collection of fibers which represent the muscle's motor unit. Contraction may be one of the following:

- isometric: when the length (*metric*) remains the same (*iso*) while the fibers contract and increase the tension in the muscle. In muscle testing this is achieved through the practitioner providing a static resistance against which the patient contracts the muscle under test
- concentric: where the length of the muscle shortens while the fibers contract as tension in the muscle increases to overcome or move some resistance. The ends of the muscle approximate
- eccentric: where the resistance is greater than the tension achieved within the muscle and the length of the muscle increases while it is producing tension. The ends of the muscle move apart
- econcentric: a combination of a controlled concentric and a concurrent eccentric contraction of the same muscle over two separate joints (Prentice 2001). Naturally this type of contraction is only possible in a muscle which crosses two joints, such as the hamstring. Prentice gives the example of a prone, open-kinetic chain hamstring curl, where concentric contraction flexes the knee while the hip tends to flex eccentrically, lengthening the hamstring (Prentice 2001 p. 59).

Muscle spasm is defined as a neuromuscular phenomenon relating either to an upper motor neuron disease or an acute reaction to pain or tissue injury. EMG activity is increased in these cases and any clinical protocol would be incomplete without including a diagnostic algorithm to exclude or include this source of potentially confounding data. The old idea that muscle spasms are due to a reflex activation of γ-motoneurons following a deep lesion has not been supported by the results of animal studies (Mense 1991).

Muscle strength

Muscle strength is defined as the ability of a muscle to generate force against resistance. All muscles have a normal level of strength which allows normal healthy living. Abnormal posture, movement, and gait arise from muscle weakness and may impair normal functional movement. Muscular strength is closely associated with muscle endurance, which is the ability to perform repetitive muscular contractions against some resistance for an extended period of time. It is thought that muscle endurance is more important than strength in carrying out the activities of daily living, particularly as one ages (Prentice 2001).

The quantification of muscle strength and endurance is a sophisticated process utilizing purpose-built mechanical devices which can be adapted to provide specific patterns of resistance to certain muscles and groups of muscles. There are times when quantified muscle strength is useful and it is ideally suited to rehabilitation assessment and outcome measurement. In the typical clinical situation the use of manual muscle testing has greater flexibility and usefulness.

Manual muscle testing requires the subject to apply an isometric contraction against a constant resistance provided by the practitioner. Skeletal muscle which is functioning normally will demonstrate two specific characteristics with manual muscle testing in addition to allowing the practitioner to make an estimate of strength or power.

The first is the reaction time of the muscle to the verbal command "resist". A patient with normally functioning cognitive and neural pathways will demonstrate an equal and rapid response for the same muscle on each side of the body. This response is termed the "leading edge of the force pulses" and most practitioners report they derive most of their assessment from this initial interaction (Caruso & Leisman 2000). Any unilateral delay may suggest compromise of the cognitive, neural, and/or muscle contracting processes. A bilateral delay suggests a central disorder which should then be tested to determine whether it is affecting either the lower or the upper body only, or both.

The second is the ability to maintain isometric contraction for the duration of applied resistance, normally no more than 6 s. The muscle is observed during the application of resistance to determine whether it moves from isometric to eccentric contraction. This is where the test muscle will lengthen or "break way" against the practitioner's resistance while still contracting. A muscle is perceived to be inhibited or weak when this change occurs within about 6 s. A force/displacement analysis demonstrates there is a distance vs force slope magnitude of difference between a conditionally inhibited (weak) muscle and a conditionally facilitated (strong) muscle and that this corresponds to a trained practitioner's subjective muscle-testing judgment (Caruso & Leisman 2001).

Muscle power is not "strength" in the sense of quantifying the amount of resistance which can be provided by a particular muscle. The power-rating scale (Box 6.1) rates the ability of a muscle to perform in the zone of function up to where normal power is demonstrated and strength, per se, can thereafter be quantified. This "zone of function" ranges from grade 0, which is no movement at all within the muscle, to grade 5, which represents normal power for the particular individual. Muscle strength in ambulatory practice will usually lie in the range of 4− and above, with an occasional 3.

It is well accepted that a nerve root for which compromise can be demonstrated by diagnostic imaging will have some effect on the muscle it supplies. What is less accepted outside the field of manual medicine is that minor irritations to the same nerve root will have similar effects but to a lesser degree. The skill of the practitioner lies in being sufficiently competent to identify these small changes for which blatant causes are not obviously demonstrated on imaging.

The nerve supply to muscles is quite variable and may range over one or two nerve roots above and below what is typically cited in textbooks. This is all part of the diagnostic challenge which faces practitioners. The important relationships to remember are given in Table 6.1, where the most common muscles to test as indicators of specific spinal level dysfunction are given.

Table 6.1 Muscles indicative of specific spinal level function

Action	Muscle tested	Indicative spinal level
Ipsilateral lateral flexion and contralateral rotation of the head	Upper trapezius	C3, C4
Early shoulder abduction	Supraspinatus	C5
Elbow flexion	Biceps brachii	C5, C6
Elbow extension	Triceps	C7
Finger flexion	Flexor digitorum superficialis and profundus	C8
Finger abduction	First dorsal interosseus	T1
Hip flexion	Iliopsoas	L1, L2
Hip adduction	Adductors	L2, L3
Knee extension	Quadriceps femoris	L3, L4
Foot inversion	Tibialis posterior	L4, L5
Dorsiflexion of the foot	Tibialis anterior	L4, L5
Hip extension	Gluteus maximus	L5, S1
Knee flexion	Hamstrings	
Plantar flexion of the foot	Gastrocnemius	S1

In essence, this is a table of myotomes for the body, where a myotome consists of all muscles which are derived from one somite and are innervated by one segmental spinal nerve. It is clear that, in most instances, especially lower-limb motor function, movement arises from two spinal levels. Hence hip flexion, for example, is innervated by both the L1 and L2 myotomes. It must also be appreciated that, just as authors differ in mapping the dermatomes of the body, they may also differ in associating myotomes with actions.

Symmetry

Asymmetry of muscle is a regional observation given that there is no "global" muscle of the body. The basic assessment is of the physical characteristics of paired muscles, looking for comparable left right size. Muscles of the trunk are assessed for bulk, in particular the muscles about the shoulder. There is usually a slightly greater bulkiness in the muscles of the dominant side.

Muscles of the extremities are assessed for girth as measured by a soft tape measure. The diameter of the upper limb is measured at the greatest dimension of the relaxed biceps and about the proximal forearm. The lower limb is measured about the midpoint of the thigh and notation should be made in the file of the distance of the tape measure from the superior margin of the patella. The leg is also measured at the greatest dimension of the relaxed gastrocnemius in the seated patient.

A left/right difference in diameter greater than 1 cm should be noted. The next step is to determine whether the muscle with the lesser diameter is exhibiting atrophy or whether the muscle with the greater diameter is exhibiting hypertrophy. This judgment is made with consideration of other clinical findings, such as pain or changes in sensation.

A smaller thigh in a leg which has obvious signs of spinal nerve irritation such as nerve root pain, reflex change, and sensory change will be suggestive of atrophy. A larger biceps in a tennis player in the presence of normal strength and function of the smaller biceps is more likely to be indicative of task-specific hypertrophy.

Left/right comparisons are also made for strength which, like bulk, should be approximately symmetrical, taking account of the dominant side. A footballer, for example, would be expected to have greater strength and responsiveness in the preferred kicking leg. Strength may be assessed by manual muscle testing but the asymmetry this reveals may be more representative of functional weakness than structural weakness. A dynamometer is useful for quantifying the strength of muscle groups and a "grip dynamometer" can be used for this purpose to assess the muscles of the forearm.

A sense of symmetry is also gained by observation from the side of the patient, in particular looking for suggestions of the upper crossed and/or lower crossed syndromes, as discussed earlier (Fig. 6.2). Gait is also assessed for symmetry and important clues for muscle dysfunction may be evident by changes to the rhythm of the patient's gait (Fig. 4.6).

Functional asymmetry may also be found in the order in which certain muscles are recruited to perform a defined task. The act of prone hip extension involves a number of muscles and muscle groups about the low back and pelvis. Their recruitment sequence is ipsilateral erector spinae, semitendinosus, contralateral erector spinae, tensor fascia latae, then gluteus maximus (Vogt & Banzer 1997). A unilateral alteration to this sequence suggests inhibition of one or more muscles such that other muscles must fire first either to provide support and stabilization or to initiate and conduct the task. A bilaterally altered activation sequence suggests chronic muscle insufficiency and a need for closer investigation and rehabilitation.

Myofascial pain syndrome

The myofascial pain syndrome has been discussed in Chapter 5 with regard to the fascial involvement and further comment will be given here to address the muscle or "myo" component.

It must be appreciated that the clinical characteristics of a myofascial pain syndrome include the complaint of pain localized to a specific region of the body. The syndrome is not a global disorder. The pain is typically associated with a tense, shortened muscle which would usually test as weak, due to it being either inhibited or to pain which may arise from a trigger point (TrP) within the muscle.

The TrP is an exquisitely tender spot found within a taut band of muscle fibers and is thought to cause the increased muscle tension and also to limit its range of motion (Simons 1991). The patient's pain complaint may be reproduced by digital pressure on this spot. The pain may include a local component but is typically referred to a distant site, hence the name of the hyperirritable spot being trigger point; irritation of the spot triggers a pain response elsewhere, in a fairly predictable location and pattern.

The TrP may be active and generate the clinical complaint of pain, or it may be latent and less irritable and not be actively causing pain (Simons 1991). Latent trigger points produce dysfunction of the muscle, but not pain and the patient may typically experience referred tenderness, stiffness, and restricted ROM (Simons 1991).

Five neurologic mechanisms have been proposed to explain the phenomenon of referred pain (Simons 1991). In summary, they are convergence projection and peripheral branching of

---

Box 6.2 Clinical criteria for the diagnosis of myofascial pain syndrome

Major criteria
1. A regional pain complaint
2. A pain complaint or altered sensation in the expected distribution of referred pain from a myofascial trigger point
3. A taut band palpable in an accessible muscle
4. Exquisite spot tenderness at one point along the length of the taut band
5. Some degree of restricted range of motion, when measurable.

Minor criteria
1. Reproduction of the clinical pain complaint, or altered sensation, by pressure on the tender spot
2. Elicitation of a local twitch response by transverse snapping palpation at the tender spot
3. Pain alleviated by elongation or stretching the muscle.

The clinical diagnosis of myofascial pain syndrome is made when the findings include all of the five major criteria and at least one of the minor criteria.

From Simons (1991), with permission.

---

primary afferent nociceptors, which are both anatomical mechanisms, and convergence facilitation, sympathetic nervous system activity, and convergence or image projection at the supraspinal level, which are functional mechanisms. Each is discussed in detail in the next chapter.

The anatomical mechanisms of convergence projection and peripheral branching do not require any afferent input from the zone to which the pain is referred. Therefore if the reference zone is anesthetized and the pain persists, then the mechanism is most likely one of these two. If the pain ceases, Simons (1991) suggests the mechanism is likely to be one of the latter three functional mechanisms. He also makes the point that several mechanisms may operate simultaneously.

The mechanisms are somewhat academic and it is more important for the practitioner to be aware of the nature and patterns of referred pain and be able to locate the source. The active TrP is palpable within the taut band and, apart from being tender to palpation and triggering a referred pain pattern, it typically demonstrates a local twitch response. This is a sudden burst of local electrical activity in response to specific irritation by palpation and represents an abnormal reactivity of these muscle fibers (Simons 1991).

An acute myofascial pain syndrome may be initiated by a single instance of muscle overload, typically as a traumatic event. These are prone to regress to become a latent TrP with residual dysfunction on the resolution of pain from the event. In some patients the condition may multiply and involve other muscles in the region, thus becoming a regional complaint. Depending on the response of the patient, the problem may progress to become chronic (Simons 1991). Simons has identified major and minor criteria for the diagnosis of myofascial pain syndrome and these are given in Box 6.2.

Neurolymphatic points

The concept of neurolymphatic points was introduced in Chapter 5 and will be further discussed in Chapter 8. The relevance to this chapter is their purported diagnostic capacity to identify dysfunctional muscle. It is thought that a neurolymphatic point becomes active when a muscle which relates to that point becomes inhibited. It is also acknowledged that any condition which puts a load on the lymphatic system may affect these points (Walther 1981 p. 220).

An active neurolymphatic point palpates as being quite tender. Careful palpation may reveal the point has a different texture to the surrounding tissue. The spinal practitioner will commonly encounter these points on the posterior aspect of the body, about the spinal column, yet they have also been mapped on the anterior of the body (Walther 1981 p. 223).

The clinical implication is that tenderness about an SMU may be more indicative of an active neurolymphatic point and its related dysfunctional muscle than of specific dysfunction within the SMU. The process of elimination is first to assess the matching neurolymphatic point on the anterior of the body as the anterior point is more tender than the posterior point. If the matching anterior point is tender, then it suggests the posterior tenderness is most likely an active neurolymphatic point.

If the anterior point is not unduly tender then the posterior point is explored further by testing the particular muscle or muscles which relate to that point. If they test weak then it is reasonable to accept the tenderness of the point as reflective of the muscle dysfunction. If the muscles test as normal, then the tenderness may reflect local dysfunction within the SMU.

It must also be appreciated that the dysfunction within the SMU may well be a *cause* of weakness in the particular muscles which refer to the neurolymphatic point at that level. It is possible for regional dysfunction to be multifactorial and for any SC within an SMU to be associated with muscle weakness which may activate neurolymphatic points and for that muscle to be the site of a TrP which refers pain elsewhere.

The neurolymphatic points according to Walther (1981) are given in Table 6.2 for the postural muscles.

Table 6.2 Posterior neurolymphatic point location for postural muscles

Muscle	Posterior point location
Upper trapezius	Posterior arch of atlas to the lateral mass
Sternocleidomastoid	Lamina of C2
Levator scapulae	Within the belly of teres minor
Deltoid	T3–4 laminae
Pectoralis major	T5–7 laminae on the left
Latissimus dorsi	T7–8 laminae on the left
Adductor longus	Below the inferior angle of the scapulae
Rectus femoris	T8–11 laminae
Quadratus lumborum	T11 lamina and distal rib 12, upper edge
Gastrocnemius, soleus, and tibialis posterior	T11–12 laminae
Iliopsoas	T12–L1 between spinous and transverse process
Sacrospinalis	L2 transverse process
Oblique abdominals and piriformis	Between PSIS and L5 spinous process
Biceps femoris and semimembranosus	Upper SIJ medial to the PSIS

PSIS, posterior superior iliac spine; SIJ, sacroiliac joint. Adapted from Walther (1981), with permission.

Feed-forward control

Feed-forward control occurs when a signal of change in the body, a perturbation, generates a response with the intent to control the reaction to that change. This is quite different to the withdrawal reflex. The feed-forward control mechanism as it relates to protect the spine is clearly demonstrated by rapidly loading the upper limbs. The concept is that the trunk will respond with supportive actions to protect the body in this circumstance. The supportive response commences with trunk muscles such as the transverse abdominal and transverse spinalis muscles contracting to maintain dynamic spine stability. These muscles are activated before the prime muscles responsible for limb movement become active. This allows the body to position itself better to receive the load (Leinonen et al 2001).

In other words, a signal is sent from receptors in the upper limbs to the stabilizing muscles of the trunk and spine for the purpose of protecting the spine, ahead of signals which allow a dynamic response to the load. It seems the peripheral sensory input from afferents in the ligaments of the upper limbs participates in a continuous control of muscle activity through feed-forward or preprogramming mechanisms (Sjolander et al 2002). The mechanism seems to be a spinal reflex mediated by a direct afferent pathway from the upper limbs or the upper spinal segment (Leinonen et al 2001). This is seen as preprogramming muscle stiffness through reflex modulation of the gamma-muscle system (Sjolander et al 2002).

It has also been shown that feed-forward control of lumbar muscles is impaired in patients with sciatica (Leinonen et al 2001). The clinical implications are potentially quite dramatic. Measurement of these responses should theoretically enable a practitioner to identify individuals with impaired "safety" mechanisms and apply a corrective treatment protocol while ensuring that the individual is not placed in an environment where there is likelihood that the mechanism may be tested, with resultant injury. These concepts remain developmental at this time but are expected to become a practical part of clinical practice over the next decade.

Spine position sense

It has recently been reported that lumbosacral position sense is altered in individuals with low-back pain (Brumagne et al 1999, Newcomer et al 2000a, b). This means that scientifically conducted tests of the ability of subjects to sense the position of their low back in various positions show a decrease in those with low-back pain. Fatigue seems to diminish the accuracy of repositioning in both low-back pain and control subjects (Taimela et al 1999).

This newly reported ability of the lumbosacral spine to sense its position is independent of the magnitude of movement (Swinkels et al 2000) and is reproducible (Swinkels & Dolan 1998). It confirms a role for the ligamentomuscular stabilizing system of the spine (Solomonow et al 1998) and demonstrates the importance of the intersegmental trunk muscles in stabilizing the lumbar spine (Quint et al 1998).

The practical application of this knowledge in the clinical setting is yet to be determined and early studies are not very encouraging (Koumantakis et al 2002), but the findings in general are an exciting endorsement of those disciplines such as chiropractic and osteopathy which have long accepted that small dysfunction within the SMU has profound effects. It is now clearly apparent that the lumbar SMUs monitor sensory information as well as act to control spinal muscles and probably provide kinesthetic perception to the sensory cortex (Holm et al 2002).

The clinical implication as it can be interpreted at this time is that the small muscles and ligaments of the SMU play a vital role in normal spinal kinematics. The scientific evidence is that pain (Newcomer et al 2000a, b) causes changes in the tissues about the SMU (Brumagne et al 1999). A proprioceptive effect is generated at the local level and, while fatigue of those tissues impairs this ability (Taimela et al 1999), the spinal structures overall are well suited to monitor sensory information and control muscles (Holm et al 2002).

The main application of this knowledge is to improve spinal assessment and rehabilitation. A relationship exists between poor postural control of the lumbar spine and larger postural sway while standing (Radebold et al 2001). There is poorer postural control of the lumbar spine and a longer trunk muscle response in subjects with low-back pain than in healthy controls (Radebold et al 2001). This may allow observation of the size of postural sway while standing to become a clinical indicator of poor lumbar muscle function.

A relevant question is whether this sensorimotor control of the spine is affected by the SC, functional spinal lesion, or other segmental entity. The collective experience of chiropractors, osteopaths, and other practitioners of manual healthcare is in the affirmative and it now remains for science to demonstrate these relationships.

SEGMENTAL CONSIDERATIONS

Small changes within the SMU are known to affect the proprioception about the region and, given they are projected to the sensory cortex (Holm et al 2002), may have a global effect on the body. This increases the importance of the practitioner having a structured approach to the assessment of the spine which encompasses all possibilities. The sequence of global/regional/segmental as adopted in this text must remain open and fluid to link global effects with segmental dysfunction while assisting the practitioner to proceed in a logical and complete manner.

This is particularly true at the segmental level of assessment of muscle change. The small muscles of the SMU cannot be independently assessed, therefore assessment at this level must rely heavily on meshing palpatory and other findings with the mental images the practitioner has developed. It is easy to palpate the biceps brachii; it is challenging to palpate the multifidi and distinguish them from the rotatores; and impossible to palpate the intertransversarii. Therefore muscle assessment at the segmental level can only proceed with a strong conceptual understanding of the structure and function of the intrinsic muscles.

Further, the relationship between these small muscles and the larger regional muscles must also be appreciated. Pickar & Kang (2001) summarize the need for an appropriate distribution of the low forces generated by the small, multisegmental muscles of the spine, the multifidi, and rotatores (Fig. 6.3B), and the stronger forces generated by the larger multisegmental muscles (iliocostalis, longissimus), in order to prevent the stronger forces

placing the spine at risk of buckling. They found that small, sustained vertebral displacements from the neutral position could affect muscle spindle feedback by altering stretch sensitivity (Pickar & Kang 2001) which in turn affected this fine level of force balance.

The clinical relevance is the understanding that errors in neural control of paraspinal muscles due to static changes in vertebral position, as is believed to be found in the SC, could adversely affect spinal stability and contribute to low-back pain of mechanical origin (Pickar & Kang 2001). It also underscores the point that any clinical assessment of muscle change must be in conjunction with the clinical assessment of neural change as these two dimensions of the SC are intimately related. Clearly, the balance of the body is not only a matter of balance between the larger forces of the postural agonists and antagonists, but a matter of balance amongst the intrinsic muscles of the SMU.

The multifidus

The intrinsic muscles of the typical SMU are depicted in Figure 6.3. The multifidi are perhaps the most studied small muscle.

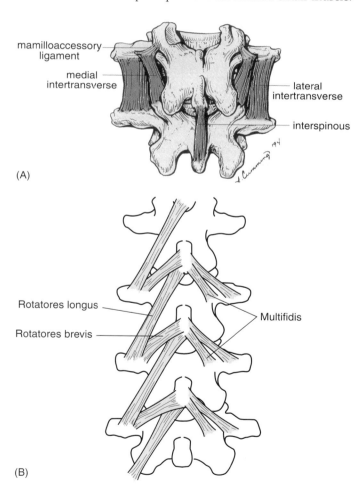

(A)

(B)

Figure 6.3 The intrinsic musculature of a typical lumbar spinal motion unit. (A) Posterior view showing the intersegmental muscles; (B) posterior view showing the multisegmental muscles. (A, B) After Cramer & Darby (1995), with permission.

They attach posterior spines of adjacent vertebrae and may span two or three segments (Herzog 2000 p. 34). Their line of action tends to be parallel to the compressive axis, particularly in the lumbar spine, and in some cases runs anterior caudal in obliquity. Even though the muscle spans only a few joints, it is considered intrinsic in that it only affects local areas of the spine. It is involved in producing extensor torque but only provides the ability for corrections or moment support at specific joints that may be the foci of stress (Herzog 2000).

Prolonged flexion of the lumbar spine results in tension-relaxation and laxity of its viscoelastic structures, including the multifidi. After about 3 mins there are random and unpredictable EMG discharges from the multifidus (Williams et al 2000). When the multifidus is injured, its recovery is not spontaneous, even with the remission of painful symptoms. Individuals who receive exercise therapy demonstrate a more rapid and complete return to muscle recovery (Hides et al 1996).

Movement and exercise are important components of recovery and rehabilitation programs for patients with low-back pain. Rehabilitation should be directed to the medial back muscles because they provide the most effective support for intervertebral motion and because mild disturbances appear to be associated with their innervation in recurrent low-back pain. The low-back EMG of those with radiating or referred pain was abnormal in about three-fourths of subjects and this is consistent with a mild degree of axonal damage in the posterior branch of the lumbar nerve innervating the medial paraspinal muscles (Sihvonen et al 1997).

The clinical implication is that dysfunction in the small muscles of the SMU, particularly the multifidus, may be detectable through careful palpation of the kinematics of the SMU and of the muscles themselves. As postural muscles, the multifidi shorten when stressed. Bilaterally they will fix the SMU in extension and limit flexion, while unilateral contraction will tend to flex and contralaterally rotate the SMU (Chaitow & DeLany 2002 p. 272) and again this should be detectable on palpation for kinematic change.

Myotenones

A myotenone consists of a clinical unit of muscle which can independently contract, and its tendons. Broad, flat muscle may comprise several myotenones while small, slender muscles represent a single myotenone (Dvořák & Dvořák 1990 pp. 64–67).

When myotenones within a large muscle become dysfunctional they demonstrate increased tone, elevated consistency, resistance, and decreased plasticity. These changes are palpable and, when present in the small muscles of the SMU, may contribute to the tenderness which is associated with the SC.

Dvořák & Dvořák have observed a relationship between certain axial skeleton parts and certain myotenones and suggest that a functional disturbance (SC) in one SMU will initiate myotendinoses simultaneously in the empirically correlated myotenones. Their published texts (1984, 1990) contain an atlas of putative relationships. They propose the "rule of eight" to suggest that each myotenone of, for example, semispinalis capitis generates dysfunction at an SMU eight levels below (Dvořák & Dvořák 1990 p. 256). This may be interpreted as suggesting a SC at L3 may produce myotendinoses about T7 and again at its insertion area on the occiput.

The clinical implication is that when tenderness is palpated about a specific SMU then further assessment should be made of other levels of the spine, perhaps some eight spinal levels apart. Dvořák & Dvořák's findings are both complex and putative, but provide justification for a broader assessment of the spine by the practitioner with an awareness to observe and record relationships as they may be found. It remains important to consider all findings in developing the rationale for mechanical intervention.

CONCLUSION

The assessment of muscle change represents a clinical challenge as any change may be either a cause or an effect of spinal dysfunction. A thoughtful, structured approach is useful first to identify and assess those muscles about the SMU which may reflect local involvement, and then those muscles innervated from a suspect spinal level which may demonstrate findings which implicate a particular SMU.

Muscle change may therefore be mechanical and part of a global postural or functional presentation of the patient, or neurological and a discrete indicator of either systemic or segmental dysfunction. Generic descriptive phrases such as "hypertonic and tender paraspinal muscles" serve little clinical use and practitioners must be concise in their identification of particular muscles which may be clinically involved in a particular presentation, and should also be careful with the words chosen to describe that dysfunction in the patient record.

7

Assessment of neural change

KEY CONCEPTS

Neural change may be considered in terms of three dimensions: objective, subjective, and abstract. Each dimension has several vectors which represent assessable components or functions. The objective dimensions are more Newtonian and the abstract dimensions more quantum in character.

Objective dimensions of neural change include motor, reflex, and sensory functions. These are the tried and true, evidence-based components of the neurological examination.

Subjective dimensions include the patient's embodied experiences of sensation, pain, autonomic function, and neurocognitive phenomena. The lived kinesthetic experience of the patient is incorporated within the biopsychosocial considerations of pain.

There is a reasonable body of evidence which demonstrates that changes in autonomic function are associated with somatic stimulation. There is a neurophysiologic rationale for the concept that aberrant stimulation of spinal or paraspinal structures may lead to segmentally organized reflex responses of the autonomic nervous system which in turn may alter visceral function.

Abstract dimensions represent the qualitative component of the pain experience and other changes in neural function, including coping strategies. The cognitive, affective, and evaluative vectors are valuable inclusions within the neural assessment process.

There are at least five known mechanisms for generating referred pain. Two are anatomical and represent pain pathways while three are functional and represent the manner in which the brain may interpret the source of pain. More than one mechanism may be involved in a particular pain experience.

INTRODUCTION

Neurology is a vast and complex topic and it is not the intent of this chapter to mimic or replace any of the excellent texts on this topic. The reader is assumed to have or be developing a comprehensive knowledge of the neurological system and to know its basic structure and function. Each chapter of Part 2 presents a structured approach to the assessment of neural change relevant to each specific spinal level. This chapter aims to provide an overall context for the assessment of neural change and presents a structured approach which may assist the budding practitioner.

Neural change is an important dimension of the subluxation complex (SC). It is neurologic dysfunction, typically perceived by the patient as pain and discomfort, which remains the most common reason patients seek consultation and treatment (Ebrall 1992a). The most obvious clinical question is whether the practitioner can replicate the pain experienced by the patient and demonstrate a mechanical cause. The location and distribution of pain are therefore important clinical clues.

However the assessment of neural change must go well beyond pain. It is not unusual for an incidental discovery to be made during a program of treatment for a purported mechanical problem. Patients often report other health improvements, some of which are reflective of change in neural function. This is indicative of a broader scope of manual practice beyond the identification and correction of mechanical dysfunction and pain (Coulter 1999).

The scheme of relationships shown in Figure 7.1 demonstrates a ranking of neural change from objective to abstract dimensions. The objective dimensions may be considered Newtonian in character and include objective findings such as a bulging disk compressing a motor nerve axon and mechanically decreasing motor function. In many respects objective neural change is evidenced by changes in the other dimensions of the SC, especially muscle change, often global kinematic change, and sometimes regional or segmental vascular change, mostly with mechanical causation.

The abstract dimensions are more quantum in character and include cognitive, affective, and evaluative effects. Whilst ample evidence can be found for the disk bulge and its effects, the evidence for quantum change is much more subtle. The subjective dimensions lie on the continuum between the two and incorporate the biopsychosocial considerations (Fig. 4.1).

Every patient encounter delivers a complex puzzle to the practitioner, especially with respect to determining the status of the neurologic system and identifying any abnormal function. The manual practitioner must then search to determine if there is any relationship between identifiable neural change and spinal dysfunction. The aim is to relate any neural change to dysfunction within a specific spinal motion unit (SMU) and

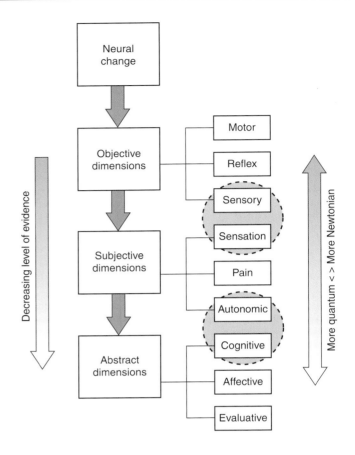

Figure 7.1 A graphic depiction of ranking and relationships of neural change. The dashed circles indicate transitional vectors between dimensions.

then to use that change as a component of the working diagnosis which leads to the diagnostic statement, selection of treatment, and outcome measurements.

The sequence of global/regional/segmental applies to the assessment of neural change; however, this will play out as a second game under the ranking of objective, subjective, and abstract dimensions. Each subdivision of those dimensions must be explored in global, regional, and segmental terms. The findings from the assessment of neural change are to be incorporated with the findings from the assessment of changes in kinematics, connective tissue, musculature, and the vascular system.

CLINICAL ANATOMY

The investigation of neural change demands a high level of knowledge of neuroanatomy. Each chapter in Part 2 reviews the relevant clinical anatomy for each spinal region. This section provides an overview of the neural elements in each of the typical cervical, thoracic, and lumbar regions of the spine. The neuroanatomy of each level is relatively consistent but the

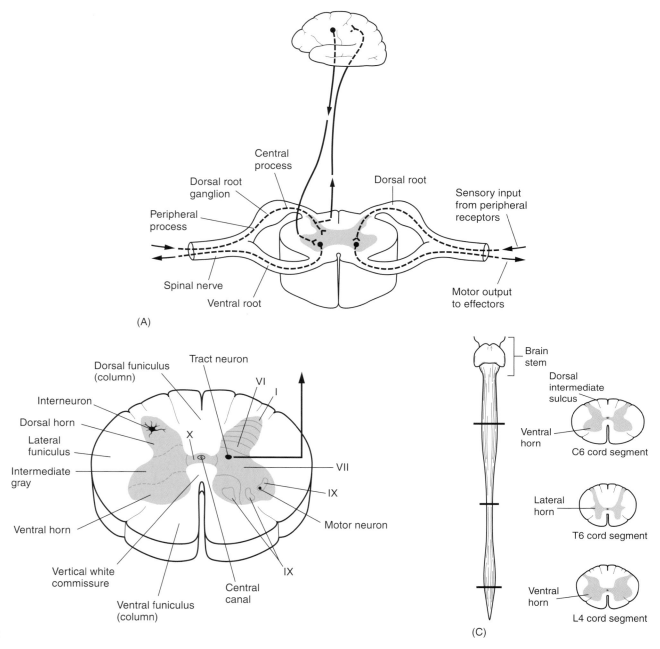

Figure 7.2 The general scheme of the spinal cord. (A) A typical section showing communication paths. (B) A section of cord showing the organization of gray matter into regions (left) and the lamination of the gray matter (right). (C) Sections of the cord from each spinal region showing regional characteristics. The cervical enlargement lies between levels C4 and T1 and the lumbar enlargement between L1 and S3. The enlargements represent the greater number of neuron cell bodies needed to manage the input and output related to the extremities at those levels. From Cramer & Darby (1995), with permission.

environmental relationships are quite variable. These are depicted in Figures 7.2–7.5 and readers are encouraged to match the following descriptions with each image in order to develop perceptual symbols in their long-term memory. This will better aid the visualization of the SMU and the potential neural effects of any SC. Cramer & Darby (1995 pp. 52–71; 251–354) provide

the appropriate level of anatomy of the spinal cord and autonomic nervous system and should be read in conjunction with the following brief summary:

● Spinal cord: an organization of central gray matter surrounded by white matter as a cylindrical structure running caudad from the medulla oblongata. Clinically the cord commences at the level of the foramen magnum and terminates about the level of the L1–2 disk (range T12–L3). It is surrounded, protected, and supported by the meninges which is continuous with the covering of the brain and tethered caudally by the filum terminale.

- Meninges: the covering of the cord and spinal nerves as the dura mater, arachnoid mater, and pia mater. The dura is the outermost layer.
- Gray matter: the central area of the cord, shaped like the letter H or a butterfly, and consisting of motor neurons, tract neurons, interneurons, propriospinal neurons, primary cell bodies, neuroglia, and capillaries. The butterfly shape results in a ventral and a dorsal horn of gray matter in each half of the cord, joined centrally by dorsal and ventral commissures.
- Ventral horn: a concentration of gray matter extending to the anterolateral portions of the cord and containing the anterior

horn cells, the axons of which leave via the ventral roots to act as motor for skeletal muscle.

- Intermediate region of gray matter: the central core of each half of the gray matter, joining the ventral and dorsal horns and receiving proprioceptive input from, and allowing interaction among, sensory afferents and descending pathways. This region becomes a lateral horn between T1 and L2–3 to innervate smooth muscle, cardiac muscle, glands, and blood vessels by sympathetic, autonomic nerves.
- Dorsal horn: a concentration of gray matter extending to the posterolateral portions of the cord and functioning to receive descending information from higher centers and sensory afferents from the dorsal roots.
- White matter: the peripheral area of the cord, consisting of white myelinated axons, neuroglia, and blood vessels. It forms a dorsal column between the dorsal horns, a lateral column between the dorsal and ventral horns, and an anterior column lying anterior and medial to the ventral horn. The axons are long and ascend and descend in roughly organized bundles called tracts.
- Ventral root: the means of conveying motor and autonomic afferents from the cord to the body's muscles, tissues, and glands to effect function. It is a paired structure and arises as a collection of rootlets from the anterolateral aspects of the cord.
- Dorsal root: the means of sensory information entering the spinal cord. It is a paired structure and the bodies of the sensory nerve cells are collected within the dorsal root ganglia which lie between the cord and the spinal nerve. The cells have a peripheral process which travels to a peripheral receptor and a central process which enters the cord as one of a collection of rootlets on the posterolateral aspect. There are many types of peripheral receptors to gather a range of sensory data.
- Spinal nerve: a paired structure on either side of the cord, formed by the merger of a dorsal and a ventral root in the intervertebral canal (IVC).
- Ventral ramus: the anterior primary division of the spinal nerve, arising from the spinal nerve at the intervertebral foramen (IVF) and turning to travel anteriorly and further

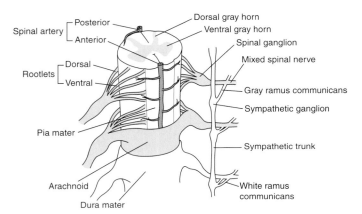

Figure 7.3 A typical spinal region. Oblique view of and about a typical spinal motion unit. After Cramer & Darby (1995), with permission.

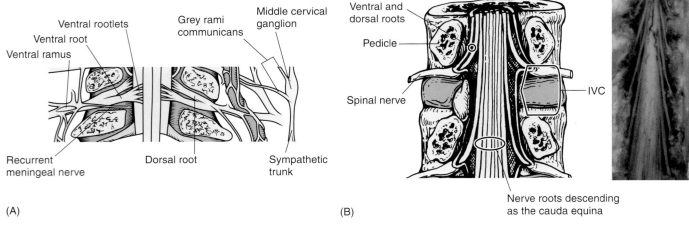

(A)

(B)

Figure 7.4 Frontal plane view of typical spinal regions. (A) The cervical region; (B) the lumbar region. IVC, intervertebral canal. After Cramer & Darby (1995), with permission.

subdivide. This is now a mixed nerve conveying both sensory and motor information. The ventral rami form the intercostal nerves in the thoracic region and contribute to a number of plexuses along the spinal column.

- Dorsal ramus: the posterior primary division of the spinal nerve, arising from the spinal nerve at the IVF and turning to

travel posteriorly and further subdivide. This is now a mixed nerve conveying both sensory and motor information to paraspinal and other tissues.

- Sympathetic division: primarily concerned with helping the body respond to stress. The ganglia lie in the sympathetic trunk which runs on each anterolateral surface of the vertebral

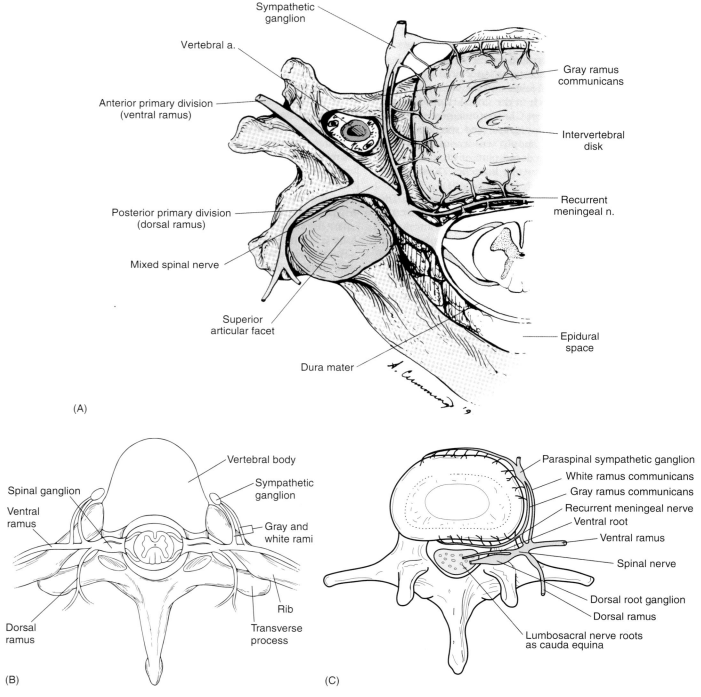

Figure 7.5 Transverse plane view of each typical spinal region. (A) The cervical region, left side; (B) the thoracic region; (C) the lumbar region, right side. (A) From Cramer & Darby (1995), with permission; (B) after Greenstein (1997), with permission; (C) from Giles & Singer (1997), with permission.

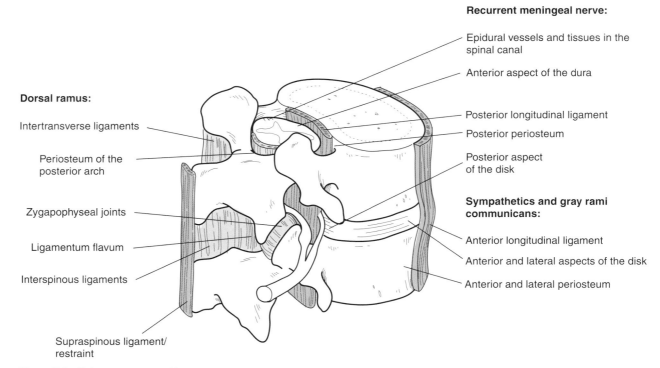

Figure 7.6 Pain generators and innervation about the spinal motion unit (SMU). The SMU is richly innervated and nearly all structures are capable of generating pain.

column from the base of the skull to the coccyx. The cell bodies of the preganglionic sympathetic neurons lie in the intermediate gray matter at each level of the cord from T1 to L2 or L3.

- White rami communicans: the preganglionic sympathetic axons travel with the ventral root and leave the spinal nerve in a white (myelinated) ramus communicans to reach the sympathetic trunk where they may enter a ganglion and synapse, or travel in various directions up, down, or through the trunk.
- Gray rami communicans: postganglionic sympathetic fibers leave the ganglion and sympathetic trunk in a gray (unmyelinated) ramus communicans and enter the spinal nerve where they travel to the relevant autonomic nervous system effector.
- Recurrent meningeal nerve: arises outside the IVF and re-enters the spinal canal to innervate the anterior aspect of the spinal dura mater, posterior longitudinal ligament, posterior aspect of the disk, the epidural contents, and the periosteum of the posterior aspect of the vertebral bodies. All of these structures are potential pain generators mediated by this nerve (Fig. 7.6).
- Parasympathetic division: primarily concerned with conserving and restoring energy, the parasympathetic cell bodies are located in autonomic nuclei of the brainstem (cranial nerves III, VII, IX, X) and the second, third, and fourth sacral cord segments. They act in coordination with the sympathetic division for the dual and antagonistic innervation of autonomic effectors. Parasympathetic neurons synthesize nerve growth factor (NGF) which is transported anterogradely to fiber terminals where it may be available to sympathetic axons. Parasympathetic NGF expression is augmented by impulse

activity within, and presumably transmitter release from, sympathetic axons (Hasan & Smith 2000).
- Cranial division: 10 pairs of nerves arising from the brainstem plus two pairs associated with the brain and innervating structures primarily in the head and neck. The vagus nerve (cranial nerve X) runs in the carotid sheath and enters the thorax and abdomen. As part of the peripheral nervous system the cranial nerves also convey special sensory information and autonomic fibers.

The above is a cursory overview of relevant components of the nervous system for the purpose of succinctly identifying relationships and functions which may be affected by change in the SMU. The reader will appreciate the complexity of the nervous system as a whole through studying the peripheral and central nervous systems, the autonomic nervous system, and the organization of the spinal cord.

NEURAL CHANGE

The question of what constitutes neural change is very broad and open. The scheme depicted in Figure 7.1 provides one structure for clinical assessment. The further one moves into and beyond subjective dimensions, the more the questions become of a quantum nature and the lower the level of available evidence. The emphasis of this text is on gathering clinical evidence in a structured manner to support a working diagnosis of SC within a particular SMU. The greater emphasis is therefore placed on those neural changes which lie at the objective end of the continuum; however, healthy respect is shown for both the historical concepts of the chiropractic profession and the emerging knowledge related to abstract dimensions.

If neural function equates to tone then a certain congruence is found with Palmer's original concepts of altered tone and altered spinal function (Masarsky & Todres-Masarsky 2001); however, the weakness remains the a priori assumption that a clinical state can occur (the subluxation) which imparts a clinical effect on the patient.

Homewood (1981) critically appraised the theories of the subluxation and, while commending DD Palmer's *The Science, Art and Philosophy of Chiropractic* (1910), lamented the loss of Palmer's essential concepts of too much or too little tone. Homewood established the richness of the neurological dimensions associated with the SC and set them within the context of patients and their variability of response, a concept now understood as a holistic approach to healing. He even discussed psychosomatics and psychogenic subluxation, a forerunner to the mind–body medicine concept of chiropractic today (Jamison 1998).

Contemporary work continues to expand on those basic neurological concepts. The SMU has been shown in preceding chapters to generate proprioceptive input which is used as a control mechanism locally about the spine and which also projects as kinesthetic data to the sensory cortex. It is now known that small vertebral displacements, such as extension of the spine by only tenths of a millimeter, are sufficient to load and unload muscle spindles in the multifidus and longissimus muscles (Pickar & Kang 2001). It is also known that there is a direct neural connection between this mechanical activity and the sympathetic nervous system; further, this neural interchange may occur within the facet joint.

The SMU is certainly an important converter of mechanical data to a wide range of neural input. In some respects the attempt to separate out the various dimensions of the SC for assessment is overtaken by the reality that the body functions as an integrated whole. The individuation of the elements of the SC does not imply that they exist as separate and distinct entities. Each will always impact on the others to a varying extent and can only be understood and interpreted in association with all clinical findings.

OBJECTIVE DIMENSIONS

An objective dimension is one which can be independently observed by more than one practitioner. It may be quantifiable through measurements which can be recorded in the patient file, but it is a fallacy to think that objectivity equates to quantification.

There are a number of objective changes which can only be qualified, for example the color of a lesion. There are also changes which can be accepted as objective if two or more experts agree on qualitative data alone. This method utilizes the consensus of experts approach in determining the presence or absence of the categorical variable. This approach has been found valid and appropriate in clinical practice where there are no gold standards available to quantify the clinical entity (Walter 1984). In the absence of objective methods to identify and describe an entity, it can be considered to exist with agreement among experts based on empirical, clinical cause and effect, or intervention and response observations.

This process is commonly used in the clinical practice of many disciplines, including pathology (Morrison et al 2002),

ophthalmology (Stanford et al 2002), obstetrics (Blix et al 2003), and gastroenterology (Neumann et al 2002). It is the bridge between expert opinion and qualitative data where interpretation directs subsequent clinical actions. The ranking step between objective and subjective dimensions is thus not as clear-cut as suggested in Figure 7.1.

Motor change

Motor change is alteration to function, commonly of skeletal muscle but also of smooth muscle, cardiac muscle, and glands. It reflects dysfunction in an upper (UMN) or lower motor neuron (LMN) or its axon on the way to the effector. In muscle, changes at the neuromuscular junction are suggested by normal or decreased tone with normal reflexes and fatigable weakness. Changes within the muscle itself have been discussed in the preceding chapter.

Muscle weakness is the initial indicator of motor change and is obvious when the patient rates 3 or less on the common power scale (Box 6.1). Global motor change, as with myasthenia gravis and motor neuron disease, grossly affects the body and the patient is typically more suited to rehabilitation and supportive therapy.

The first clinical observations flow from postural and gait assessment and the practitioner should compare sides of the body and then proximal muscle groups with distal groups. UMN lesions may affect an entire limb and are suggested by weakness of arm extensors with weak leg flexors (a pyramidal pattern), with increased resting tone and increased reflexes.

An LMN lesion is more likely to affect an individual muscle or group and is suggested by weakness with decreased tone and absent reflexes and perhaps with wasting and fasciculation. Dysfunction about the SMU may affect several muscles while entrapment of a motor nerve away from the spine may affect only the muscle it supplies. The motor change typically seen in manual practice is of a regional nature and suggests involvement of a particular LMN, usually secondary to dysfunction about a particular SMU.

The mechanisms are many, ranging from frank mechanical compromise of motor axons by disk protrusion, to altered motor activity secondary to modulation by internuncial neurons within the spinal cord. Motor change is documented by quantifying the size of its effect on the muscle and describing its clinical features and impact.

Reflex change

Reflexes test both sensory input and motor output for various spinal levels. The tendon jerk is a phasic stretch reflex characterized as being short and intense. It is elicited by a sharp striking of a particular tendon which physically stretches the tendon and stimulates a stretch-sensitive receptor within a neuromuscular spindle to fire an afferent impulse which, via a single synapse, stimulates a motor nerve leading to contraction of the muscle (Fuller 1999).

The reflex is termed either the deep tendon reflex (DTR) or muscle stretch reflex (MSR) depending on whether one considers it is elicited by the physical action on the tendon or the neurologic action of the stretch receptor which is probably within the myotendinous junction. The reflexes must be compared left and right for each level to be indicative of unilateral change. Bilateral absence is not so much a concern in the absence of other findings; however it is expected that bilaterally equal reflexes will be found for at least one level in each of the upper and lower limbs.

The reflex is subjectively graded and has limited interrater reliability (Marshall & Little 2002). The grading scale is from 0 to 4 (Box 7.1) and the locations and spinal levels are given in Table 7.1. As usual, there is some variance between authors as to the spinal levels associated with a particular reflex. Also, some authors describe a finger reflex for C8 and either a hamstring or an ankle reflex for L5, but these are somewhat unreliable.

The art of consistently eliciting a reflex is based on two skills. The first is palpation which allows the tendons to be identified, isolated, then struck. The second is the ability to swing the plessor or reflex hammer so that it strikes the tendon with a sharp, clean action which quickly rebounds. The reflex hammer is not used as a hatchet to chop away at a tendon with slow, heavy strokes in the vague hope of seeing some reaction.

An increased reflex or clonus suggests a UMN lesion above the root of the level of reflex. A pendular reflex, usually seen at the knee, is associated with cerebellar disease; the leg will swing for several beats. A slow relaxing reflex at the ankle suggests hypothyroidism. An isolated absent reflex suggests a root lesion or compromise of the peripheral nerve, while generalized absent reflexes indicate peripheral neuropathy (Fuller 1999).

The cutaneous reflexes are used as indicators of UMN lesion and changes secondary to UMNs may be associated with diminished or absent cutaneous reflexes. It is important to assess the abdominal (T8–12) and plantar reflexes (S1 and S2). An absent abdominal reflex suggests either a pyramidal tract involvement above the tested level or a peripheral nerve abnormality. A positive plantar reflex is the Babinski's sign, where the big toe extends and the others spread, and indicates UMN lesion. The normal response is for all toes to flex, and if this is absent then there may be a sensory abnormality interfering with the afferent part of the reflex (Fuller 1999).

Sensory change

Sensory change is discussed at this point in terms of the sensory input from cutaneous receptors which include mechanoreceptors, thermoreceptors, and nociceptors. These provide data on touch, pressure, vibration, temperature, and pain. There is a degree of overlap of cutaneous receptors and their density and variety vary depending on the region. The modalities can be easily tested and include:

- Pain, which in this context is the response to a stimulus. An opened safety pin is used to provide a sensation of "sharp" from the pointed end of the clasp, and "dull" from the rounded end of the safety cap. Inability to determine sharp from dull implicates the contralateral spinothalamic tract.
- Touch or tactile sensation: simple touch provides a localization of an area of changed sensation. This follows from sharp/dull discrimination and an inability to sense any touch suggests neural loss. The area may be mapped by overlaying the skin with a sheet of clear plastic and localizing it by using a felt pen to trace two bony landmarks. A pin prick will be felt through the plastic and will allow an outline to be constructed identifying the margin of sensory change. The points can then be joined by felt pen drawing on the plastic and the sheet can be retained in the patient file for future comparison.
- Light touch: an inability to sense light touch in the form of a wisp of cotton or a tissue paper lightly touching the skin implicates the spinothalamic tract or the dorsal column–medial lemniscus system (Cramer & Darby 1995).
- Temperature: tested by using objects no more than 10° colder and warmer than the skin. Warm receptors are C fibers only while cold receptors are supplied by both A-delta and C fibers. An inability to sense a difference between hot and cold implicates the lateral spinothalamic tracts. The thresholds of cold and warmth are significantly increased in the dermatome of a compressed nerve root (Nygaard & Mellgren 1998). The thresholds are also increased to some extent in the neighboring dermatomes in both the symptomatic and asymptomatic leg, suggesting synaptic interaction at the cord or higher levels between nociceptive pathways and other somatosensory channels (Nygaard & Mellgren 1998).
- Vibration: using a low-frequency (128 Hz) tuning fork on a bony prominence, loss of vibration sense implicates the dorsal column–medial lemniscus system. The tuning fork is placed first on the side of suspected involvement and when the patient reports he or she no longer senses the vibration the fork is quickly placed on the contralateral equivalent site. Vibration should be sensed for a short time from that side which demonstrates deficit in the initial side. The threshold is increased in the dermatome of a compressed nerve root (Nygaard & Mellgren 1998).

It is important to distinguish between tests of the complete central nervous system and tests which are intended to point towards altered spinal function. There are many other tests which may be applied to assess changes in the sensory system of the body but they may not be relevant to this discussion.

Box 7.1 Grading of deep tendon (muscle stretch) reflexes

0	Absent
±	Present only with reinforcement
1+	Present but depressed
2+	Normal
3+	Increased
4+	Increased and associated with pathological signs such as clonus

After Fuller (1999), with permission.

Table 7.1 Summary of deep tendon/muscle stretch reflexes

Location	Nerve roots	Nerve
Biceps tendon, antecubital fossa	C5 (C6)	Musculocutaneous
Supinator tendon, radial styloid	C6 (C5)	Radial
Triceps tendon, olecranon fossa	C7	Radial
Infrapatellar tendon; anterior knee	L3, L4	Femoral
Achilles tendon; posterior ankle	S1, S2	Tibial

What is relevant are findings which point to a lesion of a dorsal or ventral root as opposed to a UMN lesion.

A key indicator of nerve root involvement is change within a dermatomal distribution. This includes sensory change which does not implicate a UMN lesion, and changes in motor function, perhaps supported by altered reflexes. There is no one sign which is pathognomonic of spinal dysfunction with nerve root involvement and the practitioner must carefully undertake a series of tests and interpret the results in conjunction with other data obtained during the assessment.

SUBJECTIVE DIMENSIONS

Subjective dimensions rely on patients communicating their experience to the practitioner. This introduces complexities of linguistic meaning. Any set of words which records the human experience will be interpreted in accord with the individual's intuitions about and immediate understanding of the meaning of various words, phrases, and linguistic expressions (Gibbs 2003).

Patients' subjective, felt experience of their body in dysfunction secondary to the SC provides part of the fundamental grounding for language and thought about pain, spinal dysfunction, and the SC. These are embodied experiences for the patient and any attempt to link language with brain function must also respect the lived kinesthetic experience. Failure to do this ignores the biopsychosocial dimensions of pain and may begin the cycle into chronicity.

Patients' embodied representation of sensation and pain not only shapes their understanding of the clinical interaction; it influences their understanding of the practitioner's actions and gives rise to their own metaphorical structuring of the often abstract concepts of manual treatment. The simple example occurs when the practitioner asks "does it hurt here?" Not only must patients seek a common agreement with the practitioner as to what is conveyed by the word "hurt", they must attempt to determine the practitioner's preferred response. If the patient responds "yes" and the practitioner reacts positively then the patient has learned a favoring response within a dynamic interaction. If they respond "no" then there is a fear they may not be successfully treated.

The extent of the truthfulness of the patient's responses will never be known. Patients construct embodied representation of sensation changes and pain to the extent that inferences enable them to respond to practitioner questioning and understand the clinical interaction.

This problem has long been recognized and certain English words have been identified and tested as to the meaning they convey and their descriptive capacity for a range of clinical possibilities. A well-validated and commonly used instrument for recording the patient's pain experience is the McGill pain questionnaire (MPQ) (Melzack 1975, 1982). It is available in a range of languages (Marques et al 2001) but has suffered disagreement about its vocabulary of pain (Fernandez & Towery 1996). The following words taken from the MPQ have been found to be used frequently and unambiguously in the communication of pain. They are grouped in sensory subcategories:

- temporal: pulsing, throbbing, pounding, beating
- spatial: radiating, spreading

- punctate pressure: drilling, penetrating, stabbing, piercing, pricking
- incisive pressure: cutting, lacerating
- constrictive pressure: pressing, crushing, squeezing, tight
- traction: tugging, pulling, drawing
- hotness: burning, hot, scalding, searing
- coldness: cool, freezing, cold
- brightness: smarting, blinding
- dullness: aching, dull, sore (Fernandez & Towery 1996).

The practitioner should use these words when taking the pain history of the patient. A measurement of the pain experience may be recorded using the visual analog scale (VAS). This is an established, validated, self-report instrument usually consisting of a 10-cm line on paper with verbal anchors labeling the ends. Patients are asked to mark the line at the point which best represents their response to the particular dimension being measured. For example, the question may be "rate the intensity of your pain" with the anchor words "no pain" at one end and "worst possible pain" at the other. There is no significant difference between completing the VAS on paper or in electronic form (Jamison et al 2002).

Sensation

This is a crossover vector between objective and subjective data. Strictly speaking, most sensory tests can only be subjective in that they rely upon the patient to verbalize a response. They are classified as objective in the belief that different practitioners should be able to elicit the same or similar responses, thus conferring a degree of objectivity.

Sensation changes as discussed here move beyond the objective to those which are interpreted by patients in terms of their own lived experience and then verbalized in the process of communication to the practitioner. Sensations associated with neuropathic pain include paresthesia, dysesthesia, and hyperpathia (Seaman & Cleveland 1999).

Paresthesia is an abnormal sensation, such as of burning, pricking, tickling, or tingling. Dysesthesia is an impairment of sensation short of anesthesia and may include an abnormal sensation in the absence of stimulation. It also refers to the case where an ordinary stimulus produces a disagreeable sensation. It is indicative of a lesion of the sensory pathways. Hyperpathia is an exaggerated subjective response to painful stimuli, with a continuing sensation of pain after the stimulation has ceased (definitions from *Stedman's Medical Dictionary* 2000).

Pain

Pain may be categorized as mechanical, neuropathic, or visceral (Putzke et al 2002). Mechanical pain is typically described as being aching and/or dull. Neuropathic pain is most strongly described as burning and also as tingling, electric, shooting, and stabbing. Visceral pain is typically described as cramping and/or dull, and to some extent, burning. It may also give a sensation of fullness (Putzke et al 2002).

Neuropathic pain arises as a result of damage to any part of the sensory system, either peripheral or central, and may be associated with some sensory deficit (Seaman & Cleveland 1999). Nociceptive pain is the most common type of pain seen in clinical practice and arises due to active nociceptors. Nociceptors are widespread throughout the body and are stimulated by noxious mechanical and chemical stimuli that typically are associated with tissue injury. The disruption of the integrity of local structures is accompanied by noxious mechanical irritation and the release of various chemical mediators of inflammation and nociception (Seaman & Cleveland 1999).

Cramer & Darby (1995 p. 358) have described the sensory innervation of the SMU and identified the various tissues which are capable of generating pain (Fig. 7.6). After innervating posterior structures of the SMU the dorsal ramus branches and innervates the deepest back muscles; the lateral branch innervates the erector spinae.

Under normal conditions the intervertebral disk is only innervated about its periphery; however as the disk undergoes internal disruption, there is an ingrowth of nerve fibers deeper into the annulus (Coppes et al 1997) and the nucleus (Freemont et al 1997). Mast cells are involved in repair of the disk and the induction of angiogenesis, and the neural ingrowth is accompanied by the neovascularization of damaged disk tissue (Freemont et al 2002b). This may be a response to neurotrophic stimuli such as NGF which is released from the autonomic system (Hasan & Smith 2000).

Referred pain

Pain felt in an area remote to the actual pain generator is termed referred pain. Simons (1991) describes five neurologic mechanisms which explain the phenomenon of referred pain:

1. Convergence projection: a single nerve cell in the spinal cord receives nociceptive input from skin, muscle, and viscera. When this signal reaches the brain there is no mechanism for distinguishing the actual pain source so the brain interprets these messages as coming from the somatic structures. It is thought the nociceptive signal from a trigger point may be referred to the somatic areas which also converge on to the same nerve cell in the spinothalamic tract. The brain is thus misled to perceive the pain as arising from the second somatic area instead of from the actual somatic source.

2. Peripheral branching of primary afferent nociceptors: one nerve may branch and supply different structures, in which case the brain may not be able to identify correctly which specific structure among all of those supplied by the nerve is the cause of the pain. It may therefore perceive the pain as coming from structures which are actually functioning normally but which are feeding into the same branch network.

3. Convergence facilitation: it is already noted that a single cell in the spinothalamic tract may receive nociceptive input from viscera as well as skin and muscle. The background neural activity at a remote site, which may include a viscus, may be insufficient to be perceived by the brain until further signals are received on to that same cell from a trigger point. These additional signals modulate the background signals and allow them to be perceived.

4. Sympathetic nervous system activity: sympathetic nerves appear capable of releasing nociceptive substances and these may sensitize primary afferent nerve endings in the region of perceived referred pain. They may also constrict blood flow in the vessels which nourish the sensory nerve fiber itself. These actions of the sympathetic nerves may occur due to modulation by a trigger point.

5. Convergence or image projection at the supraspinal level: it is thought that pain pathways may converge at the thalamic or cortical level in the same manner as they converge peripherally. The cortex is responsible for formulating and projecting images and may make errors due to the convergence of nociceptive signals and its inability to separate them.

The anatomical mechanisms of convergence projection and peripheral branching do not require any afferent input from the zone to which the pain is referred. Therefore if the reference zone is anesthetized and the pain persists, then the mechanism is most likely one of these two. If the pain ceases, Simons (1991) suggests the mechanism is likely to be one of the latter three functional mechanisms. He also makes the point that several mechanisms may operate simultaneously.

Phantom pain

Pain without accompanying tissue pathology is phantom pain and is represented in its extreme form by a non-existent amputated limb being perceived as painful by the patient (Harris 1999). It is experienced by 60–80% of patients following limb amputation but is only severe in about 5–10% of cases (Nikolajsen & Staehelin Jensen 2000). The mechanisms are poorly understood and there is little evidence from randomized trials to guide practitioners (Halbert et al 2002). Treatment is not very successful.

Some forms of sensory reorganization may be associated with phantom pain. Neurons may store information for prolonged periods of time and this may account for clinical problems such as hyperalgesia (extreme sensitivity to painful stimuli) and allodynia (pain in response to a normal stimulus), as well as phantom pain (Rygh et al 2002).

The motor and somatosensory cortex is quite plastic and the relationship between plastic changes occurring in the sensorimotor cortex and phantom pain is complex (Schwenkreis et al 2001). There is considerable evidence that cortical representation of body parts is continuously modulated in response to activity, behavior, and skill acquisition (Chen et al 2002). There is also a region of cortex which is active in response to incongruence between motor intention, awareness of movement, and visual feedback (Harris 1999). It may be that disorganized or inappropriate cortical representation of proprioception may falsely signal incongruence between motor intention and movement in the same way that incongruence between vestibular and visual sensation results in motion sickness (Harris 1999).

The clinical implication is that patients who are amputees with phantom pain have poorer health-related quality of life than amputees without phantom pain (van der Schans et al 2002) and present a significant challenge for the effective management of spinal pain.

Dyskinesia

Dyskinesia may be an effect of pain. The aberrant movement within an SMU may reflect restriction due to reflex muscle contraction secondary to excitation of nociceptive fibers within the disk and joint capsule (Rahlmann 1987). Therefore nociceptive impulses, which may or may not be felt and reported as pain by the patient, may have a local effect within the SMU.

Causes of restriction in one or more vectors of SMU movement, as outlined by Rahlmann (1987), include meniscoid entrapment, displaced disk fragments, muscle spasm, and periarticular connective tissue adhesions. The effects of dyskinesia are speculated to be quite varied and occur at the spinal cord and supraspinal level with regard to effects on bodily function.

Dysafferentation

Aberrant muscle spindle input has been proposed as a driving mechanism for joint and muscle dysfunction by Korr (1975), Johansson & Sojka (1991), and Donaldson et al (1998). Knutson (1999) presents two mechanisms: nociception which causes muscle contraction which in turn can cause lasting increases in muscle spindle output, and nociceptor fatigue.

The term "dysafferentation" was used by Seaman & Winterstein (1998) to describe an imbalance in afferent input to the SMU such that there is an increase in nociceptor input and a reduction in mechanoreceptor input. They describe numerous cerebellar and cortical regions reliant on mechanoreceptive input in order to function properly and suggest that nociceptive input into the central nervous system is increased (but may often remain subclinical) following decreased mechanoreceptive input due to kinematic change.

The changes associated with dysafferentation are difficult to quantify but the symptoms include increased secretion of catecholamines, increases in cardiac output, blood pressure and peripheral resistance, increased secretion of cortisol, antidiuretic hormone, glucagon, and concomitant decreases in insulin levels (Seaman & Winterstein 1998). Such responses may play a role in the pathogenesis of degenerative diseases such as cardiovascular disease, cancer, diabetes, and Alzheimer's disease.

Autonomic

The findings of Suseki et al (1997) support the hypothesis that sensory pathways from the L5–6 facet joint in rats go through the paravertebral sympathetic trunk to the dorsal root ganglia of spinal nerves L1 or L2. It is also known that some nerve fibers in the dorsal ramus go directly into rami communicantes without entering the dorsal root ganglia and it is thought that these arise from postganglionic neurons regulating blood vessels. The clinical relevance is that the assessment of the spine must include assessment of the autonomic nervous system as well as the peripheral and central nervous systems.

Dysautonomia

The term "dysautonomia" refers to a change in autonomic nervous system function that adversely affects health (Goldstein et al 2002). It incorporates the concepts of the somatovisceral reflex whereby somatic stimulation such as nociception associated with spinal dyskinesia may result in effects on the autonomic nervous system.

There is a differentiation of cause between the central nervous system and the peripheral autonomic nervous system. The peripheral neuropathies most likely to cause severe autonomic disturbance are those in which small myelinated and unmyelinated fibers are affected in the baroreflex afferents, the vagal afferents to the heart, and the sympathetic efferent pathways to the mesenteric vascular bed (McLeod & Tuck 1987). Dysautonomia is associated with the postural orthostatic tachycardia syndrome and the chronic fatigue syndrome (CFS) in adolescents (Stewart 2000). A postviral idiopathic autonomic neuropathy may be involved with CFS (Freeman & Komaroff 1997).

While dysautonomia is an important subject in clinical neurocardiology (Goldstein et al 2002), it remains controversial in manual medicine at this time. Sato (1992) and Sato & Swenson (1984) have experimentally demonstrated the effects of somatic stimulation on the autonomic nervous system. Changes range from transient, occasional episodes of neurally mediated hypotension to progressive neurodegenerative diseases (Goldstein et al 2002).

Sato (1992) demonstrated the effect of somatic stimulation on visceral function varied according to the region or spinal segments stimulated, and the extent to which the autonomic response was spinally or supraspinally mediated. Effects occurred within the sympathetic and parasympathetic divisions of the autonomic nervous system. In general, spinally mediated reflex responses exhibit more specific characteristics (Dishman et al 2002). These include reflex inhibition of micturition contractures of the urinary bladder following noxious stimulation of the abdominal skin in anesthetized rats (Budgell et al 1998).

Sato & Swenson (1984) found that, by laterally stressing lower spinal segments (T11–12, L3–4), they could affect the heart rate of anesthetized rats temporarily, and that this effect was dependent on intact articular afferent fibers (Slosberg 1988). This response was equal regardless of the direction of force applied to the spinal segments, or the level (thoracic vs lumbar) and demonstrates that mechanoreceptor afferents can reduce sympathetic hyperactivity.

Decreases in mechanoreceptor input may be observed when there is kinematic change within the SMU. Igarashi & Budgell (2000) observed such effects which suggest that spinal manipulative therapy may produce somatic stimulation which in turn may have an effect in some instances of clinically diagnosed cardiac arrhythmia. These effects occur through modification of the activity of the autonomic nervous system after normalizing segmental mobility.

Recent neuroscience research supports a neurophysiologic rationale for the concept that aberrant stimulation of spinal or paraspinal structures may lead to segmentally organized reflex responses of the autonomic nervous system, which in turn may alter visceral function (Budgell 2000). The question is not so much whether or not mechanical events within the body in general and the spine in particular result in activity within the autonomic nervous system, but rather the extent to which such activity may affect visceral function and modulate activity in afferent nerves (Bolton 2000).

It is yet to be demonstrated conclusively that clinical changes in the SMU can induce dysautonomia and, more importantly, whether manipulation of the SMU can reverse such changes; however, early findings are quite promising. It is known that cervical spine manipulation produces significant alterations in both heart rate and measures of heart-rate variability (Budgell &

Hirano 2001) which may reflect a shift in balance between sympathetic and parasympathetic output to the heart. Heart-rate variability analysis allows a quantitative index of autonomic function, accurately reflecting the sympathetic and parasympathetic tone and the sympathovagal balance (Eingorn & Muhs 1999).

Arterial tonometry can now measure heart rate, systolic pressure, and diastolic pressure. The pressure variables have been shown to decrease significantly with stimuli which involved full rotation of the neck (Fujimoto et al 1999). In rats, a noxious stimulation of the mid to lower thoracic interspinous tissues is accompanied by a pronounced increase in gastric sympathetic nerve activity and inhibition of gastric motility (Budgell & Suzuki 2000). Noxious stimulation of the lower lumbar or the lower thoracic segments also produces protracted increases in adrenal nerve activity and catecholamine secretion (Budgell et al 1997).

Spinal manipulation produces a transient but significant facilitation of central motor neuron pool excitability (Fishman et al 2002a). Spinal manipulation (and mobilization) has also been shown to produce short-term inhibitory effects on the human motor system (Dishman & Bulbulian 2000).

The clinical implication is the need to explore the status of autonomic function in the patient with a view to observing and recording any changes which may or may not be associated with treatment. Some subjective reports by the patient of changes in autonomic function may be quantified, such as blood pressure and heart rate; however many of the effects of autonomic change may be subclinical. This vector forms the transition link to the abstract dimensions where cognitive, affective, and evaluative components can be identified.

ABSTRACT DIMENSIONS

It is obvious that a score on a pain rating scale is far from being a pure measure of the patient's pain, but is heavily influenced in unknown ways by the patient's emotion and motivational state (Clark et al 2001).

These abstract dimensions include the psychosomatic responses which seem to be related to physiological and musculoskeletal support for the expression of the emotions. Behavior occurs in fairly patterned responses involving motor, autonomic, and neuroendocrine activity and preprogrammed patterns can be seen in emotions such as happiness, sadness, anger, and fear (Lederman 1997 p. 192). Exaggerated psychosomatic responses may become pathological and may also generate an adaptive response.

Manipulation is appropriate in such patients as a supportive therapy, behavioral therapy and physical therapy (Lederman 1997 p. 196), and consideration of these dimensions is warranted in clinical practice.

The most important reason for considering abstract dimensions in the assessment of the spine is their usefulness as outcomes measures, particularly for qualify of life (QoL) questionnaires. It is not only pain which impacts on QoL; there is a range of cognitive, affective, and evaluative behaviors which drive an individual's response to the pain experience and ultimately impact on QoL. As Waddell (1998) has demonstrated, failure to consider adequately the biopsychosocial aspects of pain is the sure path to chronicity and disablement.

Underlying theories

Positive changes in non-mechanical disorders of the body are common occurrences in the practice of manual medicine (Jamison 1991, Jamison et al 1992, Budgell 1999). Jamison et al (1992) surveyed all registered practitioners in Australia and found that over 50% of respondents ($n = 288$) considered that chiropractic adjustments of subluxation were of benefit in treating visceral conditions, but that the perceived level of (potential) benefit varied with the visceral complaint being treated.

There are numerous theoretical models of the SC and its potential effects on function. These include dysponesis and diaschisis.

Dysponesis

Dysponesis is a neurophysiologic factor in functional disorders (Whatmore & Kohi 1968) and is seen as a reversible pathophysiological state consisting of unnoticed, misdirected neurophysiologic reactions to various agents and the repercussions of these reactions throughout the organism. These include covert errors in action-potential output from the motor and premotor areas of the cortex and the consequences of that output.

Smart & Smith (2001) incorporate the concept of dysponesis into the concept of the SC and argue that the SC represents an imbalance in symmetry within the spine, allowing for the adoption of inefficient movement patterns/behaviors, using posture as an example. As such, subluxation is considered to have similar effects or, indeed, be a form of dysponesis with regard to being a reversible state of error in energy expenditure with subsequent global effects on the organism. Moreover, it is possible that the dysafferent input, which occurs with spinal subluxation, affects the motor and premotor areas of the cortex, leading to a state of dysponesis.

They allude to the effects of subluxation and postural inefficiency as a result of dysponesis as having the ability to give rise to a variety of widespread health conditions, and having the capacity to interfere with many aspects of neural function, including the regulation of various bodily organs. However no specific effect on visceral function is outlined, nor are the effects of poor posture (due to dysponesis or otherwise) on visceral function adequately delineated.

Dysponesis is seen as one of three psychosomatic pathways to musculoskeletal pain, the others being conversion and neurotransmitter disturbance (Large et al 1990). The abstract concept is the construing of the self as being "ill" or "an invalid" and this is a crucial step in the development of chronicity. Biofeedback therapies appear useful for treating anxious patients who may exhibit a trend towards dysponesis (Hauri 1975).

Diaschisis

Diaschisis literally means the loss of function and electrical activity caused by cerebral lesions in areas which are remote from the lesion. The mechanism is secondary hypoperfusion due to neural deactivation (Ito et al 2002). Diaschisis may be transhemispheric, crossed within the cerebellum, or involve relationships between the cerebellum and the cortex or thalamus, as well as the basal ganglia (Nguyen & Botez 1998). Diaschisis results in neurobehavioral and neuropsychological findings (Nguyen & Botez 1998).

There is also dynamic diaschisis where posterior temporal responses while viewing words depend on inputs from the damaged inferior frontal cortex. This is a brain lesion which is both anatomically remote and context-sensitive and represents an abnormality of functional integration with implications for cognitive rehabilitation (Price et al 2001). Diaschisis may be a defense mechanism of the damaged brain (Pietrzykowski et al 1997).

Given that the mechanism is secondary hypoperfusion due to neural deactivation (Ito et al 2002), it can be argued that a range of cognitive functions and other symptoms could be associated with varying degrees of hypoperfusion. Terrett (1995a) refers to this as hibernation accompanied by a drop in electrical activity of neurons following a decrease of cerebral blood flow levels. Symptoms include visual disturbances, diminished concentration span, and learning difficulties. It should be noted that, while neural deactivation primarily causes vasoconstriction rather than a reduction of oxygen metabolism (Ito et al 2002), the lesion may demonstrate augmented instead of reduced blood flow (Sanchez-Chavez 1999).

Terrett (1995a) proposed that the relief of a range of symptoms experienced by patients following spinal manipulation may be due to an increase in cerebral blood flow reversing any such state of hibernation within the cerebral cortex. He considers that disorders which may respond to manipulation of the spine restoring normal cerebral blood flow include depression, poor concentration, auditory difficulty, loss of interest in sex, problems with memory, learning disability, and changes in visual acuity. Carrick (1997) suggests that non-visual variables that alter thalamic impulse trains may alter visual perception. The cerebral dysfunction theory and functional diaschisis may provide such a non-visual variable.

Cattley & Tuchin (1999) offer a mechanism for subluxation-induced cerebral ischemia when reviewing the pathogenesis of migraine. They purport that somatic dysfunction between the vertebral levels C7 and T4 results in a sustained discharge from sympathetic neurons affected by these levels, resulting in cerebral ischemia. It is possible that by manipulating these spinal levels, sympathetic tone may be normalized, reducing cerebral ischemia and returning any region of hibernation within the brain to normal status.

The question of whether subluxation in the cervical spine can be a primary cause of cerebral ischemia strong enough to induce functional cortical changes which result in changes in visceral function remains a matter of conjecture. It is known that unilateral and limited inferior brainstem lesions can have ipsi- or contralateral consequences of the regional cerebral blood flow in the cerebellum and cerebral hemispheres (Rousseaux & Steinling 1999).

Cognitive

Cognition is what occurs when the body engages the physical, cultural world. It represents the dynamic interaction between the individual and the environment. Cognition is not purely internal, symbolic, computational, and disembodied. Rather, it is a living expression of the ways that language and thought are inextricably shaped by embodied action (Gibbs 2003).

It has been argued above that variable cerebral blood flow may produce cognitive signs and symptoms. Diaschisis may therefore affect cognition. Dynamic diaschisis has been shown to affect context-sensitive tasks (Price et al 2001).

Cognitive functions include planning, verbal fluency, abstract reasoning, prosody (speech rhythms), and use of correct grammar and are influenced by the cerebellum (Middleton & Strick 1994, 2000, Dreher & Grafman 2002, Fine et al 2002, Mathiak et al 2002). Changes in cognitive functions may be non-specific, as with concentration and memory, and are seen in patients with cervical acceleration/deceleration (whiplash) syndrome (Otte et al 1997). This may indicate bilateral hypometabolism in addition to hypoperfusion in the parieto-occipital regions of the brain. Otte et al (1997) consider that these findings may be caused by activation of nociceptive afferents from the upper cervical spine.

Affective

The affective vector reports how patients feel about their situation and has particular relevance when the patient is experiencing pain. Characteristics such as tolerability, minor emotional reaction, and focus of attention are affective descriptors (Morley & Pallin 1995). The pain experience is commonly associated with depression and anxiety, and patients must develop their own coping strategies to manage these unwanted side-effects.

Coping strategies include reinterpreting the pain experience or ignoring the pain sensations. Some patients may catastrophize their pain while others will act to control or divert attention. A subset will resort to prayer and hope (Morley & Pallin 1995). These are all valid affective responses and the practitioner must be alert to this layer of humanism within patients while assessing them and determining the preferred treatment plan.

Affective descriptors include sickening, tiring, and grueling. These three terms are commonly used by patients with low-back pain to describe their experience. Patients with osteoarthritis commonly use the descriptors tiring, sickening, and punishing. Those with fibromyalgia use the most descriptors, namely sickening, grueling, tiring, vicious, wretched, blinding, and exhausting (Marques et al 2001).

Evaluative

Evaluative descriptors of pain include annoying, troublesome, and miserable. Different words are selected by patients with different types of pain. Those with fibromyalgia found it more troublesome, miserable, and unbearable. Patients with osteoarthritis found it most troublesome, then somewhat annoying and intense. Those with low-back pain found it troublesome, unbearable, and annoying (Marques et al 2001).

There are gender differences in the use of evaluative words. In patients with myocardial infarction, women characterized their symptoms through stronger emotive words than men, such as worrying, frightening, and intolerable (Albarran et al 2000).

CONCLUSION

This chapter has attempted to provide a structured overview to guide the assessment of the most complex component of the SC, neural change. The objective dimensions essentially represent the "tried and true" neurological assessment and the subjective dimensions explore the effects of dysfunction on the patient in terms of altered sensation, various pain experiences, autonomic changes, and altered neurocognitive functions.

The abstract dimensions represent a most exciting component of spinal assessment as they force the practitioner to look at the patient in a holistic manner. This area is receiving the greatest amount of attention in the current literature, which may reflect both a growing awareness of its importance and the increasing sophistication of imaging modalities to help investigators see deeper into the functioning body.

Health is a finely tuned balance of many factors, not the least among which is the ability of the body optimally to control the many functions of the nervous system in order to maintain homeostasis. The assessment of the many aspects of the nervous system to identify change is an essential component of the assessment of the spine.

8

Assessment of vascular change

KEY CONCEPTS

The vascular system includes the arteries and arterioles, the venous system, the lymphatic system, and the cerebrospinal fluid (CSF). Homeostasis includes the maintenance of a balance among all fluid systems.

CSF is an important protective mechanism for the brain, spinal cord, and cauda equina and appears to demonstrate a rhythmic pulsation.

The lymphatic system is a complex arrangement of precollectors, collectors, ducts, and nodes which return interstitial fluid to the vascular system. Lymph ducts consist of contractile tissue and are mediated by the nervous system.

The incidence of a vertebrobasilar accident causing permanent neurologic damage following skilled manipulation of the neck is estimated to be about one in 2 million procedures.

Cerebrovascular accident (CVA) after manipulation appears to be an unpredictable event and should be considered an inherent, idiosyncratic, and rare complication of cervical spine manipulation and adjustment by experienced practitioners. A simple cause-and-effect relationship does not exist between neck manipulation and subsequent patient injury.

Edema results from an imbalance between arteriolar blood flow to a region and the venous drainage of that region and may be associated with inflammation. The use of cryotherapy in the form of wet ice is a useful means of reducing posttraumatic edema and to limit tissue damage.

The term "complex regional pain syndrome" (CRPS) replaces reflex sympathetic dystrophy and involves vasculature and temperature changes in a limb or limbs associated with pain. Infrared thermography is a useful clinical imaging method for a number of disorders but its validity in patients with low-back pain is lower than other technologies and even lower than clinical examination.

Paraspinal skin temperature as measured by a contact thermocouple device may indicate levels of dynamic thermal asymmetry which are thought to be associated with dysfunction in a spinal motion unit.

Neurolymphatic points are small, palpable areas about the body which appear to have a reflex effect on the lymphatic drainage of certain muscles and other structures.

INTRODUCTION

The term "vascular" literally means a small vessel (*vasculum*, L.) and conventionally relates to blood vessels. A much broader approach is taken in this chapter in an attempt to draw together a number of other elements of spinal dysfunction which involve fluids, including blood. These incorporate the lymphatic system in its conventional sense, the neurolymphatic points about the body as a clinical indication of lymphatic function, and the CSF, which is an integral component of the central nervous system (CNS).

Osteopathy and chiropractic both have a tradition of assessing craniosacral movement on the premise that altered movement may impact upon the normal fluid dynamics of the CSF as it relates to the functional status of the CNS. Further, both disciplines have developed and adopted the concept of neurolymphatic reflexes which integrates neural, muscle, and lymphatic function into a collection of diagnostic and therapeutic points about the body. In the most holistic sense, the vascular system of the body preserves a homeostatic balance with the CSF and lymphatic systems. These maintain tissue fluid and macromolecular balance at the local level (von der Weid 2001, Gashev 2002) by removing fluid, protein, and other particles from the interstitium back to the blood stream (Johnston et al 1986).

A range of abstract dimensions were presented in the preceding chapter which associate neurocognitive changes with altered perfusion. The point is that alterations in fluid flow to and from the CNS have the capacity to alter its function. While it is not possible to separate blood vessel function from neural influence, there are other mechanisms which affect local perfusion. These include an intrinsic myogenic reactivity of epineural arterioles which confers the potential for these vessels to participate in local regulation of neural hemodynamics independently of their innervation (Wang et al 1999). This ability allows a basal level of tone that enables arterioles to adjust diameter appropriately (by vasodilation, vasoconstriction) in response to local factors, for example, metabolic and mechanical stimuli (Potocnik & Hill 2001) and neurohumoral mediators (Davis & Hill 1999, Hill et al 2001). This level of control enables a tissue

to maintain appropriate local perfusion in a manner somewhat independent of systemic events.

The most extreme instance of altered neural function secondary to vascular change is CVA. It would be remiss of any text on spinal assessment not to include a discussion on the potential vascular complications of head and neck movement, even during the supposedly innocuous process of assessment.

The model of the subluxation complex (SC) presented in this text (Fig. 3.1) collects these multiple dimensions under the singular term "vascular change" and this chapter covers a wide range of concepts. The clinical relevance is the need for the practitioner to be thorough and extensive in the assessment of vascular change and to appreciate that the dimensions of this assessment go well beyond the basics of pulse and blood pressure.

CLINICAL ANATOMY

A thorough understanding of the vascular anatomy of the spinal motion unit (SMU), spinal cord, and autonomic nervous system is essential for providing an informed framework for the assessment of other dimensions of the SC. Cramer & Darby (1995 pp. 39–41, 66–71) provide the appropriate level of anatomy and should be read in conjunction with the following brief overview.

The vertebral arteries arise from the subclavian arteries. Each lies within the intertransverse foramen on each side of the cervical spine from C6 upwards and turns medially and sharply around the lateral mass of C1 to enter the cranium through the foramen magnum.

Small branches from each vertebral artery join together to form the anterior spinal artery which runs the length of the cord (Fig. 8.1A). The branches arise within the posterior fossa and run inferiorly to join and form the artery, usually at the level of the upper cervical segments, but at times as low as the C5 cord level. The anterior spinal artery vascularizes the anterior two-thirds of the cord (Fig. 8.1B). A posterior spinal artery usually also arises from each vertebral artery but may arise from the posterior inferior cerebellar artery. Each forms two irregular anastomotic channels which descend beside the dorsal rootlet attachments to the spinal cord and supply the posterior one-third of the cord. There are numerous small vessels connecting these channels across the midline and which also anastomose with the anterior spinal artery.

The capacity of this system is only sufficient for the upper cervical segments of the cord. As the three spinal arteries descend they are joined by many radicular arteries which arise from spinal branches of the vertebral, deep cervical, ascending cervical, posterior intercostal, lumbar, and lateral sacral arteries (Moore 1980 p. 653). These give rise to 31 pairs of spinal branches which enter the spinal canal through the intervertebral canal (IVC) and divide into anterior and posterior radicular arteries. These in turn divide to vascularize the meninges, ligaments, osseous structures, nerve roots and rootlets, and act to reinforce the spinal arteries. They also give rise to anterior and posterior radicular branches which vascularize their corresponding nerve root. The main blood supply to the lower two-thirds of the cord is by a large radicular artery called the artery of Adamkiewicz which typically arises on the left from a lower intercostal or an upper lumbar artery (T6–L3).

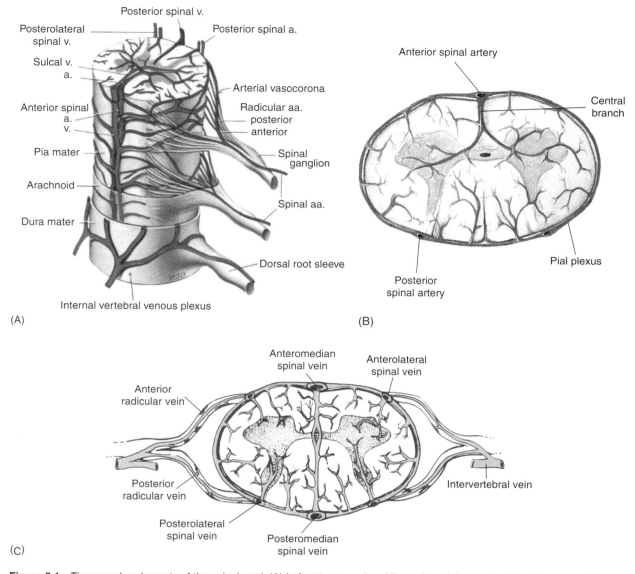

Figure 8.1 The vascular elements of the spinal cord. (A) Left anterosuperior oblique view of the cord and spinal nerves. After Moore (1980), with permission; (B) transverse view of the arterial distribution within the cord; (C) transverse view of the venous system within the cord. After Cramer & Darby (1995), with permission.

The cord is also invested with an extensive venous drainage system (Fig. 8.1C). Other veins form an internal vertebral plexus in the epidural space and an irregular plexus lying on the cord (Fig. 8.2). The internal epidural plexus is embedded in a layer of loose areolar tissue and is also referred to as Batson's plexus or Batson's channels, after the surgeon Batson, who published his observations in 1940. It is a longitudinal plexus, continuous with the sinuses and venous channels above the foramen magnum. The anterior epidural venous plexus may enlarge secondary to vessel wall abnormality in patients with Marfan syndrome, and cause headache and neck pain (Chun et al 2002). There are also three longitudinal veins running the length of each of the anterior and posterior aspects of the cord which collect into posterior radicular veins that empty into the epidural venous plexus.

The intervertebral disk is the largest avascular structure in the adult human body (Kurunlahti et al 2001). It has a blood supply while young; however, the vascular structures in the vertebral endplates regress (Chandraraj et al 1998). The network of arteries and veins within the vertebral body (Fig. 8.3) is retained and they are responsible for disk nutrition. These vessels may cause an infarct of the body which produces clinical signs and symptoms of spontaneous spinal cord ischemic stroke (Bornke et al 2002).

The disk, particularly the healthy nucleus, relies on the blood supply from the vertebral bodies for the supply of nutrients and removal of waste by diffusion through the endplates (Urban et al 2001). A reduced flow in the lumbar arteries is markedly associated with decreased diffusion in the lumbar disks and this may promote degeneration (Kurunlahti et al 2001). Endplate

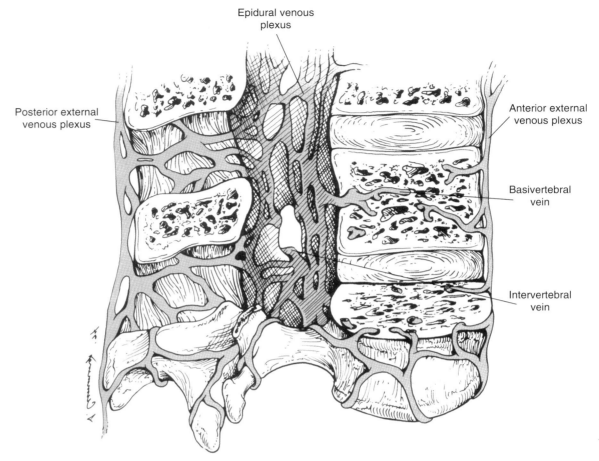

Figure 8.2 The venous system of the spinal motion unit. After Cramer & Darby (1995), with permission.

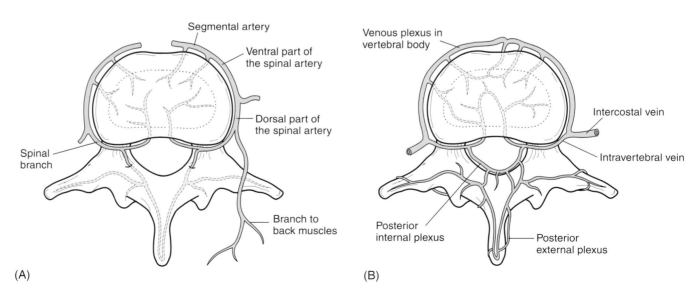

Figure 8.3 The vasculature of the vertebral body. (A) The typical arterial system; (B) the typical venous system. From Schafer (1983), with permission.

calcification may also limit solute diffusion (Urban et al 2001). In the historical context of the patient, factors such as regression of the vascular structures in the vertebral endplates (Chandraraj et al 1998) may be implicated in the contemporary clinical presentation. In some cases these may be inferred from the changes seen on plain radiograph, such as Schmorl's nodes.

The vascular system of the spinal column is an easy route for hematogenous spread of systemic neoplasms. This may occur through arterial emboli to the abundant bone marrow of the vertebral bodies and subsequently into the anterior or posterior extradural space through venous channels, or by retrograde spread through the valveless extradural Batson's venous plexus (Jacobs & Perrin 2001). Cancers from breast, lung, prostate, hemopoietic (for example, lymphoma or multiple myeloma), and renal origins account for the vast majority of extradural spinal metastases. The spinal lesion represents the first manifestation of cancer in 12–20% of patients who present with symptoms related to spinal metastases (Jacobs & Perrin 2001).

The arterial and venous dynamics within the SMU are generally unable to be assessed clinically, although shifts in tissue planes and vascular densities may at times be seen on magnetic resonance imaging (Demondion et al 2000). Their involvement must therefore be inferred through careful observation, thoughtful palpation, and reflection on the nature of any adjustment. It is thought that when a degree of edema is present about a particular SMU, perhaps within the facet joint, the cavitation resulting from adjustment may be muffled or dull as opposed to sounding sharp and crisp.

CLINICAL CONSIDERATIONS

In the global context of clinical assessment the essential vascular parameters are blood pressure and pulse. In the regional and segmental context the assessment of vascular change must include consideration of the arterial flow to an SMU, the venous drainage about and within the spine, and both the intrinsic lymphatic clearance and any extrinsic involvement of regional lymph nodes.

A generalized pain may be caused by pressure on small nerves in bone, the annulus, or ligaments, by venous hypertension. It may also compromise nerves within the IVC or about the cauda equina in the lower spinal canal and produce unusual sensations in the legs of the patient with spinal stenosis. Any reduction in space within the IVC, typically from a foraminal or extraforaminal disk protrusion (Fig. 14.14) may also compress the associated veins and cause venous stasis and ischemia which may contribute to the development of perineural and intraneural fibrosis (Gatterman 1990 p. 169).

The spinal nerve roots are susceptible to the effects of altered blood flow and venous drainage. Compressive pressure about a nerve can induce ischemia in the arterioles supplying the nerve, may degrade the intraneural transport of nutrients, and may restrict the flow of CSF about the nerve root. According to Cox (1999 pp. 148–150), the effect is worsened when there are two sites of compression on a single nerve.

The permeability of the endoneurial capillaries under compression quickly alters to allow intraneural edema which may increase the endoneurial fluid pressure. The dorsal root ganglion appears susceptible to these compressive effects (Cox 1999).

This in turn may generate pain perceived by the patient as nerve root (radicular) pain from the leg.

Kirkaldy-Willis (1992c) considers vasoconstriction within muscle as an important etiological factor in producing back pain. He describes the cycle as impaired or decreased circulation arising from vasoconstriction leading to edema as the accumulation of metabolites in the muscle, which then produces minor structural changes which in turn result in major structural changes, pain, and abnormal contraction. Given the proprioceptive and nociceptive data generated by the tissues of the SMU, the loop may commence with dysfunction in an SMU stimulating contraction of paraspinal muscles to stabilize the region which, after a period of time, results in internal vasoconstriction which then progresses to perpetuate a pain loop mediated by the muscle.

Wedge & Tchang (1992) identify abdominal aortic aneurysm (AAA) as a vascular cause of nagging, chronic back pain. The practitioner must examine and rule out AAA in presentations of this nature (Fig. 13.15). Peripheral vascular disease with claudication is a differential diagnosis of neurogenic claudication (secondary to spinal stenosis). The practitioner may rule in vascular claudication when the pain is not relieved by any particular spinal position but typically resolves quickly with rest. Neurogenic claudication is typically worsened with spinal flexion during lower-limb activity and may actually be temporarily reduced by walking without bending forward (Wedge & Tchang 1992).

EVIDENCE OF VASCULAR CHANGE

Pulse and blood pressure are two common clinical measurements which are considered indicators of vascular change secondary to SC. The relationship of the pulse is quite straightforward as its rate may increase when the patient is in pain. The question of blood pressure is another matter. The manual healthcare professions are empirically convinced that hypertension in particular may be secondary to spinal dysfunction (Gatterman 1990, pp. 384–389; Wurster 1992, Plaugher 1993 pp. 366–368); however, the evidence is yet to be convincing.

New instruments and new measurement parameters (Fujimoto et al 1999) are allowing investigators to examine more closely the autonomic nervous system and its reflex change secondary to subluxation (Budgell 2000). It may well be that in the not too distant future a range of autonomic effects, including blood pressure, will be shown to reflect segmental spinal dysfunction.

Edema and inflammation

A delicate balance between arteriolar blood flow to a region and the venous drainage of that region is maintained by the body in order to prevent edema. Edema is a collection of fluid beyond that which is normally found in cells or intercellular tissues and typically represents altered dynamics associated with inflammation following trauma or other pathological processes. The fluid dynamics may also be altered by pathological processes such as intraspinal tumor growth. There are many subcategories of edema, each reflective of different processes, including hereditary factors.

An understanding of the inflammation cycle is important to inform the process of clinical assessment. It is also important in the

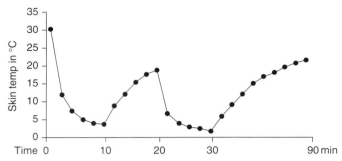

Figure 8.4 Skin temperature changes during cryotherapy. The skin temperature of the ankle was recorded during the application and removal of a wet ice pack. The temperature fell to below 5°C in the first 10 min but rose quite quickly during the 10-min period of no ice while staying below 20°. The second 10 min of ice application, between 20 and 30 min, brought the temperature down to well below 5°C and slowed the subsequent recovery time to about 60 min within the therapeutic range below 20°. From Ebrall et al (1992), with permission.

management of acute injury where ice may be used to limit tissue damage by causing vasoconstriction and then vasodilatation to improve the removal of posttraumatic debris and metabolites.

The purpose of posttraumatic ice application is to lower the temperature of the cells in the damaged area so that their metabolism slows and inflammatory damage is contained (Ebrall et al 1992). There is a normal oscillation between vasoconstriction secondary to cooling, and vasodilation as a reactive response, but as the tissues are cooled with ice the response slows. When the ice is removed there is a rise in temperature associated with increased fluid flow to purge the area. The ideal application of ice to an injured area is for 10 min followed by 10 min off and then 10 min on again (Fig. 8.4). This protocol produces about 90 min of local-tissue cooling below the temperature at which cell metabolism is active, thus reducing the production of inflammatory metabolites and ensuring the flushing of waste products from the area (Ebrall et al 1992). The body recovers quickly from an initial application and a single period of 20 min fails to extend the recovery time as long as the "10 on, 10 off, 10 on" protocol.

The practitioner must determine the cause of edema and should only select ice as a therapeutic intervention when the edema is secondary to inflammation and associated with tissue damage. These conditions generally suggest ice application as appropriate for acute strain/sprain injury to paraspinal muscles and other muscles and joints as indicated. As described above, any reduction in paraspinal edema associated with the inflammation of tissue damage will have positive clinical effects through numerous mechanisms.

All strain/sprain injury and traumatic damage to tissue is associated with the inflammatory response and the clinical question is simply one of degree. The probability of an inflammatory response is determined from a thorough history. Inflammation and edema may be palpated in severe cases where the superficial paraspinal muscles are involved, but typically the condition is subclinical and exists about the damaged SMU to a degree not palpable or directly observable, except by advanced imaging.

The classic situation is associated with disk protrusion where inflammatory metabolites secondary to damaged annular fibers

act as nociceptors. The presence of edema within and about the SMU will alter the palpatory findings and the practitioner must be aware of this. Typical findings include a spongy end-feel (Fig. 4.4). Pain on all movements is typically present in the acute presentation. Chronic edema about an SMU may be painless to palpation while generating pain through other mechanisms, such as neural compromise. Inflammation is an acute phenomenon but can be considered chronic when it is recurrent or cyclical, as in many inflammatory arthritides.

Thermal asymmetry

In addition to these basic clinical findings, practitioners have long held that thermal asymmetry about the spine is indicative of altered cutaneous blood flow, either as a unilateral increase secondary to arteriolar vasodilation or as a decrease secondary to arteriolar constriction. The clinical significance of a paraspinal temperature differential became part of chiropractic practice in the early 1920s when Evins, an electrical engineer and chiropractic student, developed a contact thermocouple which used an analog needle and dial as an indicator (Christiansen & Mueller 1990). This primitive method became entrenched in the then major paradigm of chiropractic practice and has become a component of spinal analysis in the Gonstead paradigm of practice (Plaugher 1993).

There have been sufficient technical advances to infrared telethermography to allow it to become an affordable clinical procedure, yet its use is now minimal within manual healthcare. On the other hand the neurocalometer remains a mainstay of Gonstead technique. The clinical intent is to detect thermal asymmetry about the spine which is thought to be secondary to the SC. The mechanism is thought to be altered neural control of the fine vasculature as the amount of radiated heat is a function of blood flow. Yet again the intimacy between neural regulation of such basic body functions as blood flow is evident.

Several devices exist which claim to identify other characteristics of the subluxation, including the thermal asymmetry said to accompany altered capillary hemodynamics. It is argued that variances in the autonomic nervous system are part of the neuropathophysiology of the subluxation and these alter capillary flow (Herbst 1968). Such changes are identified by contact thermography using a neurocalometer. Neuromuscular thermography is considered an accurate, sensitive method of determining cutaneous temperatures (Hubbard 1990); however, its clinical interpretation needs further investigation.

The thermal characteristics of the spinal region identified through empirical instrumentation have been measured and described using infrared telethermography under controlled laboratory conditions (Ebrall et al 1994a). The skin temperature from the left and right paraspinal areas of a typical subject are shown in Figure 8.5. There is a normal fluctuation of temperature on either side along the 15 cm region of the thoracic spine which was measured. The left varied between 34.8 and 35.5°C and the right between 34.3 and 35.4°C. These are small fluctuations, of about 1°C. The rapid deflection of the neurocalometer needle is termed a break and is thought to indicate spinal dysfunction at that spinal level. It is thought that spinal dysfunction alters local neural control such that arteriolar blood flow in the paraspinal tissues differs, thus creating a thermal differential.

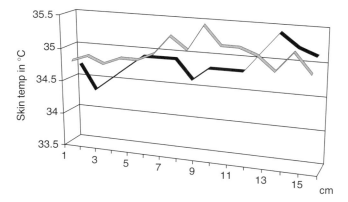

Figure 8.5 Paraspinal skin temperature profiles. The skin temperatures from the left and right paraspinal areas are plotted as strips. The x-axis represents a 15-cm length of the thoracic spine. The level of interest is about point 12, where the temperature on one side falls, whilst that on the other rises, producing a crossover effect. It is thought that this thermal crossover is the effect identified as a "break" by the neurocalometer. From Ebrall et al (1994a), with permission.

The paraspinal thermal profiles of subjects with and without breaks were obtained by infrared telethermography and those subjects in which a break was found and agreed on by a panel of experts all demonstrated a dynamic thermal crossover of the type depicted in Figure 8.5. The interpretation is that the thermal characteristics about the spine which may indicate dysfunction are not as simple as left/right thermal asymmetry. Rather, there seems to be a dynamic bilateral thermal gradient asymmetry. This means that the temperature gradient on one side moves rapidly in the opposite direction to the gradient of the other side within the space of a few millimeters along the spine, at the level of the putative SC.

The remaining data points in the paraspinal thermal scans reveal that, while a left/right asymmetry is present, the temperature gradients of both sides either fall or rise in unison between the measured points, and this does not seem to stimulate the neurocalometer to indicate a break suggestive of SC (Ebrall et al 1994b). Further investigation of this phenomenon is warranted as contact thermography is a useful clinical tool.

The American Medical Association's Council on Scientific Affairs (1987) reports that thermography may facilitate the determination of spinal root and peripheral nerve dysfunction and of spinal disorders, and may also be useful in documenting peripheral nerve and soft-tissue injuries, such as muscle and ligament sprain/strain, inflammation, muscle spasm, and myositis. Thermography has been widely reported in the literature as being a useful indicator for diagnosis of a number of clinical presentations. These include:

- peripheral nerve injuries (Brelsford & Uematsu 1985, Dudley 1987, Meyers et al 1989, So et al 1989a, Dankiw 1990, Herrick 1990)
- radiculopathies (Raskin et al 1976, Pochaczevsky et al 1982, Newman et al 1984, Green et al 1986, AMA Council on Scientific Affairs Report 1987, So et al 1989b, Dankiw 1990, Conwell 1991b, Hoffman et al 1991, Vlasuk 1991)

- vertebral joint dysfunction (Brand & Gizoni 1982, Diakow et al 1988, BenEliyahu 1992, Stillwagon et al 1992)
- reflex sympathetic dystrophy (Kobrossi & Steiman 1986, AMA Council on Scientific Affairs Report 1987, BenEliyahu 1989, Dankiw 1990)
- lumbar/low-back pain (Green et al 1986, Ellis et al 1989, So et al 1989b, Conwell 1991a)
- headache (BenEliyahu 1989)
- myofascial pain syndromes (Brelsford & Uematsu 1985, AMA Council on Scientific Affairs Report 1987, Diakow 1988, Conwell 1990)
- deep venous thrombosis (Cooke & Pilcher 1973, Ritchie et al 1979, Pochaczevsky et al 1982)
- spinal cord lesions (AMA Council on Scientific Affairs Report 1987).

Interest in the application of spinal thermography seemed to peak in the late 1980s/early 1990s and it is no longer considered a useful clinical tool for assessing pain associated with spinal dysfunction. The diagnostic accuracy of technologies used in the assessment of low-back pain has been tested and thermography performed poorly (Leclaire et al 1996). The results clearly indicated that the diagnostic accuracy of infrared telethermography failed to reach the level of other technologies, including clinical examination.

Complex regional pain syndrome

CRPS is a regional, posttraumatic, neuropathic pain problem that most often affects one or more limbs (Rho et al 2002). Normalization of temperature and blood flow is associated with the relief of pain (Cooke et al 1995). The condition was formerly known as reflex sympathetic dystrophy. Pain is typically present in the initial stage when the limb is hypothermic and vasoconstricted and recurs when the limb becomes hyperthermic and vasodilated.

The vascular changes are largely mediated by the sympathetic nervous system and the CRPS could equally be considered as a component of the assessment of neural change. This illustrates the intimate relationship among the dimensions of the SC and the need for the practitioner to have a structured approach which integrates all findings. In the case of CRPS, the vascular findings, which include edema, are a result of neural dysfunction which produces sensory and motor changes (de la Calle-Reviriego 2000).

Sympathetic failure is a unique indicator of CRPS (Birklein et al 2001) and may be due to thermoregulatory and emotional stimuli generated in the CNS. Vascular changes may also reflect altered vascular sensitivity to cold temperature and circulating catecholamines (Baron & Maier 1996). A small percentage of patients develop refractory, chronic pain (Rho et al 2002). A positive response has been reported to manual therapy of the spine in a child with chronic inversion and plantar flexion of the foot associated with a diagnosis of reflex sympathetic dystrophy (Ellis & Ebrall 1991).

CEREBROSPINAL FLUID

CSF is largely formed by the choroid plexuses of the lateral, third, and fourth ventricles. It flows from the lateral to the third ventricle through interventricular foramina and then into the fourth ventricle through the cerebral aqueduct of the midbrain (Fig. 8.6). It then passes through the median and possibly lateral apertures of the fourth ventricle into the cerebromedullary and pontine cisterns, and then into the subarachnoid space around the brain, spinal cord, and cauda equina (Moore 1980 pp. 941–947).

The CSF is absorbed into venous blood by the arachnoid villi in the dural venous sinuses. It may also be absorbed by the ependymal lining of the ventricles, in the subarachnoid space, through the walls of capillaries in the pia mater, and probably into the lymphatics adjacent to the subarachnoid space around

cerebrospinal nerves, such as the optic nerves. The cervical lymphatic vessels play an important role in the transport of CSF from the cranial vault when the intracranial pressure is elevated (Silver et al 1999).

A function of the CSF is to protect the neural tissue, including the brain, by providing a fluid cushion to absorb shock. When standing erect, the brain is in contact with the cranial fossae in the floor of the cranial cavity. The CSF separates the upper surface of the brain from the cranial bones (Moore 1980). The Monro–Keller doctrine states that any change in the volume of the intracranial contents (brain, ventricular fluid, and blood) will be reflected by a change in intracranial pressure.

The bones of the cranium are claimed by some to demonstrate a low-frequency rhythm and this has led to a subset of manual therapy which places great emphasis on assessing and normalizing these pulsations. The phenomenon is termed the cranial rhythmic impulse (CRI), in the original belief that the pulsating brain moved the cranial bones, thus imparting the rhythm to the craniosacral mechanism (Chaitow 1999 pp. 5–48).

Chaitow notes that considerable disagreement is voiced by experts in the field, even about the frequency of the rhythm, which is argued by some to be 6–12 cycles/min, others as 10–14 cycles/min, and yet others who consider it to be much slower. There is also much discussion as to the mechanism of the CRI and whether or not it relates to the CSF fluctuations and flow.

There seems little doubt that a CRI exists, although as yet it is not clear what this represents or what drives it. There are many hypotheses, including that of the lymphatic pump described by Degenhardt & Kuchera (1996). Given the interrelationships between blood, lymph, and CSF, and the many neuro-immunoregulatory actions within these fluids which are now being described in the literature, a reasonable position is to appreciate that a CRI exists and that it is likely to be associated with the homeostatic maintenance of the body's fluid systems.

Another central concept is that rhythmic involuntary motion of the sacrum is related to the involuntary motion of the occiput (Moran & Gibbons 2001). This is termed the "core-link" and represents the essence of craniosacral therapy. The involuntary motion of the sacrum is thought to be synchronous with that of the occiput. Chaitow (1999) argues that the core-link hypothesis is probably seriously flawed. Moran & Gibbons (2001) studied the intraexaminer and interexaminer reliability for palpation of the CRI at the head and sacrum and reported results that failed to support the construct validity of the core-link hypothesis. How individual practitioners identify and interpret the CRI and its putative effects on the function of the body remains their clinical prerogative.

THE LYMPHATIC SYSTEM

The assessment of the spine must include palpation of the superficial regional lymph nodes. A tender, swollen lymph node is indicative of infection or a pathological process. The practitioner needs to differentiate between nodes which have suddenly become tender and palpable, suggesting inflammation and infection, and those which are chronically or recurrently enlarged, suggesting a connective tissue disorder or neoplasia (Souza 2001 p. 532). The normal lymph node should not be palpable.

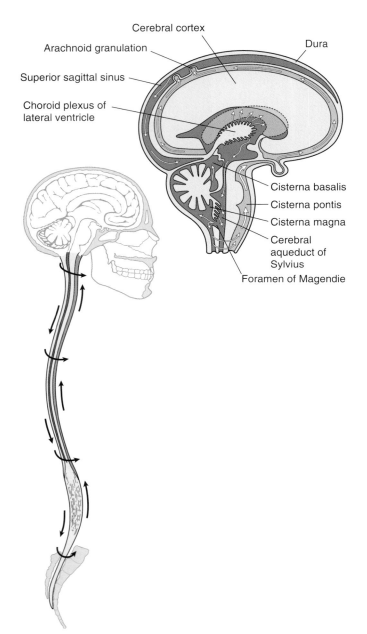

Cerebral cortex

Arachnoid granulation

Dura

Superior sagittal sinus

Choroid plexus of lateral ventricle

Cisterna basalis

Cisterna pontis

Cisterna magna

Cerebral aqueduct of Sylvius

Foramen of Magendie

Figure 8.6 Cerebrospinal fluid circulation and landmarks. From Chaitow (1999), with permission.

The clinically relevant nodes which are palpable when involved, and the regions they drain, are depicted in Figure 8.7 and include:

- occipital, postauricular and posterior cervical nodes: the scalp
- preauricular: the face and eye
- high superficial and deep cervical nodes, submaxillary and submental: the pharynx and mouth
- supraclavicular and scalene nodes: the head and neck, arms, mediastinum, and abdomen
- axillary nodes: the arm and breast
- epitrochlear nodes: the arm and hand
- inguinal-femoral nodes: most of the lower extremity and buttocks, lower anus, genitalia, perineum, and lower abdominal wall (Souza 2001).

The skin lymphatic system is the initial drainage point, and this converges into lymphatic precollectors, collectors, and lymphatic ducts. In turn these convey the lymph to the regional lymph nodes (Szuba & Rockson 1997) and eventually into the blood of the great veins. The system is far from a static network of collecting ducts and nodes. It is now known that lymphatic vessels from a number of different human tissues demonstrate both tonic and phasic changes in contractility. These changes are presumably involved in the generation and regulation of lymph flow and it has been shown that human lymphatic contractility can be influenced by a number of neural and humoral agents as a means of controlling lymph transport (Gashev & Zawieja 2001). Swollen lymph nodes may therefore indicate impaired drainage of the chain which may in turn reflect altered neural function, given that any tissue which is neurally mediated is dependent on normal spinal function.

There is a rhythmical contractile mechanism intrinsic to the smooth muscle of the lymphangions (the section of a lymphatic vessel between two adjacent valves) and the pumping activity adapts to changes in fluid load (von der Weid 2001). This intrinsic contractile capability provides a major part of the propulsive force of lymph fluid (Johnston et al 1986, Olszewski 2002). There are also extrinsic driving forces such as lymph formation itself, arterial pulsations, skeletal muscle contractions, fluctuations of central venous pressure, gastrointestinal peristalsis, and respiration (Gashev 2002).

Consideration of the lymphatic system cannot be isolated from the assessment of the other dimensions of the spine, most notably the neural component. Osteopaths have long recognized the importance of lymph circulation and consider that manipulative techniques directed at influencing the autonomic nervous system are an important means of relieving tissue congestion (Degenhardt & Kuchera 1996).

The autonomic regulation of lymphatic flow in the lower extremity has been demonstrated by lymphoscintigraphy in patients with CRPS (Howarth et al 1999). The influence of the

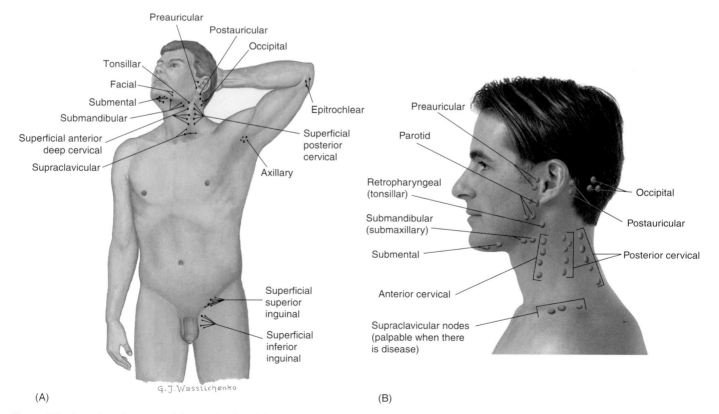

Figure 8.7 Lymph nodes accessible to palpation. (A) An overview of the body; (B) the head and neck in detail. From Seidel et al (1999), with permission.

lymph system with neural-immune reactions is well described by Ader et al (1995). It is claimed that there are two pathways which link the brain and the immune system, namely the autonomic nervous system and the neuroendocrine outflow via the pituitary. The presence of chemical-specific nerve fibers associated with primary and secondary lymphoid tissues, the release and availability of neurally derived substances for interaction with immune cells, and identification of immunoregulatory effects are criteria for neurotransmission which have been satisfied for several transmitters, such as norepinephrine (noradrenaline) and substance P (Zawieja 1996).

Di Sebastiano et al (1999) investigated the cause of pain in appendectomies where no pathology was demonstrated. They found larger amounts of immunoreactive nerves in these appendices and describe the relationship of nerve fibers and lymphoid cells as creating increased pain. This leads to the suggestion that neuroimmune appendicitis is a distinct pathological entity accounting for up to a quarter of appendectomies where no pathology is demonstrated. Further, it seems the sympathetic skin response can be used to verify the integrity of the lumbar sympathetic chains after retroperitoneal lymphadenectomy (Siracusano et al 1994).

Neurolymphatic reflex points

The concept of neurolymphatic reflex points and their clinical relevance has been described in previous chapters. The following is based on notes from Dr Donald McDowall and is presented as an attempt to reach an appreciation of this empirical phenomenon by understanding its historical context.

The neurolymphatic reflex points are termed Chapman's reflexes after Chapman, an entrant to the 1897 class of the American School of Osteopathy. After 30 years of practice, he realized that some 20% of the ailments he saw were probably related to bony lesions. He observed lymphatic congestion in many disease states and theorized that if he could find a way to unblock this congestion the body would find a quicker way to return to normal.

Osteopathic treatments at that time were typically lengthy and time-consuming. Chapman wanted to identify and locate what he considered to be the most likely cause of the problem and then to treat it specifically. He acknowledged that the lymphatic aspects of disease could originate from bony lesions, infections, toxins, or other causes.

Chapman described his reflexes as "gangliform contractions" that were tender when palpated but which then relaxed with palpatory stimulation. He felt they often needed only one or two treatments for correction. Small, a student of the Chicago College of Osteopathy in 1937, completed a report of a dissection showing the relation of the Chapman reflexes to the spinal and sympathetic nerves, the intercostal arteries, veins, and lymph nodes (Owens 1937).

Through dissection Small, quoted in Owens (1937), observed that the intercostal branch of the anterior spinal division of the spinal nerve continued around the thorax as the intercostal nerve and communicated with the sympathetic ganglion located on the anterolateral side of the bodies of the thoracic vertebra. The intercostal nerve innervates the external and internal intercostal muscles and, with its sympathetic fibers, the

intercostal arteries, veins, and lymph nodes. Small argued that some lymphoid tissue was located in the intercostal space between the anterior and posterior layers of the anterior intercostal fascia and felt that the Chapman's reflex would be found within this tissue. He reported that this tissue was drained by the anterior group of the pectoral lymph glands into the thoracic duct on the left and the right jugular duct.

Small continued by reporting that the posterior primary division further branched into a lateral and medial cutaneous branch which innervated the skin on either side of the spine for about 15 cm. He argued that stimulation of these receptor organs would cause the afferent and efferent vessels draining these tissues to increase or decrease, permitting the lymph flow to be increased or diminished, thus affecting the drainage of the entire lymph system of this area. He also thought that the lymph nodes of the vital organs, such as the heart, kidneys, liver, spleen, and pancreas, could be affected through the sympathetic fibers of this tissue. These receptor areas represent the points identified as Chapman's reflex points.

It is important to note that these reflexes were originally used to decongest the related organs. No comment was made in Chapman's work concerning muscle–organ relationships, although he did recommend structural pelvic balance for enhanced function of the reflexes. Goodheart (1965), a chiropractor, correlated Chapman's reflexes to specific muscles. His clinical observations could reasonably be extended to muscle innervation using the same anatomical reasoning for the spinal nerve–sympathetic correlation that Small attributed to Chapman.

VERTEBROBASILAR INSUFFICIENCY

The question of vertebrobasilar insufficiency (VBI) or cerebrovascular ischemia (CVI) and its sometimes clinical sequel of vertebrobasilar accident (VBA) or CVA or stroke as they may relate to manipulation of the neck has received unreasonable emphasis, due largely to medical bias against chiropractic and a serious misuse of terminology by medical writers (Terrett 1995b).

A review of the literature estimates the risk to be between five and 10 events per 10 million manipulations (Hurwitz et al 1996) and an authoritative assessment can be drawn from the records of the largest insurer of practitioners in the USA, the NCMIC Group, Inc. Their estimate of a serious complication such as a vertebrobasilar stroke causing permanent neurologic deficit following cervical manipulation is approximately one in 2 million procedures (Chapman-Smith 2001).

Misinformation about chiropractic practice may also reflect incompetence. A medical witness at an inquest into the death of a chiropractic patient in Canada has been described by an expert witness as being "scientifically irresponsible" and "incompetent as a scientist in the study of causation" (Sackett 2002, Chapman-Smith 2003). There also seems to be a sense of hysteria in parts of the medical community. In spite of acknowledging that estimates of serious complications associated with spinal manipulation range from one per 2 million manipulations to one per 400 000, Stevinson & Ernst (2002) make the odd suggestion that the safety of spinal manipulation requires rigorous investigation. In medical terms an adverse incident rate of one in 400 000 is extraordinarily low and represents a very safe intervention.

There are a number of simple facts:

- VBAs do occur throughout the population secondary to a number of causative factors
- the incidence of CVI or CVA following skilled manipulation of the neck is at least an order of magnitude lower than the complications associated with non-steroidal anti-inflammatory drug (NSAID) use (Dabbs & Lauretti 1995)
- the likelihood of CVI and/or CVA is unpredictable
- there is very little evidence associating CVA with skilled manipulation of the neck.

Manipulation of the cervical spine is a high-order psychomotor skill requiring extensive training, a period of supervision under an experienced practitioner, and frequent utilization to maintain skills and judgment. At least one jurisdiction has enacted legislation (Public Health Act, State of New South Wales, 1991) which restricts the performance of spinal manipulation to members of certain professional groupings, although there is no assurance that all members of any one professional group are appropriately trained (Refshauge et al 2002). It may well be of benefit to the public for all jurisdictions and relevant professional groupings to reconsider the training and practice requirements of those who include spinal manipulation or adjustment within their scope of clinical practice (Vautravers & Maigne 2000).

This is not to suggest that manipulation of the cervical spine is inherently dangerous; rather it acknowledges that, while the risk is so low, the consequences may be catastrophic. The risk is actually hard to measure and statistical manipulation such as bootstrapping is needed in order to achieve sufficient data to generate estimates (Rothwell et al 2001). Such rate estimates can easily be overemphasized and the association of chiropractic therapy with VBA is acknowledged to be exceedingly difficult to study (Rothwell et al 2001).

Not only is the risk of an event induced by manipulation extremely low, there is a background level of spontaneous carotid and vertebral artery dissection. Young people seem particularly susceptible to a spontaneous event. One paper reports spontaneous events in children under 15 years (Camacho et al 2001), while another reports events in young adults which were associated with indirect and subtle neck trauma (Prabhakar et al 2001).

While there are warning signs of stroke such as neck pain and headache (Saeed et al 2000), including occipital headache (Krespi et al 2002), these complaints are actually a driver of patients to seek manual treatment. A retrospective review of the records of 26 patients (Saeed et al 2000) found the most common clinical features also included vertigo (57%), unilateral facial paresthesia (46%), cerebellar signs (33%), lateral medullary signs (26%), and visual field defects (15%).

A thorough review of the literature relating to risk factors thought to be associated with neck movements causing vertebrobasilar artery dissection found no assistance to identify any offending mechanical trauma, neck movement, or type of manipulation precipitating vertebral artery dissection (Haldeman et al 1999). A subsequent study concludes that CVA after manipulation appears to be an unpredictable event and should be considered an inherent, idiosyncratic, and rare complication of cervical spine manipulation and adjustment by experienced practitioners (Haldeman et al 2002a). A simple cause-and-effect relationship

does not exist between neck manipulation and subsequent patient injury (Terrett 2002).

It is known that screening procedures are, in the main, unreliable and of little clinical use (Côté et al 1996). It is also reported that the common premanipulative tests which produce findings considered positive do not represent an absolute contraindication (Licht et al 2000). There are a number of similar clinical signs and symptoms elicited during the testing maneuvers which are perceived as being indicators for adjustment as opposed to contraindications (Ebrall & Ellis 2000). It is also known that the adjustment can be safely delivered in the presence of damaged arteries (Rubinstein & Haldeman 2001).

The failure of the screening procedures to predict altered blood flow may arise from a misunderstanding of their mechanism. It has been thought that rotation of the cervical spine occluded the contralateral artery, which then placed an emphasis on the patency of the ipsilateral artery. Any pre-existing decrease in patency of that artery would then reasonably generate signs and symptoms of VBI. This process has been thoroughly investigated by Haynes who, after extensive studies, considers that only about 5% of vertebral arteries from the general population may be severely stenosed or occluded with rotational movements of the cervical spine (Haynes 1996).

The duplex ultrasound scanning studies by Haynes & Milne (2001) found that most of the 39 vertebral arteries they examined displayed no marked changes in their blood velocities during contralateral cervical rotation, and that when the blood velocities were averaged for the whole sample of arteries, no statistically significant changes were observed during rotation. This provides further evidence that the majority of vertebral arteries are usually unaffected in a major way by contralateral cervical rotation. No change was found in the lumen dimensions of 16 vertebral arteries with full rotation as observed in the magnetic resonance angiographic studies of Haynes et al (2002). Other investigators found no change in peak flow in the vertebral artery immediately after uncomplicated spinal manipulative therapy (Licht et al 1998). The same investigators also found there were no significant changes in volume flow during premanipulative testing of the vertebral artery in pigs, but observed that the volume blood flow did increase significantly for 40 s, before returning to baseline values in less than 3 min after cervical manipulation (Licht et al 1999).

Haynes is an advocate of Doppler ultrasound assessment of vertebral artery blood flow in patients prior to cervical manipulation. There is evidence that the manual provocational tests lack validity (Haynes 2002); however, some groups of practitioners consider that their use is reliable and supported (Rivett et al 1999). Refshauge (1994) and Rivett et al (1999) suggested that the results of their duplex scanning studies provided support for the usefulness of the manual provocational tests, but Haynes (2002) has questioned their interpretation of their own data. There is evidence that bidirectional Doppler velocimeter testing is valid (Haynes 2000) and that it has strong interexaminer reliability (Haynes et al 2000).

The issue of the safety of the chiropractic adjustment, particularly in the cervical spine, is one which must be considered in terms of the risks and benefits to the patient. An authoritative review of the research evidence supporting behavioral and physical treatments for headache concludes: "manipulation is effective in patients with cervicogenic headache" (McCrory et al 2001).

The internal forces sustained by the vertebral artery during skilled spinal manipulation are known to be almost an order of magnitude lower than the strains required to disrupt the artery mechanically (Symons et al 2002). Chiropractors and osteopaths are highly skilled in the delivery of manipulation and there seems no question that the risk–benefit ratio of chiropractic spinal adjustment is acceptable (Haldeman et al 2001). This is especially so in patients for whom the history and examination lead to a working diagnosis which includes cervical subluxation with or without headache.

The bottom line is that the clinical outcomes generally outweigh the risks, and skilled manipulation or adjustment of the cervical spine is a low-risk clinical intervention. This is not to reduce in any way the importance of informed consent in the face of understanding the material risks, nor does it imply that spinal adjusting is an innocuous clinical procedure. On the contrary, the use of spinal manipulation in general, and the adjustment of the cervical spine in particular, is a most potent clinical intervention which is safely practiced thousands of times daily around the globe to produce marked improvement in patient function and quality of life for those with acute neck pain (Hurwitz et al 1996).

CONCLUSION

The vascular dimensions of the SC are diverse and present a challenge to the practitioner for their meaningful assessment and subsequent integration and interpretation within the full context of the patient. All assessment procedures involve intrusion into the homeostatic envelope of the patient. In particular, the provocative assessment of the patency and integrity of the vertebral arteries, while essentially invalid, may initiate other responses of the patient which could be interpreted as indicators for therapeutic intervention in the form of spinal manipulation or adjustment.

It is suggested that the practitioner record and carefully consider any previous unwanted effects of either assessment or treatment (Vautravers & Maigne 2000), and that a thorough assessment be undertaken prior to considering manipulation or adjustment.

Assessment of the spine by region

All are but parts of one stupendous whole, Whose body Nature is, and God the soul

Source: Alexander Pope (1688–1744), *Essay on Man.* Epistle i, 267

9

The upper cervical spine

KEY CONCEPTS

The upper cervical spine is a neurologically complex region and there is a gamut of signs and symptoms, including pain, headache, dizziness, ataxia, nystagmus, visual disturbances, and vertigo, that can be associated with dysfunction at this level.

Head pain may arise from mechanical dysfunction of the upper cervical spine as well as from active trigger points in the musculature of the head and neck.

In addition to signalling nociception, the somatosensory system of the neck may influence the motor control of the neck, eyes, limbs, respiratory muscles, and possibly the activity of some preganglionic nerves. There are reflex connections between receptors in cervical facet joints and fusimotorneurones of posterior neck muscles, which may explain the pathophysiology associated with whiplash-induced disorders.

Effective assessment, treatment, and management of disorders of the upper cervical spine require a thorough knowledge of its clinical anatomy and a deep understanding of its functional neurology. The atypical anatomy of the atlanto-occipital and atlantoaxial articulations requires a specific and structured approach to the assessment of kinematic change at this level.

The ligamentum nuchae includes extensions of the aponeuroses of the trapezius, rhomboid minor, serratus posterior superior, and splenius capitis, and has connective tissue attachments to the dura mater of the spine at the atlanto-occipital junction.

The rectus capitis posterior major and minor muscles have connective tissue bridges to the dura mater of the spinal cord which may help resist dural infolding during head and neck extension and which may also be implicated in some forms of headache.

The clinical outcomes of adjusting the upper cervical complex generally outweigh the risks and skilled manipulation or adjustment of the cervical spine is, in medical terms, an extremely low-risk clinical intervention. This is not to reduce in any way the importance of a thorough patient assessment and the recording of informed consent in the face of understanding the material risks, nor does it imply that adjusting the cervical spine is an innocuous clinical procedure.

CLINICAL ANATOMY

A posterior view of the upper cervical complex with its intrinsic ligaments is shown in Figure 9.1 and includes the following major articulations:

- occiput–C1 left and right
- C1–2
- C2–3.

Cramer & Darby (1995 pp. 109–155) provide the appropriate level of anatomy of this region for the student and can be read in conjunction with this chapter. They identify (p. 10) the following clinically important relationships:

- C1 – transition of medulla into the spinal cord; the hard palate
- C2 – inferior border of the free edge of the soft palate; the junction of the nasopharynx and oropharynx
- C2 disk – superior cervical ganglion.

Occiput–C1

The occiput and C1 form the atlanto-occipital junction, the superior components of which are the occipital condyles and the inferior components are the superior aspect of the C1 lateral masses. Each occipital condyle is a convex process with one to the left and one to the right of the foramen magnum. The condyles follow the contour of the foramen magnum and are angled anteromedially. The long axis of the resultant joint can be considered as lying about 30–40° anteromedially, thus converging towards the front of the patient.

The clinical implication of this angulation is that the patient's head must be rotated about 30–40° ipsilaterally so that the long axis of the joint being assessed lies in the sagittal plane, allowing a concentration of the applied testing vector to cause rotation about the x-axis in the joint and thus more accurate assessment of any flexion and extension fixation in the sagittal plane. The movement does not follow the usual flexion/extension arc found in typical spinal motion units (SMUs) where the arc is concave inferiorly. Rather, the arc is concave superiorly, to match the shape of the facet on C1 which receives the convex occipital condyle, and the movement is more an anterosuperior and posterosuperior glide which can be considered as a rotation about the x-axis with some glide along the z-axis. Kapandji (1974 p. 184) gives the total range of flexion and extension as 15° at the atlanto-occipital joint.

Each condyle rests in a matching concavity on the superior aspect of the lateral mass of C1 (Fig. 9.2). The depth of this concavity is responsible for the stability of the atlanto-occipital joint. The side walls prevent the occiput from slipping sideways and the anterior and posterior walls prevent translation (Bogduk & Mercer 2000). A reasonable degree of left–right asymmetry has been reported in C1 (Van Roy et al 1997), most frequently in the posterior arch and the grooves for the vertebral artery. Asymmetry or tropism of the superior facets is caused by differences in shape, size, surface area, curvature, inclination relative to the sagittal plane, implantation into the lateral mass, and unilateral subdivision of the concavity into more than one joint. The asymmetries of the inferior facets are more due to degenerative change (Van Roy et al 1997). Notwithstanding these common anatomical variants, the articular surfaces and vertebral foramina of isolated specimens of C1 can be used to estimate the race of the individual with about 70% accuracy (Marino 1997).

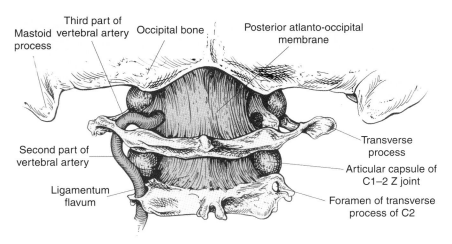

Figure 9.1 Posterior view of the upper cervical spine. From Cramer & Darby (1995), with permission.

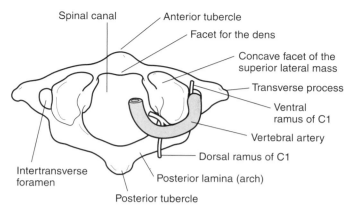

Figure 9.2 Superior view of C1. Note the anteromedial angulation of the long axis of the facet which receives the occipital condyle. Also note the intimate relationship of the intertransverse foramen to the superior lateral mass and atlanto-occipital articulation. The vertebral artery rises through this foramen and winds posteriorly then medially about the joint and then ascends into the cranium through the foramen magnum. Modified from Cramer & Darby (1995), with permission.

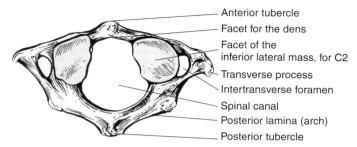

Figure 9.3 Inferior view of C1. From Cramer & Darby (1995), with permission.

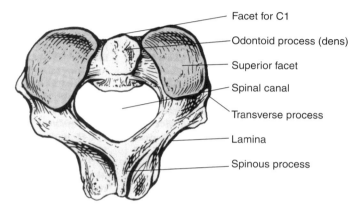

Figure 9.4 Superior view of C2. From Cramer & Darby (1995), with permission.

Lateral flexion is minimal in the atlanto-occipital articulation and occurs as a lateral slide or slip in the condyles. There is a minimal amount of rotation about the y-axis, which is a combination of anterosuperior glide on the contralateral side of rotation and a posterosuperior glide of the condyle on the ipsilateral side, and is measured as being about 3° to the left and to the right, or about 6° in total (Pfirrmann et al 2000). It occurs at the end of rotation of the upper cervical complex within the elastic zone of the supportive ligaments which induce ipsilateral lateral translation and contralateral lateral flexion of the occiput as they tighten (Kapandji 1974 p. 182).

The initial and greater rotation of the complex occurs between C1 and C2 and is about 38° to the left and to the right (Pfirrmann et al 2000). Passive rotation of the head causes C1 to follow the occiput and the rotary movement of occiput on C1 occurs as C1 reaches the end of its rotation on C2. The upper cervical complex accounts for about 70% of the total axial rotation of the cervical spine (Mimura et al 1989).

The atlanto-occipital junction is considered as a two-joint complex consisting of the left occiput–C1 and the right occiput–C1 articulations. Each occiput–C1 joint is bound by a fibrous capsule and C1 is bound to the occiput by the anterior and posterior atlanto-occipital membranes (Fig. 9.1). The anterior membrane is difficult to image with magnetic resonance imaging (MRI) (Krakenes et al 2001) and its median portion is continuous with the anterior longitudinal ligament. There is also a lateral atlanto-occipital ligament running from the jugular process of the occiput to the lateral mass of C1.

The posterior atlanto-occipital membrane is known either to merge with the dura or to be partly or totally separated from it by a fat layer (Krakenes et al 2001). It arches over the vertebral artery and in 15% of normal persons may calcify in these arcuate fibers to form a posterior ponticulus (Taylor & Resnick 2000 pp. 46, 51). This is seen as a part or complete arcuate foramen on the lateral arch of C1 in the lateral cervical radiograph and may be uni- or bilateral.

A significant association has been found between the presence of posterior ponticulus and migraine without aura, with an odds ratio of 2.19:1 in favor of this complaint being present with the osseous anomaly (Wight et al 1999). The complete foramen is significantly more common in males, without any racial predilection, and the partial foramen is commonest in white females (Stubbs 1992). While it is a normal occurrence in monkeys and other lower animals (Hasan et al 2001), it is considered by some practitioners to be a relative contraindication to forceful cervical manipulation in the human (Buna et al 1984).

The transverse fibers of the posterior atlanto-occipital membrane are attached by connective tissue to the deep surface of the rectus capitis posterior minor muscle (Dean & Mitchell 2002). This connective tissue also invests the perivascular tissue about the vertebral arteries at this level. The deep aspect of the nuchal ligament, formed from bilateral contributions from rhomboid minor, serratus posterior superior, splenius capitis, and trapezius (Johnson et al 2000), attaches to the dorsal cervical spinal dura in the interspace between the occiput and C1 (Dean & Mitchell 2002).

The inferior view of C1 is shown in Figure 9.3. The laminae, which form the posterior arch, are quite fine in their depth and form a posterior tubercle in the midline. The posterior gap between C1 and C2 seen in dry specimens is filled, in vivo, by the ligamenta flava on either side of the posterior tubercle (C1) and spinous process (C2). At this level the ligamentum flavum has been shown to consist of three tough fibrous

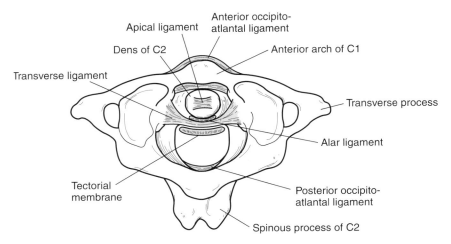

Figure 9.5 Superior view of ligaments about the C1–2 complex. From Cramer & Darby (1995), with permission.

columns attaching to the inferior border of C1 and the superior border of C2 (Dean & Mitchell 2002).

The inferior surface of each lateral mass of C1 is flat or slightly concave, to form an articulation with the superior facet of C2 (Fig. 9.4). These zygapophyseal joints have menisci as synovial folds which project into the joint. Cramer & Darby note these are type II at this level and are relatively large wedges which protrude a significant distance into the joint space (Cramer & Darby 1995 p. 115). The meniscoids are composed of fine fibrillar connective tissue with a large amount of fat and vessels and their collagenous base merges into the articular capsule (Ibatullin et al 1987).

C1–2

While the atlanto-occipital joint (occiput–C1) is technically a two-joint complex, the atlanto-odontoid articulation is intimately involved in its movement and it is clinically appropriate to consider the upper cervical complex as an interrelated, interdependent SMU of three bony structures (occiput, C1 or atlas, and C2 or axis) and at least five articulations (left occiput–C1, right occiput–C1, dens–C1, left C1–2, right C1–2). There is no intervertebral disk in this complex and its integrity is largely due to the ligamentous network (Fig. 9.5), including the transverse ligament which arches across the posterior border of the dens and inserts into a small tubercle on the medial surface of each lateral mass of C1. Its purpose is to retain the dens (of C2) in contact with the anterior arch of C1. Its superficial fibers project upwards to the occiput and blend with the apical ligament, and sometimes they project downwards to the posterior surface of C2, thus forming a cross-shaped cruciate ligament of the atlas. The transverse ligament is subject to degeneration in some patients (Cai et al 2001).

The anterior surface of the odontoid process (dens) of C2 has a hyaline-lined facet which articulates with a facet on the posterior surface of the anterior arch of C1, with its own loose synovial capsule. The posterior aspect of the dens has a larger articulation with the transverse ligament and the joint space is often continuous with one of the lateral joints. The atlantoaxial articulation is thus a three-joint complex and these joints may be partly or freely communicating.

There are two alar ligaments which run obliquely upwards and laterally from the lateral border of the upper dens to the medial aspects of the occipital condyles. These may be round, ovoid, or wing-like in cross-section and broaden from lateral to medial in the frontal plane (Krakenes at al 2001). These ligaments are covered by the tectorial membrane which has a median portion merging with the dura (Krakenes et al 2001). The tectorial membrane between C2 and occiput appears to be a continuation of the posterior longitudinal ligament which runs downwards from the posterior body of C2. There is also an apical ligament which runs from the tip of the dens to the anterior margin of the foramen magnum; it blends with the anterior atlanto-occipital membrane.

The C2 laminae are taller and thicker than those found in other cervical vertebrae. The transverse processes are small but have a number of muscle insertions. They lack distinct tubercles and face obliquely superior and anterior. The vertebral arteries pass laterally through a foramen in each transverse process. The spinous process is bifid with many muscle attachments. The lateral profile of C2 has been used with those of C3 and C4 to develop a cervical maturation index of growth potential in the adolescent (Hassel & Farman 1995) and C2 alone can be used to estimate sex with 83% accuracy in unidentified human skeletal remains (Westcott 2000).

The inferior surface of C2 (Fig. 9.6) forms a three-joint complex with the superior surface of C3. This complex includes the uppermost intervertebral disk of the spine. The lateral facets arise at the junction of the lamina and pedicle and face anteriorly, inferiorly, and a little laterally, and are of the smaller size typical in the cervical spine. The resultant zygapophyseal joints have type III menisci which are rather small nubs common to the remaining levels of the cervical spine (Cramer & Darby 1995 p. 115).

The C2–3 complex may also have uncovertebral joints formed by the uncinate processes which arise from the lateral and posterior margins of the superior surface of the C3 body. These may form synovial articulations with small indentations on the inferior surface of C2. These uncovertebral joints are also known as the joints of von Luschka and become more prominent in the lower cervical spine. They seem to allow flexion and extension

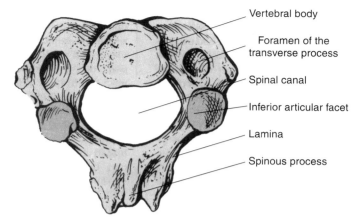

Figure 9.6 Inferior view of C2. From Cramer & Darby (1995), with permission.

while limiting lateral flexion, and provide a barrier to lateral and posterior disk protrusion. These joints appear in the second decade and are frequently subject to later degeneration. Authors differ in their opinion as to whether they are a normal progressive developmental change or a consequence of degenerative change.

ASSESSMENT OF KINEMATIC CHANGE

Postural assessment

The postural assessment will emphasize head alignment relative to the shoulders, both in the frontal plane as assessed from behind the patient and in the sagittal plane as assessed from beside the patient; however, it must be undertaken within the context of the global assessment of the patient. It is important to identify postural change which reflects a segmental or regional cause as opposed to change being a correction or compensation for significant dysfunction lower in the spine and pelvis. This is achieved by examining the full spine of the patient in the global/regional/segmental sequence, then by seeking the segmental and regional evidence of cervical involvement, and finally by interpreting these findings in the global context of the patient and the spinal condition.

Typical findings and their interpretation in terms of spinal fixation are given in Figure 9.7. The role of muscle must also be carefully assessed, as a high mastoid may be indicative of a hypertonic or shortened contralateral trapezius. The assessment is not quite this simple, however, as components of head rotation must be carefully noted as well as head carriage from the side-view. Chin tucking or elevation while the cervical curve appears normal is suggestive of upper cervical dysfunction. Head rotation may reflect weakness in the ipsilateral sternomastoid and cleidomastoid muscles, and head tilt may suggest weak contralateral scalenes.

Static palpation

The occiput and mastoid processes form the initial landmark. If the patient is seated, the examiner's position is posterolateral to the patient, using the indifferent hand on the vertex as a support and the thumb and fingers of the contact hand for palpation. The practitioner slides the contacts medially and anteroinferiorly from the mastoids into the space between the mastoid and C1. With the assumption of structural symmetry, an increased muscle/tissue bulging may be palpated on the side of posterior rotation or fixation.

The key principle is to palpate for the differences in tissue tension *between* the bony landmarks. This is more indicative of dysfunction than any perceived malposition of bony structures which may, after all, be normal bony asymmetry (Ross et al 1999). The same principle applies to dynamic palpation; the qualitative changes in the tissues as they are moved *between* segments is as important as the quantitative and qualitative assessment of the actual segment's movement. The palpatory findings must, as always, be considered within the total patient context.

When using a thumb and finger to palpate for the symmetry of structures, remember the thumb is usually larger and presents a greater data-gathering surface than the opposing finger which will be palpating the opposite side. Assess the symmetry of tissue tone in the atlanto-occipital space and about the upper cervical complex and note any tenderness and/or hypertonicity of the soft-tissue structures.

Radiographic analysis

The upper cervical spine complex is best seen on the lateral cervical and the anterior-posterior open-mouth (APOM) plain films. The lateral view demonstrates changes about the x-axis (Fig. 9.8). A line (c–c') perpendicular to the odontoid line (line a–a' drawn through the vertical axis of the dens) is extended though the body and posterior arch of C2. A line (b–b') drawn between the anterior and posterior tubercles of C1 represents the atlas plane line. A further line (not shown) drawn through the anterior and posterior aspects of the foramen magnum represents the foramen magnum line. It is considered that optimal relationships are present in the upper cervical complex when the three plane lines are parallel (Herbst 1968). These lines are not really subject to meaningful errors of projectional distortion.

The APOM view may demonstrate the lateral and rotary position of C1; however, these observations are subject to projectional distortion. It is thought that when C1 is rotated, the projected image of the more posterior lateral mass (Fig. 9.9, line a–a') appears narrower than that of the more anterior lateral mass (Fig. 9.9, line b–b'). This reflects the crescent shape of the lateral mass and the angulation of its long axis which converges medially towards the anterior. Posterior rotation brings the long axis of the lateral mass to a more sagittal alignment, thus its projected outline appears to narrow.

It is thought the radiolucent zone between the medial border of the lateral mass and the lateral border of the dens will appear to widen on the side of posterior rotation of C1 (Taylor & Resnick 2000 p. 82); however, this lucency is also affected by putative laterality of C1 which would also appear to widen the paraodontoid zone. The system of Gonstead radiographic analysis addresses this by comparing the planes of the C1 and C2 segments as they appear on the APOM view, to determine which lateral mass is elevated (Herbst 1968).

The relationships of the upper cervical complex in the frontal plane as projected on plain radiograph are represented in

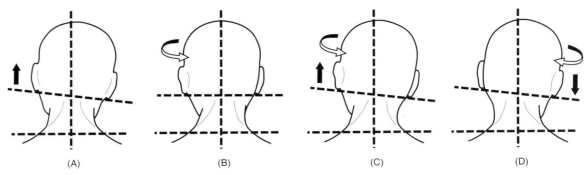

(A)   (B)   (C)   (D)

Figure 9.7 Postural findings suggestive of upper cervical fixation. (A) A high mastoid with level shoulders and no head rotation suggests a superior occiput on the high side or a sunken condyle (inferior occiput) on the low side. This may also be suggestive of a lateral fixation of the atlas on the side of the high mastoid. (B) A level head with rotation (left rotation is shown) with level shoulders suggests the occiput may be posterior on the side of rotation. There may be some contralateral translation. (C) A high mastoid with ipsilateral rotation with level shoulders suggests an ipsilateral posteriority of C1. This may also be interpreted as a contralateral anteriority of C1. The atlas may also rotate posteriorly without occipital tilt. (D) A low mastoid with ipsilateral head rotation is suggestive of C2 involvement, listed as posterior and inferior on the same side as the low mastoid and head rotation. A more prominent jaw angle on the low side is thought to be particularly suggestive of a C2 involvement, either on its own or associated with C1. After Schafer (1983), with permission.

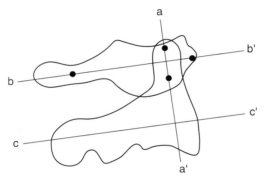

Figure 9.8 Lateral radiographic view of C1 on C2. Line a–a′ = the odontoid line; b–b′ = the plane line of the atlas (C1); c–c′ = the reference line of C2 for comparison with C1, drawn perpendicular to the odontoid line. After course notes, RMIT, with permission.

Figure 9.10. Plane lines are drawn to allow observation of changes to the normal relationships which are parallel. When the occiput appears raised on the atlas (which remains parallel to C2) it is thought the occiput is "lateral" on that side. Anterior and posterior rotation of the occiput is said to be accompanied by compensation of C1 which rotates in the opposite direction, hence the "lateral and posterior" occiput will appear to be wedged higher and is considered "posterior" as the ipsilateral lateral mass of C1 rotates anteriorly to compensate, and also appears wider in its projected image.

C2 is also assessed on whichever view shows it most clearly, usually the APOM, or perhaps the AP lower cervical. A plane line is drawn between two identifiable bilateral landmarks and compared for signs of lateral tilt or wedging, with a similar line drawn through C3.

Objective structural change of SMU mechanics

A number of anomalies are found about the upper cervical complex. A common finding is the posterior ponticulus, described

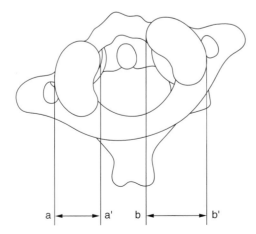

Figure 9.9 Superior (axial) view of C1 in left rotation on C2. The projected outline of the left lateral mass, which is more posterior than the right, will be narrower than that of the right (anterior) lateral mass. After course notes, RMIT, with permission.

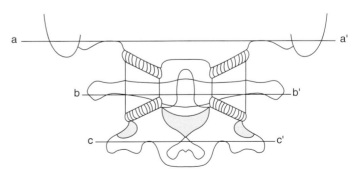

Figure 9.10 Posterior view of occiput on C1 on C2. Line a–a′ represents the level of the occiput in the frontal plane; b–b′ represents the level of the atlas in the frontal plane; and c–c′ represents the axis. Similar lines may also be drawn on the lower segments of the cervical spine. After course notes, RMIT, with permission.

earlier. More significant findings include agenesis or non-union of the dens, as os odontoideum (Taylor & Resnick 2000 p. 56). The adult X-ray will show a smooth, wide, lucent defect separating the odontoid process from the C2 body at the level of the superior articular processes. There may be associated stress hypertrophy of the anterior tubercle of the atlas. Flexion/extension radiographs of the lateral cervical spine are required in the patient under 5 years of age to demonstrate hypermobility of the odontoid process of the C2 body. This defect may be associated with Down's syndrome, Klippel–Feil syndrome, and Morquio's syndrome. The patient may demonstrate clinical findings such as syncope from compression of the vertebral artery where there is instability of the atlantoaxial joint such as os odontoideum (Moser et al 1993, Sasaki et al 2000).

Other anomalies about C1 include ossiculum terminale persistens of Bergman (Taylor & Resnick 2000 p. 54), agenesis of the posterior arch (p. 49), agenesis of the anterior arch, and spina bifida occulta.

There may be fusion anomalies secondary to ossification variations, such as occipitalization of the atlas. Failure of normal fusion may also lead to occipital vertebrae, such as a third condyle, paracondyloid process, paramastoid process, or epitransverse process. Anomalies about the occiput include accessory ossicles and platybasia/basilar impression. All are described and illustrated in radiographic atlases such as Taylor & Resnick (2000) and Yochum & Rowe (1996). These anomalies allow patterns of movement which are normal to the individual but different in comparison to patients without such structural change.

Articular pillar fracture may be associated with trauma, usually seen as a chip fracture of a superior articular facet. It is frequently undetected and may produce transient radicular pain followed by mild to intense neck pain and, if the radicular pain persists, it may suggest displacement of the fragment on to the dorsal root (Cramer & Darby 1995 p. 115).

The arch of C1 may fracture, either uni- or bilaterally (Jefferson's fracture, Taylor & Resnick 2000 p. 83) and this needs to be differentiated from a failure of ossification. The APOM view may show lateral displacement of the lateral mass or masses.

A more serious fracture is that of the dens from the body of C2, or of the body and dens from the posterior elements (hangman's fracture, Yochum & Rowe 1996 pp. 672–673). It is not appropriate to request radiographic stress views of this region when trauma is reported until fracture has been clearly ruled out, as the act of flexion or extension may shift fragments and compromise the cord. Avulsion may be seen in the lateral view as a "teardrop" fracture of the anteroinferior margin of the C2 body (Yochum & Rowe 1996 pp. 674, 678–679).

Dislocation in the C1–2 complex is usually associated with fracture. The C2–3 zygapophyseal joints may be dislocated either uni- or bilaterally. A unilateral dislocation is more stable than bilateral; however, both require immediate orthopedic referral.

Reactive osseous hypertrophy may be seen on the radiograph as increased density and bony enlargement about the uncovertebral and zygapophyseal joints. This may alter movement patterns at the particular level (Yochum & Rowe 1996 pp. 807–810). Pathological hypertrophy is not common in this region but may be seen in C1 or C2 with Paget's disease (Yochum & Rowe 1996 p. 1144).

Other diagnostic imaging assessment

The axial computed tomography (CT) scan has been described as demonstrating the relative positions of rotation of the occiput, C1, and C2 (Ebrall & Molyneux 1993). While CT images are able to demonstrate relative rotation of spinal segments about the y-axis, their clinical usefulness is limited to empirical observation as the research has not yet been undertaken to demonstrate any correction of such rotational misalignment after adjustment.

The MRI is useful to demonstrate soft-tissue relationships, including ossification or other change of the transverse ligament, and plays a vital role in demonstrating neoplastic infiltration and changes in neural tissue.

Subjective nature of movement

The active movement by the patient is assessed for both quantity and quality. Quantity is observed in terms of what is probably normal for each particular patient and is very dependent on a side-to-side comparison. The quality of movement is also compared bilaterally and is an assessment of the manner in which the movement is occurring, with a particular emphasis on smoothness. Jerky movements may be reflective of kinematic change secondary to muscle involvement as well as SC. It is important to maintain an interactive dialogue with the patient regarding the presence and nature of any pain associated with movement.

The active range of motion of the region is assessed with the patient seated and with the head and cervical spine in neutral. The patient is asked to rotate the head fully towards one shoulder, back to the midline, and then to the other, while the practitioner stands behind the patient, supporting the patient's shoulders with both hands. Normal rotation is about 70–80° left and right, from neutral.

Lateral flexion left and right is then assessed by asking the patient to lean each ear towards the respective shoulder. Normal lateral flexion of the cervical spine is about 45–55° left and right, from neutral; however, only about 5° arises from the atlanto-occipital joint and a further 5° from the atlantoaxial joint.

Flexion and extension are assessed with the practitioner to the side of the patient, and then by asking the patient to look all the way to the ceiling and to return to neutral. Normal extension is about 75–90°. In the neutral position the patient is asked to tuck the chin in. This should isolate flexion to the upper cervical complex as opposed to flexing the whole neck. Normal chin-tuck is 20–30°. Flexion/extension restriction in the upper cervical complex is manifested by pain or discomfort as reported by the patient with chin-tuck, or stiffness observed by the practitioner as restriction or asymmetry.

Rotation within the upper cervical complex is then specifically assessed from behind by asking the patient to flex the neck fully and then to look left and right. Flexion locks the lower cervical spine, limiting its contribution to rotation and emphasizing the rotation of C1 on C2. The range of motion is normally about 45°. The examiner's index finger may be placed on the patient's vertex to stabilize the head and help maintain a neutral axis. End-feel may be assessed by gently drawing the contralateral side of the chin towards the side of rotation at the end of the

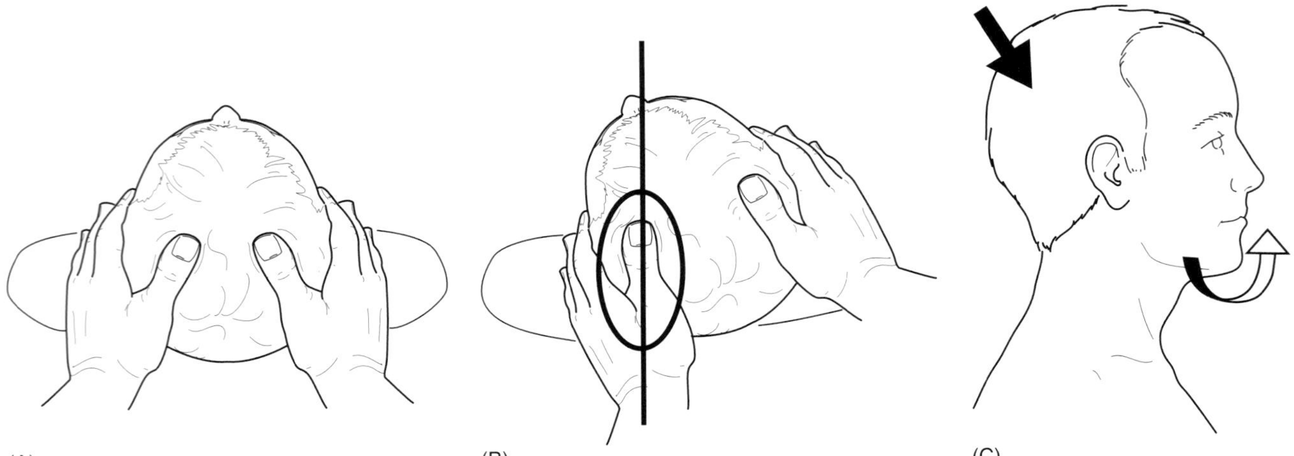

Figure 9.11 Assessment of the atlanto-occipital joint. (A) Both hands are placed in a palmar grip over the parietal bones with each thumb angled 30–40° anteromedially to replicate the angle of the long axis of the atlanto-occipital joint. (B) The head is turned 30–40° ipsilaterally so the thumb and the long axis of the joint are aligned in the sagittal plane. The position for the left joint is shown. (C) An anterior and inferior vector is provided by the ipsilateral thumb and palm and the chin is expected to scoop smoothly anteriorly and superiorly.

movement while stabilizing the parietal surface with the palm of the indifferent hand.

The above movements may be repeated passively by supporting the head with two hands and working through each of the six movements. End-feel is particularly useful with rotation, but more so when the head is rotated with the neck in full flexion. End-feel is less useful with the spine in neutral due to the difficulty in determining the spinal level associated with any alteration.

Pain-sensitive structures such as menisci may be irritated with cervical compression, and existing pain due to these structures may be relieved by cervical distraction. The compression may be as simple as the approximation of surfaces during lateral flexion, and the upper cervical complex is implicated when the patient can specifically touch the area of discomfort. On the other hand, cervical distraction may be quite painful when there is ligamentous involvement. Axial cervical compression will also affect structures in the subaxial spine and these assessment processes are discussed in detail in Chapter 10.

Assessment of the individual joints

Occiput–C1 left

The patient is seated and the practitioner position is standing behind the patient. A light bilateral palmar grip is taken over the parietal areas of the patient with the thumbs angled anteromedially about 30–40° (Fig. 9.11A). The patient's head is turned about 30–40° to the left so the left thumb is parallel with the sagittal plane (Fig. 9.11B).

The act of turning the head draws C1 in the same direction, bringing the long axis of the ipsilateral (in this case, the left) joint into the sagittal plane. The purpose is to maximize the diagnostic movements of flexion and extension which are induced into the joint.

A downwards and frontwards scooping movement is then applied through the ipsilateral palm in a vector directed towards

the joint (Fig. 9.11C). The contralateral hand does not apply any force but acts to stabilize the head. The movement of the patient's chin is observed and it should smoothly glide superiorly and anteriorly. Aberrant movement or a resistance to movement felt by the examiner may reflect kinematic change in the left occiput–C1 joint, which is then investigated further with rotation and lateral flexion.

Rotation may be assessed with the examiner in this position but with the hands rotated so the little fingers point down the neck and the index and middle fingers rest in the suboccipital space (Fig. 9.12A). A transverse view depicting left rotation is given in Figure 9.12B. As C1 moves into the elastic end-zone on C2, the occiput continues and rotates a little further, about 3°, and translates a little to the left. This is due to the tightening of the lateral atlanto-occipital ligament (Kapandji 1974 p. 182). This causes a little lateral flexion to the right at the end of rotation.

The palpating fingers will interpret these biomechanical actions as changes in the tone of the suboccipital tissues. In particular, the left transverse process of C1 will seem to glide under the occiput as the occiput rotates a little further posteriorly and rises slightly, while the right transverse process will appear to become slightly more prominent as the right occiput closes down. These findings are normal and occur as rotation moves into the elastic end-zone. A restricted feeling of the right C1 transverse process in the end-zone of left rotation where the occiput does not glide away suggests posterior fixation of C1, which may be listed as a right posterior atlas. Further investigation is needed to determine if the fixation is in the left or right joint, or both.

Some practitioners attempt to palpate the changing relationship between the end of the transverse process of C1 and the angle of the jaw. The reliability of this method is low due to the inclusion of the temporomandibular joint. Further, the patient with an atlas subluxation is usually quite tender on the tip of the transverse process.

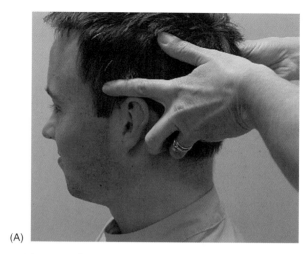
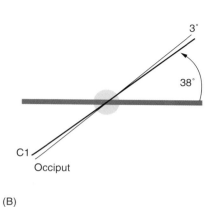

(A)   (B)

Figure 9.12 Assessment for rotary fixation at the atlanto-occipital joint. (A) Placement of the fingers for palpating rotation at the atlanto-occipital junction in the seated patient. The thumb and first finger support the head, the middle finger is placed with the distal lateral aspect palpating the atlanto-occipital interspace, and the ring and little fingers support the neck. The distal anterolateral tip of the middle finger is palpating for occipital movement while the distal lateral tip palpates the transverse process of C1. (B) A transverse view depicting left rotation. C1 rotates on C2 and follows the occiput to provide the majority of rotation, about 38°. As C1 moves into the elastic end-zone on C2, the occiput continues and rotates a little further, about 3°. It also translates a little ipsilaterally (to the left) and this causes slight contralateral lateral flexion (to the right).

Lateral flexion is assessed by standing behind and to the side of the patient and palpating the atlanto-occipital spaces bilaterally to feel for closure on ipsilateral lateral flexion and opening on contralateral lateral flexion. The indifferent hand is placed on the vertex and the head laterally flexed over the palpating digits. Assessment is made of the tissue response on the left in a comparative manner with that on the right.

The decision of whether or not to adjust the complex with a left-sided contact is made within the context of the particular paradigm of practice and with consideration of all clinical findings.

Occiput–C1 right

The above is repeated for the right joint, with reversal of left to right. That is, the head is turned 30–40° to the right so it is the right thumb which comes to lie in the sagittal plane and it is the right joint into which the test vectors are directed.

When the patient is in the supine position, the comparative posterior to anterior glide for each joint is assessed by placing the fingers on the left and right sides of the posterior arch of C1 and gently drawing it upwards. Restriction may be felt. Rotation, lateral flexion, and lateral glide of C1 under the occiput are then assessed with subtle variations of this contact. It is important to repeat the posterior-anterior glide, rotation, and lateral flexion movements while palpating in the suboccipital space between C1 and the occiput. Much clinical information is gained by assessing the tissue tension and its responses to movement in this area. Unilateral restriction is suggestive of ipsilateral posterior rotation and fixation of the joint.

C1–2

Rotation is the major movement at the atlantoaxial junction. The global rotation of the cervical spine is about 70° (range 61–84°,

occiput to T1) and about half that, or 40° (range 29–46°) occurs at this junction (Giles & Singer 1998 p. 59). The examiner's position is posterolateral to the seated patient with the indifferent hand stabilizing and rotating the head while the palpating fingers feel for movement of the posterior tubercle of C1 in relation to the spinous process of C2. It must be noted that rotation and lateral flexion are coupled movements from C2 to T1 and care must be taken to induce rotation with the head remaining neutral with respect to lateral flexion and flexion/extension.

The C1 vertebra follows the occiput in rotation, thus the posterior tubercle of C1 moves contralaterally to the rotation of the patient's face. The palpating digits are best placed towards the transverse processes of C1 to assess for any restriction in rotation in the seated patient. Supine assessment is particularly effective for C1 rotation as the doctor can efficiently assess the subtle initial changes to movement by applying a bilateral posterior-anterior gliding contact. The examiner can also assess the nature of movement during passive rotation and end-feel in each of maximal left and right rotation. The findings are considered in terms of quantity of movement with notation of any restriction; quality of movement within the normal range with the notation of variation; and quality of movement into the elastic barrier, or end-feel.

The C1 posterior tubercle may also be palpated during flexion and extension to identify whether there may be an extension fixation (reduced superior movement of the tubercle in flexion; normal closure on to C2 in extension). It is common for the atlas to be fixed in extension and for the posterior tubercle to be closed down on the C2 spinous, making it difficult to distinguish C1 from C2; however, these findings must be considered in light of the information gained from the lateral cervical radiograph. It is also effective to palpate broadly over the region to sense the relative movements of all segments.

Any suggestion of unilateral superiority (lateral wedging) of C1 may be sensed through assessment of its movement during lateral flexion. The palpating digits should be placed more laterally, over the space between the C1–2 transverse processes, remembering the increasing shift towards the midline of the lateral structures in this region. Feel for restricted motion in lateral flexion. There may be a palpable sensation of blockage or restriction on lateral flexion of C1. This may be felt as a lack of close-down motion on the side ipsilateral to the lateral flexion of the head, suggesting a superiority of C1 on C2 on that side.

A judgment has to be made as to whether this represents a contralateral close-down as an inferiority about the z-axis due to contraction of the contralateral soft-tissue structures, or an increased opening (superiority) due to ipsilateral hypotonicity secondary to pathological change in the soft tissues. Usually the posterior side will be listed and will thus be either superior or inferior. As with all clinical decision making, a working diagnosis is never made on the call of one finding; all findings must be integrated by the practitioner so the most appropriate working diagnosis can be synthesized and then supported by relevant clinical evidence.

The final assessment should rule out any perceived laterality of C1, although it is difficult to distinguish between lateral wedging and laterality, as the two exist together. Further, these movements of occiput and C1 result in coupled rotation of C2 (Giles & Singer 1998 p. 61). It is thought the atlas may translate laterally without any commensurate rotation about the y-axis or the z-axis. The findings most useful in this scenario are those of pain and tenderness over the lateral aspect of the transverse process on the ipsilateral side of lateral translation, and a sensation of restricted lateral glide away from the side of laterality. These findings may be evident while palpating slightly under the transverse processes of C1 with the thumb and finger in the tissue space between C1 and C2, while laterally flexing the head with the indifferent hand on the vertex. Comparison of symmetry may suggest more tissue bulk about the transverse process on the side of laterality.

C2–3

C2 is the most superior vertebra of the spine to have an intervertebral disk below its body, hence the C2–3 SMU carries those characteristics typical of the three-joint SMU which consists of a disk and two zygapophyseal joints.

Consideration must remain, however, for the unique relationship of C2–3 with C1 above. It is not possible or sensible to isolate this SMU to only two vertebrae and the three-joint complex between them; C1 is affected by the occiput above as well as by C2 below. The astute practitioner attempts to find a position of "most likely" as opposed to "truth" by assessing these intricate interdependent relationships.

The C2 spinous moves contralaterally to the rotation of the C2 body which follows the patient's face. As the face is rotated to the left, the C2 spinous process will move to the right. The C2 spinous process is also palpated during flexion and extension to identify whether there may be an extension fixation palpated as reduced superior movement of the spinous process in flexion with the feeling of normal closure in extension.

Any suggestion of unilateral superiority (lateral wedging) of C2 may be sensed through assessment of the spinous process movement during lateral flexion. Normal movement is for the spinous process to shift to the side of spinal convexity in lateral

flexion. This means the spinous should move to the right with left lateral flexion. The coupling between C2 and C3 creates rotary movement and the spinous process will also arc upwards as it moves to the right with left lateral flexion. The practitioner must feel for the quality of these expected movements.

The direction of lateral flexion which produces altered movement of the spinous suggests the side of fixation: restricted or aberrant movement, mainly to the left, of the spinous process during right lateral flexion suggests a right fixation of C2 on C3, perhaps listed as a right posterior superior C2.

The palpating digits may also be placed more laterally over the C2–3 articular pillars to identify any restricted motion. Lateral flexion of the segment should feel smoother, easier, and more complete to the side opposite any putative superiority. For example, if the C2 segment is perceived to be fixated as superior on the right, then lateral flexion to the left would feel normal and lateral flexion to the right would feel restricted.

The final assessment should rule out any perceived laterality of C2. The toggle-recoil system of analysis and adjustment considers that this segment may shift entirely laterally, giving the listings entire segment left (ESL) and its complement, ESR. Comparison of symmetry may suggest more tissue bulk about the transverse process on the side of putative laterality, and there should be no detectable aberrations in rotation, flexion/extension, or lateral flexion.

Plaugher echoes the Gonstead belief that the upper cervical complex is likely to act to compensate for fixation elsewhere due to the "righting reflex". He suggests that pain and tenderness in the upper cervical musculature could be due to a subluxation complex in the lower cervical or upper thoracic regions creating a cervical hypolordosis or kyphosis, in turn causing added tension in the neck extensors from anterior carriage of the head (Plaugher 1993 p. 303). Other practitioners generally place great emphasis on the upper cervical complex as the location of the primary fixation in the spine (Palmer 1966).

ASSESSMENT OF CONNECTIVE TISSUE CHANGE

There are significant challenges in demonstrating an involvement of any specific ligament of the upper cervical complex from clinical assessment. Basic imaging such as the lateral cervical radiograph can provide limited quantitative data and, while advanced imaging modalities such as MRI may be useful, the clinical relevance of MR findings remains limited in the identification of the source of neck pain in symptomatic patients (Pfirrmann et al 2000), although progress continues to be made in refining the imaging techniques (Krakenes et al 2001).

Pragmatically, various ligaments will be injured with any trauma to the cervical spine which produces a rapid strain of the structures and must be considered when determining treatment protocols and outcomes measurements. The non-acute patient is more challenging; however, the practitioner is usually able to apply a range of tests which may implicate some deep structures, although it remains difficult to identify specific involvement concisely. Notwithstanding these challenges, the effective practitioner will have a thorough knowledge of the ligamentous anatomy and their respective roles in the function of the upper cervical complex.

The following soft-tissue dimensions should be measured on the lateral cervical neutral radiograph:

- Atlantodental interspace (ADI) measured from the posterior border of the anterior arch of atlas to the anterior margin of the dens of C2 and normally 1–3 mm in adults and up to 5 mm in children. An increase suggests a decrease in support of the transverse ligament (see below) and may be accompanied by atlantoaxial instability sufficient to affect the spinal cord.
- Retropharyngeal interspace (RPI) measured from the anteroinferior margin of C2 and C3 to the contour representing the posterior wall of the pharynx and normally up to 5 mm at C2 and up to 7 mm at C3. An increase suggests swelling of the tissues anterior to the vertebral column. This finding may follow trauma such as cervical acceleration/deceleration (whiplash) in a motor vehicle accident, or may be associated with neoplasia.

Ligaments of the complex

The ligaments of the atlanto-occipital joint capsules are thin and may be non-existent medially, allowing the synovial cavity of the joint about the occipital condyle and C1 lateral mass to connect with the joint cavity between the dens and the transverse atlantal ligament (Cramer & Darby 1995 p. 127). This anatomical possibility reinforces the clinical wisdom of considering the atlanto-occipital joint as more than a simple two-joint articulation. Iatrogenic irritation of the atlanto-occipital joint capsule has been shown to refer pain ipsilaterally about the occiput, extending up behind the ear and down to the mid-neck, and described as deep, boring, and aching (Dreyfuss et al 1994).

The articular capsules at C2–3 are thin and loose and are collagen fibers which run inferiorly from around the articular facet of the inferior process of C2 to around the facet of the superior process (on C3), below. They lie perpendicular to the plane of the zygapophyseal joint. The involvement of ligaments is suggested when localized pain is produced with movements which produce strain within the ligament, such as contralateral lateral flexion or cervical distraction. Iatrogenic irritation of the lateral atlantoaxial joint capsule has been shown to refer pain ipsilaterally in the suboccipital region (Dreyfuss et al 1994).

The zygapophyseal menisci are quite large at the C2–3 articulation and their involvement is suspected when localized pain is produced with movements which compress the joint surfaces and the meniscus, such as ipsilateral lateral flexion or cervical compression.

The ligaments within the upper cervical complex (Fig. 9.5) include the transverse ligament, cruciform ligament with a superior and (often) an inferior longitudinal band, the alar ligaments, and the accessory atlantoaxial ligaments. The contributions of these ligaments to the kinematics of the complex are partly known (Kapandji 1974) and their involvement is suspected with aberrant patterns of movement, particularly of occiput on C1 in rotation and lateral flexion.

The transverse ligament may soften and become lax or rupture in patients with rheumatoid arthritis, Reiter's syndrome, Down's syndrome, ankylosing spondylitis, and psoriatic arthritis. Conversely, it may calcify as part of the degenerative process of osteoarthritis (Zapletal et al 1995, Hayashi et al 1998).

The alar ligaments may also be torn in a rear-end motor vehicle collision where the head is rotated. A torn alar ligament increases the rotation of occiput on C1 and of C1 on C2 to the contralateral side (Pfirrmann et al 2000).

The anterior longitudinal ligament attaches to the inferior border of C2 in close association with the fibers of the annulus of the C2–3 disk and the posterior longitudinal ligament attaches to the posterior aspect of the C2 body before continuing superiorly as the tectorial membrane. Involvement of these ligaments usually follows trauma and they will contribute to a deep pain worsened by resisted flexion or extension. Ossification of the posterior longitudinal ligament and its rare association with atlantoaxial subluxation sufficient to cause spastic quadriplegia has been documented (Takasita et al 2000).

The lateral and posterolateral fibers of the disk may be protected by the uncinate processes and joints (Giles & Singer 1998 p. 32). They provide a bulwark of bone which may protect against disk protrusion. The C2–3 disk exhibits the same characteristics as the remaining cervical disks and, while the nucleus is present at birth, it becomes less evident through adolescence and has mainly disappeared above the age of 40 years. The adult disk is ligamentous and dry and is composed of fibrocartilage and islands of hyaline cartilage (Giles & Singer 1998 p. 30).

C2 disk protrusion is uncommon and when it does occur it is usually secondary to trauma with forced movements of flexion, extension, and rotation which cause discoligamentary shearing and the sudden ejection of disk material into the spinal canal (Chen 2000). Radicular symptoms above C3–4 are difficult to identify clinically; however, a C2–3 disk injury sufficient to impinge on the cord is thought to impair motor and sensory function more in the upper extremities and may alter facial and perioral sensation. The signs of less serious C2 disk involvement are non-focal and include headache, tinnitus, and dizziness. There is a predominant suboccipital discomfort as opposed to middle- and lower-neck pain (Chen 2000).

Ligamentum nuchae

Perhaps the most clinically relevant connective tissue about the upper cervical complex is that constructing the ligamentum nuchae, which extends in the posterior midline from the spinous process of C7 to the external occipital protuberance (EOP). Johnson et al (2000) have demonstrated that the dorsal portion of the ligamentum nuchae is formed by the bilateral aponeuroses of four muscles:

1. trapezius
2. rhomboid minor
3. serratus posterior superior
4. splenius capitis.

Their respective levels of spinal attachment create a layered arrangement of aponeuroses running within the dorsal portion of the ligament. These muscular aponeurotic fibers are bilaminar and make a substantial contribution to the fine connective architecture of the ligamentum nuchae (Johnson et al 2000).

It has earlier been reported (Mitchell at al 1998) that continuity was observed between the ligamentum nuchae and the posterior cervical dura as the latter passed deeply from the midline toward the dura at the levels of C1 and C2. However, Johnson et al (2000) feel their results strongly contradict this finding. They argue that the posterior midline space in the upper cervical region is occupied largely by loose connective tissue that bridges the midline and continues laterally with the investing layer of deep cervical fascia. On the other hand, a recent study has again demonstrated continuity in the midline between the nuchal ligament and the posterior spinal dura at the atlanto-occipital and atlantoaxial intervals (Dean & Mitchell 2002). While more work is needed to clarify the fine relations of the ligamentum nuchae and the spinal dura, it is also known that there are connective tissue bridges between the rectus capitis superior minor and the dorsal spinal dura (Hack et al 1995).

The clinical relevance is straightforward: there is evidence that the spinal dura about the suboccipital region is linked by connective tissue to muscles about the spine, hence any assessment of the upper cervical complex is incomplete without assessment of the suboccipital muscles and of the muscles which contribute to the ligamentum nuchae.

ASSESSMENT OF MUSCLE CHANGE
The small intrinsic muscles of the complex

The rectus capitis posterior major arises from the spinous process of C2 and inserts into the lateral part of the inferior nuchal line of the occipital bone (Fig. 9.13). It crosses two joint complexes (atlanto-occipital and atlantoaxial) and extends and somewhat laterally flexes the head, and ipsilaterally rotates the face. The rectus capitis posterior minor arises from the posterior tubercle of C1 and inserts into the occipital bone below the inferior nuchal line (Fig. 9.13). It crosses the atlanto-occipital joint complex and acts to extend the head.

The anterior fascia of the rectus capitis posterior minor passes around the anterior side of the posterior arch of the atlas to reach the spinal dura mater (Kahn et al 1992), thus forming a connective tissue bridge between the muscle and the dorsal spinal dura at the atlanto-occipital junction (Hack et al 1995). Kahn et al (1992) also found the anterior fasciae of the rectus capitis posterior major and of the inferior oblique muscle to

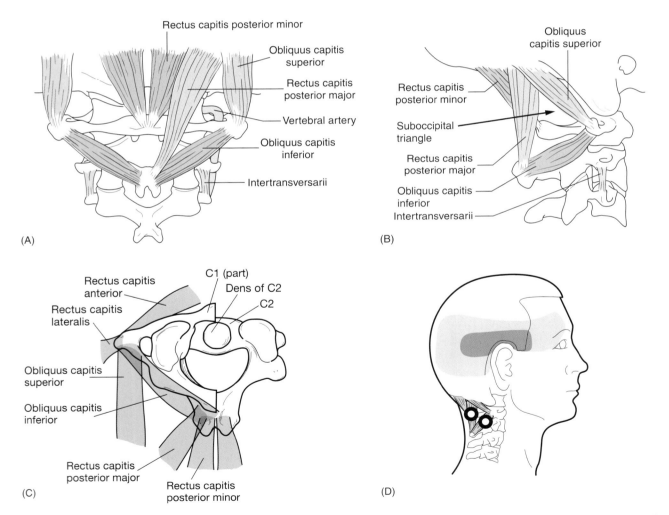

Figure 9.13 The suboccipital muscles. (A) Posterior view demonstrating the positioning of the inferior oblique for sensing rotation of C1 on C2. (B) Lateral view demonstrating the positioning of the rectus capitis posterior major and the superior oblique for flexion and extension of the head. (C) Superior view demonstrating the axial relationship. (D) The accepted trigger point location and pattern of pain referral. (A, B, D) From Chaitow & DeLany (2000), with permission; (C) modified from Giles & Singer (1998), with permission.

extend to the spinal dura mater at the atlantoaxial space. The manner in which the fibers are arranged suggest that the purpose is to resist movement of the dura toward the spinal cord and it is felt this relationship may allow anatomic and physiologic causes of cervicogenic headache (Alix & Bates 1999).

The obliquus capitis superior arises from the transverse process of C1 and inserts into the occipital bone above the inferior nuchal line (Fig. 9.13). It crosses the atlanto-occipital joint complex and extends and ipsilaterally laterally flexes the head. The obliquus capitis inferior arises from the spinous process of C2 and inserts into the transverse process of C1 (Fig. 9.13). It crosses the atlantoaxial joint complex and ipsilaterally rotates C1 and the head around the odontoid process of C2.

Together, the rectus capitis posterior major, rectus capitis posterior minor, obliquus capitis superior, and obliquus capitis inferior are referred to as the suboccipital muscles and each is supplied by muscular branches of the posterior primary rami of the first (suboccipital) nerve and the blood supply is from muscular branches of the vertebral artery and the descending branch of the occipital artery. The communicating branches between the C1 and C2 spinal nerves may allow some innervation also by the second cervical nerve (Blume 2000).

They are assessed by careful palpation and resistance to their individual movements and they may be painful on chin-tuck. When the four muscles on one side contract together they produce slight lateral flexion of the head with associated ipsilateral head rotation accompanied with extension (Chaitow & DeLany 2000). They are implicated when there is a loss of rotation, as in looking over the shoulder, and by deep-seated posterior neck pain. Patients may complain of a distressing headache caused promptly when the weight of the occiput presses against the pillow at night (Simons et al 1999 pp. 472–483).

The suboccipital trigger points (Fig. 9.13D) refer pain which is difficult to localize but seems to penetrate into the skull, extending forward unilaterally to the occiput, to the eye and the forehead, with a lack of clearly defined limits (Simons et al 1999). The headache is described as wrapping around the side of the head to the eyes (Chaitow & DeLany 2000).

The muscles, particularly the obliques, have a very high spindle receptor content, which suggests they are involved in proprioception (Kulkarni et al 2001). The inferior oblique muscle is diagonally inserted from the spine of C2 to the lateral tubercle of C1, which subjects it to stretch during almost the entire range of rotation of C1 on C2. The proprioceptive afferents from these muscles converge with vestibular and ocular inputs at various levels of the neuroaxis (Kulkarni et al 2001). The recti demonstrate marked atrophy on MRI in patients with chronic neck pain who in turn show a decrease in balance when standing (McPartland et al 1997).

There are two more small intrinsic muscles within the upper cervical complex. The rectus capitis anterior arises from the anterosuperior aspect of the lateral mass of C1 and inserts into the base of the occiput, anterior to the foramen magnum. It is supplied by anterior branches of C1 and C2, and perhaps C3 spinal nerves. It flexes the head. The rectus capitis lateralis arises from the upper surface of the C1 transverse process and inserts into the inferior surface of the jugular process on the occiput. It is supplied by branches of the anterior rami of C1 and C2 spinal nerves and ipsilaterally laterally flexes the head. Palpation and

treatment of this muscle is an advanced technique to be performed with extreme care (Chaitow & DeLany 2000 p. 226).

Muscles affecting the complex

The suboccipital muscles are deep-seated and intrinsic within the upper cervical complex. The remaining muscles which cross the complex arise from lower in the spine and attach about the complex or on to the occiput. Given that these muscles also act on lower cervical segments, they will be discussed in Chapter 10, with the exception of those muscles which specifically contribute to the ligamentum nuchae, namely the trapezius, rhomboid minor, serratus posterior superior, and the splenii (capitis and cervicis).

The trapezius

The upper or ascending fibers of the trapezius (Fig. 9.14A) attach from the external occipital protuberance, the medial third of the superior nuchal line, the ligamentum nuchae, and the spinous process of C7, and insert into the lateral third of the clavicle and the acromion process. It is commonly understood that it is supplied by the spinal accessory nerve (SAN as cranial nerve XI) and ventral rami of C2, C3, and C4; however, this is not straightforward. The transverse and ascending fibers are innervated by the SAN and the trapezius branches of the cervical plexus; however, the descending (lower) fibers, which run as low as T12, are claimed by one investigative team to be innervated solely by a single fine branch of the SAN (Kierner et al 2001) and by another as receiving motor supply from the cervical plexus (Routal & Pal 2000).

The complexity of the question increases when the spinal nerve accessory nucleus (SNAN) is considered. The nucleus is a column in the cord running a curved route in the ventral horn from the lower medulla to mid-C5 (Routal & Pal 2000). The more cranial neurons of the nucleus receive maximal input from the ipsilateral cerebral hemisphere and a minimal input from the contralateral hemisphere and project to the sternomastoid with a major motor supply to the ipsilateral muscle and a minor supply to the contralateral muscle (DeToledo & Dow 1998, DeToledo & David 2001). It is the more caudal neurons of the SNAN which receive input from the contralateral hemisphere alone and innervate both the trapezius (Routal & Pal 2000) and the ipsilateral cleidomastoid (DeToledo & Dow 1998, DeToledo & David 2001). Further, stimulation of the muscle spindle afferents in the ipsilateral trapezius monosynaptically activate the motor neurons in the contralateral muscle.

The clinical relevance is greatest for stroke patients who lose hemispheric innervation of the cleidomastoid or sternomastoid and present with confusing symptoms. The relevance when assessing the spine is more straightforward; the trapezius is co-functional with the sternomastoid and cleidomastoid muscles and they have a high degree of bilaterality. When the upper cervical complex is implicated with subluxation complex then all relevant muscles must be assessed, including the trapezius bilaterally, the remaining muscles associated with the ligamentum nuchae, the remaining muscles innervated by the SNAN, and those muscles either intrinsic to the complex or crossing it.

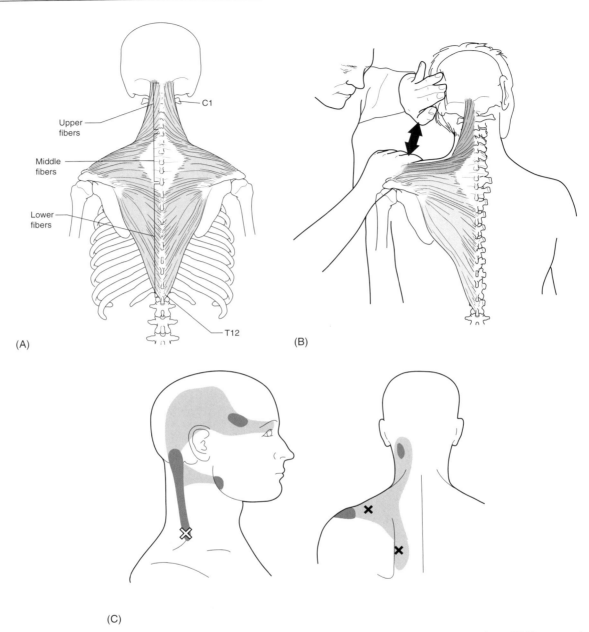

Figure 9.14 The trapezius muscle. (A) Posterior view showing the extent of the attachments and the three divisions. (B) The manual muscle test of the left upper trapezius. The double arrow illustrates the test vector. (C) Trigger point locations and pain referral patterns. (A, C) From Chaitow & DeLany (2000), with permission.

In simple terms the upper trapezius acts on the neck and head when the shoulder is stabilized and is the strongest contralateral rotator of the head (Vasavada & Delp 1998). Bilaterally it acts to extend the cervical spine. When the neck is stable the actions on the scapula are elevation and assistance to rotate the glenoid fossa upward. It is tested with the patient seated with the head laterally flexed a little with some contralateral rotation. The shoulder is also raised a little and the practitioner attempts to draw the head away from the shoulder (Fig. 9.14B).

The medial trigger point in the upper trapezius is found by pincer palpation in the fibers at the lateral base of the neck as they ascend from the clavicle. It refers pain to the temporal area, lateral upper neck to the mastoid process, and maybe to the angle of the jaw and perhaps the teeth (Fig. 9.14C left). The lateral point is found over the supraspinous fossa and it refers pain to the base of the occiput and behind the ear and perhaps to the medial border of the scapula (Fig. 9.14C right).

The rhomboid minor

The rhomboid minor originates from the ligamentum nuchae and the spinous processes of C7 and T1 and has a double fold

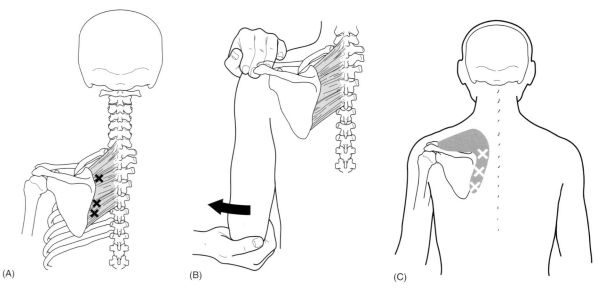

Figure 9.15 The rhomboid minor muscle. (A) Posterior view showing the left rhomboid minor (superior band) and major (inferior band). (B) The manual muscle test of the left rhomboids. The curved arrow illustrates the test vector. (C) Trigger point locations and pain referral patterns.

which inserts about the medial border of the scapula at the root of the spine (Fig. 9.15A). The posterior fold attaches to the dorsal surface of the border and the anterior fold attaches to the costal surface (Bharihoke & Gupta 1986). A rare muscular variant is for slips of the rhomboid to attach cranially as high as the occiput (Rogawski 1990). It is supplied by C4 and C5 as the dorsal scapula nerve and acts to adduct and slightly elevate the scapula and rotate it medially to tilt the glenoid fossa downwards. It is assessed and tested together with its companion, the rhomboid major (Ch. 11). The patient is seated with the elbow flexed by the side. The shoulder is stabilized while the testing hand draws the elbow outwards (Fig. 9.15B). Observe for abduction of the scapula as an indicator of weakness.

Trigger points are rare in the rhomboids. When they are present they are found towards the medial border of the scapula (Fig. 9.15C). Patients may complain of pain between the shoulder blades when they lie on the affected side or try to reach forward. The pain feels like it itches and can be rubbed by the patient and this differentiates it from the pain of serratus posterior superior, which feels too deep-seated to rub (Simons et al 1999 p. 616). A significant association has been reported between the presence of trigger points in rhomboid minor and disk lesions at C4–5, C5–6, and C6–7 (Hsueh et al 1998).

For assessment and treatment the patient lies prone with the ipsilateral forearm and wrist placed in the small of the back to abduct the scapula and expose the rhomboids and the underlying serratus posterior superior. The practitioner stands contralaterally and palpation is across the fibers and laterally towards the border of the scapula.

The serratus posterior superior

The serratus posterior superior originates in the lower portion of the ligamentum nuchae and from the spinous processes of C7

through T3 or T4 and inserts into the upper border of ribs 2 through 5 (Fig. 9.16A). It is innervated by the anterior primary rami (intercostal nerve) of T1 through T4 and its action has traditionally been thought of as elevating the ribs and assisting inspiration; however, this is challenged by Vilensky et al (2001), who propose that this muscle, together with serratus posterior inferior, primarily act as proprioceptors. They argue that there is no electromyogram evidence to support any role in respiration and consider that the muscle spindle density of 14.3/g of muscle tissue categorizes it as a muscle capable of providing proprioceptive input (Vilensky et al 2001). They also note that it has been reported that the muscle is innervated at a higher segmental level than commonly reported in textbooks (C8 vs T1) and consider this is consistent with the referred-pain pattern (Fig. 9.16B).

The trigger point is sought with the patient either prone with the ipsilateral hand in the small of the back, or seated with the ipsilateral hand on the contralateral shoulder. The purpose is to abduct the scapula as the trigger point lies about the insertion and is palpated against the ribs through the trapezius and rhomboids. The pain referral pattern is local and along the back of the arm and about the medial border of the wrist and hand (Fig. 9.16B).

The splenii

The splenius capitis arises from the lower half of the ligamentum nuchae, the spinous processes of the lower four cervical and upper three or four thoracic vertebrae, and inserts into the lateral part of the superior nuchal line, crossing the suture between the occiput and the temporal bone (Fig. 9.17A). The splenius cervicis arises from spinous processes of T3 or T4 to T6, courses around and under splenius capitis, and inserts in the transverse process of C2 and the posterior tubercles of the transverse processes of C3 and maybe C4. They are supplied by

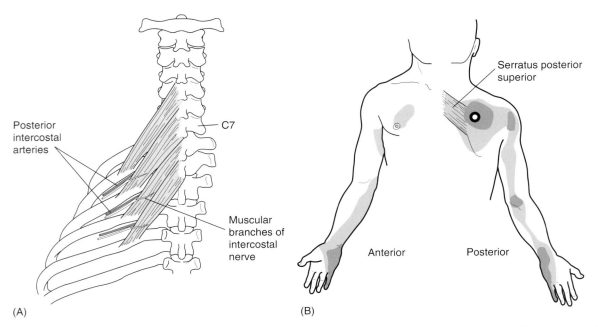

(A)

(B)

Figure 9.16 The serratus posterior superior muscle. (A) Posterior view showing the attachments between the ligamentum nuchae and the spinous processes from C7 to T3, to ribs 2 though 5 just beyond their angles. These levels are variable. (B) The trigger point lies under the scapula and refers pain posteriorly (right) and anteriorly (left). From Chaitow & DeLany (2000), with permission.

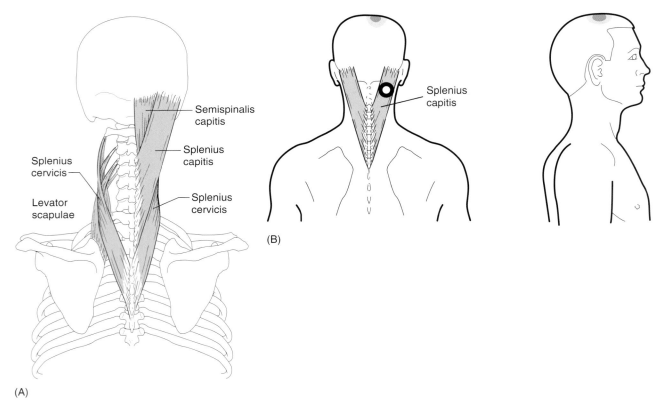

(A)

(B)

Figure 9.17 The splenii muscles. (A) Posterior view showing the attachments of splenius capitis from the ligamentum nuchae and the spinous processes of lower cervical and upper three to four thoracic vertebrae to the lateral part of the superior nuchal line. The diagonal direction of its fibers is distinctive on palpation. (B) The splenius capitis trigger point lies in the upper part of the muscle above where it emerges from under the upper trapezius. (A, B) From Chaitow & DeLany (2000), with permission.

lateral branches of posterior primary rami of middle and low cervical nerves and splenius capitis acts as a strong extensor of the neck and to rotate the head ipsilaterally. It has a subordinate role in ipsilateral lateral flexion (Mayoux-Benhamou et al 1997).

The trigger point in the splenius cervicis is difficult to palpate as it lies deep to trapezius and is bordered laterally by levator scapula. It is palpated in the superior aspect of the muscle as it emerges from under the trapezius. A flat contact is used across the fibers. The patient complains of pain to the top of the head and usually with a stiff neck. The trigger point is perpetuated by postural stress, such as working at a computer with the head turned to read documents and by sleeping with poor head support (Simons et al 1999). A significant association has been reported between the presence of trigger points in splenius capitis and disk lesions at C4–5 and C5–6 (Hsueh et al 1998).

ASSESSMENT OF NEURAL CHANGE

There is a gamut of signs and symptoms, including pain, headache, dizziness, ataxia, nystagmus, visual disturbances, and vertigo, that can be associated with the neck (Bolton 1998). Mild mechanical irritation of the upper cervical region in infants has been linked with heart rate changes (Koch et al 2002) and apnea (Koch et al 1998).

While the positive response of these to manual intervention has been observed by all spinal practitioners for centuries, our collective understanding of mechanisms is still in its infancy. We know that, in addition to signalling nociception, the somatosensory system of the neck may influence the motor control of the neck, eyes, limbs, respiratory muscles, and possibly the activity of some preganglionic nerves (Bolton 1998, Bolton et al 1998). It has also been shown that reflex connections exist between receptors in cervical facet joints and fusimotoneurons of posterior neck muscles, which may explain the pathophysiology associated with whiplash-induced disorders (Thunberg et al 2001). The following comments are a mix of what is known in the scientific sense to underpin what is empirically seen on a day-to-day basis in clinical practice.

The C1 spinal nerve exits the vertebral canal by passing over the posterior arch of the atlas and divides into a ventral and a dorsal ramus (the suboccipital nerve) which is the motor nerve to the suboccipital muscles. It also communicates with the C2 dorsal ramus. The ventral rami innervate the atlanto-occipital joint while the ventral rami of C2 assist innervation of the atlantoaxial joint. Fibers from both the ventral rami of C1 and C2 join with the hypoglossal nerve. Some fibers from C1 travel upwards with the hypoglossal nerve to help provide sensation to the dura mater in the posterior fossa.

The ventral rami of C1 and C2 join with those of C3 to form the ansa cervicalis, which is the motor component of the cervical plexus, providing innervation to the infrahyoid muscles. The cervical plexus includes the ventral rami of C4 and supplies cutaneous innervation to the posterolateral part of the head, neck, and shoulder (Cramer & Darby 1995 p. 254). It is clinically relevant to note that motor fibers from this plexus course as low as the diaphragm.

The ventral ramus of C2 exits by passing posterior to the vertebral artery and through the anterior muscles, innervating them. Dysfunctional movement of the atlantoaxial joint may laterally compress the C2 ventral ramus, perhaps resulting in the "neck–tongue syndrome" where there is suboccipital pain with ipsilateral numbness of the tongue (Cramer & Darby 1995 p. 143).

The C2 dorsal root ganglia are located posteromedially to the lateral atlantoaxial joint and their sensory fibers innervate the medial and lateral zones of the joint. This dorsal root ganglion also has sensory fibers extending to the neck and scalp from the posterior occipital region to the vertex. Its motor function includes longissimus capitis, splenius capitis, and semispinalis capitis.

The median branch of the dorsal ramus of C2 is the greater occipital nerve and it runs through the semispinalis capitis muscle and a "sling" formed around the insertions of the upper trapezius and sternocleidomastoid muscles on to the superior nuchal line. Its terminal branches provide diffuse sensory innervation to the occiput, around the mastoid process and posterior to the ear, and up to the coronal suture and anteriorly through sensory branches to the occipital and transverse facial arteries.

Local pain

Local pain usually reflects local trauma, such as capsular strain. Diffuse local pain may be referred from viscera; in particular, pain which is felt at the angle of the jaw may reflect cardiac involvement. The rich anastomoses among adjacent spinal cord segments allow for nociceptive impulses through the dorsal root ganglion of one spinal level to enter the cord at the level above or below, making it difficult to localize. These anastomoses also disrupt the dermatomal patterns of innervation, resulting in numerous patterns of referred pain from the neck, reflecting the complexity of the pain generators in the region.

Referred pain

The typical nature and patterns of pain referred from trigger points in muscles of the region are given in Table 9.1. Noxious stimulation of the greater occipital nerve can arise from irritation to the nerve as it arises or of the ganglion, particularly through hyperextension injury. Distal interference can arise from hypertonicity of the muscles though which it passes. Noxious stimulation of the superior posterior rootlets of C1 is reported to cause orbital pain; of the middle rootlets, frontal pain; and of the inferior rootlets, vertex pain (Cramer & Darby 1995 p. 140).

Stimulation of the greater occipital nerve induces increased excitability of dural afferent input (Bartsch & Goadsby 2002). A considerable population of neurons has been identified in the superficial and deep layers of the C2 spinal dorsal horn which show a convergent input from the dura as well as from cervical cutaneous and muscle territories. This supports the view of a functional continuum between the caudal trigeminal nucleus and upper cervical segments involved in cranial nociception. Bartsch & Goadsby (2002) demonstrated a facilitatory effect of greater occipital nerve stimulation on dural stimulation, perhaps through a central mechanism at the second-order neuron level, and suggest this mechanism may be important in pain referral from cervical structures to the head. The mechanism is known as nociceptive convergence and it leads to a loss of somatosensory spatial specificity (Piovesan et al 2001).

Table 9.1 Pain patterns arising from trigger points of the region

Description of pain	Probable trigger point location
An ache inside the skull about the vertex	Splenius capitis, lateral to the suboccipital space. Also consider sternomastoid
A shooting pain to the posterior orbit	Splenius cervicis, about the mid to lower cervical spine. Also consider sternomastoid, temporalis, and masseter
Ipsilateral temporal pain	Trapezius, at the base of the neck. Also consider sternomastoid and temporalis
Hat-banding pain	Semispinalis capitis, at its insertion into the occiput. Also consider the suboccipitals
Ipsilateral posterior head pain	Semispinalis cervicis, lateral to the C1–2 transverse processes. Also consider trapezius, sternomastoid, cleidomastoid, suboccipitals
Ipsilateral suboccipital pain	Multifidus, deep about the C4, C5 level
Poorly defined, deep head pain	Suboccipitals, within the medial suboccipital and C1–2 spaces
Pain about the forehead	Cleidomastoid, sternomastoid. Also consider semispinalis capitis and frontalis
Pain in the ear	Cleidomastoid. Also consider masseter and the pterygoids

Medical practitioners have used nerve blocks of the greater occipital nerve in patients with cervicogenic headache and report a long-lasting effect from repeated blocks (Inan et al 2001). They also report the same results from nerve blocks of C2–3.

The C2–3 zygapophyseal joints also refer neck pain and headache and the C3 spinal nerve, the most superior to pass through an intervertebral canal, branches into a dorsal and a ventral ramus in the lateral aspect of the intervertebral canal. The dorsal ramus passes between the transverse processes of C2–3 and branches, one forming the third occipital nerve which passes closely around the lower part of the zygapophyseal joint, providing articular branches to the joints. This close relationship is thought to implicate this nerve in headache secondary to bony degeneration at the C2–3 level. After the joint it pierces semispinalis capitis, splenius capitis, and trapezius, and assists the greater occipital nerve with sensory innervation of the scalp. The deep branch of the C3 spinal nerve is motor to the upper multifidi.

There are sensory nerve fibers throughout the annulus fibrosus of the C2–3 disk, but none in the healthy nucleus pulposus. A large number are consistent with those which transmit pain and it is reported that the annulus is pain-sensitive as well as contributing to proprioception (Cramer & Darby 1995 p. 135). Proprioceptive input from the atlanto-occipital and atlantoaxial joints, along with proprioceptive input from the suboccipital muscles, is responsible for the control of head posture.

There are no specific motor weaknesses or reflex abnormalities associated with a C2 disk lesion. The patient may report difficulty walking, loss of balance, ascending tingling and numbness in the fingers, dysesthesia, or hypesthesia to pinprick stimulation over varied dermatomes (Chen 2000). There may also be sharp pain radiating down the spine and into the upper or lower limbs with head flexion (Lhermitte's sign) and increased symptoms with cervical compression (Spurling's maneuver). Pain may also refer to the vertex, temporal region, around the eyes and retro-orbital region in the presence of a C2 disk lesion (Blume 2000); however, it is not yet known whether this is pain generated and referred from the disk itself or from concomitant trigger points in the surrounding musculature.

Upper cervical injury can also refer pain into the regions of the head supplied by the trigeminal nerve. The central processes of C1–3 converge into the upper spinal cord and on to neurons of the spinal tract and the spinal nucleus of the trigeminal nerve. This is known as the trigeminocervical nucleus. The resultant pain can be felt in the anterior head or from the suboccipital region to the vertex.

The recurrent meningeal nerves of C1, C2, and C3 have relatively large branches which ascend to the posterior cranial fossa (Cramer & Darby 1995 p. 144). They supply the atlantoaxial joint, the tectorial membrane, components of the cruciate ligament of the atlas, and the transverse ligament. Within the fossa they supply the cranial dura mater and are probably related to occipital headaches.

Sensory change

The basic assessment includes recording the bilaterally comparative responses to crude touch and further assessment can include pain or sharp touch, temperature, and vibration. The cutaneous peripheral nerve distributions are:

- greater occipital nerve (C2, C3) to the posteromedial head to the vertex
- lesser occipital nerve (C2) to the posterolateral head
- dorsal rami C3–5 to the posteromedial neck extending to the spine of the scapulae.

The general dermatomal distributions are:

- C2: the posterior head above the nuchal line, to the vertex
- C3: the posterior neck, postauricular, lateral mandible to anterior midline.

Hyperesthesia may be seen in a specific facial distribution as a herpes zoster or trigeminal neuralgia distribution.

Motor function

The basic assessment of the lower motor neuron function includes recording muscle weakness, absent or diminished tone, fasciculations, neurogenic atrophy, and altered deep tendon reflexes. The individual C1–3 spinal nerve root motor function cannot be assessed. Typically, if a patient can demonstrate strong neck movements in flexion, extension, and shoulder shrugging, then the cervical nerve roots and plexuses are likely to be unaffected.

Autonomic effects

The preganglionic sympathetic neurons lie in the thoracic and upper lumbar levels of the spinal cord. Their fibers leave the cord in the ventral roots from T1 to L2 or L3 and reach postganglionic neurons which form a sympathetic trunk on the anterolateral vertebral column, from the upper cervical complex to the sacrum. There are 22 ganglia in each trunk with extensive interconnections, including the autonomic nerve plexuses. Autonomic fibers travel with the spinal nerves and then peripheral nerves, and innervate peripheral blood vessels, including those in skeletal muscle and skin, sweat glands, and erector pili muscles.

The cervical sympathetic chain lies anterior to longus capitis and posterior to the carotid sheath. The preganglionic bodies for the head and neck are found in the spinal cord at levels T1–3, and maybe T4 and T5. Branches from the cervical chain form the plexus about the vertebral artery. The superior cervical ganglion is at the level of the transverse processes of C2–3 and the cervical part of the internal carotid (Cramer & Darby 1995 pp. 144, 313). It lies closely with the internal jugular vein and the glossopharyngeal, vagus, spinal accessory, and hypoglossal cranial nerves. It is thought this close relationship may account for the autonomic effects seen with lesions of those nerves in this location.

Branches from the superior cervical ganglion form the internal carotid plexus and some sympathetic vasoconstrictor fibers innervate cerebral branches of the internal carotid artery. Lateral branches travel with cervical spinal nerves 1 through 4. Medial branches include laryngopharyngeal and cardiac branches. Anterior branches travel with the common and external carotid arteries and are vasomotor and secretomotor to structures such as the facial sweat glands (Cramer & Darby 1995 pp. 314, 334).

The parasympathetic fibers are secretomotor to the lacrimal, mucosal, and salivary glands while the sympathetic fibers act as vasoconstrictors. The autonomic nervous system plays an important role with structures of the orbit, such as smooth-muscle function, which can be assessed during neurological examination. Sympathetic activation causes vasoconstriction of the choroidal arterioles while parasympathetic stimulation, via the facial nerve, results in vasodilatation (Cramer & Darby 1995 p. 334). Changes to these functions may alter visual performance and may have some involvement with the visual changes reported after cervical adjustment (Stephens & Gorman 1997).

Atlas subluxations are thought to have a greater effect on the parasympathetic division than the sympathetic division (Plaugher 1993 pp. 303, 307). The parasympathetic division (rest and digest) are also known as the craniosacral division. The preganglionic cell bodies lie in the brainstem within the cranium, and in the second, third, and fourth sacral segments. The cranial sympathetic fibers travel with the oculomotor, facial, glossopharyngeal, and vagus cranial nerves (III, VII, IX, X) and innervate glandular tissue and smooth muscle.

Functional disorders of the upper cervical spine have been found in association with symptoms of fullness in the ear, episodic vertigo, fluctuating hearing, and tinnitus (Franz et al 1999). Other findings include a mild eustachian tube dysfunction and mydriasis on the side of the affected ear. A positive response following physiotherapy was recorded in some patients and it is suspected that mild levels of dysfunction of this nature, which form a cervicogenic oto-ocular syndrome, may be a forerunner of the more sinister presentation of Ménière's disease (Franz et al 1999).

Some practitioners talk of "cord compression" secondary to upper cervical fixation, especially counterrotation; however, Plaugher considers this is unlikely to be due entirely to rotation of the bony elements (Plaugher 1993 p. 307). Plaugher refers to Grostic who proposed that the dentate ligaments may have a restraining function on the cord and restrict vertical movement, thus perhaps "distorting the cord" by mechanical tensions in the area. As discussed earlier, we now know of the connections to the spinal dura mater at the atlanto-occipital and atlantoaxial spaces from the suboccipital muscles and at the atlanto-occipital space by the ligamentum nuchae. It appears that subluxation within the upper cervical complex could include a tensile effect on the spinal dura through these connections.

ASSESSMENT OF VASCULAR CHANGE

Apart from the effects of injury noted below, consideration must be given to variations as evidenced on diagnostic images which relate to vascularization of the region. In particular, the posterior atlanto-occipital membrane is pierced by the vertebral artery as it ascends and curves lateromedially over the posterior arch of C1. The inferior border of the membrane, as it curves over the artery, forms an arcuate foramen which may ossify and be noted on the lateral X-ray as a posterior ponticulus. As discussed earlier, it is thought that these may have an association with headache and its presence is considered by some practitioners to be a relative contraindication to forceful cervical manipulation in the human (Buna et al 1984). The radiograph may also demonstrate calcific densities within the carotid arteries; this is a contraindication to cervical manipulation.

The pericervical lymphatic collar lies in this region and includes the occipital nodes, postauricular nodes, preauricular nodes, submandibular nodes, and submental nodes. These drain into the deep cervical nodes which lie along the internal jugular vein. Consideration must be given to the nodes of the region during assessment and palpation, and when taking adjustive contact.

A traumatic sprain of the capsular ligaments or supporting ligaments may result in inflammation and edema and, given the close relationships among the joints, may affect the kinematics of the complex. Edema is palpated as focal tenderness and bogginess. Inflammation is generally a contraindication to adjustment and may be associated with arthritides or posttraumatic injury.

Areas of colder temperature may be palpated about the region and also about the occiput and parietal areas, suggestive of vasoconstriction secondary to altered joint mechanics and subsequent neural reflexes constricting the arterial supply. More work needs to be undertaken on this type of finding and any relationship with the subluxation complex.

Vertebrobasilar insufficiency

The issues surrounding vertebrobasilar insufficiency (VBI) have been discussed in Chapter 8. It is not known whether upper cervical dysfunction or subluxation has any causal relationship with VBI. It has been reported that patients attending for chiropractic treatment of the neck exhibit signs and symptoms similar to those which may suggest VBI, including transient syncope (Ebrall & Ellis 2000). It is also known that "manipulation is effective in patients with cervicogenic headache" (McCrory et al 2001).

Cerebrovascular ischemia associated with manipulation of the cervical spine is an unpredictable event (Haldeman et al 2002a) and does not seem to be associated with any particular form of standard cervical manipulative technique (Haldeman et al 2002b). Further, the literature does not assist in identifying the patient at risk (Haldeman et al 1999) and a simple cause-and-effect relationship does not exist between neck manipulation and subsequent patient injury (Terrett 2002). The internal forces sustained by the vertebral artery during skilled spinal manipulation are known to be almost an order of magnitude lower than the strains required to disrupt the artery mechanically (Symons et al 2002).

A review of the literature estimates the risk to be between five and 10 events per 10 million manipulations (Hurwitz et al 1996) and an authoritative assessment can be drawn from the records of the largest insurer of practitioners in the USA, the NCMIC Group, Inc. Their estimate of a serious complication such as a vertebrobasilar stroke causing permanent neurologic deficit following cervical manipulation is approximately one in 2 million procedures (Chapman-Smith 2001).

Another way of expressing the risk is to think of "about 1 case of serious neurovascular complication for cervical manipulation for each 25 practitioners who all practice for a 40 year period" (Chapman-Smith 2001); in medical terms this is extraordinarily low.

While chiropractors have questioned the value of the cervical extension-rotation test for screening patients at risk of stroke after cervical manipulation (Côté et al 1996), the test is commonly used by chiropractors and osteopaths to identify patients who may present with positional VBI (Ivancic et al 1993). Physiotherapists consider it may be a useful test of the adequacy of collateral circulation by causing significant changes in flow velocity of the vertebral artery in the end-range position of rotation and extension (Rivett et al 1999), despite the fact that the lumen of the vertebral arteries is usually unaffected by atlantoaxial rotation (Haynes et al 2002).

The prudent practitioner could be expected to take the patient's blood pressure to identify the presence of hypertension (a possible risk factor), auscultate the carotid arteries to rule out bruits, and conduct a cervical extension-rotation test to rule out positional VBI and other factors causative of transient syncope or a neurological reaction. The patient history and physical exam should be complete and include assessment of currently known risk factors, including smoking, atrial fibrillation, previous transient ischemic attack, physical inactivity, diabetes mellitus, and obesity (Côté 1999) and any use of oral contraception in the female patient (Haldeman et al 1999). The purpose is to provide the practitioner with a clear understanding of the patient's clinical profile and to allow the practitioner better to inform the patient of any material risk in order to gain appropriate informed consent.

The fact remains that the clinical outcomes generally outweigh the risks and skilled manipulation or adjustment of the cervical spine is, in medical terms, an extremely low-risk clinical intervention. This is not to reduce in any way the importance of a thorough patient assessment and the recording of informed consent in the face of understanding the material risks. While there seems no question that the risk–benefit ratio of chiropractic spinal adjustment is acceptable (Haldeman et al 2001), there is no implication that adjusting the cervical spine is an innocuous clinical procedure.

CONCLUSION

The upper cervical spine is likely to be involved in a wide variety of presentations, from straightforward, localized cervicogenic headache to presentations of complex autonomic dysfunction. There is also clinical evidence that it may have involvement with dysfunction at other spinal levels.

While it is a difficult area to assess thoroughly, most problems seem to stem from incomplete protocols. It is particularly important to be thorough in the assessment of kinematic change and then equally as thorough in the assessment of the remaining elements of the subluxation complex.

The risks to the patient from skilled manipulation and adjustment of this region are extremely low, even though the outcomes of associated events may be catastrophic.

10

The mid cervical spine

KEY CONCEPTS

There is an intimate physical relationship and an almost seamless functional relationship between the ventral and dorsal rami, the sympathetic ganglia, and the structures they innervate, including the disk and the vertebral artery.

The practitioner must learn to distinguish between nerve root pain and cervical myelopathy by appreciating the gamut of signs and symptoms which accompany each pathological process.

Acute nerve root pain is typically associated with disk damage and subacute pain is more likely to be secondary to degenerative changes and spondylosis. Chronic nerve root pain also tends to involve musculature about the thoracic outlet and other long-term changes.

The clinical evidence of C5 involvement includes pain in the neck, tip of the shoulder, and anterior arm; sensory change about the deltoid; motor change in the deltoid and biceps; and reflex change at the biceps tendon.

The clinical evidence of C6 involvement is pain in the neck, shoulder, medial border of the scapula, lateral arm, and back of the forearm; sensory change about the thumb and index finger; motor change in the biceps; and reflex change at the brachioradialis tendon.

The complaint of headache may also reflect a referred pain from the mid cervical spine as degenerative changes of the spine have been reported as causing about one-third of all cases of headache and the zygapophyseal joints are known to be a cause of neck pain and headache.

The morphology of the cervical disk is distinctly different from that of the lumbar disk and a fluid nucleus pulposus is non-existent in the adult. There are sensory nerves in the annulus fibers and it is considered to be a pain generator. When a cervical disk is damaged, the sinuvertebral nerve may sprout and grow new nerves into the central region where they may be exposed to inflammatory and algogenic chemicals.

The mid cervical spine is best visualized on the lateral cervical neutral and the anteroposterior (AP) lower cervical plain films and the relationship of one segment to another on the lateral view is thought to be normal when the plane lines of each segment slowly converge towards the posterior.

CLINICAL ANATOMY

The mid cervical spine (Fig. 10.1) includes the following spinal motion units (SMUs):

- C3–4
- C4–5
- C5–6.

Cramer & Darby (1995 pp. 109–118, 134–155) provide the appropriate level of anatomy of this region for the student and can be read in conjunction with this chapter. They (p. 10) and others identify the following clinically important relationships:

- C3: epiglottis; hyoid; oropharynx becomes laryngopharynx
- C3 spinous: greater cornua of the hyoid bone
- C3–4 disk: common carotids divide into internal and external carotid arteries; carotid sinus
- C4–5 disk: laryngeal prominence
- C5: vocal folds
- C5–6: superior margin of lobes of thyroid gland; Erb's point, which lies posterior to sternocleidomastoid and stimulation of which contracts various arm muscles.

The anterior structures of the neck in the supine patient form landmarks for each SMU (Fig. 10.2). Gentle palpation is used: the

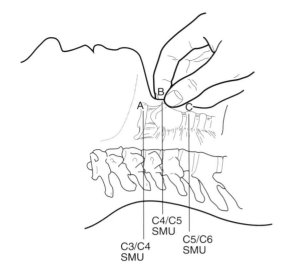

Figure 10.2 Landmarks for the mid cervical spine. (A) The hyoid bone forms a landmark for the C3–4 spinal motion unit (SMU). (B) The laryngeal prominence of the thyroid cartilage forms a landmark for the C4–5 SMU. (C) The commencement of the cricoid cartilage forms a landmark for the C5–6 SMU.

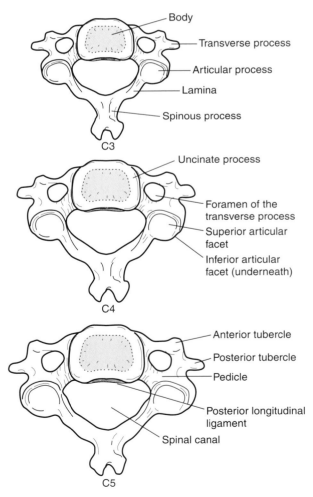

Figure 10.3 Superior view of mid cervical vertebrae.

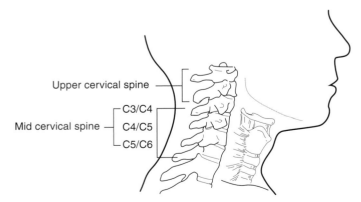

Figure 10.1 Right lateral view of the mid cervical spine.

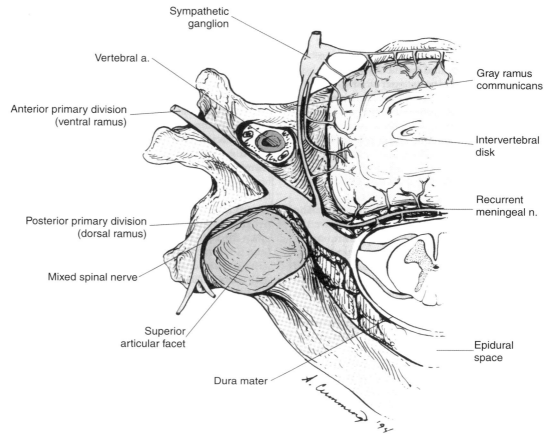

Sympathetic
ganglion

Vertebral a.

Anterior primary division
(ventral ramus)

Gray ramus
communicans

Intervertebral
disk

Posterior primary division
(dorsal ramus)

Recurrent
meningeal n.

Mixed spinal nerve

Superior
articular facet

Epidural
space

Dura mater

Figure 10.4 Superior view of the left side of a typical mid cervical segment. Note the innervation of the disk by the gray rami communicantes and the relationships of the sympathetic ganglion to the segment and the intimacy of its plexus with the vertebral artery. The dorsal ramus travels posteriorly around the articular pillar and zygapophyseal joint to innervate the muscles of the neck. The ventral ramus extends anteriorly along the transverse process to exit between the anterior and posterior tubercles on its way to the ansa cervicalis at the level of C4 or the brachial plexus (C5, C6). From Cramer & Darby (1995), with permission.

thumb and finger for the hyoid; the index finger for the laryngeal prominence; and thumb and finger for the transition to the cricoid. The greater cornua or horn of the hyoid is about the level of the C3 spinous and the cricoid lies about C6. The thyroid cartilage lies anterior to the bodies of C4 and C5 (Hoppenfeld 1976). These relationships are important for understanding the AP lower cervical radiograph which may demonstrate varying degrees of calcification of these structures.

The growth and development of the pediatric cervical spine have been documented radiographically (Wang et al 2001) and the assessment of skeletal maturity from cervical vertebrae (Hassel & Farman 1995) has been shown to be reliable, reproducible, and valid (Chang et al 2001) and significantly related to estimates of skeletal maturity made from hand–wrist radiographs (Kucukkeles et al 1999).

The gradually changing structure of the C3, C4, and C5 vertebrae must be appreciated to facilitate the level of palpation required in clinicial practice (Fig. 10.3). Comparative illustrations demonstrate the obvious anatomical changes to the size and shape of the spinal canal, from a more semicircular profile at C3 to a more triangular profile at C5. Also note the anterolateral angulation of the intervertebral canal (IVC) which runs

along the transverse process; the close approximation the neural contents of the IVC have with the vertebral artery (Fig. 10.4); and the anterior and posterior tubercles at the distal transverse process for the attachment of supportive muscles.

Another feature of clinical significance is the angulation of the posterior laminae, both in the transverse view (Fig. 10.3) and the lateral view (Fig. 10.5). It is particularly important to integrate smoothly palpation of the zygapophyseal joints, posterior laminae, and spinous process of a particular segment in relation to the structures above and below, in both static position and with movement, and also comparing bilaterally.

The intimacy of the neural, vascular, and muscular structures, particularly in the intervertebral foramina (IVF), is shown in Figure 10.4. While the cord appears to float in the spinal canal, recognition must be given to the surrounding soft-tissue contents, in particular the vascular structures and adipose tissue. The sympathetic ganglion embraces the vertebral artery, a reminder of the autonomic contribution to the neural plexus about this artery. The dorsal ramus is clearly shown extending posteriorly to innervate the muscles of the neck and the ventral ramus is shown extending anteriorly on its way to the ansa cervicalis at the level of C4 or the brachial plexus (C5, C6).

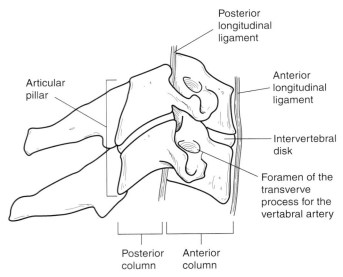

Figure 10.5 Right lateral view of a typical mid cervical spinal motion unit.

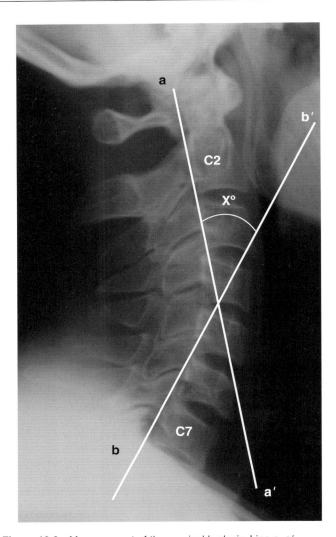

Figure 10.6 Measurement of the cervical lordosis. Line a–a' is drawn tangential to the posterior border of the body of C2 and extended downwards. Line b–b' is drawn tangential to the posterior border of the body of C7 and extended upwards. The resultant angle (X°) is a reliable measure of cervical lordosis.

The lateral view of a typical mid cervical SMU is shown in Figure 10.5. Note the decrease in bony height which is palpated as the fingers move posteromedially from the articular pillars to the spinous process. Note also the relationship of the spinous process to the disk, but place this in context with the normal angulation of the segments as they reflect the sagittal curve of the cervical spine, which is normally a lordosis.

The cervical lordosis has traditionally been measured from the lateral cervical neutral radiograph by extending a plane line through C1 and at the inferior border of C7, and then measuring the angle formed by the intersection of perpendicular lines drawn from each plane line. This method provides an average value of 40°, range 35–45° (Yochum & Rowe 1996 p. 153). Other practitioners have demonstrated a high degree of variability in the value of the cervical lordosis when it includes the upper cervical complex (Harrison et al 1996a, 2002c) and have developed a tangential marking procedure based on the orthopedic lines of Ruth Jackson (Yochum & Rowe 1996 p. 154). One line is drawn to extend the posterior border of C2 downwards and another to extend the posterior border of C7 upwards, and the value of the lordosis is taken from the angle formed at the intersection of these two lines (Fig. 10.6). Using this method the average lordosis in an asymptomatic North American population is about 42° (Harrison et al 1996a, 2002c). Given that the reliability of this method over time has been shown to be acceptable (Harrison 2002c), and given the distinctive nature of the upper cervical complex, which some consider may more represent a kyphosis, it is appropriate for the tangential method of Harrison to be considered the preferred method of measuring the cervical lordosis.

The clinical relevance of the cervical lordosis remains unclear, as any relationship between altered or even reversed lordosis and clinical symptoms has yet to be demonstrated satisfactorily. On the other hand, evidence is starting to appear which associates a restoration of cervical lordosis with a reduction in visual analog pain scores (Harrison et al 2002a).

ASSESSMENT OF KINEMATIC CHANGE

Postural assessment

Care must be taken with making inference to the mid cervical spine from postural presentations due to the greater role played by the upper cervical complex. Global malpositions, as in torticollis, may reflect a gross, regional involvement which may include a specific subluxation complex (SC) at C3–4, C4–5, or C5–6. Significant findings such as anterior head carriage may reflect more the dynamics associated with alterations to the cervical curve, such as reduced lordosis, than dysfunction at a particular level. In short, there are no specific postural findings indicative solely of dysfunction of the mid cervical spine and this region must be subsumed into the regional and global findings.

Static palpation

Static palpation is performed with the patient either seated or supine, and as an extension from static palpation of the upper cervical complex.

Typically there is less asymmetry in the mid cervical spine. The most bifid spinous process is that of C2 and, while C3 may be bifid, it generally extends less posteriorly and is often palpated inferiorly and deeper to that of C2. The C3 and C4 spinous processes are generally the least prominent in that they lie deeply given their placement about the apex of the lordosis. The C5 spinous process may palpate quite seamlessly with that of C6, making particular identification of this level difficult.

The laterality of the articular pillars (the z-joint or posterior column) is relatively consistent after narrowing towards the midline, in comparison with C2. The transverse processes are palpated with an approach from the anterior with a lateral to medial contact; however, the tubercles are attachment points for muscles and they may be quite tender and painful to touch. Palpation from the anterior requires great care to avoid the vasculature and skill to work through muscle layers to locate the tubercles. Generally, the most useful information is found from palpation about the articular pillars and posterior elements.

Radiographic analysis

The mid cervical spine complex is best seen on the lateral cervical neutral and the AP lower cervical plain films. The relationship of one segment to another on the lateral view is thought to be normal when the plane lines slowly converge towards the posterior (Fig. 10.7A). While they appear to be parallel in this extracted image, they do converge at a point some distance behind the patient. This represents the nature of the normal lordosis.

The plane line for each segment is constructed by placing a pencil dot at the inferior anterior margin of the body and at the inferior posterior margin. A line parallel to a line through these dots is drawn through the lower part of the body and extended posteriorly through the lamina. This method is used within the Gonstead system of radiographic analysis and it provides useful information for general practice.

Where these lines steeply converge posteriorly, as in Figure 10.7B, it is thought to be an indicator of an extension fixation of the superior segment on the one below. The segment is considered to be in a position of extension fixation and this will be accompanied by specific findings from dynamic palpation. Conversely, where the lines diverge posteriorly, it is thought to indicate a flexion malposition of the segment.

The segments are also assessed on the lateral radiograph for antero- and retrolisthesis. These changes are indicated by interruption to George's line, a continuous line drawn along and connecting the posterior vertebral bodies. It should be smooth and continuous and provides an indicator of any listhesis of a segment. The Ruth Jackson stress lines are the tangential lines shown in Figure 10.6. Normally they should cross about the level of the C4 disk. It is particularly important also to note any change in the space representing the height of the disk at each SMU. Decreased disk height is indicative of internal disk derangement.

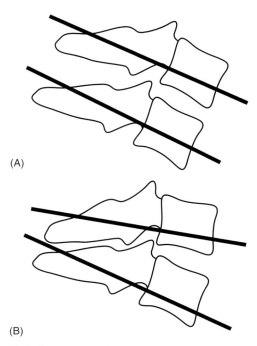

(A)

(B)

Figure 10.7 Assessment of the lateral radiograph. (A) The expected finding in a normal spinal motion unit. The plane line of the superior segment converges gently towards that of the inferior segment at a point posterior to the patient. (B) A depiction of extension fixation where the plane line of the superior segment converges sharply toward that of the segment below.

Plane lines drawn on the AP view may be useful to demonstrate any relative loss of a normal-level, parallel relationship among segments. In one context any tilt of the plane line is thought to represent an open wedge on the side of superiority; however, care must be taken to place any such segmental finding in the context of the entire cervical spine, and often the thoracic spine as well.

It is imperative to place such objective data in the context of all clinical findings from the patient. It must be emphasized that the data from a radiograph is only one piece of clinical data, and while the radiograph is particularly important for depicting the structural architecture of the cervical spine, the information it provides must be incorporated into the wider clinical decision-making process.

Objective structural change of SMU mechanics

The major anomalies of this region are block vertebrae, where two or more vertebrae fail to separate and thus do not form a normal disk joint (Taylor & Resnick 2000 p. 69). This is a congenital anomaly where the two become as one. The zygapophyseal joints also fuse in about 50% of cases. Vertebrae may also fuse due to degeneration or secondary to surgical intervention. Generally there is little clinical significance associated with congenital block vertebrae; however, movement will be aberrant and there may or may not be diminished IVCs. The practitioner needs to be aware of this anomaly when palpating the patient in order to establish the parameters of normal movement for that individual at that particular level. Block vertebrae may be associated with Klippel–Feil syndrome, in which the patient has a short, webbed neck, a low hairline, and a reduced cervical range of motion (ROM) (Yochum & Rowe 1996, 218, Taylor & Resnick 2000 p. 70).

The cervical pedicle may be unilaterally congenitally absent. Yochum & Rowe (1996 p. 220) report C4 and C5 as least common, each accounting for about 12.5% of such cases. Cervical spondylolisthesis is a rare anomaly.

Fracture in this region is as described for the upper cervical spine complex. Articular pillar fracture may be seen as a chip fracture of a superior articular facet (Cramer & Darby 1995 p. 115). It may produce transient radicular pain followed by mild to intense neck pain. If the radicular pain persists, it may suggest displacement of the fragment on to the dorsal root. Dislocation will occur either bilaterally or unilaterally and involves the zygapophyseal joints. It is typically secondary to accidental trauma. Avulsion suggests trauma and such patients require thorough assessment and evaluation of the associated soft-tissue damage.

Reactive osseous hypertrophy is commonly seen as increased density about the articular pillars on the lateral radiograph and is considered a component of degenerative change. The maximal cervical compression test may cause compromise between these bony changes and a spinal nerve root, resulting in nerve root pain.

Other diagnostic imaging assessment

The computed tomography (CT) scan provides useful axial images as well as sagittal reconstructions to demonstrate fracture and other bony changes. A little-used feature of CT is the ability to generate a three-dimensional reconstruction which may provide useful documentation of structural relationships, particularly when facet involvement is suspected. The magnetic resonance imaging (MRI) is useful for demonstrating soft-tissue relationships and plays a vital role in identifying neoplastic infiltration and changes in neural tissue. Advanced ultrasound techniques can document the real-time flow patterns within the cervical arterial system; however, they are not yet routinely used in clinical practice.

Subjective nature of movement

The assessment of movement of the mid cervical spine is subsumed within the regional ROM of the cervical spine. The active ROM is assessed with the patient seated and with the head and cervical spine in neutral. The patient is asked to rotate the head fully towards one shoulder, back to the midline, and then to the other shoulder, while the practitioner stands behind the patient supporting the shoulders with both hands. The normal axial rotation in neutral is about 70° (SD about 10°) left and right, from neutral, for the whole cervical spine, and these values decrease with age but are not related to gender (Trott et al 1996, Feipel et al 1999). The segments from C3 to C6 contribute about 24% of total rotation (Dumas et al 1993). The mean value of axial rotation as determined by CT at C3–4, C4–5, and C5–6 is between 6° and 7° (Penning & Wilmink 1987); however, these

values are influenced by the manner in which the coupled movement varies when the patient is placed in the horizontal plane for measurement by CT (Bogduk & Mercer 2000). Corrected data suggest the segmental range of rotation in the plane of the zygapophyseal joints would be about 8° (Bogduk & Mercer 2000).

The regional assessment procedures are the same as used with the upper cervical complex and will not be repeated here in detail. Remember to assess lateral flexion left and right, and then flexion with the chin to the chest as opposed to chin-tuck, and extension. The range and nature of movement may also be assessed passively by supporting the head with two hands and working through each of the six directions.

Rotation within the mid and lower cervical spine is then specifically assessed from behind the patient. The patient is asked to extend the neck and look to the ceiling and then to turn the head fully to the left and then to the right. When the neck is extended, the upper cervical complex is locked and its contribution to rotation is limited, while the facets of the zygapophyseal joints are approximated and movement about them is emphasized. The facets guide rotation and their involvement can be identified by aberrant movement as qualitative change, and restricted movement as quantitative change. It is important to support the patient during this procedure.

The ROM of rotation in extension is normally about 60° to each side. The examiner's hands may be placed over the parietal eminences to support the patient, control the movement, and to assess for end-feel. An interactive dialogue is maintained with the patient regarding the nature of any pain associated with these movements as well as to reassure the patient. Placement of the neck in extension and rotation is a position in which the patient feels particularly vulnerable. It is also the position which is thought to be a provocative test for vertebrobasilar insuffiency, as discussed earlier, and the practitioner must be alert to any indicative signs or symptoms which may arise during the assessment of ROM.

The quantity and quality of regional movement are assessed as described above, with notation of areas of restriction. Movement is then induced into each individual joint with an awareness of the effects of coupling between the segments. In lateral flexion the typical movement of the spinous process is towards the convexity or the contralateral side (Fig. 10.8) and it occurs due to the shape and profile of the zygapophyseal joint surfaces and contraction of the connective tissues.

The assessment of the SMU motion must take this coupled movement into consideration with the realization that pure lateral flexion cannot be distinguished, nor can pure rotation. The coupling is largely due to the profile and orientation of the facets. The superior articular facets are flat and lie obliquely and superiorly and their movement in rotation and lateral flexion is relative, where one facet moves superiorly and anteriorly as the other moves posteriorly and inferiorly (Kapandji 1974 pp. 200, 201).

It is this *relative* movement which induces a coupled movement of rotation with lateral flexion and lateral flexion with rotation (Fig. 10.9). The result is the body rotates towards the side of lateral flexion, or into the resultant concavity of the spine, and the spinous process rotates towards the side of convexity, or away from the side of lateral flexion. The second movement is a *combined* movement, with both the inferior facets of the superior segment (the superior facets of the zygapophyseal joints) sliding

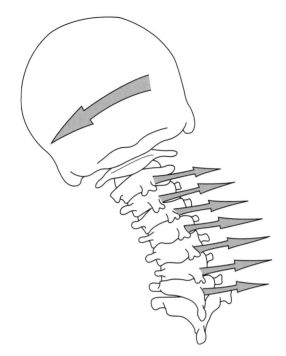

Figure 10.8 Posterior view of the cervical spine in left lateral flexion. The vertebral body rotates to the side of lateral flexion, causing the spinous process to move towards the contralateral side, the side of convexity. From Peterson & Bergmann (2002), with permission.

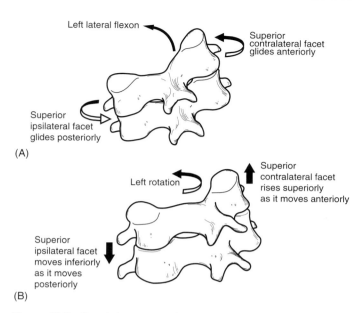

(A)

Left lateral flexon

Superior contralateral facet glides anteriorly

Superior ipsilateral facet glides posteriorly

Left rotation

Superior contralateral facet rises superiorly as it moves anteriorly

Superior ipsilateral facet moves inferiorly as it moves posteriorly

(B)

Figure 10.9 Coupled movement in a typical mid cervical spinal motion unit. (A) Lateral flexion induces ipsilateral rotation due to the orientation of the facets which draw the contralateral side anteriorly and the ipsilateral side posteriorly. (B) Rotation induces lateral flexion as the orientation of the facets forces the contralateral side to glide superiorly and the ipsilateral side to glide inferiorly. (A, B) After Bergmann et al (1993), with permission.

superiorly during flexion or inferiorly during extension; however, during flexion extension there is also around 11–18° of rotation about the *x*-axis by each segment (Frobin et al 2002).

The nature of the movement during each degree of freedom within the zone of the normal ROM is assessed using observation and palpation at the segmental level. The nature of the active regional ROM assessment may have demonstrated jerky movements reflective of kinematic change secondary to muscle involvement as well as SC, and this information is used to guide the segmental palpation. The regional end-feel within the elastic zone is assessed, particularly in rotation with the neck in extension, and provides a further context for the subsequent assessment of end-feel within each SMU.

Pain-generating structures may be irritated with cervical compression and existing pain arising from these structures may be relieved by cervical distraction. These movements will also affect structures around the C2–3 complex as well as in those below the mid cervical spine, hence the practitioner must be specific in exploring the nature of any resultant pain. The most obvious characteristic is whether the test replicates the pain experience of the patient, or perchance, creates a new pain. The location and distribution of the pain are most important clinical clues and this topic is explored under Assessment of neural change, below. The clinical outcome is that more complete information about any kinematic change of the SMU at the C3–4, C4–5, and C5–6 levels is derived from interpreting the characteristics of movement within the context of the patient's reported pain experience, together with palpable soft-tissue findings such as the state of the capsule around a particular zygapophyseal joint.

Assessment of the individual joints

The assessment of individual joints may be undertaken with the patient seated or supine. There are some movements best demonstrated with the patient seated, such as rotation with the neck in extension, and others with the patient supine, such as posterior to anterior glide. A thorough assessment requires data to be gathered from the patient in both positions.

C3–4

With the patient seated, the practitioner stands posterolaterally to the patient with the indifferent hand on the patient's vertex to induce movements of lateral flexion, rotation, and flexion/extension in each specific SMU. The contact hand palpates with a thumb and finger contact over the articular pillars.

Alternatively, the practitioner may take a standing position squarely behind the patient and palpate with a bilateral finger contact, modified from that shown in Figure 9.12A. The palmar surface of each hand is placed over each parietal eminence with the index fingers pointing inferiorly and lying anterior to the ear. The ring fingers support the middle fingers, which provide the palpatory pads.

Rotation is the first movement to assess, as the typical fixations of this region tend to have a more observable effect on rotation, notwithstanding that flexion and extension are the cardinal movements of the lower cervical spine (Bogduk & Mercer 2000). Lateral flexion is then assessed with contact over the zygapophyseal joints and the articular pillars. The nature of the coupling between rotation and lateral flexion means that both movements should identify a common side of fixation; however, this is a theoretical construct based on the supposition that fixation is unilateral. It may well be bilateral at a particular level and expressed by different kinematic changes on each side. Typically the articular pillar will feel restricted in contralateral rotation. For example, fixation of the right zygapophyseal joint is more palpable with left rotation. The same zygapophyseal joint should feel restricted in ipsilateral lateral flexion and in this example restriction and limited closure will be felt in the right articular pillars with right lateral flexion.

Segmental movement and end-feel in rotation may also be assessed with the practitioner standing to the side of the patient with a thumb and index finger contact laterally about the spinous process. This allows for assessment of end-feel by a push–pull, medial–lateral movement of the thumb and finger. The distal lateral index finger pad may also be placed horizontally between two spinous processes so that movement of the superior spinous process can be felt and compared to that of the inferior. The C3 spinous process may be quite challenging to identify by palpation due to the overlying ligamentum nuchae and the relative prominence of C2, therefore contacts on the posterolateral laminae usually provide more clinically useful data. The technique chosen by the practitioner will reflect his or her individual approach to practice. For some it is imperative to describe fixation with reference to altered movements of the spinous process, while others prefer to identify specific zygapophyseal joints which exhibit restriction.

Movement in flexion and extension is assessed while standing more beside the patient and placing the palpating finger pads into the two spaces between three consecutive spinous processes. In flexion the interspace between the spinous processes should appear to open or separate, while on extension the processes should appear to close or approximate. A posteriority of any segment, palpated at either or both articular pillars, is considered an extension fixation. In this condition the sense of tissue resiliency is lost as the spinous processes attempt to open as the neck is moved into flexion.

Palpation in the supine position requires the patient to lie on a flat table with little or no neck flexion. The practitioner's position is square at the head of the table and may be seated or squatting. Alternatively, the table may be raised to about the height of the standing practitioner's waist. The comparative posterior to anterior glide of the segment is assessed in the supine position by placing the fingers on the left and right sides of the posterior arch of C3 and gently drawing it upwards. Restriction may be felt on either or both sides. This process can be commenced at occiput–C1 and applied as low as C7–T1. It is a "stair-stepping" procedure where the head is held off the table and, as each lower joint is assessed, the head is raised a little higher. The movement can be assessed as end-feel with micromovement at the end of the anterior glide as well as during the anterior movement.

Rotation, lateral flexion, and lateral glide or translation of C3 on C4 can also be assessed in the supine patient with subtle variations of the finger contact, bearing in mind the comments above that rotation and lateral flexion are coupled. An index finger contact along the posterolateral lamina of the segment provides patient comfort while assessing movements of the body as opposed to specific movement of the zygapophyseal joint. It is

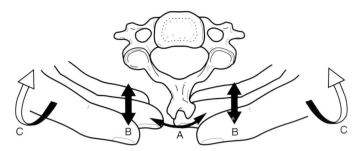

Figure 10.10 Palpation in the supine patient. Alternating lateral to medial palpation is applied about the spinous process to assess the quality of segmental rotation (arrow A). Bilateral posterior to anterior palpation is applied over the articular pillars to assess the quality of anterior glide or translation, a component of extension (arrows B). Unilateral posterior to anterior palpation provides further information on the quality of segmental rotation. The palpation is also applied during left and right lateral flexion of the spinal motion unit to assess the quality of segmental lateral flexion (arrows C), which is coupled with rotation. Modified from Chaitow & Delany (2000), with permission.

easy and efficient to move between posterior to anterior glide, an assessment of rotary motion by the push–pull, lateral–medial movement of the spinous process, and lateral flexion assessment in the supine patient (Fig. 10.10).

Valuable clinical information is also gained by assessing the tissue tension about each SMU and its responses to palpation and movement. Unilateral restriction and tenderness may suggest ipsilateral posterior rotation of the underlying segment.

C4–5

The above is repeated for the C4–5 SMU, with an appreciation for the changing angulation of the facets as well as the disk.

C5–6

The above is repeated for the C5–6 SMU, also with an appreciation for further changes in the angulation of the facets and disk.

Palpation errors are often made in this region of the spine, perhaps due to the inaccessibility of the C3 spinous and inaccurate palpation about C1–2. The landmarks given in Figure 10.2 should be borne in mind, especially during supine palpation. The mid cervical spine is often the site of restriction due to compensation as opposed to primary fixation. The compensation typically suggests a prime SC in either the upper cervical spine or the cervicothoracic spine. Care must be taken to determine the dimensions of any suspected SC in the mid cervical segments by first ruling out any subtle kinematic changes in the spine above or below.

A rule of thumb when SC is suspected in the mid cervical spine is to recheck the upper cervical complex and the cervicothoracic spine to see what may have been missed. Remember specifically to assess for quantity of movement and to identify any restriction; quality of movement within the normal range; and quality of movement into the elastic barrier, or end-feel.

ASSESSMENT OF CONNECTIVE TISSUE CHANGE

The following soft-tissue dimensions should be measured on the lateral cervical neutral radiograph, especially in the post-trauma patient:

- Retropharyngeal interspace (RPI) measured from the anteroinferior margin of C3 and C4 to the contour representing the posterior wall of the pharynx and normally up to 7 mm at these levels. An increase suggests swelling of the tissues anterior to the vertebral column. This finding may follow trauma such as cervical acceleration/deceleration (whiplash) in a motor vehicle accident.
- The retrotracheal interspace (RTI), measured from the anteroinferior margin of C5 to the contour representing the posterior wall of the trachea which is normally up to about 20 mm.

Ligaments of the region

The anterior longitudinal ligament firmly attaches to the anterior aspect of each body in this region (C3, C4, C5) and loosely about the disk (Bland 1991), where it intermingles with the anterior fibers of the annulus of each disk. It broadens as it descends and acts to limit extension. It is often implicated in acceleration/deceleration injury such as traumatic extension from a rear-end motor vehicle accident and may tear at the level of the inferior margin of the disk/superior margin of the body (Foreman & Croft 2002 p. 336). This injury may include some avulsion of the body margin.

The posterior longitudinal ligament continues inferiorly from its attachment on the posterior aspect of the C2 body and is the extension of the tectorial membrane. It is a wide ligament and is thickest in this region. It attaches to the posterior aspect of each body, somewhat loosely in the mid-portion to allow venous drainage, but quite strongly to the posterior aspect of each disk. This ligament may demonstrate ossification on X-ray, particularly in the Japanese (Takasita et al 2000).

The ligamentum flavum is paired left and right and each runs between the laminae at each level. It is thin in this region and contains elastin which may assist with extension and limit the extremes of flexion. Cramer & Darby (1995 p. 134) suggest the main function of the elastin is to prevent buckling into the spinal canal during extension. It may degenerate with age and lose its elastic qualities, and it may (uncommonly) ossify in Caucasians (Hankey & Khangure 1988) and Blacks (Cabre et al 2001) and develop a ganglion cyst within (Yamamoto et al 2001), causing myelopathy.

The ligamentum nuchae runs between the spinous processes of this region and its importance has been discussed in the preceding chapter. It may be tender to palpation in and about the midline. Its anterior aspect may be considered as an interspinous ligament, although these are poorly developed in this region. The ligament has reasonable anterior to posterior depth at these levels due to the lordosis which reduces the palpatory feel of the tip of the spinous processes of these segments. The intertransverse ligaments are poorly defined and may exist more as the posterior intertransverse musculature.

The zygapophyseal joints

The articular capsules of the zygapophyseal joint capsules are quite thin and, in comparison with those in the thoracic and lumbar region, are longer and looser (Cramer & Darby 1995 p. 113). They include collagen fibers and run inferiorly from around the inferior articular facet of the segment above to around the superior facet of the segment below, thus being somewhat at right angles to the plane of the joint.

The capsule may be implicated by local pain secondary to movements which stretch or compress the fibers. These include cervical distraction (stretch), rotation and/or flexion (stretch), and localized palpation (lateral to medial compression).

The zygapophyseal menisci are described as type III at these levels, being "rather small nubs" (Cramer & Darby 1995 p. 115). The meniscus may be implicated by local pain secondary to movements which compress the zygapophyseal joint, such as cervical compression and/or maximal cervical compression. Cervical extension, with a combination of lateral flexion and rotation (producing compression), may also irritate the meniscus. The joints contain nociceptive, proprioceptive, vasomotor, and vasosensory nerve functions (Blume 2000).

The intervertebral disk

The intervertebral disk is considered to be a major focus of the connective tissue assessment. The morphology of the cervical disk is distinctly different from that of the lumbar disk (Mercer & Jull 1996). It lacks a concentric annulus fibrosis around the entire perimeter and it tapers laterally and posteriorly towards the anterior edge of the uncinate processes on each side (Bogduk & Mercer 2000). The criss-cross arrangement of collagen fibers seen in the lumbar disks is absent and the fibers of the anterior annulus converge upwards towards the anterior end of the upper vertebra and form an interosseous ligament in the shape of an inverted V, whose apex points to the axis of rotation (Bogduk & Mercer 2000).

There are sensory nerves in the annulus fibers and it is considered to be a pain generator. They are interwoven with the nerve root and ganglion and connect the sympathetic chain, the rami communicantes, and the perivascular nerve plexus of the vertebral artery (Blume 2000). It is thought the sinuvertebral nerve will sprout when a cervical disk is injured and grow new nerves into the central region where they may be exposed to inflammatory and algogenic chemicals such as stromelysin, metalloproteinase, creatine phosphokinase, and phospholipase A_2 (Blume 2000). The resultant pain is a type of sympathetically maintained pain. The disk may thus be implicated by local or diffuse referred pain with cervical compression. If the nature of disk damage is such that compression increases irritation of the nerve root then upper-quadrant nerve root pain may be reported by the patient.

There is an important interplay between the disk and the uncinate processes in this region. Cramer & Darby (1995 p. 135) note that, by the age of 40, the uncinate processes have enlarged to the point of forming a significant posterior and lateral barrier which limits disk displacement. The uncinate processes act as stabilizers with respect to motion within the SMU and, where an articulation about them has developed as a Luschka joint, there is an increase in motion (Clausen et al 1997). The uncinate process and any subsequent articulation thus complement each other.

Giles & Singer (1998 p. 24) describe the nucleus pulposus as being present from birth to about age 14, from which time it gradually disappears. They report it to be dry and fibrous and functioning more like a ligament in the adult. Disk space narrowing as seen on the lateral cervical radiograph is an indicator of degenerative change and is usually associated with adjacent end-plate sclerosis and marginal osteophyte formation (Pelz & Fox 1990). The decrease in disk height is considered severe degeneration and is accompanied by a dehydrated nucleus and disintegrated annulus (Kumaresan et al 2001). Giles & Singer (1998) find it to be fibrous and breaking up and ultra-low-field MRI has demonstrated the nature of posterior disk displacement. Degeneration appears to decrease the stress and strain on the annulus but increase the strain energy density and stress in the vertebral cortex adjacent to the degenerated disk and this may be the mechanism of osteophyte formation (Kumaresan et al 2001). The C5–6 (Aker et al 1989) disk among others (Bagatur et al 2001, Gerlach et al 2001) has been reported to calcify in children.

The lack of a gelatinous nucleus pulposus in persons other than children and very young adults calls into question those conceptual models of clinical practice which assume the cervical and lumbar disks are virtually similar (Mercer & Jull 1996). The current knowledge of the morphology and biomechanics of the disk in the cervical spine suggests it is time to re-examine these clinical models, including the model of McKenzie (1990), which purports to correct any disturbance of the position of the nucleus in the cervical spine; of Gonstead (Herbst 1968), which purports to reposition the cervical vertebra on its disk; and of others, who argue an active role for the nucleus in the symptomatic adult patient. These comments certainly do not negate the importance of the adult disk in the kinematics of the cervical spine; they simply make us reconsider it in terms other than having a fluid and mobile nucleus.

ASSESSMENT OF MUSCLE CHANGE

There are many directly attached muscles and muscles which cross multiple segments in the mid cervical spine, innervated by the spinal nerves which originate at this level. These nerves typically intermingle with nerves above and below to provide motor function. The mid cervical spine is the transitional zone between spinal nerve roots which are difficult to assess by individual muscle test (C1, C2, C3) and those which can be relatively isolated (from C5).

The splenii, upper trapezius, and rhomboid minor have been discussed in Chapter 9. Cramer & Darby (1995 pp. 106, 107) summarize the cervical muscles by their actions, while Chaitow & DeLany (2000 p. 187) group them in planes from superficial to deep. This discussion will group them in a sequence based on a clinical approach to their assessment and testing.

Muscles assessed with the patient supine

The sternocleidomastoid

This muscle is typically considered as a two-headed sternocleidomastoid muscle; however, from the clinical perspective it is better considered as two separate muscles given their differences in innervation, force generation, and trigger point activities.

The sternomastoid arises from the anterior surface of the manubrium and ascends to the mastoid, and the cleidomastoid arises from the superior surface of the medial half of the clavicle and ascends to the lateral surface of the mastoid process and the lateral half of the superior nuchal line (Fig. 10.11A).

The sternomastoid receives bilateral hemispheric motor innervation via the spinal root of the accessory nerve (Routal & Pal 2000) with the maximal input from the ipsilateral hemisphere (DeToledo & Dow 1998). The cleidomastoid is innervated via the spinal root of the accessory nerve arising from the caudal portion of the spinal accessory nucleus. This caudal portion of the nucleus is innervated preferentially by the contralateral hemisphere (DeToledo & David 2001).

The muscles typically function as one except in patients with certain patterns of hemispheric damage following stroke. The sternomastoid is much stronger, generating some 69 N of peak force, compared to the 34 N generated by the cleidomastoid (Vasavada & Delp 1998). The two muscles are well positioned to generate lateral flexion, are weak contributors to contralateral axial rotation after the trapezius, and, when acting bilaterally, contribute to flexion and a little extension (Vasavada & Delp 1998).

As postural muscles they will shorten when stressed. The muscle is tested with the patient supine with the head fully rotated contralaterally. It is important that the patient places the hands with the palms up, towards the ears, as shown in Figure 10.11B, to remove synergists and any counter balance. The head is raised off the table and held by the patient and then the patient attempts to raise the head a little more into the examiner's hand. Gentle posterolateral force may be applied by the examiner on the temporal area. The examiner's fingers should be placed in line with the long axes of the muscles. Weakness is indicated by the patient attempting to turn the head medially (Walther 1981 p. 432).

They are a complex pair of muscles and must be examined in all patients with head pain. The sternomastoid trigger points mainly project pain to the cheek, temple, and orbit (Fig. 10.11C right) and may generate autonomic phenomena such as tearing of the eye. The cleidomastoid trigger points project more as frontal headache (Fig. 10.11C left) and may generate postural dizziness (Simons et al 1999 p. 314).

The indications for assessment include referred pain as well as visual disturbances, blurred vision, persistent dry cough or sore throat, congested sinuses, hearing loss, and disturbances to orientation (Chaitow & DeLany 2000). The trigger points are treated with the patient supine and the head contralaterally rotated. The muscle bellies are exposed when the muscles contract as the patient raises the head from the bench, and a gentle squeezing or milking action is applied by the thumb and index finger as the patient relaxes the head back to the bench. This process is repeated.

The scalenes

The scalenus medius arises from the transverse process of C2 and the posterior tubercles of C3–7 and inserts into the upper surface of rib 1, posterior to the subclavian groove (Fig. 10.12A).

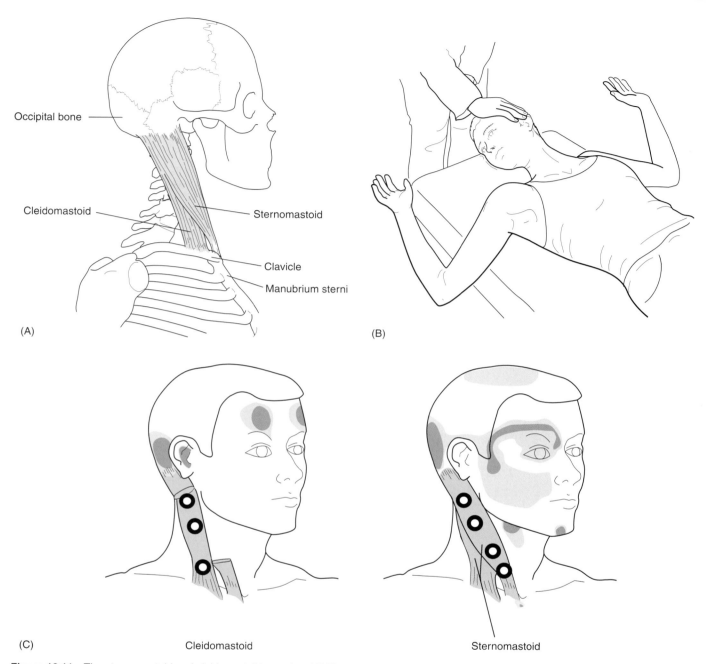

(A)

Occipital bone

Cleidomastoid

Sternomastoid

Clavicle

Manubrium sterni

(B)

(C)   Cleidomastoid   Sternomastoid

Figure 10.11 The sternomastoid and cleidomastoid muscles. (A) The sternomastoid muscle lies anterior to and over the cleidomastoid muscle. (B) The manual muscle test of the left muscles. The test force is provided by the patient raising the head into the examiner's hand. (C) The pain referral from trigger points in the sternomastoid (right) project more about the face, cheek, and jaw, while those of the cleidomastoid (left) are more focal to the forehead. From Chaitow & DeLany (2000), with permission.

It is supplied by the anterior primary rami of C3–8. It is the largest of the scalene muscles and acts as a lateral stabilizer of the neck, being involved in flexion and lateral flexion of the cervical spine. When the neck is fixed, it also assists in elevating rib 1.

The scalenus posterior arises from the posterior tubercles of the transverse processes of C4–6 and inserts into the outer surface of rib 2, posterior to the attachment of serratus anterior. It is supplied by the anterior primary rami of C6–8 and acts to flex and laterally flex the cervical spine. With the neck is fixed, it acts to elevate rib 2, thus having a role in inspiration.

The scalenus anterior arises from the anterior tubercles of the transverse processes of C3–6 and travels inferiorly to insert into the scalene tubercle and ridge on the upper surface of rib 1. It is supplied by anterior branches of C4–6 and acts to flex and laterally flex the neck and, when the neck is fixed, to elevate rib 1.

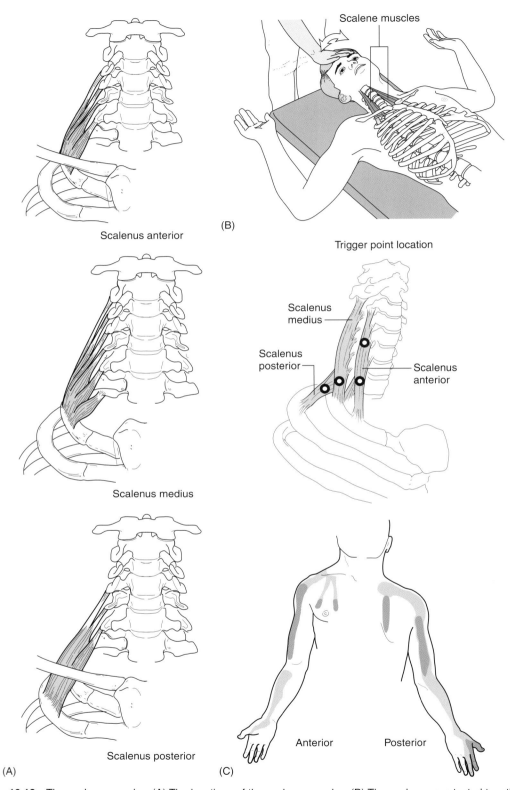

Figure 10.12 The scalene muscles. (A) The locations of the scalene muscles. (B) The scalenes are tested together, with the supine patient rotating the head no more than 20° contralaterally. The position is similar to that for testing the sternomastoid and cleidomastoid but with far less rotation. The test also includes longus colli and capitis and can be further modified to be a bilateral test of medial neck flexors by placing the head in neutral with no rotation. The patient raises the head from the bench, and then attempts to raise the head further against the resistance of the examiner's hand. (C) The trigger points lie deep about the base of the neck and refer pain into the arm and back of hand. From Chaitow & DeLany (2000), with permission.

It has been thought that the scalenes assist with contralateral rotation of the head; however, the model of Vasavada & Delp (1998) does not demonstrate any moment arm for the scalenes to participate in axial rotation with the head and neck in the upright neutral position. They are tested with the patient supine and with the head rotated about 20°. The patient raises the head into the resistance of the examiner's hand (Fig. 10.12B).

The scalenes are important muscles to assess in patients presenting with signs and symptoms of thoracic outlet syndrome. They should be assessed when the patient complains of tingling and numbness in the hand, carpal tunnel syndrome, cervical acceleration/deceleration syndromes, dysfunctional breathing, loss of cervical disk height, and chest, back, or arm pain (Chaitow & DeLany 2000). Their trigger points lie deep about attachments to rib 1 and maybe about the C5–6 transverse processes and refer pain along the medial scapula, posterolateral arm, and in and about the posterior thumb, with maybe some radiation to above the nipple (Fig. 10.12C).

They are palpated with the thumb as the neck is cradled in the examiner's hand. The thumb takes a deep, sweeping contact laterally to medially over the trapezius web and nestled into the tissue about the very low cervical segments and upper ribs, angled towards the opposite nipple. Sufficient pressure for ischemic compression is achieved by laterally flexing the neck over the contact thumb.

The longus colli and capitis

The longus colli has vertical, inferior oblique and superior oblique fibers which generally arise from the anterior bodies of C5–7 and T1–3 and ascend to the anterior bodies of C3–4 with slips to their anterior tubercles. The superior oblique fibers insert at the anterior tubercle of C1, providing an intimate relationship between C1 and the mid cervical segments. All are supplied by the anterior primary rami of C2–8 and together they act as neck flexors and assist with lateral flexion.

The muscle has a high density of muscle spindles which are clustered and concentrated anterolaterally, away from the vertebral body (Boyd-Clark et al 2002). It has a postural function on cervical curvature and its cross-sectional area correlates to the lordosis index (Mayoux-Benhamou et al 1994), although its number of type II fibers suggests it responds equally to postural and phasic demands (Boyd-Clark et al 2001). The adult phenotype of longus colli starts during postnatal life following the development of the mechanisms holding up the head and neck which lead to the development of the lordosis (Hannecke et al 2001).

The longus capitis originates from the anterior tubercles of the transverse processes of C3–6 and inserts into the inferior surface of the basilar (anterior) occiput. It is supplied by the muscular branches of C1–4 and acts with longus colli.

The muscles lie deeply and their physical treatment is an advanced technique requiring great skill and care. They should be assessed in patients complaining of difficulty swallowing and may be involved with the loss of cervical lordosis, chronic dysfunction of the cervical musculature, recurrent atlas subluxation, loss of cervical disk height, and posterior protrusion of cervical disks (Chaitow & DeLany 2000). They are tested as medial neck flexors with the scalenes, either unilaterally with the head turned about 20° contralaterally, or bilaterally with the head in neutral rotation (Fig. 10.12B).

Muscles assessed with the patient prone

The posterior cervical muscles are best considered as lying in planes. The trapezius and splenii are superficial and second-plane muscles respectively and have been discussed in the preceding chapter. The third plane of muscles includes the semispinalis capitis and cervicis and those muscles broadly grouped as the erector spinae or sacrospinalis (Fig. 10.13A). These are the spinalis as the medial column, the longissimus as an intermediate column, and the iliocostalis as the more lateral column. The muscle bands are further subdivided as "capitis" where the fibers reach the head and "cervicis" where they run to the cervical spine. The deepest muscle plane includes the rotatores, multifidi, and interspinales muscles. The posterior muscles are tested with the patient prone, raising the head into the examiner's hand (Fig. 10.13B). All muscles are tested with the head in neutral, and isolated to the ipsilateral muscles only when the head is rotated.

The semispinalis and spinalis

The semispinalis capitis arises from the articular processes of the low cervical and upper thoracic segments (C4 through T6) and inserts into the occiput at the medial impression between the superior and inferior nuchal lines. The semispinalis cervicis arises from the articular processes of the lower cervical and upper thoracic segments and inserts into the spinous processes of C2–5. The muscles are supplied by posterior rami of the cervical nerves and their main action is to extend the neck and head. They make a reasonable contribution to lateral flexion and a small contribution to contralateral rotation (Vasavada & Delp 1998).

They are postural muscles and shorten when stressed. Trigger points are found lateral to the C1–2 transverse process to produce ipsilateral head pain as a band which projects to the temple and over the eye (Fig. 10.13C). There is also a trigger point lower in the neck which produces posterior head pain. The indications for assessment include a hat-band headache into the eye, restricted neck flexion, and cervical subluxation.

The medial column theoretically formed by the spinalis capitis and cervicis is usually indistinct from the semispinalis. Further, the capitis and cervicis fibers are usually inseparable. When the column is present the fibers arise from the spinous processes of C7–T2 and ascend to the spinous processes of C2–4. The capitis fibers blend with semispinalis capitis to ascend to the occiput. They are supplied by posterior primary rami of spinal nerves and act together to assist extension of the neck. Acting unilaterally, they assist with ipsilateral lateral flexion of the neck. They are postural muscles and shorten when dysfunctional and are implicated in patients with restricted flexion of the neck and altered lateral flexion.

The longissimus

The longissimus capitis crosses the mid cervical spine as it arises from transverse processes of the upper thoracic segments and the articular pillars of the lower cervical segments, and inserts the posterior margin of the mastoid process. The longissimus cervicis fibers arise only from the transverse processes of the upper thoracic segments and insert into the transverse processes

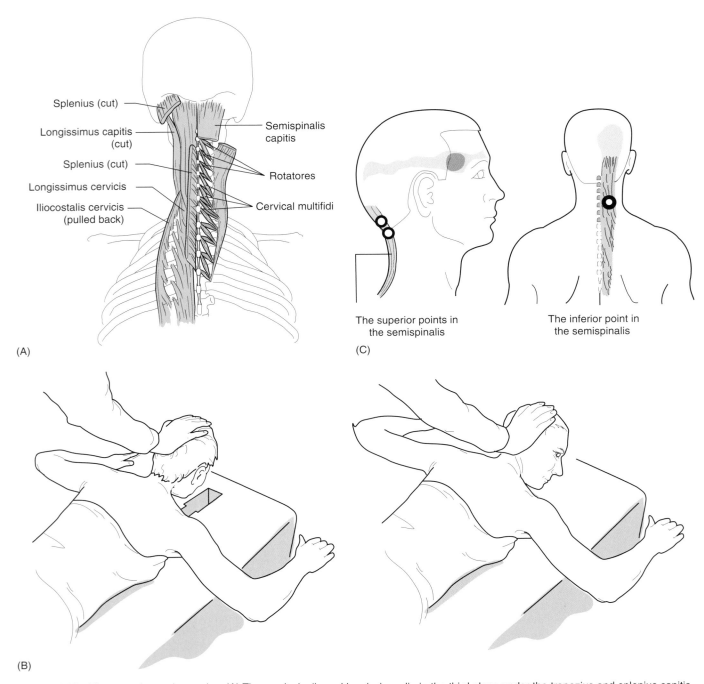

Figure 10.13 The posterior neck muscles. (A) The semispinalis and longissimus lie in the third plane under the trapezius and splenius capitis. The most lateral bands are the iliocostalis and the rotatores and multifidi lie in the deep plane. (B) The posterior neck muscles are tested bilaterally with the head in neutral (left) or unilaterally when the head is rotated towards the side being tested (right). (C) The superior trigger points within the semispinalis muscles refer ipsilateral head pain in a hat-band manner concentrating around the temple. The inferior trigger point refers pain to the back of the head. (A, C) From Chaitow & DeLany (2000), with permission.

of C2 through C6. They are supplied by posterior primary rami of spinal nerves and they act bilaterally to extend the neck. Acting unilaterally, they assist with ipsilateral lateral flexion and rotation.

The muscle should be considered in patients with kinematic change of the neck, particularly in rotation and flexion, and in patients complaining of general neck pain, and/or pain around the ear and maybe around the eye. The trigger points seem to be diffuse within the muscle.

The iliocostalis cervicis is the most lateral column (Fig. 10.13A) and is more a muscle of the cervicothoracic spine. It is discussed in the next chapter.

It is supplied by ventral rami of C3 and C4 and the dorsal scapula nerve from C5. When acting bilaterally with the scapulae fixed it acts to extend the head. When acting unilaterally with the scapulae fixed it is a strong lateral flexor of the head and neck and assists with ipsilateral rotation. When the head and neck are fixed it acts to raise the medial scapulae, thus rotating the glenoid fossa downwards.

It is a postural muscle and shortens when stressed. The muscle is tested with the patient seated with the elbow flexed and held by the side (Fig. 10.14B). The patient laterally flexes to lower the elbow to the level of the iliac crest to align the fibers vertically. The examiner stabilizes the shoulder while attempting to draw the elbow laterally while observing for inferior rotation of the superior angle of the scapula. This test is similar to that for the rhomboid minor (Fig. 9.15B), except for the lateral flexion of the patient.

The levator scapulae is typically associated with a stiff neck and is usually involved with torticollis. The postural assessment may reveal ipsilateral head tilt and a high shoulder. The trigger points are located about the attachment to the scapula with another lateral to the C7 transverse process (Fig. 10.14C). They refer pain about the base of the neck to the superior medial border of the scapula, with perhaps some spillover to the posterior shoulder and along the medial border. The presence of a tenoperiosteal zone of tenderness at the superior medial border of the scapulae, about the insertion of the levator scapulae, is thought to indicate SC at the C4–5 SMU (Maigne 1996 pp. 362–363).

The small muscles

The small muscles are not able to be individually tested and their dysfunction is mainly inferential, based on pain and tenderness about specific cervical SMUs and alterations to movement, particularly reduced flexion and rotation (Fig. 10.15). They are implicated with chronic instability of spinal segments and will be associated with altered movements, both of several segments and of a specific SMU. They are all postural muscles which shorten when dysfunctional.

The intertransversarii are slender muscular slips between the transverse processes of each cervical segment below C2 or C3. They are most highly developed in the cervical region and consist of anterior and posterior subdivisions that run between adjacent anterior and posterior tubercles. The ventral ramus of the mixed spinal nerve exits between each pair of anterior and posterior muscles and provides innervation to the anterior muscle. The medial part of the posterior muscle at each level is innervated by the dorsal ramus (posterior primary division) and the lateral part by the ventral ramus (Cramer & Darby 1995 pp. 88, 89).

There are also rotatores (longus and brevis) and interspinales muscles between each segment and they are supplied by the medial branches of the posterior primary rami of the spinal nerves. The interspinales lie either side of the interspinous ligament. The rotatores lie deep to the multifidi and the brevis muscle attaches between the transverse process of one segment and the root of the spinous process of the segment above. The rotatores longus originate in the same region but ascend to the root of the spinous process two segments above. They are poorly developed in this region (Cramer & Darby 1995 p. 86).

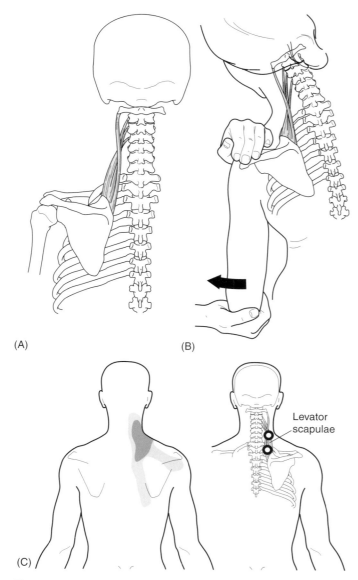

(A) (B)

(C)

Levator scapulae

Figure 10.14 The levator scapulae. (A) The levator scapulae turns on itself as it ascends from the superomedial angle of the scapula to attach on to the transverse process of C1 and the posterior tubercles of C2–4. (B) The seated patient leans ipsilaterally to bring the levator scapulae fibers into the vertical plane for testing. The test vector is in the direction of the arrow and the examiner looks for rotation of the scapula. (C) The trigger point location and pattern of referred pain. From Chaitow & DeLany (2000), with permission.

Muscles tested with the patient seated

The levator scapulae

The levator scapulae attaches to the transverse processes of C1 and the posterior tubercles of the transverse processes of C2–4 and inserts to the medial border of the scapula between the superior angle and the level of the root of the spine (Fig. 10.14A). The fibers twist on themselves so that the highest originating fibers from C1 attach to the scapula as the lowest fibers on the medial border (Simons et al 1999).

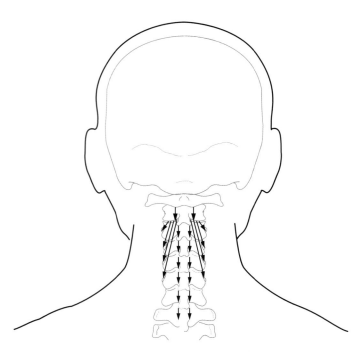

Figure 10.15 The small muscles. The arrangement of the deep, small muscles is to cross two or three segments and run an oblique course inferiorly, laterally, and anteriorly. From Kapandji (1974), with permission.

These small muscles are thought to rotate and extend the superior vertebral segment on its inferior partner; however, Herzog considers they are poorly placed to provide sufficient moment to induce movement (Herzog 2000 p. 32). He notes they are highly rich in muscle spindles and are more likely to act as length transducers or vertebral position sensors within the SMU. His comments specifically relate to the thoracic and lumbar spine. Herzog suggests the rotatores have a minimal contribution as lateral flexors and contralateral rotators (Herzog 2000 pp. 32, 71).

The multifidi arise from the articular processes of the lower four cervical vertebrae and the fascicles each ascend a varying number of segments as high as C2 to insert into the spinous processes (Cramer & Darby 1995 p. 84). They are innervated by the dorsal ramus and act as extensors and assist lateral flexion and contralateral rotation of the cervical spine. They are antagonists to the longus colli and have a low density of muscle spindles (Boyd-Clark et al 2002) and a greater proportion of type I than type II fibers, suggesting it is a predominantly postural muscle (Boyd-Clark et al 2001).

The multifidi are implicated with chronic instability of the SMU, kinematic change in flexion and perhaps rotation, and pain about the suboccipital region and medial scapula. The multifidus trigger points are deep about the C4, C5 level and refer ipsilateral suboccipital pain. They are especially prone to fixation in this region (Schafer 1983).

Extrinsic muscles

The following muscles are extrinsic to the mid cervical spine but receive their innervation from this level. They are assessed as part of the clinical process of seeking evidence supportive of the

SC in this region of the spine. Any weakness or hypertonicity may suggest spinal dysfunction or perhaps interference to the relevant peripheral nerve. The typical tests of motor function and strength are described for each.

Biceps brachii

The biceps brachii originates as a short head from the tip of the coracoid process and a long head from the supraglenoid tubercle of the scapula and inserts into the radial tuberosity and the deep fascia about the flexors of the forearm. It is supplied by C6 (with some C5) as the musculocutaneous nerve which gives a branch to each belly. It acts as a powerful supinator and is a flexor of the forearm, especially when in supination.

The muscle is tested with the patient seated or supine and the elbow flexed to 90° with the forearm in supination and the elbow supported in the indifferent hand. The test force aims to draw the distal forearm into extension and derives from the contact hand being applied across the volar surface of the distal forearm.

Pronators

The pronator teres originates as a humeral head from the medial epicondylar ridge and common flexor tendon and as an ulnar head from the medial side of the coronoid process, and inserts into the medial lateral border of the radius. The pronator quadratus originates from the distal volar surface of the ulna and inserts into the volar surface of the distal lateral border of the radius. Pronator teres is supplied by C6 and C7 and pronator quadratus by C8 and T1 as the median nerve and they act to pronate the forearm.

Both muscles are tested together with the patient seated or supine and the elbow flexed to remove the elbow flexion function of the pronator teres. The forearm is held in neutral with the thumb up and the elbow is held close to the patient's body. The indifferent hand supports the elbow while the contact hand takes a 'handshake' grip to supinate the forearm while the patient resists with pronation.

Wrist extensors

The wrist extensors include the extensor carpi radialis longus and brevis and the extensor carpi ulnaris. Their action is aided by the other smaller extensors about the hand. The extension action at the wrist is innervated by C6 as the radial nerve.

They are classified as phasic muscles and weaken when stressed. The extensors are tested with the patient seated with the wrist extended and fingers flexed to weaken the long finger extensors. The forearm is supported by the indifferent hand while the test force is applied by the contact hand to flex the wrist.

ASSESSMENT OF NEURAL CHANGE

The spinal nerves

The spinal nerves of the mid cervical spine, and the levels at which they exit, are:

- spinal nerve C4 from the C3–4 SMU
- spinal nerve C5 from the C4–5 SMU
- spinal nerve C6 from the C5–6 SMU.

The assessment for signs and symptoms of neural change must include sensory, motor, deep or muscle tendon reflexes, and autonomic functions, and consider distributions in terms of dermatomes (Fig. 10.16), myotomes, and sclerotomes.

C4 spinal nerve

The C4 spinal nerve exits the IVC and divides with the dorsal ramus looping posteriorly about the anterolateral aspect of the articular pillar, where it may leave a groove. It divides to a medial branch which innervates the deep muscles and the zygapophyseal joints, and a lateral branch which is motor to the more superficial muscles.

The ventral ramus passes posterior to the vertebral artery and between the anterior and posterior intertransversarii muscles to innervate the anterior muscles about the neck. It is sensory to the anterior vertebral body, anterior longitudinal ligament, and the anterior disk, along with sensory fibers from the sympathetic chain and autonomic fibers about the vertebral artery. The recurrent meningeal nerve arises from the ventral ramus and links with these fibers and provides sensation about the posterior vertebral body and disk and related structures at this level.

The C4 ventral ramus contributes motor function to the ansa cervicalis and forms the supraclavicular nerve with C3. The phrenic nerve, which is motor and sensory to the diaphragm, arises from the ventral rami of C3 and chiefly C4, with some C5.

C5 spinal nerve

The C5 spinal nerve exits the IVC and divides with the dorsal ramus looping posteriorly about the anterolateral aspect of the articular pillar, where it too may leave a groove. It divides to a medial branch which innervates the deep muscles and the zygapophyseal joints, and a lateral branch which is motor to more superficial muscles, and sensory to the skin about the lateral shoulder and arm (brachium), and along the clavicle.

The ventral ramus passes posteriorly in the same manner as C4. It provides motor function as the dorsal scapular nerve to the rhomboids, joins with C6 to provide motor function as the suprascapular nerve, and contributes to the upper trunk of the brachial plexus which provides motor function as the musculocutaneous and axillary nerves, and contributes to the median and radial nerves. Some C5 fibers contribute to the phrenic nerve.

The clinical evidence of C5 involvement includes pain in the neck, tip of the shoulder and anterior arm; sensory change about the deltoid; motor change in the deltoid and biceps; and reflex change at the biceps tendon. Cold stimulation of the forearm below the inside of the elbow has been shown on functional MRI (fMRI) to produce activation around the C5 cervical cord segment (Stroman et al 2002).

C6 spinal nerve

The C6 spinal nerve exits the IVC and divides with the dorsal ramus looping posteriorly close to the anterolateral aspect of the articular pillar. Usually, the dorsal ramus itself does not divide, giving only a deep medial branch which innervates the deep muscles including multifidi, and the zygapophyseal joints with a branch to the joint above and a branch to the joint below.

Usually the dorsal ramus does not have cutaneous branches (Cramer & Darby 1995 p. 142).

The ventral ramus passes posteriorly in the same manner as C4 and C5. It joins with C5 to provide motor function as the suprascapular nerve and contributes to the upper trunk of the brachial plexus which provides motor function as the musculocutaneous and axillary nerves, and contributes to the median and radial nerves.

The clinical evidence of C6 involvement is pain in the neck, shoulder, medial border of the scapula, lateral arm, and back of the forearm; sensory change about the thumb and index finger; motor change in the biceps; and reflex change at the brachioradialis tendon. Cold stimulation of the thumb side of the palm has been shown on fMRI to produce activation at the C6 cervical cord segment (Stroman et al 2002).

Local pain

Acute pain usually reflects local trauma and a thorough patient history is crucial to direct the examination and working diagnoses. Acute pain may be associated with a torticollis and may involve SC and/or muscle change. Torticollis secondary to trauma requires radiographs to rule out fracture before further assessment.

Acute pain may also arise from synovitis, when it is important to exclude other inflammatory processes, and from capsular strain. The rich anastomoses among adjacent spinal cord segments allow for nociceptive impulses through the dorsal root ganglion of one spinal level to enter the cord at the level above or below, making it difficult to localize. These anastomoses also disrupt the dermatomal patterns of innervation, presenting a further challenge to the practitioner.

The cervical disk can also be a cause of acute pain, with or without referral. There are sensory nerve fibers throughout the annulus fibrosus of the healthy disk but none in the central region. A large number of the sensory fibers are consistent with those which transmit pain and it is reported that the annulus is pain-sensitive as well as contributing to proprioception (Cramer & Darby 1995 p. 135). The localized pain will be reproduced or worsened with provocative tests such as cervical compression.

Chronic pain requires sinister causes to be ruled out during the assessment. These include intramedullary tumors such as meningiomas, neurofibromas, and ependymomas (Maigne 1996).

Referred pain

There are numerous patterns of referred pain from the neck, reflecting the complexity of the pain generators in the region. Cramer & Darby (1995 p. 358) identify the following structures innervated by nerves of the dorsal ramus and note that they are possible pain generators:

- zygapophyseal joints
- periosteum of the posterior vertebral arch
- interspinous, supraspinous, and intertransverse ligaments, ligamentum flavum
- skin (upper cervical dorsal rami)
- splenius capitis and cervicis muscles.

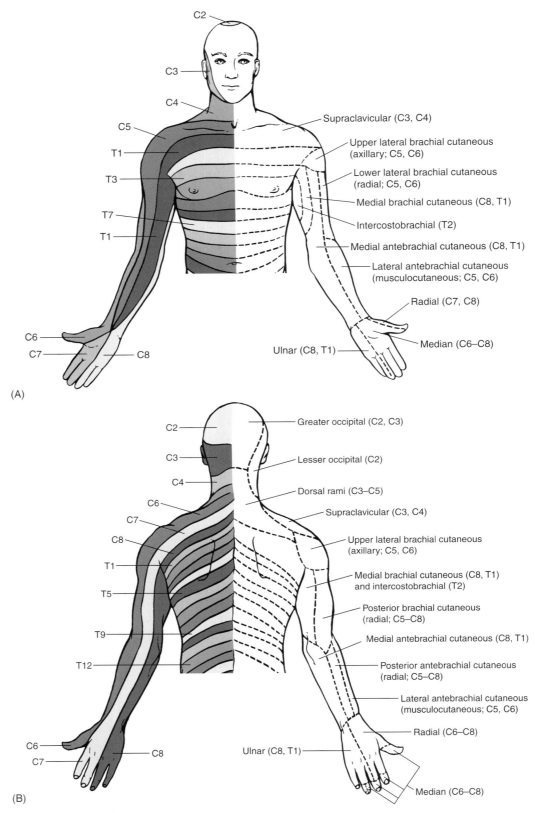

Figure 10.16 Cutaneous innervation. The cutaneous innervation of the upper body is shown by dermatome (left of each image) and cutaneous peripheral nerve (right of each image) for the anterior (A) and posterior (B). From Cramer & Darby (1995), with permission.

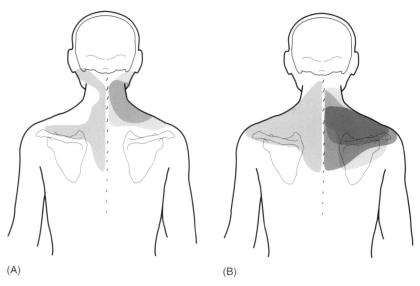

Figure 10.17 Patterns of referred pain. (A) The left side shows referred pain from irritation of the paraspinal tissues between C4 and C5 and the right side shows referred pain from irritation of the C4–5 zygapophyseal joints. (B) The left side shows referred pain from irritation of the paraspinal tissues between C5 and C6 and the right side shows referred pain from irritation of the C5–6 zygapophyseal joints. (A, B) From Terrett & Terrett (2002), with permission.

The patterns of referred pain have been documented in studies where the tissues have been irritated by the researchers injecting liquids at specific spinal levels. The patterns arising from the paraspinal tissues differ to those from the zygapophyseal joints. The findings from several studies have been compiled by Terrett & Terrett (2002) and are shown in Figure 10.17.

The practitioner should first attempt to distinguish between nerve root pain and myelopathy. Nerve root involvement may be single or multiple, unilateral or bilateral, and symmetrical or asymmetrical, and the degree to which each nerve root may be involved is variable (Lestini & Wiesel 1989). Acute nerve root pain is typically associated with disk damage and subacute pain is more likely to be secondary to degenerative changes and spondylosis. Chronic nerve root pain tends also to involve musculature about the thoracic outlet and other long-term changes.

Sensory symptoms appear more frequently with nerve root involvement and include paresthesias, hyperesthesia, or hyperalgesia which are accentuated with neck movements which irritate the affected nerve (Lestini & Wiesel 1989). The sensory changes are rarely confined to a specific nerve root and typically include a broad distribution.

While nerve root pain arises from direct mechanical mechanisms, the causes of cervical myelopathy are less defined and include spondylotic transverse bars, hypertrophic facets, preexisting and acquired changes to canal diameter, vascular changes, differences in cord sensitivity due to hypoxia, and canal shape (Lestini & Wiesel 1989). Symptom onset is increasing disability over a period of several months. Sensory changes include numbness and tingling in the tips of the fingers which may appear in a nerve root distribution. Motor signs may be present as weakness or clumsiness and the deep or muscle tendon reflex may diminish or exaggerate.

The complaint of headache may also reflect a referred pain from the mid cervical spine. Degenerative changes of the spine were thought to cause about one-third of all cases of headache in one report (Turk & Ratkolb 1987). The zygapophyseal joints are known to be a cause of neck pain and headache (Bogduk & Marsland 1988, Speldewinde et al 2001).

Sensory change

Basic assessment includes recording the bilaterally comparative responses to crude touch. Further assessment can include pain or sharp touch, temperature, and vibration. The distributions are shown in Figure 10.16. The general dermatomal distributions of the nerve roots are:

- C4: a "collar" as posteroinferior neck to anterior neck, above clavicle
- C5: lateral shoulder and arm, and along the clavicle
- C6: the lateral forearm (antebrachium), thumb and index finger.

The general dermatomal distributions of the peripheral nerves are:

- C3–4 supraclavicular nerve: skin over clavicle and proximal deltoid muscle
- C5 axillary nerve: skin on the lateral brachium about the deltoid insertion as the "axillary patch"
- C6 lateral antebrachial cutaneous nerve: skin on the lateral forearm
- C6 median nerve: skin on the lateral anterior thumb
- C6 radial nerve: skin on the posterior thumb web.

Motor function

Basic motor assessment includes recording muscle weakness, absent or diminished tone, fasciculations, neurogenic atrophy, and altered tendon reflexes. The nerve roots are difficult to assess singly due to the variability of the contribution from various levels. The peripheral nerves may be assessed and then inference made back to the root level. In general terms, the tests for motor function of individual spinal nerve roots are:

- C4: not tested singly
- C5: shoulder abduction as tested with the middle fibers of the deltoid
- C6: wrist extension, although C7 and C8 may be included.

The peripheral nerve motor function is assessed as follows:

- C3–4 spinal accessory nerve: upper trapezius – shoulder elevation
- C5 dorsal scapular nerve: rhomboid – scapula adduction
- C5 suprascapular nerve: supraspinatus – early shoulder abduction
- C5 axillary nerve: deltoid – late shoulder abduction
- C5–6 musculocutaneous nerve: biceps brachii and brachialis – elbow flexion in supination
- C6 radial nerve: wrist extensors – wrist extension. If a radial nerve lesion is suspected, work towards the midline by first testing the extensors, and then the triceps (radial nerve, elbow extension, C7, C8)
- C6 median nerve: pronator teres and pronator quadratus – forearm pronation.

The muscle tendon reflexes are assessed as follows:

- C5 (and C6): the biceps reflex; causes flexion at the elbow when the bicipital tendon is struck
- C6 (and C5): the brachioradialis reflex; causes flexion and supination of the forearm when the brachioradialis tendon is struck proximal to the radial styloid.

Autonomic effects

Autonomic fibers travel with the spinal nerves and then peripheral nerves and innervate sweat glands, erector pili muscles, and peripheral blood vessels, including those in skeletal muscle and skin.

The cervical sympathetic chain lies anterior to longus capitis and posterior to the carotid sheath. The preganglionic bodies for the head and neck are found in the spinal cord at levels T1–3, and maybe T4 and T5. Branches from the cervical chain form the plexus about the vertebral artery.

Cramer & Darby (1995 p. 359) identify the following structures innervated by nerves associated with the sympathetic trunk and the gray rami communicans and note they are possible pain generators:

- periosteum of the anterior and lateral vertebral body
- lateral aspect of the intervertebral disk
- anterior aspect of the intervertebral disk
- anterior longitudinal ligament.

Signs of abnormal sympathetic activity may be seen as the following functions: pupil dilation, increased heart rate, increased sweating, erect body hair, dry eyes, dry mouth, and vasoconstriction to the skin.

The C4 nerve root communicates with the superior cervical ganglion of the sympathetic chain and it is thought that irritation of the C4 root may produce symptoms related to the sympathetic nervous system (Tamura 1989). This could explain the symptoms of the Barré–Lieou syndrome, namely that headache could result from spasm of the internal and external carotid arteries; vertigo may be caused by ischemia of the brain produced by sympathetic vasoconstriction of the internal carotid artery and its intracerebral branches; tinnitus may be produced by sympathetic stimulation of the caroticotympanic nerve which derives from the internal carotid plexus; ocular symptoms may arise under the influence of the internal carotid plexus on the ciliary muscles or by vasoconstriction of the ophthalmic artery; and facial pain may arise through the communicating branches with the facial nerve and the trigeminal ganglion (Tamura 1989). It is known that preganglionic sympathetic neurons projecting to target organs in the head exhibit distinct reflex patterns to stimulation of various afferent systems in the rat (Bartsch et al 2000) and not just spinal nerve irritation.

The parasympathetic division (rest and digest) is also known as the craniosacral division (Cramer & Darby 1995 p. 321). The preganglionic cell bodies lie in the brainstem within the cranium and in the second, third, and fourth sacral segments. The cranial sympathetic fibers travel with the oculomotor, facial, glossopharyngeal, and vagus cranial nerves (III, VII, IX, X) and innervate glandular tissue and smooth muscle. Signs of parasympathetic activity may be seen in the following functions:

- with the oculomotor nerve: pupil constriction by the smooth muscle of the iris; accommodation–convergence reflex by contraction of the ciliary muscle
- with the facial nerve: vasodilation of and secretion from the submandibular, sublingual, and minor salivary glands; secretion from the lacrimal gland; secretion from the glands and mucous membranes of the palate and nasal mucosa
- with the glossopharyngeal nerve: vasodilation and serous secretion from the parotid gland
- with the vagus nerve: extensive function within the thorax and abdomen but not the head. Some 75% of all parasympathetic fibers travel with the vagus; however, the afferent fibers conveying sensory information in the vagus nerve outnumber the efferent fibers (Cramer & Darby 1995 pp. 321–326). The vagal afferent fibers innervate the esophagus, lower airways, heart, aorta, possibly the thymus, and via abdominal branches the entire gastrointestinal tract, liver, portal vein, billiary system, and pancreas. It also innervates numerous thoracic and abdominal paraganglia (Berthoud & Neuhuber 2000).

The afferent vagal system has also been shown to have a range of specific terminal structures and this suggests functional specializations. It is thought that the system is well placed to detect immune-related events in the periphery and generate appropriate autonomic, endocrine, and behavioral responses via central reflex pathways (Berthoud & Neuhuber 2000). The vagal afferents also seem to generate the affective-emotional responses such as increased blood pressure and tachycardia typically associated with the perception of pain.

The sympathetic and parasympathetic systems generally exist in balance to maintain homeostasis. Evidence is starting to appear which suggests this balance may be shifted by manipulation of the cervical spine. Budgell & Hirano (2001) have reported significant alterations in both heart rate and heart-rate variability, as calculated from power spectrum analysis following manipulation in health young adults.

ASSESSMENT OF VASCULAR CHANGE

Apart from the effects of injury noted below, consideration must be given to variations as evidenced on diagnostic images which relate to vascularization of the region.

The pericervical lymphatic collar lies in this region and includes the occipital nodes, postauricular nodes, preauricular nodes, submandibular nodes, and submental nodes. These drain into the deep cervical nodes which lie along the internal jugular vein. Consideration must be given to the nodes of the region during assessment and palpation and when taking adjustive contact.

Edema may result from a traumatic sprain of the capsular ligaments or supporting ligaments and, given the close relationships among the joints, may affect regional and segmental movement and palpate as focal tenderness and bogginess. Inflammation is generally a contraindication to adjustment and is associated with arthritides or posttraumatic injury. It may be indicated by swelling of the prevertebral soft tissues and quantified by measuring the RPI and/or RTI.

Areas of colder temperature may be palpated about the mid cervical region, suggestive of vasoconstriction secondary to altered joint mechanics and subsequent neural reflexes constricting the arterial supply. Thermal asymmetry may be seen on the infrared thermograph and is thought to be detected by the Nervoscope. More work needs to be undertaken on these findings and their correlation, if any, to the SC.

The most important vascular considerations are those associated with VBI, as discussed in the preceding chapter and in Chapter 8. There is nothing specific to this region of the spine associated with VBI.

CONCLUSION

The mid cervical spine is commonly overtreated due to its propensity to demonstrate kinematic change which is actually compensatory for subluxation in either the upper cervical complex or the cervicothoracic junction.

When SC is suspected in this region, the practitioner must make a special effort to identify associated elements, particularly muscle and neural change. Attention must be paid to the connective tissues, particularly in posttrauma patients, and to the same range of potential vascular complications which may be associated with upper cervical treatment.

11

The cervicothoracic spine

KEY CONCEPTS

Any assessment of the cervical spine is incomplete without thorough assessment of the cervicothoracic spine due to the relatively high prevalence of disk degeneration in the upper thoracic segments and the muscles which form the ligamentum nuchae attaching in this region.

The clinical evidence of C7 involvement is pain in the neck, shoulder, medial border of the scapula, lateral arm, and back of the forearm; sensory change about the index and middle finger; motor change in the triceps; and reflex change at the triceps tendon.

The clinical evidence of C8 involvement is pain in the neck, shoulder, medial border of the scapula and medial aspect of the forearm; sensory change about the ring and little finger; and motor change in the intrinsic muscles of the hand.

The muscles of the forearm, wrist, and hand are innervated from this region and specific muscle assessment and testing may indicate neural change arising within the spine, about the spine, or within the shoulder and arm.

In empirical terms the upper thoracic spinal motion units (SMUs) are associated with hypertension and respiratory changes such as asthma. Adjustment at these levels is thought to produce a sympathetic effect including lung dilation.

There is a relationship of the thoracic sympathetic ganglia about the head of each rib which is thought to allow the regular and rhythmic motion of the rib head during respiration to provide a local intermittent pumping action ensuring fluid movement in and about the ganglia. This normal movement may be compromised with rib fixation.

CLINICAL ANATOMY

The cervicothoracic junctional spine includes the following major articulations:

- C6–7
- C7–T1
- T1–2
- left and right rib 1 – posterior
- left and right rib 1 – anterior
- T2–3
- left and right rib 2 – posterior
- left and right rib 2 – anterior.

Cramer & Darby (1995 pp. 126–127, 144–149, 156–168) provide the appropriate level of anatomy of this region for the student and can be read in conjunction with this chapter. They (p. 10) and others identify the following clinically important relationships:

- C5–6: superior margin of lobes of thyroid gland; Erb's point (posterior to sternocleidomastoid, stimulation contracts various arm muscles)
- C6: middle cervical ganglion; cricoid cartilage; first tracheal ring; transition of larynx to trachea
- C7: inferior cervical ganglion
- T1: stellate ganglion; inferior margin of the thyroid gland; apices of lungs
- T2: brachiocephalic veins unite to form superior vena cava
- T2–3 disk: suprasternal notch (variable).

The gradually changing structure of the mid cervical vertebrae abruptly alters at C7–T1. While C6 maintains similarity with those segments above, C7 is considered atypical in that it is the interface between the highly mobile cervical spine and the much more rigid thoracic spine. The superior articular facets of C3 and C4 face posteromedially and this transitions through this region such that those from T1 and below face posterolaterally. The change may be sudden or gradual and the C5–6 articulation is the most frequent site to show the transition (Pal et al 2001). The shape of the superior articular facets was found to be circular to oval at C5 and above, gradually changing to a transversely elongated surface at C7 and T1 (Pal et al 2001). There is a relatively high incidence of left/right asymmetry and facet angle asymmetry at C6, C7, and T1 (Boyle et al 1998).

Comparative illustrations (Fig. 11.1) also demonstrate the obvious morphologic changes to the spinal canal, from the semicircular profile with a short spinous at C6 to the more smaller canal profile with a much longer spinous at C7. The spinal canal becomes more circular about T1 and T2 and the transverse processes enlarge. Note also the change from the bifid spinous of the cervical spine to the non-bifid thoracic spinous process. While T1 is considered unique, T2 is a typical thoracic vertebra.

The lateral view of T1 (Fig. 11.2) demonstrates the complexity of the joints associated with the thoracic segments. The corporal facet to receive the head of rib 1 is complete on the vertebral body in hominoids (Ohman 1986, Stern & Jungers 1990). This facet transitions in subjacent segments to be a more superior

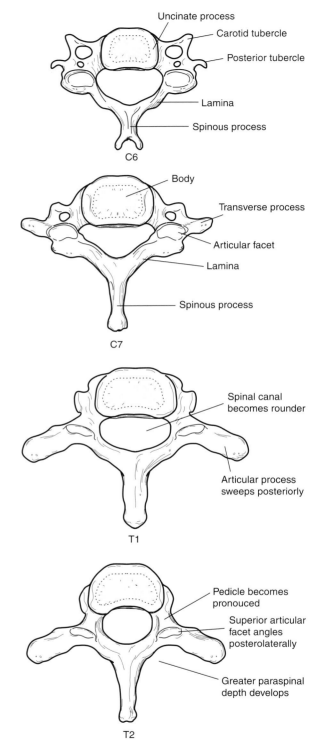

Figure 11.1 Superior view of cervicothoracic vertebrae.

demifacet and the head of the rib comes to articulate across two bodies and the disk. The inferior demifacet for the superior facet of the head of rib 2 is seen at the inferior lateral margin of the body. It is important also to note the changes in the angulation

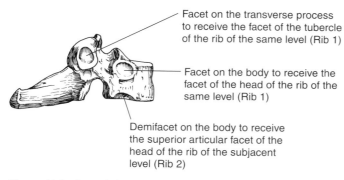

Facet on the transverse process to receive the facet of the tubercle of the rib of the same level (Rib 1)

Facet on the body to receive the facet of the head of the rib of the same level (Rib 1)

Demifacet on the body to receive the superior articular facet of the head of the rib of the subjacent level (Rib 2)

Figure 11.2 Lateral view of T1. From Bergmann et al (1993), with permission.

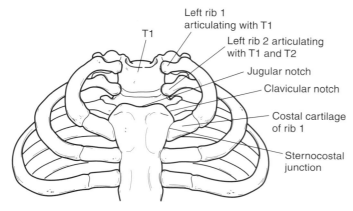

T1

Left rib 1 articulating with T1

Left rib 2 articulating with T1 and T2

Jugular notch

Clavicular notch

Costal cartilage of rib 1

Sternocostal junction

Figure 11.3 Anterior view of the rib articulations about T1 and T2. From Cramer & Darby (1995), with permission.

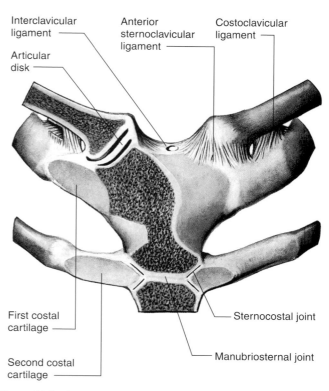

Interclavicular ligament

Anterior sternoclavicular ligament

Costoclavicular ligament

Articular disk

First costal cartilage

Second costal cartilage

Sternocostal joint

Manubriosternal joint

Figure 11.4 An anterior view of the anterior rib articulations. From Williams & Warwick (1980), with permission.

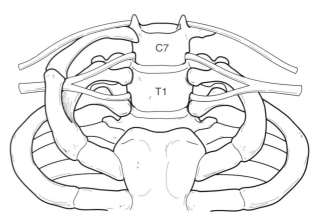

C7

T1

Figure 11.5 Cervical ribs. The transverse process of C7 may be hyperplastic and extend inferolaterally (left) or it may form an articulation with a distinct cervical rib (right).

and orientation of the zygapophyseal facets and the resultant joints when other thoracic levels are considered (Fig. 12.4).

The rigidity of the thoracic spine is enhanced by the rib articulations and these must be considered in any assessment of the SMU in this region. The cervicothoracic junction is the transition zone between the highly mobile cervical spine, based on C6–7, and the very stable thoracic spine, starting with T1 and ribs 1, then T2 with ribs 2, and so on. The practitioner must not only consider the posterior articulations of the ribs about the vertebral bodies, but also the anterior articulations, in this case about the manubrium and sternum (Fig. 11.3).

The anterior rib 1 articulation is quite intricate as the joint capsule includes the sternoclavicular articulation (Fig. 11.4). Within this joint there is a flat, nearly circular articular disk which has a broad, fibrous insertion superiorly to the articular capsule. There are blood vessels in this component; however, the inferior attachment to the cartilage of rib 1 as it joins the sternum is thinner and may be reduced to a fine, translucent pellet with or without perforations (Barbaix et al 2000). The disk can be divided into a sternal and a costal segment, separated by a vascular zone.

Rib 1 is also attached to the clavicle by the costoclavicular ligament which reaches upwards to the inferior medial clavicle. The subclavius muscle arises from rib 1 at its junction with the costal cartilage and inserts into the inferior surface of the middle third of the clavicle. Rib 2 articulates at the manubriosternal joint where

there is an intra-articular ligament extending from its costal cartilage and attaching to the fibrocartilaginous manubriosternal joint. It divides the joint cavity into two. The sternocostal joints are bound by the radiate sternocostal ligaments.

Two common anomalies about the cervicothoracic junction are hyperplastic transverse processes at C7, and cervical rib(s) (Fig. 11.5). The transverse process is considered hyperplastic when its lateral margin extends more than the lateral margin of the T1 transverse process below. It may remain a discrete bony element or it may project inferolaterally as a cartilaginous/ligamentous band, of which only part may be seen on the

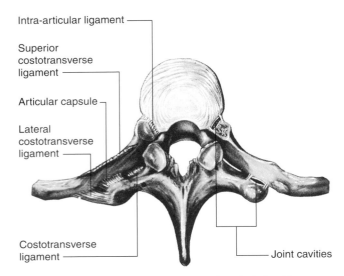

Figure 11.6 Plane view of a typical right rib articulation. From Williams & Warwick (1980), with permission.

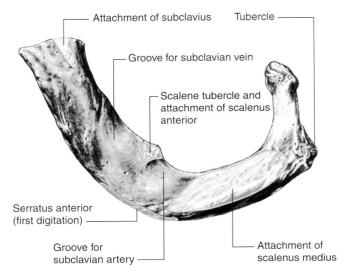

Figure 11.7 Superior view of a typical left rib 1. From Williams & Warwick (1980), with permission.

radiograph, although it is clearly demonstrated on magnetic resonance imaging (MRI) where it has been shown to distort the brachial plexus (Panegyres et al 1993). The true cervical rib is a distinct rib which articulates with C7 and which may or may not articulate with other structures such as the true rib 1. These anomalies may be seen unilaterally or in combination, as shown. They alter the kinematics of the segments and have clinical implications, not only for the assessment of kinematic change, but also for the neurovascular structures of the brachial plexus and thoracic outlet.

Another feature of clinical significance is the morphology of the spinous processes in this region. The typical facet relationship of C6 on C7 allows C6 to be relatively mobile, hence in full extension the C6 spinous process may be palpated as slipping away anteriorly. The increasing angle of the superior facets of T1, which face posteriorly, restrict the ability of C7 to glide anteriorly, hence in extension the C7 segment is less anteriorly mobile than that of C6. The C7 spinous process is also usually the largest of the spine, giving the appearance of the "vertebral prominens" when the neck is flexed; however, it must be appreciated that C6 and T1 may also have a similar appearance in some individuals, particularly ectomorphs.

The axial view of a typical rib articulation demonstrates the complex joint relationships about the vertebral bodies (Fig. 11.6). Note the articulation of the proximal rib to the posterolateral vertebral body. This is usually a full facet at T1 but there may at times be a demifacet providing articulation of rib 1 with both C7 and T1 bodies, as well as the C7–T1 disk. There is also the articulation of the tubercle of the rib with the transverse process of the same-numbered vertebra.

Rib 1 is atypical in that it lies flatter and has a tubercle on the superior surface for the insertion of the scalenus anterior and scalenus medius muscles (Fig. 11.7; see also Fig. 10.12A). The prominent tubercle of rib 1 articulates with the transverse process of T1. Rib 2 is larger and carries a tuberosity for the insertion of the serratus anterior muscle and has a longer neck than rib 1 (Fig. 11.8).

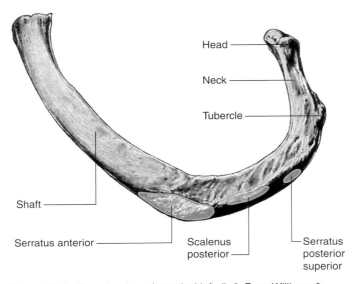

Figure 11.8 Superior view of a typical left rib 2. From Williams & Warwick (1980), with permission.

ASSESSMENT OF KINEMATIC CHANGE

Postural assessment

The nature of the base of the neck must be noted in the context of the somatotype of the patient during observation. The neck of an ectomorph, for example, will exhibit different soft- and hard-tissue relationships to that of an endomorph. Secondly, careful observation may reveal a suspicion of underlying congenital anomaly; this is usually obvious in the patient with Klippel–Feil syndrome or Sprengle's deformity. Finally, observation may reveal patients' functional response to their environment; their neck and shoulder musculature may appear bunched and tense (hypertonic secondary to stress) or asymmetrical due to chronic work postures.

Static palpation

This transitional area has been considered a difficult region in the spine (Bergmann et al 1993 p. 308); however, a thorough understanding of the region's anatomy and neurology makes it a joy to assess. Static palpation is important to demonstrate subtle changes in relationships which may result in distal neural change, for example, a hypertonic scalene muscle may elevate rib 1 and compromise the neurovascular bundle of the upper quadrant, generating signs and symptoms of arm and hand pain and weakness.

Vigorous motion palpation is not appropriate for this region and the more useful clinical information is gained through static palpation which incorporates micromovement and end-feel. For example, it is difficult to induce movement into rib 1 and the practitioner's perception of superior fixation is drawn more from the rib's resistance to specific attempts to induce small movement. If movement palpation with superior to inferior vectors produces a sensation of less or restricted movement compared to the opposite side then the rib may be considered as being fixed superiorly, and especially so if the palpation produces pain and tenderness.

All segments (C6–7, C7–T1, T1–2, T2–3) may be assessed with the patient either seated or supine. The seated position allows easy transition to dynamic palpation which may or may not be useful at or below T2 or so, while the supine position allows an easy segue from the cervical segments to both T1 and T2 in most patients and allows the assessment of ribs 1 and 2 through posterior to anterior springing.

It is reasonably assumed that the structures in this region will exhibit the same general symmetry as do the structures above; however, it must be appreciated that the thoracic spinous processes start to demonstrate a marked inferior angulation from about T2 or T3 and this may be accompanied by normal deviation to one side or the other.

C6 is typically symmetrical, while C7 may have a bulbous end to the spinous process which may give the appearance of misalignment on static palpation. Cervical ribs are commonly unilateral, while hyperplastic C7 transverse processes without fibrous extension are typically bilateral. It is not common for paired true ribs to be markedly asymmetrical.

Radiographic analysis

The cervicothoracic junction is clearly seen on the anteroposterior (AP) lower cervical plain radiograph. This view is quite useful for demonstrating levels of segmental lateral flexion which correct for unlevel segments below, perhaps associated with scoliosis or lateral flexion fixation. A plane line drawn through matching points on one particular body may help quantify any lateral flexion component in comparison with the comparable line on the bodies above and below. The AP view should also demonstrate the relationships about the ribs, although the use of radiographic line marking to attempt to quantify these relationships is not known to have any purpose.

The clinical usefulness of the lateral cervical neutral film will vary with the body type of the patient. In some, this view may clearly demonstrate segments as low as T2 or T3, but in others the muscle bulk about the shoulders and base of the neck may obscure segments from C6 or C7. On the occasions when the practitioner requires a clear depiction of relationships in the sagittal plane, a lateral cervicothoracic view is requested. This is colloquially known as the "Swimmer's" projection (Yochum & Rowe 1996 p. 37).

Objective structural change of SMU mechanics

The major anomalies of this region are block vertebrae and Klippel–Feil syndrome, both discussed previously. Klippel–Feil syndrome may present with an omovertebral bone which may project from the C7 lamina toward the superior angle of the scapula. Sprengle's deformity occurs in 20–25% of patients with Klippel–Feil syndrome, and may also present as an isolated anomaly (Yochum & Rowe 1996, p. 217, Taylor & Resnick 2000 p. 813). A 2 : 1 female predominance is reported and most cases are unilateral. It is thought to represent a failure of the scapula to descend from its level of formation at C4–5.

The cervical pedicle may be unilaterally congenitally absent. Yochum & Rowe (1996 p. 220) report C6 as most common, accounting for about 44% of such cases, and C7 as one of the least common (12.5% of such cases). Cervical spondylolisthesis, as a bilateral absence of pedicles with dysplasia of the articular pillars and spina bifida occulta, is rare. It usually affects C6. Yochum & Rowe make the point (1996 p. 218) that spina bifida occulta is rare at C6 and is usually indicative of spondylolisthesis. Flexion/extension radiographs may demonstrate altered movement and inform the practitioner prior to therapeutic intervention.

A cervical rib is described as a "separate piece of bone that articulates with the transverse processes of one or more cervical vertebrae" (Yochum & Rowe 1996 pp. 220–222) and is most common at the C7, C6, and C5 levels. They are differentiated from, and distinct to, elongated transverse processes and are found in 0.5% of the population, more commonly in females, and are bilateral in 66% of cases (Yochum & Rowe 1996 pp. 220–222).

Fracture has been discussed as an articular pillar fracture for the mid cervical spine and the same principles apply in this region. Yochum & Rowe (1996 pp. 678–684) describe a number of fractures specific to this region, including:

- vertebral body and neural arch fracture
- transverse process fractures (C7, T1)
- wedge compression fracture (C7)
- the tear-drop fracture (an avulsion of the anteroinferior body)
- the "clay-shoveler's" fracture, described below.

Signs of avulsion suggest trauma and such patients require thorough assessment and evaluation of the associated soft-tissue damage. The more common finding is known as the "clay-shoveler's" fracture and is the avulsion of the C7 spinous process (Yochum & Rowe 1996 pp. 680–681). It may involve only the tip of the spinous or, more seriously, may avulse the spinous from the laminae and pedicles.

Dislocation, either bilateral or unilateral, involves the zygapophyseal joints and those of the cervical segments more than the thoracic. It is typically seen secondary to accidental trauma. Rib dislocation is more likely to be at the posterior than the anterior articulations.

Disk space narrowing, as seen on the lateral view, is the earliest radiographic finding of disk degeneration and is usually associated with adjacent endplate sclerosis and marginal osteophyte formation (Pelz & Fox 1990). As in other levels of the spine, hypertrophy of the lower articular pillars may represent degenerative joint disorders. Pain is more likely to develop in persons with degenerative changes at C6–7 (Gore 2001).

Other diagnostic imaging assessment

The axial computed tomography (CT) scan is the imaging modality of choice as it may demonstrate both the bony and soft-tissue relationships in the various small joints about this region, although plain radiographs are the initial premanipulative image of choice. The CT scan allows the practitioner to observe and integrate the status of the articulations at the disk and zygapophyseal joints at the cervical SMUs and with the posterior and anterior aspects of the ribs about the disk and facets of the thoracic SMUs. It must be appreciated that the uncinate joints are not present in the thoracic SMU and are variable in the C7–T1 SMU. Further, the CT scan has great value in demonstrating pathology in the viscera about this region. The lung apices are at the level of T1 and may be the site of tumor.

The MRI is useful to demonstrate soft-tissue relationships and plays a vital role in demonstrating neoplastic infiltration and changes in neural tissue. It is the imaging modality of choice when there is suspicion of neural compromise such as cord compression and is particularly useful for examining thoracic outlet syndromes (Panegyres et al 1993).

Subjective nature of movement

The assessment of the active range of motion of the region is a continuation of the assessment of the upper and mid cervical spines and will not be repeated in detail here. The practitioner performs this assessment with consideration of the patient's somatotype and ability to respond to direction.

It is important to observe movement about T1, T2, and T3 in full neck flexion and extension as aberrant movement may be visible. An interactive dialogue must be maintained with the patient regarding the nature of any pain associated with these movements. Pain generated by movement about the cervicothoracic junction will likely include referred patterns, hence the practitioner must inquire for reproduction of the presenting pain symptoms, especially when they are remote from the spine.

The active assessment may be repeated passively by supporting the head with two hands and working through each of the six movements. The nature of the coupled rotation in the cervicothoracic junction is that found in the cervical segments above and the thoracic segments below; namely ipsilateral rotation of the vertebral body with lateral flexion, producing contralateral rotation of the spinous process. The size of the coupled moments varies with the nature of the relationship between the uncinate processes and Luschka joints (Clausen et al 1997).

It must also be appreciated that the introduction of ribs significantly reduces the amount of rotation available at T1–2 and T2–3. The variability of the involvement of C7 with rib 1 may similarly markedly limit the rotation available at C7–T1.

The question of the quantity of global movement is assessed as above with notation of areas of restriction; however, the concept of restriction must take into account the individual nature of the quantity of movement at individual levels. Movement is then induced into each SMU and rib joint, as described below. It is important to observe the nature of the active regional range of motion assessment as this may demonstrate jerky movements reflective of kinematic change secondary to muscle involvement as well as subluxation complex (SC).

The more appropriate segmental movement to assess in this region is that about the x-axis as flexion and extension. Flexion is to be appreciated as a movement which typically has a soft, springy end-feel which derives from the tensile resistance of soft tissues during separation of the posterior column of the spine and the compressive nature of the disk at the anterior of the anterior column. On the other hand, extension closes the zygapophyseal joints and approximates the spinous processes, giving a different, more bony type of end-feel as the normal expectation.

The better assessment of any change in movement about the thoracic segments is thus the attempt to detect any restriction in flexion. Rotation restriction remains valid for assessing C6–7, while C7–T1 is a transitional level where lateral flexion may best demonstrate any fixation. The practitioner will need to determine which movements are normally the better at this level; for example, rotation may follow C6 or be restricted by normal variation of the articulation of rib 1 or by an anomalous cervical rib, and specifically assess the particular movement which will better suggest fixation.

The changing nature of the elastic zone must be foremost in the practitioner's mind as the quality of end-feel is palpated at each level in this region. As noted above, flexion will exhibit "soft-tissue" end-feel, while extension will feel bonier due to the approximation of the zygapophyseal joints and the spinous processes. Rotation will change from a high quantity of movement at C6–7 to a more limited quantity at T2–3 due to the supportive ribs. A high level of palpatory discrimination is required in order to appreciate that the movement of a vertebral segment is not separate from the movements of the articulations about it, namely those of each rib at both the posterior and anterior articulations.

The movement available at the articulations of the rib tubercle with the transverse process and the rib head with the vertebral body are so small they are essentially palpated as end-feel. Hence the qualitative assessment of end-feel is the major palpatory finding. The anterior articulation is more cartilaginous than diarthrodial, hence again findings of tissue resilience are important, along with findings of pain and tenderness.

The assessment of the SMU movement must not only take the coupled movement into consideration but also the changing quantity of such movement. While C6 will exhibit good rotation with lateral flexion, this movement is significantly reduced, although still present, at T2. Pure movements in any one plane are not to be expected. Even flexion and extension (rotation about the x-axis) of the vertebral body are accompanied by translation along the z-axis.

The clinical outcome is that the better information about any kinematic change of the SMU at C6–7, C7–T1, T1–2, and T2–3, and the relevant rib articulation, is derived more from interpreting the characteristics of movement and end-feel within the context of pain and palpable soft-tissue findings.

Assessment of the individual joints

The upper thoracic segments and ribs may be included in the assessment of the thoracic spine which includes prone placement of the patient; however, their clinical intimacy with the lower two cervical segments, the brachial plexus, and the upper limb, suggests that the individual joints of the cervicothoracic junction are best assessed with the patient either supine or seated. Practitioners will develop their preferred method over time; however, there will be many occasions when assessment of the same segments is conducted in both the seated and then supine position. The advantages of the seated position are that it:

- facilitates a procedural flow from global cervical range of motion
- allows easy palpation of both the anterior and posterior rib articulations
- allows easy application of cervical spine compression and related tests
- allows easy procedural flow to upper-limb neurovascular integrity tests.

The advantages of assessment with the patient supine are:

- movements are often smaller, and gentler, thus appropriate for use in the patient with headache or neck pain
- posterior to anterior springing is gentle as it is against the inertia of the patient's body
- procedural flow is enhanced for the supine adjustment.

C6–7

The comparative posterior to anterior glide for each joint is assessed in the supine position by placing the fingers on the left and right sides of the posterior arch of C6 and gently drawing it upwards (Fig. 10.10). Restriction may be felt, and pain or tenderness may be reported. It is thought that tenderness suggests posteriority of the underlying segment. This process can be commenced at occiput–C1, and applied as low as C7–T1, as stairstepping (previously described).

Rotation, lateral flexion, and lateral glide of C6 on C7 are also assessed with subtle variations of this contact, bearing in mind that rotation and lateral flexion are coupled. A lateral index contact may be taken along the posterolateral lamina of the segment to provide greater patient comfort while assessing movements of the body as opposed to specific movement of the zygapophyseal joint.

With the patient seated, the examiner may palpate with a "thumb and finger" contact or a bilateral finger contact. With the former, the examiner's stance is posterolateral to the patient and the indifferent hand is placed on the vertex to induce movements of lateral flexion, rotation, and flexion/extension in each specific SMU. Flexion and extension and rotation may be assessed in this position by using two fingers, one in each interspinous space above and below the C6 spinous. In flexion the spinous processes should appear to open or separate while on extension

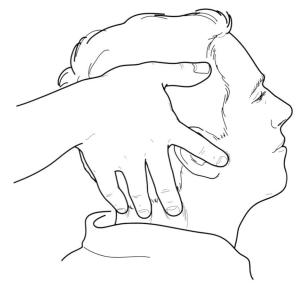

Figure 11.9 Finger placement for bilateral palpation of the mid and low cervical regions.

they should appear to close or approximate. Remember it is generally the C6 spinous which glides anteriorly or "slips away" from the palpating finger near the end-range of whole cervical spine extension.

Rotation may be assessed with a thumb and index finger contact laterally about the spinous. This allows for assessment of end-feel by a push–pull, lateral–medial–lateral movement of the thumb and finger. Also, the distal lateral index finger pad can be placed horizontally between two spinous processes so that side-to-side movement of the superior process can be felt and compared to that of the inferior spinous process.

With a bilateral finger contact the stance is behind the patient and the palmar surface of the hands is placed over the parietal eminences, with the index finger pointing inferiorly, on or anterior to the ear (Fig. 11.9). The ring finger palpates the posterior aspect of the articular pillars and provides most data during rotation, while the middle finger palpates the lateral aspect and provides most data during lateral flexion. Lateral flexion is again assessed with contact over the zygapophyseal joints and the articular pillars and also by curling the finger to give a distal lateral index contact on the posterolateral lamina.

Valuable clinical information may be gained by assessing the tissue tension about each SMU and its responses to movement. Unilateral restriction and tenderness may suggest ipsilateral posterior rotation.

C7–T1

The above is repeated for the C7–T1 SMU with an appreciation of the changing angulation of the facets as well as the disk. The C7–T1 is a transitional level and subject to anomalies and the practitioner needs to determine which movements are normally the better movement at this level. For example, in rotation, C7 may follow C6 or be restricted by normal variation of the articulation of rib 1 or by an anomalous cervical rib.

The sensation of segmental movement must also be placed within the context of the preferential movement of the soft-tissue planes about the base of the neck. This topic is discussed below under Assessment of connective tissue change and the point is made that "normal" movement is indeed a nebulous concept. Notwithstanding this, when the general nature of movement in a particular patient has been determined, the practitioner may then assess those particular movements which are considered better to suggest fixation.

T1–2

The above is repeated for the T1–2 SMU, also with an appreciation for further changes in the angulation of the facets and disk. At this level any restriction is probably best felt with flexion movements as a restriction to the T1 spinous opening on T2. There may be tenderness about the posteroinferior tip of the spinous process.

Any component of lateral flexion or a superiority of the body on one side may be better inferred from the AP radiograph; however, any such finding must be placed in the clinical context of the patient. It may be possible to visualize more of a regional loss of lateral flexion through close observation and with lateral flexion of the cervical spine which concentrates the vector into the SMU.

It is wise to consider that fixation at this level is quite complex and that any resultant listing should reflect the coupled nature of movements and therefore may not actually distinguish between a rotation fixation and a lateral flexion fixation.

T2–3

This SMU is assessed in the manner of T1–2 with an appreciation for further changes in the angulation of the facets and disk. The ribs are included, both at the posterior and anterior.

Rib 1

The left rib will be used as the example (Fig. 11.7). The putative rib fixation can be thought of in the following notional terms:

- superior when there is a discernible resistance to superior to inferior palpation
- inferior when there is a discernible resistance to inferior to superior palpation
- medial when there is a discernible resistance to medial to lateral palpation
- lateral when there is a discernible resistance to lateral to medial palpation
- posterior when there is a discernible resistance to posterior to anterior palpation
- anterior when there is acute tenderness about the anterior costochondral cartilage and unclear palpatory findings about the rib head and tubercle.

With the patient supine, the rib is assessed with posterior to anterior springing by finger contact between the head and the tubercle. A firm contact may then be taken with the index finger with medial to lateral removal of tissue slack to assess lateral

glide. The contact is lifted and retaken with lateral to medial removal of tissue slack to assess medial glide. The index finger then palpates the inferior border and assesses superior glide, and then the superior border to assess inferior glide. The cervical spine may be laterally flexed a little to assist the rib palpation.

Palpation of the insertion of the scalenus anterior is difficult and best attempted in the supine patient by using the pad of the thumb under the medial clavicle. Care must be taken not to compress the subclavian vessels unduly. The practitioner is looking for myotendinosis about the insertion which may be suggestive of rib fixation. Dvořák & Dvořák suggest the "so-called elevated rib is normally the result of myotendinosis in one part of the scalene muscles" (1990 p. 104) hence the clinical wisdom of assessing the scalenes for dysfunction in conjunction with palpation for fixation of ribs 1 and 2.

The anterior articulations about the manubrium are then palpated with the finger pads. Tenderness is a likely finding; however, side-to-side differences may be palpated with anterior to posterior springing. A painful elevation of the cartilage may be noted and is suggestive of rib fixation. Any suggestion of fixation of rib 1 must also be accompanied by assessment of the ipsilateral clavicle, in particular the sternoclavicular joint.

Restrictions and tenderness with movements are noted and interpreted in the context of other clinical findings for the patient. Again, the point must be made that fixation purely in any one plane is unlikely and that the resultant adjustive vectors will need to reflect the opposite multiple vectors of fixation.

Rib 2

The second rib is assessed in the manner of rib 1 with an appreciation of the different muscle attachments, its larger size, the differing angles of articulation by the head and the tubercle, and of the relationship between it and rib 1. This relationship is assessed with palpation of the rib 1/rib 2 interspace, such as it is, and more between the proximal posterior articulations with the transverse processes. As with the tissue between the occiput and C1, these tissues may demonstrate palpable differences in resilience and tenderness, secondary to kinematic change in the region.

Assessment of rib 2 is also made with the patient prone and the process of palpation is extended to include the lower ribs about the mid thoracic segments. The anterior articulation is palpated lateral to the junction between the manubrium and the sternum – the sternal angle.

ASSESSMENT OF CONNECTIVE TISSUE CHANGE

The following soft-tissue dimensions should be measured on the lateral cervical neutral radiograph, especially in the posttrauma patient.

The retrotracheal interspace (RTI) is measured from the anteroinferior margin of C6 to the contour representing the posterior wall of the trachea and is normally up to about 20 mm. It is included with those measurements taken in the mid cervical spine.

The tracheal shadow will be quite prominent in the AP view and should be assessed for any deviation from central alignment. The AP radiograph about this region may demonstrate shadows in the apices of the lungs as they sit within the shadows of ribs 1 and 2. These areas must always be assessed for clarity.

Tissue preference

Chaitow & DeLany (2000 pp. 7–13) suggest that the cervicothoracic spine is a crossover region for fascial chains of the body, including the superficial back line, the superficial front line, and the spiral line. They also describe patterns of fascial compensation detectable by palpation, one region of which is about the cervicothoracic junction (Fig. 5.1). The clinical relevance of determining the side of tissue preference is to establish the soft-tissue context of the individual patient within which the dynamic segmental palpation will be undertaken. Typically, the right-sided tissue is less tense and a mental compensation must be made for this by the practitioner during movement palpation.

It is suggested that the doctor stands behind the seated patient and lightly rests the hands on each shoulder, with the fingers on the clavicles. The patient actively rotates the neck and head a little to the left and right, while the doctor feels for "tightness or looseness" preferences. The tissue tension changes palpated in this manner may be reflective of asymmetrical muscle tone associated with the dominant hand.

Ligamentum nuchae

The ligamentum nuchae has been discussed in detail and the practitioner is reminded of its importance within this region due to the intimacy of the muscles which contribute their fascia to form the ligament. In particular, the serratus posterior superior has direct attachment to the vertebrae and ribs of this region and the rhomboid minor, splenius capitis, and the middle fibers of trapezius attach to the spinous processes of these segments.

Ligaments of the SMU

The anterior longitudinal ligament attaches to the anterior aspect of each body in this region and intermingles with the anterior fibers of the annulus of each disk (C6–7, C7–T1, T1–2, T2–3). The posterior longitudinal ligament also blends with the annulus fibers of each disk and takes on the morphology of two layers: a deep layer which passes downwards and also to the posterolateral perimeter of the disk, blending with the periosteum of the pedicles, and a superficial layer which blends with the deep layer at each disk level, leaving a shallow pocket (Giles & Singer 2000 p. 35). At lower levels this allows medial disk protrusions to travel laterally; however, protrusion of the thoracic disk is much less common than that of the lumbar or cervical spines (Cramer & Darby 1995 p. 159) although the frequency of disk degeneration ranges between 40% and 50% in both the low cervical and high thoracic disks (Boyle et al 1998).

The dura mater is firmly adherent to the posterior longitudinal ligament at the C5–6 and C6–7 interspaces (Iwamura et al 2001). This is thought to allow chronic irritation of the dura by a hypertrophied ligament which in turn may weaken the dura

and allow transdural perforation by herniated disk material secondary to trauma. The resultant intradural disk herniation is rare and only 17 cases have been reported (Iwamura et al 2001).

The ligamentum flavum is paired left and right and each runs between the laminae at each level. As noted by Giles & Singer (2000 p. 23) the intra-articular synovial folds of the zygapophyseal joints arise from tissue adjacent to the ligamenta flava. They have a particular function to limit forward flexion and are subject to calcification which may be associated with disk herniation (Ugarriza et al 2001) or myelopathy and, while this is recognized in the Japanese population, it has also been reported in Caucasians (Hankey & Khangure 1988) and Blacks (Cabre et al 2001). At this level the ossified ligament may grow nodular masses on both the anteromedial and posterolateral surfaces (Mak et al 2002).

The interspinous ligaments are present between each spinous process at these levels, although they are thin and membranous in structure (Cramer & Darby 1995 p. 165). They are more developed than any in the cervical segments above and run along the length of each process. Anteriorly they are continuous with the ligamentum flavum, while posteriorly the fibers combine with the supraspinous ligament which acts to limit flexion. It is a continuous band which arises from the spinous process of C7 and travels inferiorly, perhaps to the sacrum (Cramer & Darby 1995 p. 165).

The zygapophyseal joints

The articular capsules of the thoracic SMUs are less developed laterally. Giles & Singer (2000 p. 20) suggest this is to allow axial motion and they identify small intra-articular synovial folds as being found in the thoracic zygapophyseal joints, which is consistent with most synovial joints (p. 23). They identify them as arising medially from tissue adjacent to the ligamentum flavum, and extending a varying distance into the medial joint cavity.

The intervertebral disk

The disk morphology changes significantly through the cervicothoracic junction, from the thicker, broader cervical disks to the thinner, more heart-shaped, thoracic disk. As with all disks, there are sensory nerves in the annulus and it is considered to be a pain generator.

It is known that pain is more likely to develop in persons with degenerative changes at C6–7 (Gore 2001). The frequency of disk degeneration in this region has been reported as 49% at C6–7, 42% at C7–T1, 40% at T1–2, and 50% at T2–3 (Boyle et al 1998). Soft cervical disk herniation has its highest incidence at C5–6 (54%) and then C6–7 (46.6%) (Bucciero et al 1998a), while traumatic disk herniation has a much higher incidence at C5–6 (58.5%) compared to C6–7 (19.5%) and C4–5 (17.1%) (Bucciero et al 1998b).

Signs of disk involvement at C6–7 affecting the C7 nerve root or at C7–T1 affecting the C8 nerve root include pain felt in the neck, shoulder, medial border of the scapula, lateral arm, and forearm (more dorsally for C7). The C5–6 disk lesion is clinically associated with trigger points in the splenius capitis, deltoid, levator scapula, rhomboid minor, and latissimus dorsi, while the C6–7 lesion is associated with trigger points in the latissimus dorsi and rhomboid minor (Hsueh et al 1998).

Damage to the vertebral endplates which subsequently allows vertical extension of disk material is more common in lower thoracic segments and is typically not seen in this region. It is common for the C6 and C7 disks to thin with degeneration and aging.

Ligaments about the ribs

The complexity of the sternocostal joint has been discussed above. Recall that there is a largely fibrocartilage disk which divides the sternocostal joint in two and it is attached to the capsular fibers. The joint between the second costocartilage is also divided into two spaces by an intra-articular ligament which attaches to the manubriosternal articulation. The practitioner must be aware of the clinical anatomy of the ribs and their articulations and allow this knowledge to guide the assessment.

The costovertebral capsules include intra-articular bands of ligaments which provide strong attachment of the rib about the thoracic disk (from T2 through T9) and radiate ligaments about the head of the rib and the demifacet on the thoracic body. The intra-articular band is short and flat and creates distinct upper and lower articular compartments lined with synovial membrane (Cramer & Darby 1995 p. 167). The capsule around these costo-corporal articulations blends with the disk at that level. The radiate ligament of rib 1 has some superior fibers which attach to the body of C7 (Cramer & Darby 1995 p. 167).

The articulation of the tubercle of the neck and the transverse process of the thoracic segment is supported by the costotransverse ligament and lateral costotransverse ligaments. A thin synovial membrane lines the resultant thin, fibrous joint capsule.

ASSESSMENT OF MUSCLE CHANGE

Many of the muscles relevant to the cervicothoracic spine are also relevant to the upper cervical and mid cervical spines. The splenii, upper trapezius, and rhomboid minor have been discussed in Chapter 9. The sternomastoid, cleidomastoid, scalenes, longus colli and capitis, semispinalis and spinalis, longissimus capitis and cervicis, levator scapula, and the small muscles of the spine have been discussed in the preceding chapter.

Muscles about the region

The iliocostalis cervicis

This is the most lateral column of muscles about the spine (Fig. 10.13A) and it arises from the angle of ribs 3 through 6 and inserts into the transverse processes of C4 through C6. The iliocostalis thoracis fibers run between the angles of the lower six and the upper six ribs. The muscles are innervated by the posterior primary rami of spinal nerves and assist with extension and lateral flexion of the spinal column through this region. As postural muscles they shorten when stressed.

Careful bilateral, comparative palpation is required to identify the flat and atonic nature of weak fiber bundles or the ropy nature of the hypertonic fiber bundles (Walther 1981 p. 444). Dvořák & Dvořák (1984 p. 160) suggest myotenones in iliocostalis

cervicis are related to dysfunction at L5. The muscle is implicated in patients with upper-rib dysfunction.

Semispinalis thoracis

This muscle arises from the transverse processes of the lower thoracic segments and inserts into the spinous processes of C6 though T4. It is supplied by the dorsal rami of thoracic nerves and acts to assist contralateral rotation of the spine. When acting bilaterally, it assists with extension. The muscle is implicated with reduced flexion of the region or of segments within the region, and with restrictions in rotation. It seems to be associated with SC of the upper thoracic segments and Dvořák & Dvořák (1984 pp. 144–147) associate its myotenones with spondylogenic reflex syndromes of T1 through T4.

The subclavius

This muscle runs from rib 1 at its junction with the costal cartilage to a groove along the inferior clavicle. It is frequently overlooked as a participant in radiating arm pain and must be included in the assessment of the cervicothoracic spine, along with the assessment of the adjacent anterior articulations. It is supplied by C5 and C6 through the subclavian nerve from the brachial plexus and it acts to draw the clavicle anterior and inferiorly.

The muscle is palpated better when the patient elevates the ipsilateral arm. An active trigger point will refer pain along and under the clavicle, to the anterior arm, and lateral forearm and hand (Simons et al 1999 p. 823). The subclavius cannot be tested directly and within the Applied Kinesiology paradigm it is assessed through the process of therapy localization (Walther 1981 pp. 386–387). Its pain patterns mimic ischemic cardiac disease and cardiac involvement must be ruled out before the muscle is ruled in.

The levatores costarum

These arise as paired muscles from each transverse process at levels C7 through T11, and insert between the tubercle and the angle on the outer surface of the rib below the vertebral segment of origin. Thus, in this region, the levatores costarum for rib 1 arise from the transverse process of C7 and insert into rib 1; and for rib 2, from T1 with insertion into rib 2. They are supplied by lateral branches of the dorsal ramus (posterior primary division) at the relative segmental level (spinal nerve T1 supplies the muscle in the first intercostal space), and they act to rotate and laterally flex the spinal column, elevate the ribs, and assist in inspiration.

These muscles are often involved with SC and rib fixation and Dvořák & Dvořák (1984 pp. 102–103) suggest various levels reflect higher in the spine to certain vertebral levels. For example, they propose that the muscle at intercostal space 1 (rib 1) is related to fixation of the occiput, and rib 2 to fixation of C1.

The intercostales

These muscles are anatomically distinguished as three layers (external, internal, and innermost); however, clinically they are considered as one functional unit. They are muscles of respiration and act to elevate and depress the ribs during inspiration and expiration. They also provide a structural soft-tissue containment for the contents of the thorax. The fibers attach between the inferior border of one rib and the superior border of the subjacent rib and are supplied by the intercostal nerves.

The muscles are implicated in patients with breathing difficulties or respiratory dysfunction, and may be dysfunctional secondary to asthma. In general they are affected by scoliosis – more so in the lower thoracic, where scoliotic curvature may be greater. The muscles at each rib interspace are assessed for function and tonicity with careful bilateral observation and palpation and are affected by rib fixation.

Serratus anterior

The serratus anterior arises from the convex portion of the body of ribs 1–10 (Fig. 11.10A) and travels posterosuperiorly, under the scapula, to insert along its inferior angle. It is supplied by the long thoracic nerve from C5, C6, and C7 and acts to draw the scapula forward and rotate the glenoid fossa superiorly. It is an important muscle to assess with any dysfunction of the cervicothoracic junction, the rhomboids, and the scapulae.

Walther groups this as a shoulder muscle, which serves to emphasize the clinical interrelationships between function of the cervicothoracic junctional spine and the upper extremity. The muscle is tested with the patient seated, and the arm held at about 100° of flexion with slight abduction (Fig. 11.10B) (Walther 1981 pp. 372–374). Before the testing force is applied, the examiner looks for difficulty in holding the arm in the testing position. The test should not be conducted in a patient with shoulder injury or a history of shoulder dislocation.

The muscle is reflexively weak in patients with a winging scapula and may be associated with abnormal shoulder movements. It may be implicated in patients with breathing difficulties and when the trigger points are active it may restrict the rib movement required for adequate inspiration. The trigger points refer about the lateral chest wall, the medial inferior border of the scapula, and along the medial border of the arm up to and including the hand (Fig. 11.10C).

The serratus anterior is associated with stress fractures of rib 1 (Mintz et al 1990). The mechanism is thought to be a fatigue fracture caused by repeated physical forces that ultimately overcome the limit of fatigue of the bone. This type of fracture may result from overuse during gym workouts, typically using the "pec deck," which is an eccentric exercise where the external forces overcome the internal tension generated by the muscle, causing it to lengthen despite contraction. Other activities which may produce a stress fracture about the serratus insertion into rib 1 include bench press, tennis, table tennis, surfing, baseball pitching (dominant-side rib fracture), and the use of chest expanders (Mintz et al 1990). The resultant pain is deep within the anterior shoulder about the thorax and may radiate along the ulnar aspect of the arm to the little finger.

The small muscles

The intertransversarii are slender muscular slips between the transverse processes of each SMU of this region. The typical patterns of rotatores and interspinales are also present within and about each SMU. Each spinal nerve has motor fibers to these small, intrinsic muscles but their function is probably more proprioceptive than motor (Herzog 2000 p. 32). They are implicated by pain and tenderness on palpation.

The multifidi run upwards from the transverse processes to insert about the spinous process of two to four vertebrae above, filling the groove between the transverse and spinous processes and covering the rotatores and lying lateral to the interspinales.

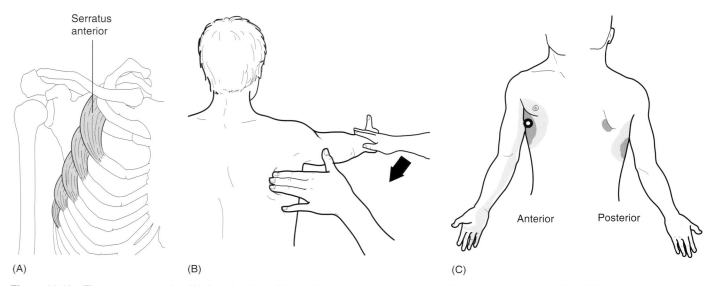

(A) (B) (C)

Figure 11.10 The serratus anterior. (A) Anterior view of the right serratus anterior showing the attachments to the ribs. (B) The seated patient's arm is held in full flexion with some abduction and the test force is applied about the distal forearm in the direction of the arrow to produce extension and adduction. The inferior angle of the scapula is palpated during the test to detect whether the scapula rotates or lifts away from the thorax. (C) The triggers points refer pain to the inferior medial border of the scapula, about the chest wall, and along the medial arm and hand. (A,C) From Chaitow & DeLany (2000), with permission.

They provide an extension torque which is localized to one or two segments (Herzog 2000 p. 34). They are innervated by medial branches of the dorsal rami and are postural muscles which shorten when stressed. They are implicated with segmental dysfunction, particularly decreased flexion and/or rotation.

Notwithstanding the above segmental concept, Dvořák & Dvořák (1984 p. 82) suggest the multifidi function as regional groups (cervical, upper thoracic, lower thoracic, lumbar), and that the myotenones can be further subgrouped over four spinal levels. They are palpated deep about the root of the spinous process as it joins the lamina, with the finger in a superomedial direction, on to the origin. The insertion is palpated with the finger in an inferolateral direction.

For completeness, the transversus thoracis are anterior, internal muscles of the thorax, arising from the xiphoid process and the sternum, to travel superolaterally and insert into the lower borders and inner surfaces of the costal cartilage extensions of ribs 2 through 6. They are supplied by anterior primary rami of the respective intercostal nerve and act to depress the costal cartilage as a muscle of expiration. As internal muscles they cannot be palpated; however, they should be considered in the assessment of the anterior rib articulations and could theoretically be associated with dysfunction about the anterior articulations.

Extrinsic muscles

These are muscles away from the spine but which are innervated by levels of this region. Their clinical usefulness lies as indicators of neural change whether centrally within the spine, such as protrusion of disk material, laterally about the spine, such as degenerative change within the intervertebral canal (IVC), or laterally from the spine, such as thoracic outlet syndrome, brachial plexus compromise, or peripheral nerve root entrapment. They are tested in the first instance to determine severe compromise, which may result in wasting of the muscles, and assessed in the second instance to determine changes in left/right function and strength.

The wrist flexors include the flexor digitorum superficialis and flexor digitorum profundus. They are supplied by C7–T1 as the median nerve and flexor digitorum superficialis acts firstly to flex the second phalanx of each finger on the proximal phalanx at the proximal interphalangeal (PIP) joints and, with continued contraction, the first phalanx at the metacarpophalangeal (MCP) joints, then the wrist. The flexor digitorum profundus acts in synergy to flex the distal phalanx. They are tested with the patient seated with the wrist in neutral and the fingers flexed at the PIP joint. The test force is applied by a matching finger of the practitioner and it acts to extend the finger at the PIP joint.

The C7 function via the median and ulnar nerves can be isolated and tested by taking a "handshake" grip with the wrist flexed and then applying the testing force to extend the wrist. This grip straightens the fingers and weakens the role of C8. When the "monkey grip" is taken (the practitioner's fingers take a curled grip into the patient's fingers, which also curl and grip) and with the wrist held in neutral, the test emphasizes the motor function of C8 through the median and ulnar nerves. A second reasonable test is to ask the patient to wrap the fingers around the practitioner's extended index and middle fingers, and then to squeeze. These last two tests can be performed bilaterally at the same time, allowing direct comparison of left and right strength and function.

The interossei test T1 as the ulnar nerve. The patient holds the hand flat and spreads the fingers. The examiner's fingers are placed between, and the patient adducts the fingers to squeeze the examiner's fingers. Individual fingers can be tested by matching the examiner's finger to the patient's finger (index to index, middle to middle), and testing individual adduction and abduction.

Atrophy secondary to neurologic compromise is assessed in relevant muscles of the upper limb and related to the spinal level servicing the particular muscle. In particular, the intrinsic muscles of the hand are carefully observed for wasting and weakness.

Finally, the neurolymphatic points of this region should be noted, as tenderness about them is not only a useful clinical indicator of particular muscle involvement, it may also be a confounder for pain secondary to local tissue involvement associated with SC. There are posterior points over the lamina of T1 for the subclavius and intrinsic spinal muscles and over the T2–3 lamina junction for subscapularis and teres minor and major. There are anterior points between rib 1 and rib 2 in the mid clavicular line for the neck flexors and extensors, and about the second sternocostal junction for levator scapula (Walther 1981).

ASSESSMENT OF NEURAL CHANGE

The spinal nerves

The spinal nerves of the cervicothoracic junctional spine and the levels at which they exit are:

- spinal nerve C7 from the C6–7 SMU
- spinal nerve C8 from the C7–T1 SMU
- spinal nerve T1 from the T1–2 SMU
- spinal nerve T2 from the T2–3 SMU.

The typical course of the cervical spinal nerves is as described in the previous materials for the mid cervical spine. The typical branching of the thoracic spinal nerves is shown in Figure 11.11. Note the course of the ventral ramus which becomes the intercostal nerve, and the posterior distribution of the dorsal ramus. Note also the segmented sources of the cutaneous branches. This is a typical distribution from T2 and, while the actual distribution varies from level to level and individually, the principle remains that the skin about the spinal column is innervated by the dorsal ramus and there is a lateral crossover zone to innervation by the lateral and anterior cutaneous nerves from the ventral ramus. The lateral cutaneous branch of the T1 ventral ramus services the axilla.

The assessment for signs and symptoms of neural change must include motor, sensory, reflex, and autonomic functions and the distribution is considered in terms of dermatomes, myotomes, and sclerotomes. The autonomic nervous system is strongly associated with the cervicothoracic junction and an appreciation of potential reflex mechanisms is valuable in aiding the understanding of various clinical presentations and their possible relationship with any SC in this region.

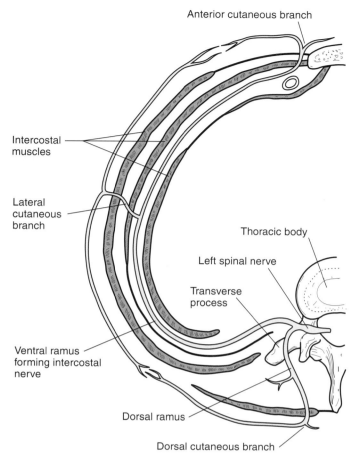

Anterior cutaneous branch

Intercostal muscles

Lateral cutaneous branch

Thoracic body

Left spinal nerve

Transverse process

Ventral ramus forming intercostal nerve

Dorsal ramus

Dorsal cutaneous branch

Figure 11.11 Typical thoracic spinal nerve distribution. The left spinal nerve is shown.

C7 spinal nerve

The C7 spinal nerve exits the C6–7 IVC and divides with the dorsal ramus, looping posteriorly about the anterolateral aspect of the articular pillar, dividing to give medial and lateral branches. As with the C6 spinal nerve, the medial branch does not divide further, being only a deep medial branch which innervates the deep muscles, specifically the multifidi, the intertransversarii, and the zygapophyseal joints. It extends upwards to the zygapophyseal joint above and downwards to the joint below, thus sharing innervation of two joints, namely, the inferior zygapophyseal joint of C6 and the superior zygapophyseal joint of C7.

It is also interesting to note that the deep medial branch of the dorsal ramus, through its motor function to the multifidus, exerts action across its SMU. Spinal nerve C7, at the C6–7 SMU, has motor fibers to the multifidus which attaches between C6 and C7, thus giving motor function to the superior vertebra, C6, on C7. The lateral branch is motor to more superficial muscles, such as the semispinalis capitis and longissimus cervicis.

The C7 ventral ramus is typical and is as previously described for the spinal nerves above. It travels between the intertransversarii to contribute, as the sole component of the middle trunk, to the brachial plexus, which innervates the anterior neck and

upper extremity. It is motor to longus capitis and longus colli and the posterior and middle scalene muscles. It joins with fibers from C5 and C6 to form the long thoracic nerve to serratus anterior and contributes, with C5 and C6, to the musculocutaneous nerve, which is motor to the arm flexors and sensory about the lateral forearm. It joins with C6 fibers, and sometimes with C5 fibers, to form the median nerve, and contributes to the radial nerve.

It gives rise to the recurrent meningeal nerve which returns though the intervertebral foramen to innervate the dura about the spinal cord at that level. The sympathetic nervous system about this level may have a middle cervical ganglion, anterior to the C6 transverse process, and anterior to longus capitis.

The clinical evidence of C7 involvement is pain in the neck, shoulder, medial border of the scapula, lateral arm, and back of the forearm; sensory change about the index and middle finger; motor change in the triceps; and reflex change at the triceps tendon.

C8 spinal nerve

The C8 spinal nerve is the transitional nerve in that those above (C1–7) exit the SMU *over* the same-numbered spinal segment while those below exit *under* the same-numbered spinal segment (from T1). C8 exits at the C7–T1 SMU.

The dorsal ramus is distributed in the same fashion as that for C7, turning posteriorly and passing medial to the intertransversarii, to innervate splenius cervicis and iliocostalis cervicis. The C8 ventral ramus is typical, as previously described, and contributes to the brachial plexus which innervates the anterior neck and upper extremity. It joins with the ventral ramus of the T1 spinal nerve to form the lower trunk. These nerves (C8) pass above and (T1) below rib 1 and, after joining, lie along the superior surface of the rib. They send a branch to the middle trunk and continue as the medial cord to become the medial antebrachial cutaneous nerve, the medial brachial cutaneous nerve, and the ulnar nerve. They branch to give motor and sensory fibers to the median nerve. The ulnar nerve is thus largely C8 and T1, but may have some C7 fibers. The C8 ventral ramus also provides motor function to the posterior and middle scalene muscles.

The sympathetics lie anterior to longus capitis, with the inferior ganglion often joining with the T1 and T2 ganglia to form the stellate (cervicothoracic) ganglion, which lies just inferior to the transverse process of C7 and thus in the important region about rib 1.

The clinical evidence of C8 involvement is pain in the neck, shoulder, medial border of the scapula, and medial aspect of the forearm; sensory change about the ring and little finger; and motor change in the intrinsic muscles of the hand. Cold stimulation of the little finger side of the hand has been shown on functional MRI (fMRI) to produce activation around the C8 cervical cord segment (Stroman et al 2002).

T1 spinal nerve

The T1 spinal nerve exits the T1–2 IVC and divides close to the anterolateral aspect of the articular pillar with the dorsal ramus looping posteriorly. The first few thoracic spinal levels lie about the level of the vertebra, but as the cord descends, the spinal levels progressively become above the respective vertebral level, such that spinal level T12 (the origin of the ventral and dorsal rootlets for spinal nerve T12) lies about the T10–11 SMU. The cord terminates with the lower sacral segments about the L1–2 SMU.

The T1 dorsal ramus, the posterior primary division, passes posteriorly across, and innervates, the zygapophyseal joint of T1–2 and then under the T1 transverse process and over the rib of the level below (rib 2), medial to the superior costotransverse ligament. The medial branch passes between the multifidi and levator costarum and the lateral branch is motor to the erector spinae. This branch has sensory fibers which vary in the area of skin they innervate on the back.

The ventral ramus joins with that of C8, as noted above. It also has a smaller branch of sensory, motor, and sympathetic fibers which becomes the intercostal nerve, with variable distribution. The ventral ramus also sends white ramus communicans to the sympathetic ganglion at this level, which, as noted above, is often coalesced with the inferior cervical and T2 ganglia to form the stellate ganglion. The sympathetic trunk and ganglia are anterior to the intercostal nerve and lie along the lateral aspect of the vertebral bodies. Thus it travels superior to inferior over the head of the rib and helps form the splanchnic nerves which innervate the abdominal viscera.

The relationship of the sympathetics about the head of the rib is thought to allow the regular and rhythmic motion of the rib head during respiration, to provide a local intermittent pumping action ensuring fluid movement in and about the ganglia (Patriquin 1992 p. 5).

T2 spinal nerve

The T2 spinal nerve exists the IVC and travels in a manner similar to T1. While it does not make a major contribution to the brachial plexus, there may be some fibers from T2 traveling up to T1 before it joins with C8. The dorsal ramus of T2 (along with those of T3 and T4) passes through the tendon of splenius cervicis, pierces the rhomboids and trapezius, and innervates the skin about the spinous process. Frequently these fibers are affected by hypertonicity in the erector spinae or splenius cervicis, giving the clinical presentation of vague discomfort about the upper mid-back.

The ventral ramus provides cutaneous innervation to the axilla by the intercostal brachial nerve, and also the intercostal nerve, which is variously distributed, in the manner of T1. It is important to note that the visceral afferents associated with the smooth muscle and glands of the head, the cutaneous effectors, the blood vessels of the upper-extremity skeletal muscle, the lungs, and the heart arise at this spinal level.

Local pain

There are sensory nerve fibers throughout the annulus fibrosus of the disk, but none in the healthy nucleus pulposus. Given the high incidence of disk degeneration at this level, and the knowledge that in the lumbar spine there is neural ingrowth into the centre of damaged disks, it is reasonable to expect all disks at this level to be pain generators. Care must be taken to distinguish between local pain of mechanical origin and pain referred about the region, either by active trigger points or by muscle dysfunction, as suggested by tonicity, tender points, and/or myotendinoses.

Typically, the pain generators within the spine will give increased nociceptive input, perceived as pain by the patient, worsened with mechanical movement. Thus the dynamic palpation must be specific and localized and must include the ribs and their anterior and posterior articulations.

Local pain usually reflects local trauma, such as capsular strain. The same principles of rich anastomoses among adjacent spinal cord segments, as previously described, apply in this region. Attention must be paid to the complex interplay of ligaments and capsules about the anteromedial attachments of ribs 1 and 2 as well as to the posterior attachments, especially of the tubercle about the transverse process.

Specific pain and tenderness may be palpated about the tip of the C7 spinous in the posttrauma patient, reflective of a strain injury of the ligamentum nuchae. Significant tenderness or specific pain in these patients warrants a request for radiographs to rule out avulsion, especially when it is worsened by flexion.

Referred pain

There are numerous patterns of referred pain from active trigger points and the relevant trigger points should always be assessed and then either included in or ruled out of the working diagnosis. It remains important to distinguish between *trigger* points and *tender* points and to use the correct descriptive terminology. Where an active trigger point is identified it should be described in the manner of Travell and Simons (Simons et al 1999), for example, trigger point 1 or trigger point 2 for a specific muscle, with both the pattern of distribution and nature of pain being identified, described, and documented. Tender points are simply noted as focal areas of tenderness within a muscle or its attachments.

Sensory change

Basic assessment includes recording the bilaterally comparative responses to crude touch. Further assessment can include pain or sharp touch, temperature, and vibration. The brachial plexus provides a reasonable degree of overlap of nerve roots; however, the locations which provide an acceptable level of consistency in the distribution of the nerve root dermatome for sensory testing purposes (Figs 10.16 and 11.12A) are described as:

- C7: the anterior or posterior surface of the middle finger, and proximally on to the skin of the hand over the respective metacarpals
- C8: the anterior or posterior surface of the ring and little finger, and proximally on to the skin of the hand over the respective metacarpals, and the medial forearm
- T1: the skin of the medial arm proximal to the elbow
- T2: the skin about the axilla.

Sensation in the peripheral nerve distribution (Fig. 11.12B) is assessed as follows:

- median nerve (C6, C7, C8): the anterolateral surface of the hand and the skin over the medial thenar pad
- radial nerve (C7, C8): the posterior thumb web and posterolateral hand
- ulnar nerve (C8, T1): the medial (ulnar) border of the hand, both anterior and posterior skin

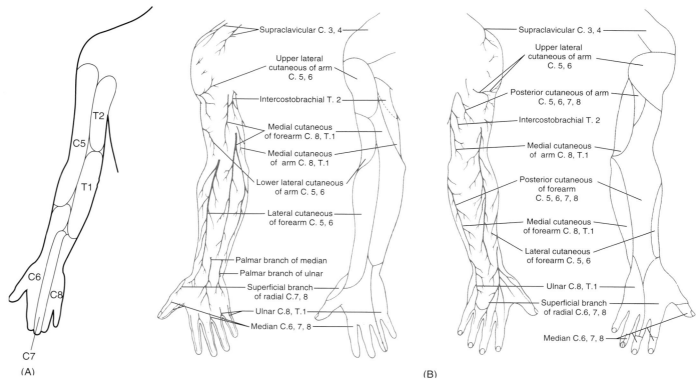

Figure 11.12 Nerve root and peripheral nerve dermatomes. (A) The typical dermatomes for nerve roots C7, C8, T1, and T2; (B) peripheral nerves arising from C7, C8, T1, and T2. From Petty & Moore (2001), with permission.

- lateral antebrachial cutaneous nerve (C5, C6): the lateral forearm
- medial antebrachial cutaneous nerve (C8, T1): the medial forearm
- intercostal brachial nerve (T2): the skin about the anterior lateral axilla and along the anterior chest at that level.

Motor function

Basic assessment includes recording muscle weakness, absent or diminished tone, fasciculations, neurogenic atrophy, and altered deep tendon reflexes. The motor distributions are given in Figure 11.13A–C. The nerve roots may be assessed as C7, C8, or T1, or the peripheral nerves may be assessed with inference back to the root. The actions to test for motor function of individual spinal nerve roots are:

- C7: wrist flexion
- C8: finger flexion
- T1: finger adduction and abduction
- T2: quite difficult to assess; however, observation during deep inspiration may reveal asymmetrical action of the intercostal muscles between ribs 2 and 3.

The peripheral nerve motor function is assessed as follows:

- C7 as median nerve: wrist flexors for wrist flexion
- C7 as radial nerve: extensor digitorum longus for finger extension

- C8 as median nerve: flexor digitorum superficialis for flexion at the proximal interphalangeal joint
- C8 as ulnar nerve: flexor digitorum profundus for flexion at the distal interphalangeal joints of the ring and little fingers
- C8 and T1 as radial nerve: abductor pollicis longus for thumb abduction
- C8 and T1 as ulnar nerve: adductor pollicis for thumb adduction
- C8 and T1 as median nerve: opponens pollicis for thumb to little finger opposition
- T1 as ulnar nerve: dorsal interossei for finger abduction or palmar interossei for finger adduction.

The muscle stretch reflexes are assessed as follows:

- C7 (and C8): the triceps reflex; causes extension at the elbow when the tendon of the triceps is struck as it passes over the olecranon fossa
- C8 (and C7): there is no reflex specific to C8. The Trömner reflex has been proposed (Dvořák 1998); however, this is accepted more as an indicator of pyramidal tract lesions with moderate spasticity. When the flexed middle or index finger is tapped into extension, the remaining fingers reflexively flex.

Autonomic effects

The cervical sympathetic chain lies anterior to longus capitis and posterior to the carotid sheath. The preganglionic bodies for

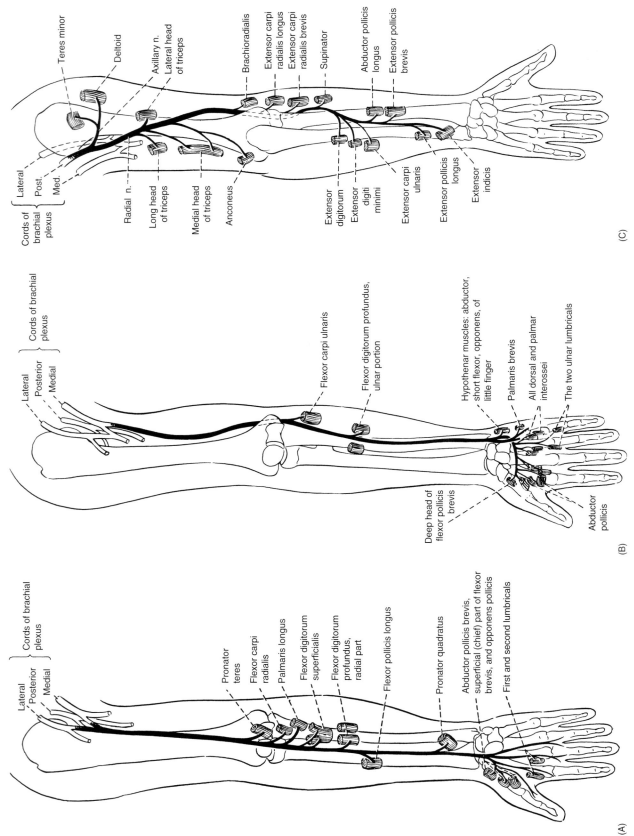

Figure 11.13 Motor distribution. (A) Distribution of the median nerve as motor to the flexor forearm; (B) distribution of the ulnar nerve as motor to the flexor forearm; (C) distribution of the radial and axillary nerves as motor to the extensor forearm. (A-C) From Jenkins (1998), with permission.

the head and neck are found in the spinal cord at levels T1–3, and maybe T4 and T5. Branches from the cervical chain form the plexus about the vertebral artery. The splanchnic nerves innervate the abdominal viscera.

Sympathetic fibers travel with each intercostal nerve to provide visceral motor to blood vessels and sweat glands about the thoracic wall. Nerves associated with the sympathetic trunk and the gray rami communicans also innervate the periosteum of the anterior and lateral aspects of the vertebral bodies, the anterior and lateral aspects of the intervertebral disk, and the anterior longitudinal ligament (Cramer & Darby 1995 p. 359).

Traditional concepts

The following comments represent traditional empirical considerations which are found within chiropractic and other manipulative disciplines. Authors are not consistent in identifying whether they refer to the vertebral segment or the spinal nerve, hence some discrepancy between precise levels is to be expected. Schafer reports the concept of stimulating a spinal center (Schafer 1983 p. 371). It is based on empirical physiological responses thought to occur after deep and rapid short-duration percussion has been applied on the spinous processes at a particular level. The percussion is applied by hand or instrument at a rate between one and two impulses per second for 20 s with a 30-s rest period and is thought to stimulate the spinal center at that level. The references below are from Schafer (1983 p. 371). The Lovett Brother relationship is a purported synchronous movement of one vertebra with another and suggests that, when fixation is found at a particular level, the related segment should also be specifically assessed. The references below are from Walther (1981 p. 67).

About C7 – the C6–7 SMU

Traditional chiropractic associates this level with the thyroid gland and bursae in shoulder and elbows. Gonstead observed subluxations at this level in patients with systolic hypertension (Plaugher 1993 p. 367). Stimulation of the spinal reflex center at this level is thought to increase generalized vasoconstriction and myocardial tone. The Lovett Brother relationship to the C6 body is movement in the opposite direction of the T12 body. Maigne suggests dysfunction at C6–7 may be associated with chronic dysfunction at L4–5 and dysfunction at C2–3 and T12–L1 (Maigne 1996 p. 102).

About C8 – the C7/T1 SMU

Gonstead observed subluxations at this level in patients with systolic hypertension (Plaugher 1993 p. 367). The Lovett Brother relationship to the C7 body is movement in the opposite direction of the T11 body. Faridi (1995) associates the C7 vertebral segment with sympathetic neural pathways to the liver and gall bladder and suggests that a recurring subluxation at C7 is the result of a viscerosomatic reflex from the liver and associates C7 with T8. The acupuncture point Du 14 Dazhui lies below the spinous process of C7 and is indicated with febrile diseases, malaria, cough, asthma, hectic fever and night sweating, epilepsy, stiffness and pain in the head and neck, and rubella (Qiu 1993 p. 156).

About T1 – the T1–2 SMU

Traditional chiropractic associates this level with the arms from the elbow down, including hands, wrists, and fingers, oesophagus, trachea. The Lovett Brother relationship to the T1 body is movement in the opposite direction of the T10 body. Subluxation at this level is thought to be associated with sympathetic disturbances (Plaugher 1993 p. 357). Efferent sympathetic preganglionic fibers to the heart arise here and Gonstead associates this level with systolic hypertension (Plaugher 1993 p. 367).

Osteopathy considers this level is a reference site for thoracic viscera and suggests that changes in the temperature, moisture, and texture reflect changes in visceral function (Beal 1989 p. 20). Faridi (1995) associates T1 with sympathetic neural pathways to the heart and cardiac plexus and suggests symptoms such as epigastric distress and difficulty swallowing implicate this level. Stimulation of the spinal reflex center is thought to initiate lung reflex dilation, relax the stomach body, contract the pylorus, and inhibit heart action (antitachycardia reflex) and gastric motility.

The posterior neurolymphatic point for the subclavius muscle lies over the T1 laminae (Walther 1981 p. 386). In acupuncture terms, the site for Du 13 Taodao lies below the spinous process of T1 and is indicated in headache, malaria, febrile disease, and stiffness of the back (Qiu 1993 p. 154). Extra 19 Jiaji (Huatuojiaji) points lie 0.5 cun lateral to the lower border of the spinous process and are used to stimulate the posterior ramus and their arterial and venous plexuses at each level from T1 to L5 (Qiu 1993 pp. 176–177).

About T2 – the T2–3 SMU

Traditional chiropractic associates this level with the heart, including valves, pericardium, and coronary arteries. The Lovett Brother relationship to the T2 body is movement in the opposite direction of the T9 body. Subluxation at this level is thought to be associated with sympathetic disturbances (Plaugher 1993 p. 357). Efferent sympathetic preganglionic fibers to the heart arise here and Gonstead associates this level with systolic hypertension (Plaugher 1993 p. 367).

Osteopathy considers this level is a reference site for thoracic viscera. Beal (1989 p. 20) reports that a study of 108 patients with cardiovascular disorders found the greatest number of spinal findings (tissue texture, joint motion) at T2 and T3 on the left. Faridi (1995) associates T2 with the myocardium and suggests that the functional symptoms include asthma, bronchitis, difficulty in breathing, fatigue, and fluid retention. Stimulation of the spinal reflex center is thought to initiate lung reflex dilation, relax the stomach body, contract the pylorus, and inhibit heart action (antitachycardia reflex) and gastric motility. The posterior neurolymphatic point for subscapularis lies between the transverse processes (Walther 1981 p. 400).

ASSESSMENT OF VASCULAR CHANGE

Apart from the effects of injury noted below, consideration must be given to variations as evidenced on diagnostic images which relate to vascularization of the region, in particular about the brachial plexus, such as a cervical rib.

A traumatic sprain of the capsular ligaments or supporting ligaments may result in oedema and, given the close relationships among the joints, may produce kinematic change and thus palpate as focal tenderness and bogginess. In particular, the rib 1 tubercle and the T1 transverse process facet joint should be assessed. The anterior costochondral capsules and the capsule about the sternoclavicular joint are indicated for assessment with upper-limb or shoulder trauma.

Inflammation is generally a contraindication to adjustment and may be associated with arthritides or posttraumatic injury. Care must be taken with the application of a wet-ice pack about the base of the neck to ensure that only the injured tissue is cooled and the arteries are not. It is preferable to use the ice massage process here, where a foam cup has been filled with water and frozen. The upper edge of the cup is peeled away to provide a knob of wet ice to contact the patient in specific muscular locations while the foam base serves as an insulated grip for the practitioner.

Vasoconstriction may palpate as areas of colder skin temperature about the cervicothoracic junctional spine and the more lateral areas about the shoulders and thorax. Mechanical constriction of the neurovascular bundles serving the upper limbs may also result in thermal asymmetry of a region in a limb. This type of thermal asymmetry is ideally demonstrated by infrared thermography; however, more work needs to be undertaken on these findings and those about the spine and their correlation, if any, to the SC.

Consideration must be given to the cervical lymph nodes of the region during assessment and palpation, and when taking adjustive contact. The posterior cervical chain of lymph nodes runs along the anterior edge of the upper trapezius. The deep cervical chain is difficult to palpate as it lies deep to the sternocleidomastoid muscles; however, careful palpation around the muscles with a hooked finger may locate them. The supraclavicular nodes are deep in the angle formed by the clavicle and the muscle attachments and care must be taken in this region with soft-tissue techniques such as the "corkscrew" for the scalenes. The infraclavicular lymph nodes lie inferior to the medial clavicle and care must be taken in palpating rib 1 in this area.

CONCLUSION

The cervicothoracic spine presents a clinical challenge due to the changing architecture of the spinal elements and the commencement of the rib cage. It is a very important region in the neurological sense, as it feeds the brachial plexus and the upper extremities. The assessment of this region clearly involves neurological and muscle function as well as vascular and connective tissue changes.

The first two thoracic SMUs are recognized as being the most difficult region of the spine to adjust. The nature of the intersegmental movement changes dramatically as one moves from the cervical spine into the thoracic spine; however, the painstaking assessment of segmental kinematics, read in conjunction with the other clinical findings, usually allows the determination of the dysfunctional SMU.

12

The mid thoracic spine

KEY CONCEPTS

An intimate understanding of the variable spatial relationship between the transverse processes and the spinous process of each vertebra throughout the mid thoracic spine is essential for accurate palpation and subsequent spinal adjustment.

The dimensions of the spinal canal are relatively smaller through the mid thoracic spine, allowing less free space for the contents of the canal about the spinal cord with an increased sensitivity of the cord to mechanical compromise.

The ganglia of the sympathetic chain lie against the anterior surface of the costovertebral joints and it is thought that the normal movement of the rib head during respiration provides a pumping effect to the substrates within the sympathetic chain.

The costovertebral joints have been shown to contain innervation within the anterior capsule and synovial tissues and the articulation certainly has the requisite innervation for pain production in a similar manner to other joints of the spine and must be considered as a pain generator.

There are differing philosophic concepts regarding the palpatory findings of anteriority of mid thoracic segments and, while some will only adjust the spine from posterior to anterior, others have developed a variety of techniques for adjusting what is considered an anterior subluxation.

Recurrent subluxation of segments in this region may be more indicative of visceral dysfunction than mechanical dysfunction and warrants a broader assessment of the patient.

The presence of a structural scoliosis is suggested by the finding of a rib hump when the patient bends forward at the waist. Quantification and progression of any scoliosis are determined from the plain anteroposterior (AP) radiograph.

Pain from a degenerated disk in the low cervical spine may refer to the mid scapular region about the mid thoracic spine. The cervical compression tests are indicated when pain is reported in this region.

CLINICAL ANATOMY

The mid thoracic spine lies between the cervicothoracic junctional spine and the thoracolumbar junctional spine and includes segments T3 through T9 inclusive. The mid thoracic spine includes the following major articulations:

- T3–4
- Left and right rib 3 – posterior
- Left and right rib 3 – anterior
- T4–5
- Left and right rib 4 – posterior
- Left and right rib 4 – anterior
- T5–6
- Left and right rib 5 – posterior
- Left and right rib 5 – anterior
- T6–7
- Left and right rib 6 – posterior
- Left and right rib 6 – anterior
- T7–8
- Left and right rib 7 – posterior
- T8–9
- Left and right rib 8 – posterior
- T9–10
- Left and right rib 9 – posterior.

Cramer & Darby (1995 pp. 156–176) provide the appropriate level of anatomy of this region for the student and can be read in conjunction with this chapter. The following spinal landmarks should be noted with an appreciation of their clinically important relationships, as shown in Figure 12.1. The relationship between the spinous process of one vertebra and the transverse processes of another must also be committed to memory to facilitate accurate palpation:

- T3 transverse process: about level with the T2 spinous process, 2–3 cm laterally
- T4 transverse process: about level with the T3 spinous process, 2–2.5 cm laterally
- T5 transverse process: about level with the upper border of the T4 spinous, 2–2.5 cm laterally
- T6 transverse process: about level with the interspinous space of T4–5, 2–2.5 cm laterally
- T6 spinous process: about level with the inferior medial border of the scapula
- T7 transverse process: about level with the interspinous space of T5–6, 2–2.5 cm laterally
- T7 spinous process: about level with the inferior angle of the scapula

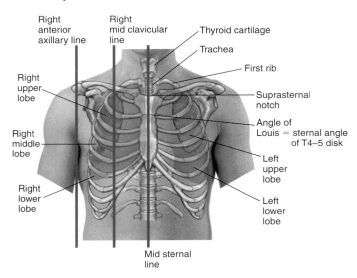

Figure 12.2 Key landmarks of the anterior thorax. From Seidel et al (1999), with permission.

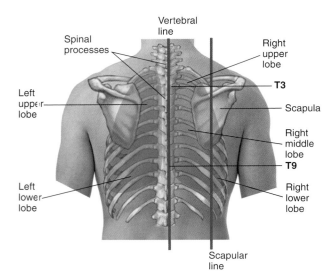

Figure 12.1 Key landmarks of the posterior thorax. From Seidel et al (1999), with permission.

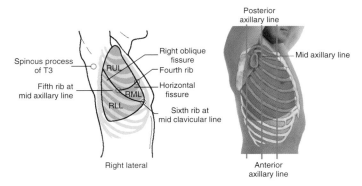

Figure 12.3 Right lateral view of the thorax showing lung landmarks. From Seidel et al (1999), with permission.

- T8 transverse process: about level with the interspinous space of T6–7, 2–2.5 cm laterally
- T9 transverse process: about level with the upper border of the T8 spinous process, 1.5–2 cm laterally
- T9 spinous process: about level with the 10th rib costovertebral articulation.

Key landmarks of the anterior and lateral thorax are shown in Figures 12.2 and 12.3 and the following relationships with spinal landmarks should be noted:

- T2–3 disk: about level with the suprasternal notch
- T4 spinous process: about level with the tracheal bifurcation

- T4 spinal nerve sensory innervation: about the nipple line
- T4–5 disk: about level with the sternal angle
- Left sixth intercostal space, mid clavicular line: gastric air bubble
- T7 spinal nerve sensory innervation: about the xiphoid process.

Thoracic vertebrae 3 through 8 are regarded as being typical (Fig. 12.4). T9 is considered atypical in that at times rib 10 may not articulate with it, in which case there is no demifacet at the inferior lateral margin of the T9 body.

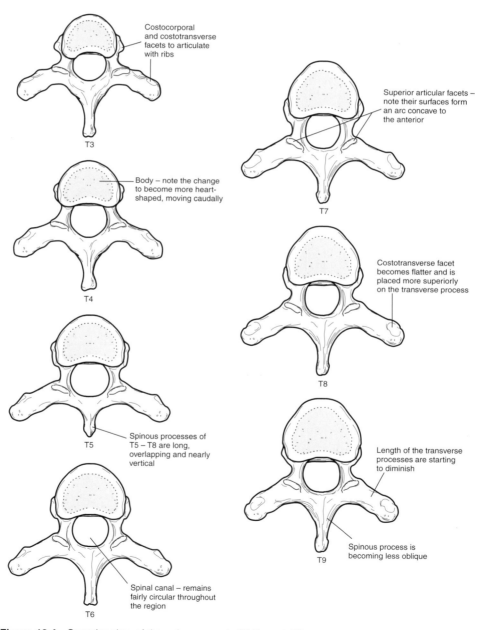

Figure 12.4   Superior view of thoracic segments T3 through T9.

The typical thoracic vertebral body is heart-shaped and increases in size downwards, reflective of the increasing load carried by the lower segments of the spine. The body of T3 is the smallest thoracic body. While the anterior aspect of T1 and T2 above is flattened, that of T3 is rounded and convex from side to side. The spinal canal is small and circular throughout the region.

The typical superior zygapophyseal facets face backwards and are angled slightly superolaterally (Fig. 12.5), while the inferior facets face frontwards, being angled slightly superomedially. The spinous processes of T3 and T4 are similar to those of T1 and T2, being more horizontal than angled. However the spinous processes of T5, T6, T7, and T8 angle sharply downwards and overlap. That of T8 is regarded as being the largest, longest, and most vertical in the region (Cramer & Darby 1995 p. 159) while that of T9 is considered to be quite small (Plaugher 1993 p. 253).

The transverse processes extend backwards and upwards in an oblique manner, lying in a more posterior plane than those of the cervical and lumbar segments. The tips of the transverse processes are most lateral at T1 in the cervicothoracic junction, and become more medial moving downwards through the mid thoracic spine. The costal facet on each transverse process faces frontwards and laterally. They also start to angle more superiorly from T6 downwards. The transverse process itself becomes progressively shorter, downwards from T3 to T9 (Fig. 12.4).

Ribs 3 through 9 are regarded as being typical, and all are quite similar in their morphology (Fig. 12.6A, B). The posterior articulations of the ribs are typical throughout the region, with the head articulating to the superior demifacet of the same-numbered vertebra and the inferior demifacet of the segment above. The tubercle, at the junction of the neck and shaft of the rib, articulates with the facet on the transverse process of the same-numbered thoracic segment.

These costovertebral articulations contain innervation within the anterior capsule and synovial tissues (Erwin et al 2000). A number of joints have also been found to have large intra-articular synovial inclusions or meniscoids which contain small bundles of axons with immune-like reactivity to substance P. The articulation certainly has the requisite innervation for pain production in a similar manner to other joints of the spine (Erwin et al 2000) and must be considered as a pain generator.

The anterior ends of ribs 3, 4, 5, 6, and sometimes 7 articulate with the sternum in a similar manner to rib 2, namely through a cartilaginous extension to the sternum. They are thus termed "true ribs". The extension of rib 7 may articulate above with that

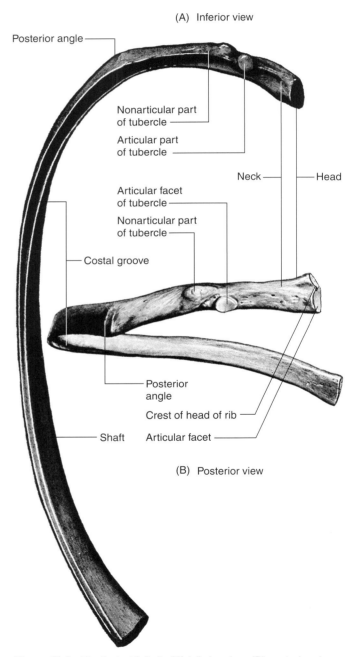

Figure 12.6 The typical left rib. (A) Inferior view; (B) posterior view. (A, B) From Williams & Warwick (1980), with permission.

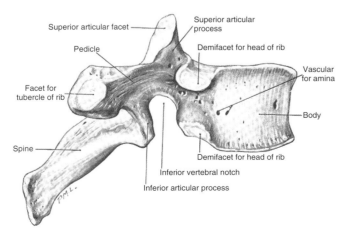

Figure 12.5 Right lateral view of a typical thoracic segment to illustrate T3 through T9. From Williams & Warwick (1980), with permission.

of rib 6, while the bony ends of ribs 8 and 9 have a short extension of cartilage which articulates with the lower border of the cartilage immediately above. This forms a common cartilaginous element as a steeply angulated, anterior inferior costal cartilage margin, extending superomedially to the inferior border of the sternum. The costal cartilage may undergo superficial ossification as part of the aging process and become brittle.

The lateral view of a typical thoracic vertebra demonstrates the superior placement of the facet for the head of the rib on the vertebral body (Fig. 12.5). This is a demifacet for the inferior facet of the head of the rib of the same number as the vertebral body. A small, transverse ridge on the head, called the *crest*, separates that inferior facet from the superior facet of the head which articulates with the inferior demifacet of the vertebral body above. Note also the posterior sweep of the transverse process and its facet which articulates with the tubercle of the rib.

The spinous process is clearly seen to extend downwards. The backwards angulation of the superior articular facet and the frontwards angulation of the inferior facet allow them to

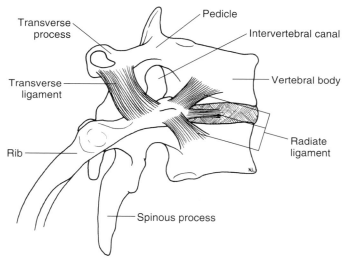

Figure 12.7 Right lateral view of a typical mid thoracic spinal motion unit. From Peterson & Bergmann (2002), with permission.

interlock as they articulate with those above and below. This significantly limits anterior to posterior glide but guides flexion/extension and the coupled movements of rotation and lateral flexion. The downwards angulation of the spinous process significantly limits extension.

Combined flexion and extension is only about 4° at T3–4, T4–5, and T5–6, increasing slightly to 6° at T9–10 (Bergmann et al 1993 p. 298). Lateral flexion to either side is about 6° and rotation to either side is about 7° or 8°. These are very small ranges within which to infer changes in the quantity and quality of movement.

Notwithstanding the small amount of movement at each spinal motion unit (SMU), the amount of forward flexion of the thoracic spine as a region appears reasonable due to the cumulative effects of the greatest number of SMUs of any spinal region, typically being between 20° and 45°. Similarly, while segmental rotation is noted as the greatest movement, the regional effect is limited due to the rigidity of the thoracic cage, being between 35° and 50° to either side. An appreciation of these paradoxes suggests there is clinical benefit in assessing segmental end-feel at the elastic limit of regional movement.

The coupling of lateral flexion and rotation is thought to follow that of the mid cervical and cervicothoracic spines to about T4, namely, the spinous will move to the contralateral side with lateral flexion. It is thought this pattern is less distinct between T5 and L1 (Bergmann et al 1993 p. 300); however, it is suggested that these patterns may be influenced by the degree of flexion or extension of the spine during assessment (Pletain 1997).

The rigidity of the mid thoracic spine is enhanced by the rib articulations and these must be considered in any assessment of the SMU in this region. The typical relationship, as seen in the transverse plane, between typical ribs and a typical thoracic segment is shown in Figure 11.6. A right lateral view is shown in Figure 12.7. It is important to understand the intimacy of the neck of the rib and the transverse process, and its relationship to the intervertebral canal (IVC). This compact region is dense with neurovascular structures. The sympathetic ganglia lie against the anterior border of the rib head and its articulation and are stimulated by normal movement of these structures during respiration (Patriquin 1992 p. 5) (Fig. 12.8).

The IVCs of the mid thoracic spine differ from those above in that they face laterally instead of angling anterolaterally (Fig. 12.7).

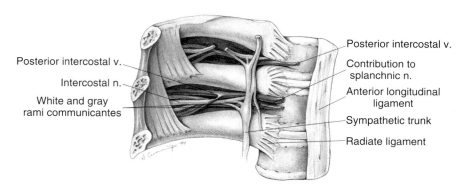

Figure 12.8 Right lateral view showing sympathetic trunk. The sympathetic trunk and its ganglia lie against the anterior surfaces of the ribs close to their articulation with the vertebral bodies and disk. From Cramer & Darby (1995), with permission.

The neurovascular bundle lies relatively high within the IVC. In this region the spinal nerve occupies only about a twelfth of the available space (Cramer & Darby 1995 p. 159) and it lies high in the IVC, posterior to the vertebral body. The disk lies lower in the IVC and the rib head articulates with it and the demifacets. The head of the rib is bound to the disk (T2 through T9) by an intra-articular ligament which arises from the crest and merges with the lateral fibers of the annulus, dividing the joint completely.

The clinical implication is the intimate relationship between the rib, vertebral bodies, disk, and sympathetic nervous system. The disk itself is quite thin in this region and protrusion is not common. Similarly, radiculopathy is also not common, although intercostal neuralgia does occur and may be seen as a form of nerve root pain.

ASSESSMENT OF KINEMATIC CHANGE
Philosophical context

An appreciation of various technique paradigms is helpful with the assessment of kinematic change in the mid thoracic spine. Bergmann et al (1993 p. 332) identify a controversy within chiropractic which surrounds the use of supine adjustive techniques for "anterior" thoracic segments. While providing little, if any, comment regarding assessment, they provide a spectrum of both supine and standing adjustive techniques (pp. 375–383; 385–390). On the other hand, Plaugher (1993 pp. 248–249) argues that a flexion fixation of a single segment (for example, of T7) produces a "compensation reaction" in multiple thoracic segments above. Plaugher suggests the compensating segments can be visualized as being "anterior" or dished and will palpate as a painful, edematous area, resilient to compressive (posterior to anterior) palpation. Plaugher argues that the adjustment must be performed with a prone, spinous contact at the one flexed segment.

Gatterman (1990 pp. 189–190) acknowledges both the flexion fixation and the related supine and standing adjustments as well as the prone adjustment. The skills required for competence with the adjustment of an anterior segment have been described in the journal literature (Fligg 1986) and Byfield provides a "single spinous–supine" adjustment specifically for the mid thoracic spine (Byfield 1996 pp. 197–201).

Walther (1981 pp. 60–62) describes the concept of the anterior thoracic subluxation in detail and provides empirical clinical assessment procedures. These include specific palpation for exquisite tenderness at the tip of the spinous process thought to be reflective of *interspinalis* muscle weakness. It is thought that the tip of the spinous process of the inferior segment in the "anterior" SMU will also be tender. The anterior thoracic has also been considered to represent a "sectional subluxation" in an attempt to understand the signs and symptoms which accompany a flattening of the thoracic kyphosis over several segments (Zachman et al 1989). The mechanism is that which Plaugher describes, namely a flexion fixation with multiple extension fixations above, and it is considered that the supine approach is more sensible.

Zachman et al (1989) also relate this sectional subluxation to many of the patient's symptoms, a clinical approach expanded by Patriquin (1992), who suggests that diminished, minor motion between two or three adjacent segments is indicative of

viscerosomatic reflex activity, secondary to visceral disease. Patriquin suggests that a finding of thinned, atrophic, fibrous deep paraspinal musculature in one area represents a long-standing problem, while vigorous edema, swelling, and tenderness, perhaps with increased local muscle tone, are more suggestive of acute visceral disease.

The pain associated with musculoskeletal problems in this region is usually localized and identified quite well by the patient, perhaps with one finger, while pain from visceral dysfunction is poorly defined, perhaps indicated by the patient moving the hand about a region. Further, the muscular hypertonicity associated with musculoskeletal dysfunction usually improves after the adjustment whereas tonicity secondary to visceral dysfunction remains or appears only slightly improved. The assessment of kinematic change must therefore include particular attention to the soft tissues of the region and allow for findings not evident in other spinal regions, namely anteriority, either of single or several segments, within the context of the visceral status of the patient.

Postural assessment

Postural assessment is particularly important in this region and will give an indication of the nature of the thoracic kyphosis and whether it is accentuated. While observing the patient an attempt is made to determine whether any underlying process affecting the posture is muscular, ligamentous, osseous, antalgic, proprioceptive, or any combination (Schafer 1983 pp. 359–366). Muscular distortion patterns start with a simple C curve with head tilt to the contralateral side of pelvic tilt, and progress to a double major S scoliosis with pelvic tilt but a level head. A third pattern has multiple curves and head tilt to the same side as the pelvic tilt (Figs 13.6, 14.5).

The lower spinous processes may deviate laterally with lower trapezius hypertonicity. The upper spinous processes (T2–4) may deviate inferolaterally with hypertonicity of the rhomboid major. Hypertonicity of the iliocostalis elevates multiple ribs and may lead to scoliosis when chronic. Unilateral hypertonicity of the multifidus imparts a rotary torque at the segmental level which may result in altered quantity and quality of motion. This may be perceived by the practitioner as the "altered position" of the vertebra and subsequently described as a "fixation".

Walther (1981 pp. 31–39) explores the postural expressions of specific muscle involvement and Schafer (1983 pp. 362–366) describes and illustrates some eight postural patterns thought to reflect subluxation in the thoracic spine. These are presented in Chapters 13 and 14 and must be reviewed and integrated into the assessment of this spinal region.

The question of scoliosis is complex and the role of postural assessment is to determine the likelihood of positive findings on further investigation by diagnostic imaging. When scoliosis is suspected, the patient is asked to stand and then flex forwards while the practitioner observes from behind. The patient's hands hang downwards towards the floor and the patient flexes the thorax and trunk to about 70–90° at the hips. This is the Adam's forward-bending test and the practitioner observes for leveling of the shoulders, rib cage, and scapulae (Fig. 12.9).

A "rib hump" will be observed in the patient with a structural scoliosis due to the fixed rotation of the vertebral bodies and the

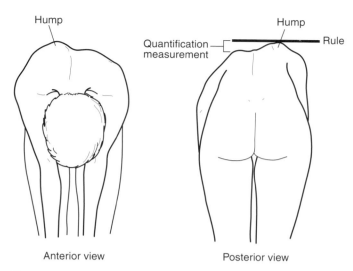

Figure 12.9 The rib hump of structural scoliosis. A structural scoliosis generates a rib hump on one side as the patient bends forwards. It may be quantified by measuring the depth of the low side below a horizontal rule placed on the hump or high side. From Gatterman (1990), with permission.

resultant posteriority of the rib cage on one side. This may be clinically quantified in linear units by measuring the variation of the lower side from a horizontal bar placed level with the higher side, or in degrees by placing a bar with a protractor so it touches both sides. A rib hump greater than 11 mm measured with the patient seated is strongly suggestive of progressive scoliosis (Duval-Beaupere 1992). The Adam's forward-bending test is quite sensitive and is the preferred non-invasive clinical test to evaluate scoliosis (Côté et al 1998). Diagnostic quantification and prognosis are made from the AP radiograph.

Assessment continues with the patient seated and the naked thoracic cage is observed from the anterior, side, and posterior during respiration, looking for symmetry of the fine "bucket handle" rib movements. The tone of the intercostal spaces is also assessed during respiration. The rib cage is expected to elevate during inspiration with a symmetrical increase in the anterior to posterior, and lateral dimensions.

The extent and symmetry of thoracic excursion are observed and may be quantified through palpation. From behind, the practitioner's hands are placed about the lower rib cage. A broad, palmar contact is taken with the fingers around the sides of the thorax over the lower ribs, with the thumbs almost meeting at about the spinous of T9 or T10. The patient is asked to breathe all the way out and the thumbs are adjusted so they lightly touch each other. The patient is then asked to breathe in deeply and the thumbs are allowed to swing lightly laterally as the thorax expands and raises. Observe for symmetry of movement and an opening between the thumbs of several centimeters.

All patients are observed for the barrel chest associated with emphysema; pectus excavatum suggestive of murmurs; pectus carinatum or "pigeon chest"; and for signs of kyphoscoliosis. The nature of the skin must be noted, including its temperature and tone. In particular, observe for lesions such as melanoma on

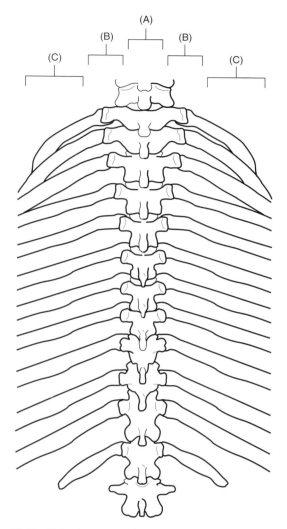

Figure 12.10 Palpation zones of the mid thoracic spine. (A) The mid sagittal zone (spinous processes, interspinous ligaments); (B) medial parasagittal zones (transverse processes and the costotransverse articulations); (C) lateral zones (rib angles, medial scapulae, intercostal muscles).

the back and for rashes and vesicular lesions. The female patient is assessed for signs of a poorly fitted bra, in particular, for constriction from the circumferential support strap and for soft-tissue indentation from narrow shoulder straps.

Static palpation

Static palpation is performed with the patient prone and the back exposed. The mid thoracic region can be considered as five parallel zones running from superior to inferior (Fig. 12.10). The mid sagittal zone (A) contains the spinous processes and interspinous ligaments and has cutaneous innervation from the medial branch of the dorsal ramus. The two most medial parasagittal zones (B) contain the transverse processes and the costotransverse articulations, while the two lateral zones (C) contain the rib angles with cutaneous innervation by the lateral branch of the dorsal ramus.

The region is systematically palpated to ensure all bony structures and the tissues between them in each zone are assessed. A sense of the tone of the skin and the subcutaneous tissues is gained through bilateral palpation at the levels of each rib and then intercostal space, firstly along the paraspinal line (zone A), then along a line covering the transverse processes and proximal ribs (B), and finally, more laterally (C).

The tonicity of muscles must be explored in detail, and palpation includes the scapula in general and its medial border in particular. The major muscles should be identified and palpated, looking for tonicity, nodularity, ropiness, and any sign of atrophy.

The anterior thorax should be palpated when indicated by either a specific complaint of pain by the patient or by identification of any involvement of posterior elements. Otherwise this assessment falls within the physical examination protocols for the respiratory and cardiovascular systems.

Radiographic analysis

The two standard plain film views are the AP thoracic and the lateral thoracic, both taken with the patient standing. The AP view typically includes some lower cervical segments and the upper lumbars and is used to identify scoliosis and congenital anomaly. The lateral allows assessment of the vertebral endplates and disk spaces. Kyphosis may also be measured on the lateral radiograph from plane lines extended anteriorly along the superior border of T1 and the inferior border of T12 if these landmarks are clearly visualized (Fig. 12.11). The typical range is around 45°, increasing with age to around 60° by the eighth decade. The morphology of the vertebral bodies accounts for over 60% of the variability in regional kyphosis (Goh et al 1999).

Scheuermann disease is clinically suspected when there is a well-circumscribed, angular thoracic kyphosis with an onset around puberty and is radiographically confirmed by the presence of anterior wedging of at least three adjacent vertebrae of 5° or more (Lowe 1990). The patient is typically taller than average with a skeletal age ahead of chronological age and is usually well-muscled compared to underdeveloped patients with postural kyphosis (Lowe 1990). Spinal osteochondrosis seems to be an important etiological factor and there is a very high incidence of disk degeneration in these patients (Paajanen et al 1989).

Scoliosis can be quantified by Cobb's method, where the plane line of each of the two end vertebrae of the curve, as seen on the AP radiograph, is extended to the concave side of the curve (Fig. 12.12). The superior plane line is extended along the superior endplate of the uppermost body, and the inferior plane line along the inferior endplate of the lower body. Perpendicular lines are extended from each plane line and the angle made at their intersection is taken as the angle of the scoliosis.

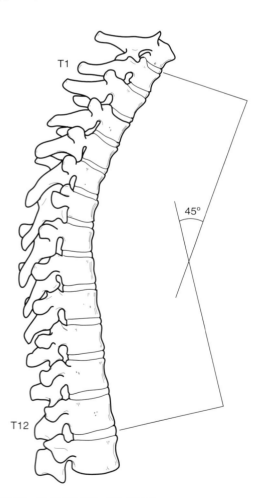

Figure 12.11 Quantification of kyphosis.

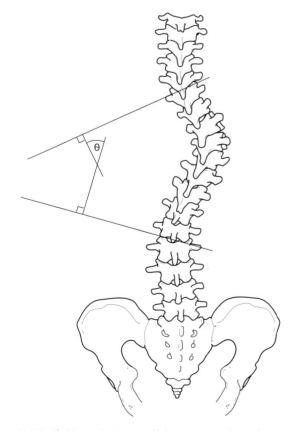

Figure 12.12 Cobb angle for quantifying scoliosis. From Cramer & Darby (1995), with permission.

Curvatures up to 20° are appropriate for conservative, manual management and may need monitoring if the patient has not reached skeletal maturity (Souza 1994). Curves up to 40° are also within the conservative management range; however, the issue of monitoring becomes more important. The point where surgical intervention is warranted is given as beyond 40° by Souza and when rapidly progressive and greater than 50° by Plaugher (1993 p. 273). Yochum & Rowe nominate a progression of 5° or more in a 3-month period as warranting referral (1996 p. 156). Progression of the curve usually ceases when the growth plates have closed.

A structural scoliosis is a permanent lateral deviation usually secondary to bony anomaly or development variance. Some 13 categories are given by Plaugher (1993 pp. 267–268). A functional scoliosis is secondary to non-structural disorders such as disk herniation, inflammation, leg-length inequality, tumor, or poor posture. The three-dimensional nature of the spine must be appreciated even though scoliosis is measured in the frontal plane from the AP radiograph and it is clinically useful to visualize the spiral nature of the affected spine from an axial perspective.

Objective structural change of SMU mechanics

Common anomalies seen on the AP radiograph include the hemivertebra and butterfly vertebra. The hemivertebra is a unilateral presentation and usually not a sole finding, appearing as a triangular body associated with lateral deviation of the spine above. The butterfly vertebra has a vertically increased central disk space created by indentation of the endplate cortices.

Common anomalies seen on the lateral radiograph include the Schmorl's node, which appears as a squared "pencil end" protrusion through the endplate, either centrally or towards the margins. Disk material has been shown to protrude into the resultant space within the body. These are to be differentiated from the nuclear impression, which is a smooth and more rounded indentation of the endplate, not commonly seen in the mid thoracic region. The giant Schmorl's node is a large node near the anterior of the body associated with significantly reduced disk space above and increased anterior to posterior dimension of the involved body (Yochum & Rowe 1996 p. 227).

There may be numerous endplate irregularities which should not be mistaken for ossification centers in the developing spine and which need to be differentiated from Schmorl's nodes and endplate fracture. Anomalous ribs may be noted within the thoracic cage, and variations such as a tortuous aorta may also be noted in soft-tissue contours.

The typical fractures of this region involve compression of the vertebral body secondary to either trauma or metabolic change. Traumatic fractures usually compress the anterior body margins and, given that a reasonable amount of force is required, may involve the ribs and other structures. The trauma is commonly a motor vehicle accident; however, metabolic fractures occur with osteoporosis in the aging patient and may involve more than one level. Typically the body collapses into itself, increasing the kyphosis. Rib fractures are rarely singular and specific radiographs must be taken to assess the complete thoracic cage.

Avulsion suggests trauma and may be seen about the anterior margins of the body, above or below the disk space. Dislocation is not common and requires reasonable traumatic force. Rib dislocation is more likely to be at the posterior than the anterior articulations. Hypertrophy of the articular pillars may represent degenerative joint disorders while hypertrophy of an individual vertebral body suggests Paget's disease.

Other diagnostic imaging assessment

The computed tomography (CT) scan is the axial imaging modality of choice and is used to identify thoracic pathology. It has little use in typical chiropractic practice for this region except in cases where lesions of or about the spinal cord are suspected. The magnetic resonance imaging (MRI) is perhaps more useful to demonstrate soft-tissue and neural relationships about the spine in this region.

Subjective nature of movement

The presence of scoliosis may vary the movement pattern of the mid thoracic spine and the following discussion applies to the patient with minimal or no scoliosis and a kyphosis within normal limits.

The range of motion of the region is assessed first. Care must be taken to stabilize the standing patient adequately and especially to limit flexion, which normally includes the hips, to the thoracic spine. Flexion, while the practitioner supports the pelvis by standing behind the patient and holding the pelvis against the practitioner's lateral thigh, is the supported Adam's test. Similarly, rotation normally includes the lumbar spine and pelvis, which again should be stabilized. Consideration is given to the patient's somatotype and ability to perform, especially if antalgic or in pain.

Lateral flexion is induced in free-standing patients by instructing them to run one hand down the side of the ipsilateral leg and then to repeat the move on the other side. Restriction can be quantified by measuring the distance from the fingertips to the floor at the end of movement; however, this may not be indicative of restriction within the mid thoracic spine; rather, it reflects regional restriction in both the thoracic and lumbar spines, and perhaps pelvis.

It is more valuable to observe the mid thoracic spine during lateral flexion as it may reveal segmental fixation. This will be seen as a kink in the spinal gutter as it laterally flexes. This is a reflection of the quality of movement within the mid thoracic region. The ribs must also be observed during lateral flexion, for both approximation on the ipsilateral side and separation on the contralateral side.

The active regional assessment may be repeated passively in the seated patient. The patient's arms are folded and the practitioner directs lateral flexion and rotation with the forearm across the posterior neck and shoulders. Passive flexion and extension are induced with the practitioner's indifferent hand under the patient's folded arms.

With the patient seated to stabilize the pelvis, the expected regional ranges of motion for the thoracic spine are:

- flexion: up to about 45°
- extension: about 25°
- rotation to one side: 35–50°
- lateral flexion to one side: typically about 20°, up to 40°.

The ranges are difficult to quantify with any degree of accuracy. Whilst the basic clinical assessment will rely on noting any unilateral restriction, with or without pain, advanced assessment, particularly in the rehabilitation setting, will require quantification, for which an inclinometer is useful.

Flexion can be clinically quantified by marking the spinous processes and, using a soft tape measure, recording the distance between them in neutral and then in flexion. The increase is normally around 2.5–3 cm for the full thoracic spine, between C7 and T12 (Mootz & Talmage 1999). The distance increases to reflect the "opening" of the spinous processes as they flex forwards. The question of the quantity of global movement is assessed as above, with notation of areas of restriction; however, the concept of restriction must take into account the individual nature of the quantity of movement at each SMU.

The multiplicity of articulations in this region highlights the importance of assessing segmental end-feel. It must also be appreciated that one effect of the ribs is significantly to reduce the amount of rotation available at the mid thoracic SMUs.

A broad, screening assessment of the region may be conducted by using the dorsal surface of the fingers of the contact hand, which is held as a clenched fist. The patient is seated with the arms folded. The practitioner takes a square stance lateral to the patient and, with the indifferent hand, supports under the patient's folded elbows. The plane of the contact fingers is horizontal and the contact arm provides a posterior to anterior movement, coordinated with the flexion and extension of the region induced by raising and lowering the indifferent hand. This assessment is useful for identifying broad areas of fixation, including any sectional subluxation above a particular flexed segment.

The more clinically useful segmental movement to assess in this region is flexion. Extension from neutral is limited by the overlocking spinous processes. Movements of rotation and lateral flexion are coupled and it must be appreciated that each of these movements is less than 10°. With the seated patient, the practitioner can readily palpate the interspinous spaces during flexion, and induce end-feel provocation of the spinous process. The movement typically has a soft, springy end-feel due to the separation of the posterior column of the spine, the subsequent stretch of the capsular ligaments about the zygapophyseal joints, and the compressive nature of the disk at the anterior border of the anterior column.

On the other hand, extension closes the zygapophyseal joints and approximates the spinous processes, giving a different, more bony type of end-feel as the normal expectation. The practitioner gains a sense of segmental movement in extension by palpating for closure of the spinous processes as the patient returns to neutral from forward flexion. The better assessment of any change in movement of the thoracic segments about the x-axis is thus the attempt to detect any restriction while moving into, and returning out of, forward flexion.

Assessment of lateral flexion and rotation is complicated both by coupling and the associated costovertebral joints. The simplistic visualization of a spinous process raising up on the side of an open disk wedge while the body has rotated to the other side presents the challenge of attempting to palpate such a small mechanical change and identify it as the primary problem within a sea of associated small joints.

The interexaminer reliability of manual end-play palpation of this region with the patient seated has been found to be poor (Haas et al 1995), suggesting two things: (1) any such findings must be considered in the complete clinical context of the patient; and (2) seated assessment may be appropriate for regional screening and for gauging the quantity of movement at segmental levels, but prone assessment may be more productive for qualitative assessment of pain and tenderness (Christensen et al 2002).

The more important clinical finding seems to be the presence or absence of tenderness over the zygapophyseal joints in a region rather than a precise anatomical level. Christensen et al (2002) report an acceptably low level of variability by trained examiners for this procedure but also found poor agreement values for sitting motion palpation and prone joint play evaluation. Further, Keating et al (2001) found that mid thoracic tenderness relative to the cervical spine is not a normal finding in asymptomatic subjects. They report statistically significant regional differences, suggesting there is real clinical value in palpating for areas of tenderness (Keating et al 2001).

Careful qualitative palpation of end-feel with the patient prone remains an appropriate clinical procedure when interpreted in the context of the patient's pain and tenderness. In the doctor–patient relationship the question is more one of intra-examiner repeatability than interexaminer agreement. The application by the practitioner of gentle springing movements bilaterally on the transverse processes may gap the zygapophyseal joints of the level above the contact segment and allow an estimate of segmental resiliency. This then informs the practitioner's subsequent decision making, especially if tender or painful.

A high level of sensitivity is required to assess each SMU completely in the mid thoracic spine. The various aspects of the spinous process (inferior tip, lateral borders, posterior border, junction with lamina) can be specifically provoked for end-feel and pain findings (Fig. 12.10 zone A). The posterior to anterior resiliency of the SMU can be assessed at each specific location, both uni- and bilaterally, with contact over the transverse processes (zone B). The movement of a particular vertebral segment must be considered in terms of the pathomechanical status of the articulations about it, namely those of each rib at both the posterior and anterior articulations. The movement available at the articulations of the rib tubercle with the transverse process, and the rib head with the vertebral body, are so small they are palpated as end-feel. Hence the qualitative assessment of end-feel is the major palpatory finding.

The clinical outcome is that the better information about any kinematic change of the SMU at the T3–4, T4–5, T5–6, T6–7, T7–8, T8–9, and T9–10 levels, and the relevant rib articulations, is mainly derived from interpreting the characteristics of movement and end-feel within the context of pain. Palpable soft-tissue findings must be included and a thorough systemic history of the patient is also required, given the nature of viscerosomatic pain distribution about the thorax.

Assessment of the individual joints

The assessment of the mid thoracic spine follows the assessment of the upper thoracic levels at the cervicothoracic junction, in both the seated and then prone patient positions.

T3–4

The patient is seated with the arms folded. The practitioner takes a square stance lateral to the patient and supports under the patient's folded elbows with the indifferent hand. The contact hand is placed with a flat digital contact between the spinous processes. The index finger palpates the T3–4 interspinous space, with the lateral border of the finger contacting the inferior margin of the T3 spinous processes, and the medial border contacting the superior margin of the T4 spinous processes. The middle finger is similarly placed at the T4–5 level.

The indifferent hand gently flexes and extends the patient, first with a small, rocking movement, which is then increased in amplitude to bring the T3–4 level into full extension, and then flexion. It is important to direct the vector of the testing force to the actual level being assessed. In the normal SMU the interspinous space will appear to open as the T3 spinous flexes forward from T4 and the space will appear to close as the spinous processes approximate as they return from flexion by moving in extension.

Perceived movements of the spinous process in both lateral flexion and rotation may be palpated with the same finger contacts and end-feel can be assessed at the elastic zone for each movement with provocation about the lateral borders of the T3 spinous. Lateral flexion is induced by the practitioner's indifferent hand on the patient's shoulder for the upper levels, and then by the forearm laying across the posterior neck and shoulders for lower levels. Again, care must be taken with the angle of the vectors so that the force is directed into the particular level being assessed. The testing movement is not a side-to-side wobbling of the spine; it is a vector of force direction into a specific SMU to induce the desired movement of lateral flexion at that specific segment.

Rotation may be guided with the forearm across the shoulders as with lateral flexion, or the practitioner may turn a little sideways and use the thigh against the shoulder to stabilize and direct rotation. It must be remembered that rotation and lateral flexion at the SMU are coupled movements and are predominantly ipsilateral (Willems et al 1996).

The patient is placed prone to continue the assessment of the SMU and to facilitate assessment of the soft tissues and ribs. Careful point-palpation is made about the complete SMU and a flat, digital contact is useful. Whereas kinematic change in other SMUs is inferred by perceived changes in movement of the superior segment on the inferior segment, both segments must be provoked in this region. Kinematic change is synthesized from the perceived responses of both the movement of the superior segment on the inferior segment, and of the inferior segment under the superior segment.

Resiliency may be assessed with bilateral contact over the transverse processes. The vector should be perpendicular to the plane of the facets (Fig. 12.13 arrow A). Recall the facet relationship at the thoracic SMU; the superior facets of the inferior segment form the anterior border of the zygapophyseal joint and the inferior facets of the superior segment form the posterior border. Thus the zygapophyseal joint is "sprung" or "gapped" by posterior to anterior contact about the transverse processes of the inferior segment. This movement stresses the capsular ligaments about the facet joints. Conversely, the joint is approximated or

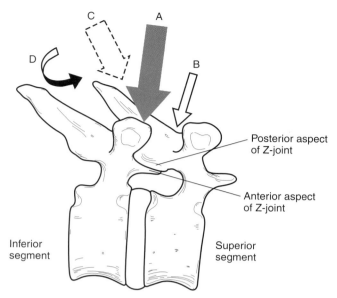

Figure 12.13 Prone palpation vectors for the mid thoracic spinal motion unit. (A) Bilateral contact over the transverse processes with the test vector perpendicular to the plane of the facets will open the Z-joint and stress the capsular ligaments; (B) contact over the lamina about the root of the spinous process of the superior segment will compress the Z-joint; (C) the inclusion of a small inferior to superior component may increase the localization of movement to a particular facet joint with consideration to changing the nature of the vector to reflect the kyphotic angulation through this region; (D) flexion of the superior segment may be induced by hooking under the inferior tip of the spinous process.

compressed by contact over the lamina about the root of the spinous process of the superior segment (arrow B).

The inclusion of a small inferior to superior component (arrow C) may increase the localization of movement to a particular facet joint with consideration given to changing the angle of the vector to reflect the changing kyphotic angulation through this region. Provocation into flexion and into coupled lateral flexion/rotation can also be made. The thumbs may be used for bilateral side to side movement of the spinous process, as well as to induce flexion of the superior segment by hooking under the inferior tip of the spinous process (arrow D).

The tissue resiliency of the intercostal space (Fig. 12.10 zone C) is assessed with a broad, flat thumb or finger-pad contact with gentle bilateral posterior to anterior movement, lateral to the erector spinae, and again, more laterally, about the mid-axillae lines. The practitioner should utilize a recording scheme which allows notation of the perceived changes in movement, as well as areas of tenderness, not only about the spinous and transverse processes but also within the interspinous and intercostal spaces.

Rib 3

The ribs of the mid thoracic spine are best assessed with the patient prone and the nature of any rib involvement is as described for ribs about the cervicothoracic junction:

- superior when there is a discernible resistance to superior to inferior palpation

- inferior when there is a discernible resistance to inferior to superior palpation
- medial when there is a discernible resistance to medial to lateral palpation
- lateral when there is a discernible resistance to lateral to medial palpation
- posterior when there is a discernible resistance to posterior to anterior palpation
- anterior when there is acute tenderness about the anterior costochondral cartilage and unclear palpatory findings about the rib head and tubercle.

The anterior costochondral cartilage is palpated in the supine or seated patient. Acute tenderness at the anterior, with unclear palpatory findings about the rib head and tubercle, suggests an "anterior rib" to be differentiated from costochondritis. Remember, a rib is not an isolated structure and its movement cannot be judged by assessing it in isolation. Each rib must be compared with both the one above and below, as well as its contralateral partner.

T4–5

Assessment is as described for T3–4, remembering that the T4 transverse processes are about level with the T3 spinous process, 2–2.5 cm laterally, and that the T5 transverse processes are about level with the upper border of the T4 spinous, 2–2.5 cm laterally. Note that the spinous process of T5 is more elongated than that of T4 and it angles inferiorly. This alters the feel of the interspinous space to being a little flatter than between T3–4.

Rib 4

Assessment is as described for rib 3.

T5–6

Assessment is as described for T3–4, remembering that the T5 transverse processes are about level with the upper border of the T4 spinous, 2–2.5 cm laterally, and that the T6 transverse processes are about level with the interspinous space of T4–5, 2–2.5 cm laterally. Note that the spinous process of T6 is also elongated and angles steeply inferiorly.

Rib 5

Assessment is as described for rib 3.

T6–7

Assessment is as described for T3–4, remembering that the T6 transverse processes are about level with the interspinous space of T4–5, 2–2.5 cm laterally, and that the T7 transverse processes are about level with the interspinous space of T5–6, 2–2.5 cm laterally. Note that the spinous process of T6 is about level with the inferior medial border of the scapula and that the spinous process of T7 is also elongated and angles steeply inferiorly.

Rib 6

Assessment is as described for rib 3.

T7–8

Assessment is as described for T3–4, remembering that the T7 transverse processes are about level with the interspinous space of T5–6, 2–2.5 cm laterally, and that the T8 transverse processes are about level with the interspinous space of T6–7, 2–2.5 cm laterally. Note the spinous process of T7 is about level with the inferior angle of the scapula and that the spinous process of T8 is a little less elongated than that of T7 and it angles a little less steeply inferiorly.

Rib 7

Assessment is as described for rib 3; however, rib 7 may not articulate with the sternum.

T8–9

Assessment is as described for T3–4, remembering that the T8 transverse processes are about level with the interspinous space of T6–7, 2–2.5 cm laterally, and that the T9 transverse processes are about level with the upper border of the T8 spinous process, 1.5–2 cm laterally. Note that the spinous process of T9 is starting to change from the elongated nature of those above, to be shorter and less angled.

Rib 8

Assessment is as described for rib 3; however, the cartilaginous extension of rib 8 integrates with that of rib 7 about the hypochondrium.

T9–10

Assessment is as described for T3–4, remembering that the T9 transverse processes are about level with the upper border of the T8 spinous process, 1.5–2 cm laterally, and the T10 transverse processes are about level with the upper border of the T9 spinous process, about 1.5–2.0 cm laterally. Note the spinous process of T10 is starting the transition to the stocky nature of those in the lumbar region.

Rib 9

Assessment is as described for rib 3; however, the cartilaginous extension of rib 9 integrates with that of rib 8 about the hypochondrium.

ASSESSMENT OF CONNECTIVE TISSUE CHANGE

The typical AP and lateral thoracic radiographs do not really allow useful soft-tissue assessment and the posteroanterior (PA) chest view is required to assess mediastinal structures and lung fields.

Ligaments of the SMU

The anterior longitudinal ligament attaches to the anterior aspect of each body in this region and intermingles with the anterior fibers of the annulus of each disk. The interspinous ligaments are present between each spinous process at these levels, although they are thin and membranous (Cramer & Darby 1995 p. 165). Anteriorly they are continuous with the ligamentum flavum, while posteriorly the fibers combine with the supraspinous ligament which acts to limit flexion. It is a continuous band which arises from the spinous process of C7 and travels inferiorly, perhaps to the sacrum.

The ligamentum flavum is paired left and right and each runs between the laminae at each level. As noted by Giles & Singer (2000), it is associated with the intra-articular synovial folds of the zygapophyseal joints. The ligamenta flava have a particular function to limit forward flexion. Ossification of the ligamentum flavum is common in Japan, rare in western countries (Akhaddar et al 2002), and is seen in the Chinese (Xiong et al 2001). It is most commonly seen in the lower thoracic spine in middle-aged men and is complicated by various other spinal lesions (Shiokawa et al 2001) including ossification of the posterior longitudinal ligament (Xiong et al 2001).

The zygapophyseal joints

The zygapophyseal joint capsules are less developed laterally. Giles & Singer (2000 p. 20) suggest this is to allow axial motion. The zygapophyseal menisci are small intra-articular synovial folds within the thoracic zygapophyseal joints which are consistent with most synovial joints. They arise medially from tissue adjacent to the ligamentum flavum and extend a varying distance into the medial joint cavity (Giles & Singer 2000 p. 23).

The intervertebral disk

The intervertebral disk functions as a major connective tissue. As with all disks, there are sensory nerves in the annulus and it is considered to be a pain generator. The disk morphology is thinner and more heart-shaped. The disk plays a small role in the normal development of kyphosis; however, the development of spinal angulation in juvenile kyphosis can be partly attributed to a loss in anterior disk height associated with herniation of disk material through the vertebral endplates (Goh et al 1999). Damage to the vertebral endplates which subsequently allows vertical extension of disk material is more common in the lower thoracic segments.

The annulus fibrosus has an intimate relationship to the posterior longitudinal ligament as they blend together. The ligament takes on the morphology of two layers; a deep layer which passes downwards and also to the posterolateral perimeter of the disk, blending with the periosteum of the pedicles, and a superficial layer which blends with the deep layer at each disk level, leaving a shallow pocket (Giles & Singer 2000 p. 35). At lower levels this allows medial disk protrusions to travel laterally;

however, protrusion of the thoracic disk is much less common than that of the lumbar or cervical spines (Cramer & Darby 1995 p. 159). The peak age for thoracic disk herniation is 40–50 years and the condition occurs more frequently in men. It is suspected that herniated disks in the lower thoracic spine may refer pain to the shoulder (Wilke et al 2000).

Ligaments about the ribs

The costovertebral capsules include intra-articular bands of ligaments which provide strong attachment of the rib about the thoracic disk, and radiate ligaments about the head of the rib and the demifacet on the thoracic body (Figs 12.7 and 12.8). The intra-articular band is short and flat and creates distinct upper and lower articular compartments lined with synovial membrane (Cramer & Darby 1995 p. 167). The capsule around these costo-corporal articulations blends with the disk and is a pain generator.

The articulation of the tubercle of the neck and the transverse process of the thoracic segment is supported by the costotransverse ligament and lateral costotransverse ligaments (Figs 11.6, 12.7, and 12.8). A thin synovial membrane lines the resultant thin, fibrous joint capsule.

ASSESSMENT OF MUSCLE CHANGE

Many of the muscles relevant to the mid thoracic spine are also relevant to the cervicothoracic and mid cervical spines and have previously been discussed. The iliocostalis cervicis, semispinalis thoracis, levatores costarum, intercostales, and serratus anterior are presented in Chapter 11. The rhomboid minor, serratus posterior superior, and splenii are integral to the ligamentum nuchae and are presented in Chapter 9. The small muscles, including the multifidi, have also been discussed in preceding chapters and the general principles and characteristics apply throughout this region.

The serratus posterior inferior and the latissimus dorsi, while relevant to this region, are perhaps more relevant to the thoracolumbar junction and will be presented in Chapter 13. Figure 12.14 illustrates the relationships within the mid thoracic spine between serratus posterior superior, the levatores costae, and the multifidi. While some of the following muscles attach about the cervicothoracic junction, they can be considered as muscles of the mid thoracic spine and are to be included in any evaluation of this region.

Middle and lower trapezius

The fibers of the middle and lower trapezius originate from the spinous processes of C7 through T12 and travel laterally to converge on the scapula. The middle fibers are more horizontal and attach about the medial margin of the acromion and superior lip of the crest of the spine of the scapula, while the lower fibers ascend superiorly and laterally to pass into an aponeurosis which attaches to a tubercle about the medial third of the spine. The arrangement of the fibers is given in Figure 12.15A. Motor innervation is by the spinal accessory nerve and the ventral rami of C3 and C4 provide sensory innervation, although some variations have been described.

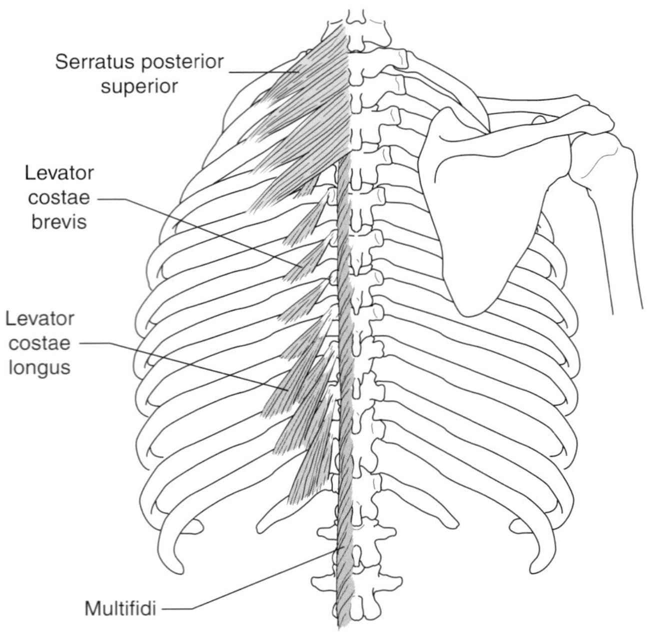

Figure 12.14 The levatores costae and multifidi. The function of the levatores costae is to elevate and rotate the ribs during inspiration. The pain from active trigger points is localized and radiates around the involved muscle. From Chaitow & DeLany (2000), with permission.

These fibers of the muscle act to adduct the scapula and draw back the acromion process. They are tested with the patient prone with the head turned ipsilaterally (Fig. 12.15B). For the middle fibers the ipsilateral arm is extended to 90° at the shoulder with the elbow extended and the thumb pointing towards the ceiling (Fig. 12.15B). The contralateral shoulder is stabilized. For the lower fibers the arm is abducted to align diagonally with the fibers (Fig. 12.15B). The patient's head may be turned ipsilateral or be straight and stabilization is provided about the contralateral flank. Weakness may allow the scapula to rise and the shoulder to roll forward; the spinal kyphosis may also increase.

The posterior neurolymphatic point is in the left seventh intercostal space, about the laminae of T7 and T8. The trigger points and their referral patterns are given in Figure 12.15C. They are numbered after the work of Simons et al (1999). Trigger point 2 refers to the suboccipital region; #3, the central trigger point in the lower fibers, is very common and refers severe pain to the high cervical region, mastoid, and acromion; #4 and #5 refer pain about the medial scapula; #6 is localized about the point of the shoulder; and #7 responds to light touch to refer a tingling sensation to the arm.

Pectoralis major

The sternal division of the pectoralis major arises from the sternum and ribs to rib 7 and inserts into the lateral lip of the bicipital groove of the humerus (Fig. 12.16A). It acts to adduct the humerus towards the opposite iliac crest and is a major anterior shoulder stabilizer. These fibers are innervated by the lateral and medial pectoral nerves from C6 to T1. The clavicular fibers are associated more with the cervicothoracic spine and run from the medial clavicle to the lateral lip of the bicipital groove of the humerus. These are innervated by the lateral pectoral nerve from C5 to C7.

The muscle is tested with the patient supine with the elbow extended and the shoulder flexed to 90° and medially rotated with the thumb pointing towards the feet. The examiner stabilizes the contralateral anterior superior iliac spine when testing the sternal division (Fig. 12.16Bii) and applies a test force to abduct the arm and increase its flexion with the vector about 45° superolaterally. This aligns the test force with the majority of fibers in this division. The clavicular division is tested in a similar manner (Fig. 12.16Bi) with the force directed laterally, perpendicular to the spine, so the test axis is again in line with the fibers of the muscle. Stabilization is over the contralateral shoulder.

Trigger points may be found in the central area of the sternal division and in the lateral free margin (Fig. 12.16Ci). They can refer intense pain to the anterior chest and down the inner aspect of the arm. The trigger points in the clavicular division refer pain more locally about the anterior shoulder (Fig. 12.16Cii).

Pectoralis minor

The pectoralis minor arises from near the costal cartilage of ribs 3 through 5 and inserts into the coracoid process (Fig. 12.16A). It is innervated by the medial pectoral nerve and acts as an anterior shoulder stabilizer by drawing the coracoid process forwards. It is often involved in patients with arm and shoulder pain and is tested in supine patients by having them raise their shoulder off the table against resistance (Fig. 12.16Biii).

Tender points are sought about the myotendinous attachment to the coracoid process and are treated with cross-friction massage. The trigger points are found in the belly of the muscle over the ribs and refer intense pain to the shoulder and diffuse pain about the thorax and into the arm, even reaching the hand and medial fingers (Fig. 12.16Ciii).

Rhomboid major

The rhomboid major pairs with rhomboid minor (Fig. 9.15). It arises from the spinous processes of T2 through T5 and attaches to the medial border of the scapula between the spine and the inferior angle. It is innervated by the dorsal scapular nerve from C4 to C5 and acts to adduct and elevate the scapula, to rotate the scapular medially so the glenoid fossa moves inferiorly, and is an important stabilizer of the scapula during arm movement.

According to Chaitow & DeLany (2000 p. 331), it is a phasic (type 2) muscle which weakens when stressed but which can modify its fiber type to be a postural (type 1) muscle under conditions of prolonged misuse. The muscle is tested in conjunction with rhomboid minor (Fig. 9.15) and its trigger points generate a similar pain about the medial border of the scapula.

The back extensors

The back extensors through this region are a combination of slips which extend cephalad and originate from transverse processes and ribs, and slips which insert into the lower borders of ribs and the transverse and spinous processes. The palpation of these slips must take into consideration structural features

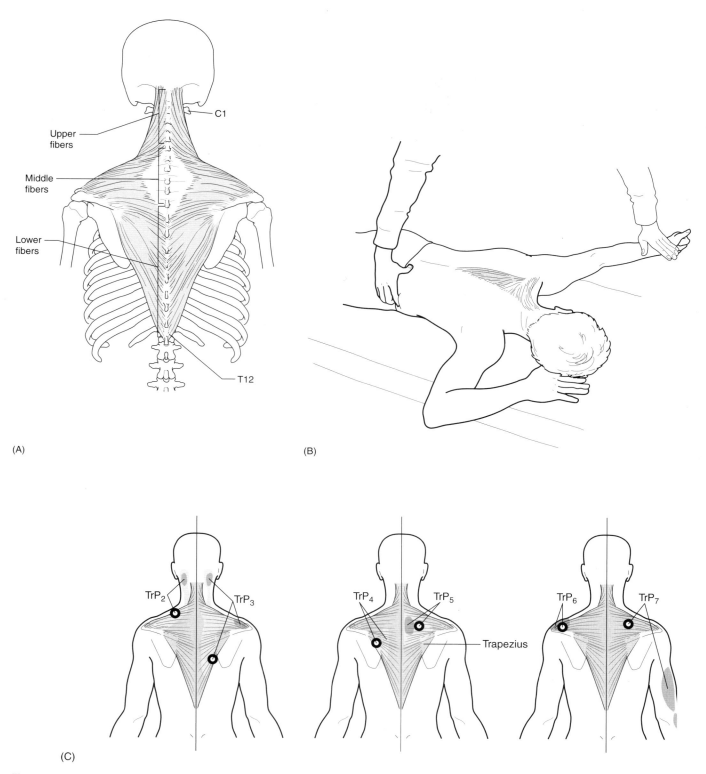

Figure 12.15 The trapezius. (A) The middle fibers lie horizontally while the lower fibers ascend superolaterally to insert about the spine of the scapula. (B) The muscle is tested with the patient prone. The arm is held in the same axis as the direction of fibers and the thumb of the patient's hand is facing upwards. (C) The trigger points (TrP). (A, C) From Chaitow & DeLany (2000), with permission.

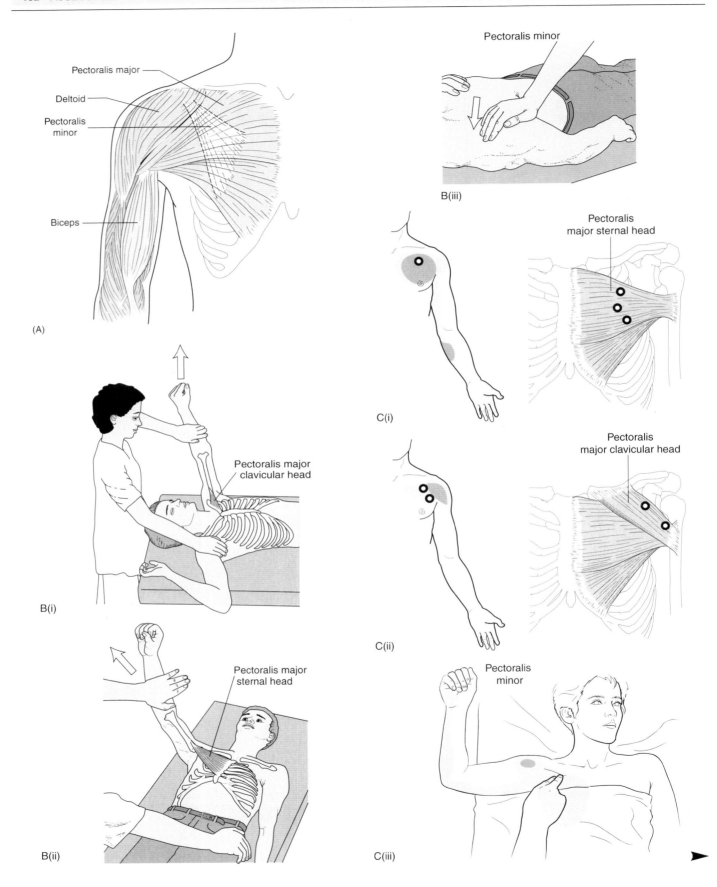

(A)

B(i)

B(ii)

B(iii)

C(i)

C(ii)

C(iii)

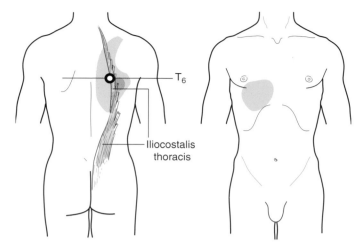

Figure 12.17 Pain referral from iliocostalis thoracis. From Chaitow & DeLany (2000), with permission.

such as whether they are fibers from below which are inserting, or new fibers which are originating to rise superiorly. A flat-finger, lateral–medial–lateral palpation perpendicular to the spine is useful to identify specific bands which may be dysfunctional, and then specific palpation either in an inferior to superior or a superior to inferior direction is applied to differentiate the particular slips which may be involved.

The spinalis thoracis arises from the spinous processes of low thoracic and upper lumbar segments and inserts into the spinous processes of the upper thoracic vertebrae, variously around T4 through T8. The fibers act to extend the spine and weakness may allow scoliosis, concave on the contralateral (strong) side.

The trigger points usually refer pain unilaterally, both cephalad and caudad, about their location; however, some, in particular those in the iliocostalis thoracis, will also refer pain to the anterior thorax (Fig. 12.17).

ASSESSMENT OF NEURAL CHANGE
The spinal nerves

The spinal nerves of the mid thoracic spine and the levels at which they exit are:

- spinal nerve T3 from the T3–4 SMU
- spinal nerve T4 from the T4–5 SMU
- spinal nerve T5 from the T5–6 SMU
- spinal nerve T6 from the T6–7 SMU
- spinal nerve T7 from the T7–8 SMU
- spinal nerve T8 from the T8–9 SMU
- spinal nerve T9 from the T9–10 SMU.

While the spinal nerves exit the spinal column as noted above, it must be appreciated that the level of the spinal cord from which they arise becomes progressively higher in relation to the vertebral level as the number of the spinal nerve increases. The typical relationship between the spinal nerve and the vertebral segment is:

- spinal nerve T3 arises about the mid level of vertebra T2
- spinal nerve T4 arises about the upper border of vertebra T3
- spinal nerve T5 arises about the upper border of vertebra T4
- spinal nerve T6 arises about the middle of vertebra T5
- spinal nerve T7 arises about the middle of vertebra T6
- spinal nerve T8 arises about the middle of vertebra T7
- spinal nerve T9 arises about the upper border of vertebra T8.

In addition to the above, the spinal nerve travels along the IVC above the level of the respective disk, hence, for example, were there to be a posterolateral disk protrusion at T7–8, it would less likely affect spinal nerve T7 and more likely affect spinal nerve T8. The clinical application is the understanding that injury or dysfunction of the spinal column and cord will be reflected in the neural distribution of much lower levels. The typical course of the thoracic spinal nerve is shown in Figure 11.11.

The assessment for signs and symptoms of localized mid thoracic neural change includes dermatomal sensory and reflex changes. Thoracic root syndromes are extremely rare; however, the clinical presentation of a herniated disk in this region can be dramatic, partly due to the smaller diameter of the spinal canal (Dvořák & Dvořák 1984). Gross motor changes of the lower limb are suggestive of significant central neural change, such as transection of the cord secondary to trauma.

Pain assessment

The pain generators about the SMU have been previously described. Care must be taken to distinguish between local pain of mechanical origin and pain referred about the region, whether by active trigger points, by muscle dysfunction, as suggested by tonicity, tender points, and/or myotendinoses, or by viscera, as described below. A hierarchy for chest and back pain presentations within ambulatory manual healthcare practice is given in Table 12.1. This must be reversed for medical practice, where all chest and thorax pain is cardiac until proved otherwise.

Mechanical pain

Typically, the pain generators within the spine will give increased nociceptive input, perceived as pain by the patient, with mechanical movement. Thus the movement palpation must be specific and localized and must include the ribs and their anterior and posterior articulations. The dysfunctional SMU may refer pain to either or both the anterior and posterior

Figure 12.16 Pectoralis major and minor. (A) Anterior view of the right thorax and shoulder showing the pectoral muscles. (B) The muscles are tested with the patient supine. The arm is held straight and flexed at 90° at the shoulder for testing pectoralis major. The test vector is in line with the fibers, being lateral for the clavicular fibers (i) and 45° superolateral for the sternal fibers (ii). Pectoralis minor is tested by the patient raising the shoulder off the bench and resisting a downwards force over the head of the humerus from the practitioner (iii). (C) The trigger points and pain referral patterns are shown for the sternal head of pectoralis major (i), the clavicular head of pectoralis major (ii), and for pectoralis minor (iii). (A, C) From Chaitow & DeLany (2000), with permission.

Table 12.1 Pain assessment

Rank	Pain generator	Characteristic	Example
1	Mechanical	Worse with movement, sharp, localized	Subluxation
2	Cervical disk	Burning, vague, between scapulae	C5 disk degeneration
3	Trigger point	Unilateral, steady, deep, aching about the thorax, shoulder, and/or arm; discomfort when the muscle is used, replicated by palpating a found trigger point	Iliocostalis thoracis trigger point
4	Muscle dysfunction	Localized ache worse with resisted movements	Pectoralis major strain
5	Other viscera	Burning, deep	Gall bladder referral to right shoulder
6	Respiratory system	Vaguely localized, worse with inspiration, difficulty breathing	Pneumonia
7	Cardiovascular	Constricting, central, crushing, burning; patient using a clenched fist to describe	Angina

The rank given represents a hierarchy of probable diagnoses within ambulatory manual therapy practice; it is reversed for medical practice, where all chest and thorax pain is cardiac until proved otherwise.

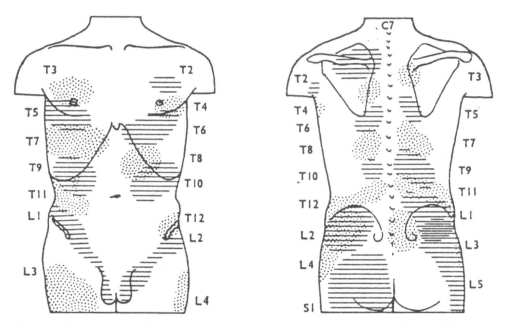

Figure 12.18 Pain referred from structures about the laminae and zygapophyseal joints. Kellgren (1977) mapped areas of deep pain resulting from stimulation of structures in the back lying deeply in the region of the lamina and zygapophyseal joints. From Kellgren (1977), with permission.

and the typical pattern is for the zone of the body where the pain is felt to lie several segments lower than the level at which it is generated. These patterns were mapped as long ago as the 1930s by Kellgren as he injected saline to irritate deep thoracic spinal structures about the laminae and zygapophyseal joints (Kellgren 1977; Fig. 12.18). These locations should be considered during the assessment of the patient.

As noted previously, the costovertebral articulations contain innervation within the anterior capsule and synovial tissues (Erwin et al 2000). The articulation has the requisite innervation for pain production in a similar manner to other joints of the spine (Erwin et al 2000). The pain generated by dysfunction in these articulations is typically intensely local, with perhaps

some unilateral radiation around the chest wall in the region of the involved rib. The pain typically worsens on inspiration.

There are also numerous patterns of referred pain from active trigger points and the relevant trigger points should always be assessed and then either included in, or ruled out of, the working diagnosis. It remains important to distinguish between *trigger* points and *tender* points and to use the correct descriptive terminology. Where an active trigger point is identified, it should be described with both the pattern of distribution and nature of pain being documented, as well as with a concise description of the location of the trigger point. The locations and pain referral patterns of relevant trigger points have been discussed with the assessment of muscle change.

Referred visceral pain

Clinical observation has resulted in known patterns of referred pain associated with visceral dysfunction. These are given to emphasize the thoroughness required with assessment of the patient presenting with pain about the thorax and mid thoracic spine. This summary includes work from Jacob et al (1992) and Murtagh (1994). The assessment must exclude the following types of pain, which require appropriate referral:

- Pain about the left breast and into the left arm, particularly the medial border, is strongly suggestive of a cardiac origin. The typical pain of myocardial ischemia is retrosternal and may also be felt about the mid thoracic spine, in the left breast and medial arm, in the throat and jaw, and about the epigastrium. The patient describes the pain as constricting and may indicate this with a clenched fist. The history and observation of the patient are crucial.
- Dramatic-onset central chest pain may also be secondary to pulmonary embolism and may be accompanied by dyspnea.
- Central chest pain also felt about the mid thoracic spine, with perhaps some pain under the left breast or referred to the left shoulder, suggests pericarditis. It may be worsened by coughing and deep breathing.
- Unilateral pain on both the anterior and posterior thorax, about the breast and scapula, suggests pneumothorax, especially if accompanied by dyspnea.
- Sudden and severe mid thoracic pain, with low central chest pain and/or pain about the epigastrium, which appears to be drawing downwards, is suggestive of dissecting aneurysm.
- Pain about the right shoulder in the gravid female may be suggestive of uterine bleeding and threatened spontaneous abortion.

Patients with the following types of pain are typically appropriate for conservative manual assessment. If the working diagnosis suggests it or the outcomes demonstrate that the pain is non-responsive to intervention, then the patient may benefit from referral and co-management.

- Pain about the sternum, anterior neck, and jaw may be referred from the esophagus. It is a burning pain, worsened by lying down or bending. It usually follows eating, and is often worse at night.
- Pain about the base of the neck on the right may be referred from the liver.
- Pain about T3 and T4 may be cardiogenic.
- Pain about T5 to T7 may be gastrogenic.
- Pain lateral to around T8 and medial to the scapula may be referred from the gall bladder.
- Pain inferior to the right scapula may be referred from the liver.
- Pain about the right hypochondrium may arise from the liver.
- Central epigastric pain arises from the stomach.

Sensory change

Basic assessment includes recording the bilateral comparative responses to crude touch. Further assessment can include pain or sharp touch and temperature sense about the thorax. The

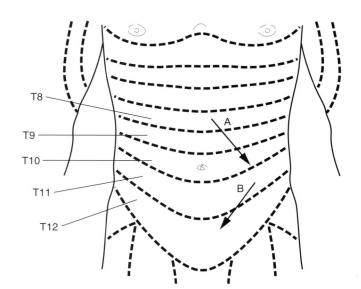

Figure 12.19 Cutaneous dermatomes about the umbilicus. A stroke with the end of the plessor in the direction of arrow A will most likely stimulate the left cutaneous dermatomes for T8, T9, and T10; similarly, stroke B will most likely stimulate those for T11 and T12. The normal response is for the umbilicus to flinch towards the stimulus.

typical dermatomal distributions for the spinal nerves of this region which are clinically useful are:

- T3: a horizontal band about the level of the axillary crease, superior to the nipple on the anterior
- T4: a horizontal band inclusive of the nipple, on the anterior
- T5: a horizontal band under the breast fold, on the anterior
- T6, T7, T8, and T9: successive horizontal bands, to above the umbilicus, on the anterior.

A paraspinal area of intense hyperesthesia may be identified. Typically it is a unilateral vertical rectangle over two or three transverse processes, which resolves with adjustment of the SMU about the level of the superior margin of the area. This finding may be identified during palpation; however, it is more clinically effective to perform skin-rolling along either side of the spine while the patient is prone. This is an effective method of identifying areas of neural change secondary to mechanical change.

Objective motor function is quite difficult to assess in this region; however, observation during deep inspiration may reveal asymmetrical action of the intercostal muscles between the ribs which may be taken as indicative of altered motor function. Further, an assessment of the resting tone of the intercostal muscles can provide similar diagnostic clues.

There are no deep tendon reflexes to assess for this region. The cutaneous reflex about the umbilicus should be assessed as it may be indicative of neural change associated with the subluxation complex. A light stroke is made with the assessment instrument, usually the end of a plessor or reflex hammer, starting about 5 cm superior and lateral to the umbilicus, in an inferolateral direction at 45°, for about 5 cm (Fig. 12.19 arrow A). This is expected to cross the T8, T9, and T10 dermatomes. Both sides are compared. The expected response is a bilaterally comparable twitching of the umbilicus towards the stimulus of the stroke.

Autonomic effects

Sympathetic fibers travel with each intercostal nerve to provide visceral motor to blood vessels and sweat glands about the thoracic wall. The posterior cutaneous distribution angles inferiorly from the spine, following the rib line. It is common to identify "zits" or pustular lesions along the distribution of a specific spinal nerve. Their relevance is hypothetical, yet they provide a useful clinical indicator which may point to a specific SMU and suggest dysfunction.

Traditional concepts

There is a considerable body of empirical opinion based on clinical observation from a variety of disciplines regarding relationships between visceral function and spinal levels of this region. The following notes attempt to present a summary as being suggestive of what may be seen in clinical practice. The references below regarding the stimulation of a spinal center are from Schafer (1983 p. 371). As in Chapter 11, the references to the Lovett Brother relationship are from Walther (1981 p. 67).

About T3 – the T3–4 SMU

Traditional chiropractic associates this level with lungs, bronchus, pleura, chest, and breast. The Lovett Brother relationship to the T3 body is movement in the opposite direction of the T8 body. Adjusting here is considered to produce a sympathetic effect; efferent sympathetic preganglionic fibers to the heart arise here and Gonstead associates this level with systolic hypertension (Plaugher 1993).

Osteopathy considers this level is a reference site for thoracic viscera (Beal 1989 p. 20) and reports that a study of 108 patients with cardiovascular disorders found the greatest number of spinal findings (tissue texture, joint motion) at T2 and T3 on the left (p. 23). Faridi (1995) associates the T3 vertebral segment with sympathetic neural pathways to the trachea and bronchi and relates this level to asthma, chronic obstructive pulmonary disease, and bronchitis. Stimulation of the spinal reflex center is thought to initiate lung reflex dilation (e.g., inspiratory dyspnea), to relax the stomach body, contract the pylorus, and inhibit heart action (i.e., antitachycardia reflex) and gastric hypermotility.

The posterior neurolymphatic point for serratus anterior lies over the T3–5 laminae (Walther 1981 p. 374); the posterior neurolymphatic point for deltoid – anterior division, deltoid – middle division, deltoid – posterior division, and coracobrachialis lies over and between the T3–4 laminae (p. 388); and the posterior neurolymphatic point for teres major and teres minor lies over the T3 laminae (pp. 398, 403). In acupuncture terms the site for Du 12 Shenzhu is below the spinous process of T3 and is indicated for cough, asthma, scrofula, stiffness, and pain in the back (Qiu 1993 p. 155).

About T4 – the T4–5 SMU

Traditional chiropractic associates this level with the gall bladder and the common bile duct. The Lovett Brother relationship to the T4 body is movement in the opposite direction of the T7 body. Adjusting here is considered to produce a sympathetic effect and this level is implicated in hypertension, as efferent sympathetic preganglionic fibers to the heart arise here (Plaugher 1993).

Osteopathy considers this level is a reference site for thoracic viscera (Beal 1989 p. 20) and suggests range of motion abnormalities at T4 to be highly indicative of coronary artery disease (Beal 1989 p. 21). Faridi (1995) associates the T4 vertebral segment with neural pathways to the gall bladder, and gallstone formation. Stimulation of the spinal reflex center is thought to initiate cardiac and aortic dilation and inhibit viscerospasms.

The posterior neurolymphatic point for serratus anterior lies over the laminae (Walther 1981 p. 374). There is no specific acupuncture point at this level; however, the generic Extra 19 Jiaji (Huatuojiaji) point applies, as it does at each spinal level, to stimulate the posterior rami and their arterial and venous plexuses at this level (Qiu 1993 pp. 176–177).

About T5 – the T5–6 SMU

Traditional chiropractic associates this level with the liver and the solar plexus. The Lovett Brother relationship to the T5 body is movement in the opposite direction of the T6 body. Adjusting here is considered to produce a sympathetic effect and this level is implicated in hypertension as efferent sympathetic preganglionic fibers to the heart arise here (Plaugher 1993).

Osteopathy considers this level is a reference site for thoracic and abdominal viscera (Beal 1989 p. 20). Faridi (1995) associates the T5 vertebral segment with sympathetic neural pathways to the esophagus and stomach and relates this level to gastric ulcer. Stimulation of the spinal reflex center is thought to initiate pyloric and duodenal dilation when applied to the right side.

The posterior neurolymphatic point for popliteus lies between the T5–6 laminae on the right (Walther 1981 p. 331). The posterior neurolymphatic point for serratus anticus lies over the T3–5 laminae (p. 374) and that for pectoralis major – sternal division, lies near the T6–7 laminae, usually on the right (p. 382). In acupuncture terms the site for Du 11 Shendao is below the spinous process of T5 and is indicated for palpitations, amnesia, cough, and stiffness and pain in the back (Qiu 1993 p. 155).

About T6 – the T6–7 SMU

Traditional chiropractic associates this level with the stomach. The Lovett Brother relationship to the T6 body is movement in the opposite direction of the T5 body. Adjusting here is considered to produce a sympathetic effect and this level is implicated in hypertension (Plaugher 1993).

Osteopathy considers this level is a reference site for abdominal viscera and Beal (1989 p. 22) reports a case of duodenal ulcer complicated by cholecystitis with a severe spinal reflex between T6 and T7 on the left, which disappeared following cholecystectomy. Faridi (1995) associates the T6 vertebral segment with sympathetic neural pathways to the pancreas and relates this level to pancreatitis. Stimulation of the spinal reflex center is thought to initiate gall bladder contraction when applied to the right side.

The posterior neurolymphatic point for rhomboid major, rhomboid minor, pectoralis major – clavicular division, and supinator lies between the T6–7 laminae on the left (Walther 1981 pp. 368, 378). The supinator may also involve the posterior neurolymphatic point for the adductors, pronator teres, and flexor pollicis longus, below the inferior angle of the scapula (Walther 1981 pp. 289, 417, 420, 428). In acupuncture terms the site for Du 10 Lingtai is below the spinous process of T6 and is indicated for cough, asthma, carbuncle and boils, stiffness and pain in the back (Qiu 1993 p. 155).

About T7 – the T7–8 SMU

Traditional chiropractic associates this level with the duodenum. The Lovett Brother relationship to the T7 body is movement in the opposite direction of the T4 body. Adjusting here is considered to produce a sympathetic effect (Plaugher 1993). Osteopathy considers this level is a reference site for abdominal viscera (Beal 1989 p. 20). Faridi (1995) associates the T7 vertebral segment with sympathetic neural pathways to the spleen and immune system and relates this level to immune deficiency disorders. Stimulation of the spinal reflex center is thought to initiate slight visceromotor renal dilation when applied bilaterally and to stimulate hepatic function.

The posterior neurolymphatic point for trapezius – middle division, trapezius – lower division, latissimus dorsi, triceps brachii and anconeus lies between the T7–8 laminae on the left (Walther 1981 pp. 364, 376, 410–411). In acupuncture terms the site for Du 9 Zhiyang is below the spinous process of T7 and is indicated for jaundice, distension, and fullness in the chest and hypochondrium, cough and asthmatic breathing, stiffness in the back, and pain in the back (Qiu 1993 p. 155).

About T8 – the T8–9 SMU

Traditional chiropractic associates this level with the spleen. The Lovett Brother relationship to the T8 body is movement in the opposite direction of the T3 body. Adjusting here is considered to produce a sympathetic effect (Plaugher 1993). Osteopathy considers this level is a reference site for abdominal viscera (Beal 1989 p. 20). Faridi (1995) associates the T8 vertebral segment with sympathetic neural pathways to the liver and gall bladder and relates this level to cirrhosis. Stimulation of the spinal reflex center is thought to initiate gall duct dilation.

The T8 lamina is within the location of the posterior neurolymphatic point for the quadriceps muscle (Walther 1981 p. 276). In acupuncture terms the site for Extra 20 Weiguanxiashu (Bashu, Cuishu) is 1.5 cun lateral to the lower border of the T8 spinous process and is indicated for diabetes and dryness of the throat (Qiu 1993 p. 177).

About T9 – the T9–10 SMU

Traditional chiropractic associates this level with the adrenal and suprarenal glands. The Lovett Brother relationship to the T9 body is movement in the opposite direction of the T2 body.

Adjusting here is considered to produce a sympathetic effect (Plaugher 1993). Osteopathy considers this level is a reference site for abdominal viscera (Beal 1989 p. 20). Faridi (1995) associates the T9 vertebral segment with sympathetic neural pathways to the adrenal glands and relates this level to adrenal adenoma. Stimulation of the spinal reflex center is thought to initiate gall duct dilation.

The T9 lamina is within the location of the posterior neurolymphatic point for the quadriceps muscle (Walther 1981 p. 276). In acupuncture terms the site for Du 9 Jinsuo is below the spinous process of T9 and is indicated for epilepsy, stiffness of the neck, and gastric pain (Qiu 1993 p. 155).

ASSESSMENT OF VASCULAR CHANGE

Cardiac function is assessed within the physical examination and must be considered in terms of understanding the nature of the patient's pain. The following comments relate to the vascular changes which may be associated with the SC.

Edema results from a traumatic sprain of the capsular ligaments or supporting ligaments and, given the close relationships among the joints, may affect kinematic change and thus palpate as focal tenderness and bogginess. The nature of the palpatory findings associated with the "sectional subluxation" or "anterior segments" must also be considered in terms of ruling out edema, as the end-feel may be similar. The anterior costochondral capsules should also be assessed, specifically for ribs 3–6. Inflammation (costochondritis) is generally a contraindication to adjustment and is associated with arthritides or posttraumatic injury.

Vasoconstriction may be manifest as areas of colder skin temperature palpated about the mid thoracic spine. Infrared images of the thorax (posterior, lateral, and anterior) are to be interpreted within the context of the underlying viscera which project their own regional heat variations. Paraspinal images appear appropriate for identifying levels of spinal dysfunction and analysis of the infrared images associated with Nervoscope findings suggest that dynamic thermal asymmetry exists and can be identified (Ebrall et al 1994a).

CONCLUSION

In some respects the mid thoracic spine is a neglected region. It is all too easy to knock down the high spots or overlook the information these segments seem desperate to reveal. In essence, this region demonstrates little evidence of muscle change; its real wonder lies in its bidirectional communication, meaning that it seems to act as an indicator of underlying visceral function.

The challenge thus becomes one of distinguishing between primary dysfunction, which may affect other body systems, or secondary dysfunction due to changes elsewhere.

The careful application of palpation, with due consideration of the arrangements of the connective tissues which intimately envelope each SMU, can reveal much to guide the thoughtful practitioner who integrates these data into the total picture of the patient and presentation.

13

The thoracolumbar spine

KEY CONCEPTS

The thoracolumbar junction between T12 and L1 gains strength from form closure due to the typical orientation of the joints towards the sagittal plane where the superior articular processes and the mamillary processes envelope the inferior articular processes.

The costocorporal rib articulations in this region are much simpler in that there are single facets on the vertebral body with no relationship of the rib head to the disk, nor does the rib articulate with the transverse process.

Disk herniation does occur at all levels in this region and, typically, herniations of the T10–11 and T11–12 disk generate upper neuron disorders, lesions of the T12–L1 disk are typically lower neuron disorders, lesions of the L1–2 disk are typically considered as mild disorders of the cauda equina and lesions of the L2–3 disk as nerve root pain or radiculopathy.

There is no clear pattern of nerve root tension tests for this level, with some patients demonstrating a positive straight leg raise (SLR) and others a positive femoral nerve tension test. Clinical findings vary according to the level but include lower-extremity weakness, altered patellar and Achilles tendon reflexes, sensory disturbances of the entire lower extremities, and severe thigh pain and sensory disturbance on the anterior or lateral aspect of the thigh.

The thoracolumbar fascia acts to transfer load from the latissimus dorsi of one side to the gluteus maximus of the other and, apart from this diagonal transmission of forces, there is a chain of communication from the biceps femoris tendon which ascends to the spine through the sacrotuberous ligament and into the aponeurosis of the erector spinae.

Postural changes about the pelvis, shoulders, and head can be indicative of several types of subluxation complex (SC) in the thoracolumbar spine.

Calcification of an abdominal aortic aneurysm has been reported in the young and consideration should be given to assessment for normal pulse profiles of the abdominal aorta in all patients before prescribing and applying manual treatment of the spine and soft tissues.

CLINICAL ANATOMY

The thoracolumbar spine consists of the three lowest thoracic segments, T10, T11, and T12, and the first three lumbar segments, L1, L2, and L3. This spinal region is a transitional zone between the complexity and rigidity of the thoracic spine lying above the diaphragm and the sturdy yet mobile lumbar spine leading to the lower lumbar spine and pelvis. The thoracolumbar spine includes the following major articulations:

- T10–11
- Left and right rib 10 – posterior
- T11–12
- Left and right rib 11 – posterior
- T12–L1
- Left and right rib 12 – posterior
- L1–2
- L2–3
- L3–4.

Cramer & Darby (1995 pp. 164–176, 177–196) provide the appropriate level of anatomy of this region for the student and can be read in conjunction with this chapter. Key landmarks of the anterior and lateral thorax are shown in Figures 13.1 and 13.2 and the following relationships with spinal landmarks should be noted:

- T10 lies around the level of the apex of the heart. It also marks the anteroinferior ends of the oblique fissures of the lungs and the esophageal hiatus of the diaphragm.
- T11 marks the lowest extent of the lungs and the level of the left suprarenal gland.
- T12 marks the aortic hiatus of the diaphragm, the inferior pole of the spleen, and the tail of the pancreas. It is about the level of the right suprarenal gland and therefore marks the superior aspect of the kidneys, with the left being a little higher.
- L1 marks the level along which the proximal duodenum lies.
- L1–2 disk: the spinal cord ends at this level as the conus medullaris. Beyond this level the spinal nerves form the cauda equina within the spinal canal.
- L2 marks the level of the head of the pancreas and the duodenal-jejunal junction.

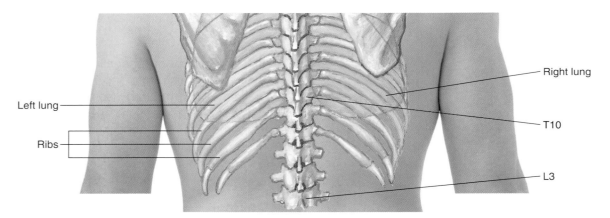

Figure 13.1 Posteroanterior view of the thoracolumbar region, showing key landmarks. From Seidel et al (1999), with permission.

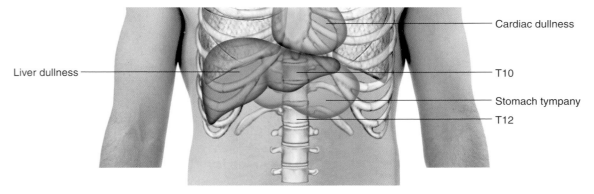

Figure 13.2 Anteroposterior view of the thoracolumbar region, showing key landmarks. From Seidel et al (1999), with permission.

● L3: the inferior margins of the costal cartilage (from rib 10) lie about this level. This is also the inferior border of the normal liver on the right, and the inferior poles of the kidneys. The right kidney is a little lower due to the liver.

The spinal cord ends in the conus medullaris around L1–2 and this means the spinal segments of the cord and their corresponding spinal nerves lie progressively above their corresponding vertebral elements. The spinal cord segments lie about the following levels:

● spinal cord level T10: about the level of the T8–9 disk
● spinal cord level T11: about the level of the T9 body
● spinal cord level T12: about the level of the superior portions of the T10 body
● spinal cord level L1: about the level of the T10–11 disk
● spinal cord level L2: about the inferior level of the T11 vertebra
● spinal cord level L3: about the level of the T11–12 disk.

The left ureter lies about the L2 and L3 transverse processes, and the right ureter about that of L3. The implication is that the application of soft-tissue technique to the fibers of the quadratus lumborum may adversely compress and damage the ureters against bony elements. There are also a number of neurolymphatic points thought to lie about the junctional area and rib 12; these are discussed under Assessment of neural change, below.

The assessment of the anterior aspect of the patient should be undertaken in the supine position with the head comfortably supported. The knees are bent to reduce tension on the anterior abdominal musculature and tissues and better allow abdominal auscultation and palpation. Soft-tissue work to the insertion of the diaphragm about the inferior costal margins and to the belly of the psoas is also undertaken with the patient's knees bent.

The morphology of the vertebral segments varies greatly through this region (Fig. 13.3). The underlying concept is one of change from where the spine acts as a mast to support the thoracic cage, with good movement about the x-axis, to one where the segments act as a column to support the increasing body mass above. This necessitates changes to the vertebral body which becomes larger in both its anteroposterior and lateral dimensions. It also becomes kidney-shaped, concave posteriorly, to increase its weight-bearing ability.

The articular pillars also change dramatically, from the typical thoracic alignment of the superior facet facing posterolateral

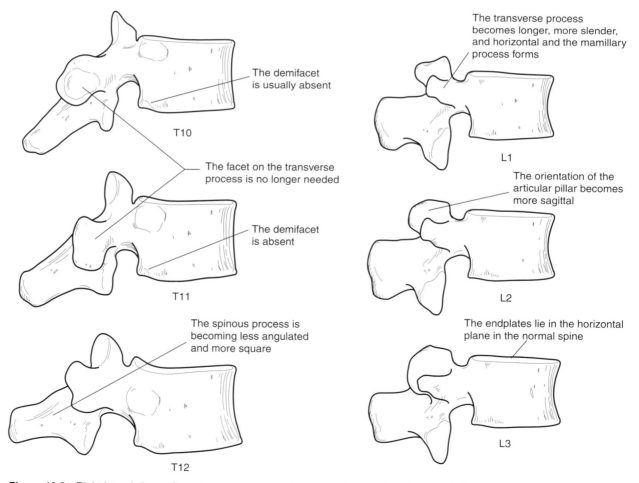

Figure 13.3 Right lateral views of the thoracolumbar vertebrae, showing the changing morphology of the vertebrae through the thoracolumbar region.

and superior at an angle of about 60° to the coronal plane, to a typical lumbar alignment of the superior facet facing postero-medial. The surface of the superior facet becomes concave better to receive the convex surface of the inferior facet. In general, the lumbar zygapophyseal joints lie more in the sagittal plane but this angulation becomes less pronounced distally, such that the L5–S1 facets are typically about 45° or midway between the sagittal and coronal planes (Fig. 2.5B).

These structural changes are accompanied by the functional changes associated with the transition from the kyphotic thoracic spine to the lordotic lumbar spine. The changing nature of the facet arrangement from coronal to sagittal creates a very strong "mortice and tenon" effect at T12–L1, which becomes the key transitional level in this region (Fig. 13.4). This structural method of obtaining strength and stability without constant muscle activity is called "form closure".

The complete thoracic spine is thought to allow for up to 35° rotation while the whole lumbar spine totals only about 5°. This demonstrates the major functional difference which occurs across the thoracolumbar junction. The typical amount of rotation to either side within a thoracic SMU is about 3° while within the lumbar SMU it is about 1°.

The thoracolumbar spine is considered to include L3 given its role as a relay station for, as Kapandji (1974) describes, "the ilio-lumbar fibers of the latissimus as they insert into the transverse processes of L3, and, on the other, the ascending fibres of the spinalis whose lowest point of origin is the spinous process of L3" (Fig. 2.10). L3 is also the apex of the lumbar lordosis and, as such, it should normally sit with both its superior and inferior surfaces in the horizontal plane.

The typical lumbar pedicle attaches closer to the superior aspect of the posterior body, allowing a greater amount of space below it to form the superior aspect of the intervertebral foramen (IVF). This, together with the greater lateral dimensions under the pedicle, creates more of a canal than a foramen, suggesting the lumbar IVF is also better thought of as being an intervertebral canal or IVC (Giles & Singer 1997). The posterolateral borders of the disk form a lower margin of the canal such that the spinal nerve, which angles obliquely inferolaterally through this canal, is typically not affected by protrusion of its co-numbered disk. This is more evident in the lower lumbar spine where, for example, an L4 posterior disk protrusion is more likely to impact on the L5 spinal nerve than that of L4. This topic is covered in more depth in Chapter 14.

T10 differs from the typical thoracic segment in that it is a transition segment for rib change (Fig. 13.3). There is usually no demifacet at the inferior margin for articulation with rib 11. The costocorporal facet is variable and may be the sole attachment for the head of rib 10 which itself is atypical; however, the head of rib 10 is variable in whether or not it articulates with any demifacet on T9 and/or the T9–10 disk. The costotransverse facet is variable and the tubercle of rib 10 may or may not articulate with the transverse process. Similarly, rib 10 is atypical in that there is no crest on its head, leaving a single facet to articulate at the costocorporal junction. It is not known whether the nature of the head of rib 10 varies to include a crest should it also articulate with either the disk or T9.

The costocorporal facet of T11 is located more on the pedicle (Cramer & Darby 1995) and there is no facet on the transverse process (Fig. 13.3). Rib 11 is atypical and does not articulate other than at the head, thus it is described as being a floating rib. The T11 segment transitions towards the morphology of typical lumbar segments, particularly in the nature of the inferior facets and the blunter spinous process.

T12 is most often the transitional segment between the thoracic and lumbar spines, although various characteristic changes can shuffle between segments about this level. A notable change at T12 is the increase of the size of the body. The transverse processes also change significantly, perhaps being better considered as three smaller processes transitioning towards the mamillary and accessory processes found on the lumbar segments (Cramer & Darby 1995). There is also only a single facet on the side of the T12 body to receive the head of rib 12, which is also a floating rib when it is present (Fig. 13.3).

The articulation of T12 with L1 is unique as the mamillary processes of L1 overlap the posterior aspect of the inferior articular processes of T12 (Cramer & Darby 1995). This type of mortice and tenon articulation represents form closure (Fig. 13.4)

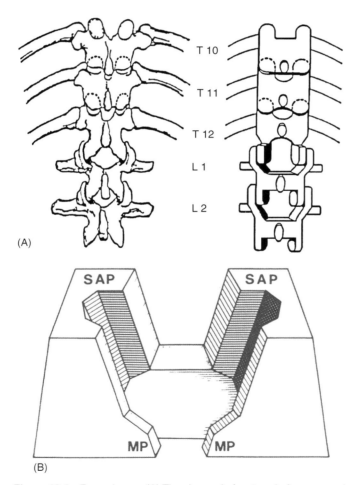

Figure 13.4 Form closure. (A) The change in facet angle from coronal to sagittal through the thoracolumbar junction creates a "mortice and tenon" effect between T12 and L1 which provides strength and stability through form closure. (B) A schematic illustration of a type I mortice emphasizing the medial taper effect of the superior articular processes (SAP) and the posterior enclosure formed by the mamillary processes (MP). (A) From Peterson & Bergmann (2002), with permission; (B) From Singer (1989), with permission.

and was first described in 1877 (Topinard). The biomechanical strength of the joint is achieved by the interlocking nature of the structures, which is the principle of form closure. These principles also apply to the sacrum as it sits within the pelvis.

Singer (1989) has described three characteristic patterns of zygapophyseal joint orientation found at the thoracolumbar junction. They are:

- Type I, where the joints are oriented towards the sagittal plane and the superior articular processes and the mamillary processes envelope the inferior articular processes. This type affords the greatest depth of form closure about the inferior articular pillars and is the most common finding (Fig. 13.4).
- Type II, where the joints are oriented between the sagittal and coronal planes and the inferior articular pillars are enclosed by prominent mamillary processes situated posteriorly.
- Type III, where there are coronally oriented facets where the inferior articular pillars are bounded posteriorly by the mamillary processes.

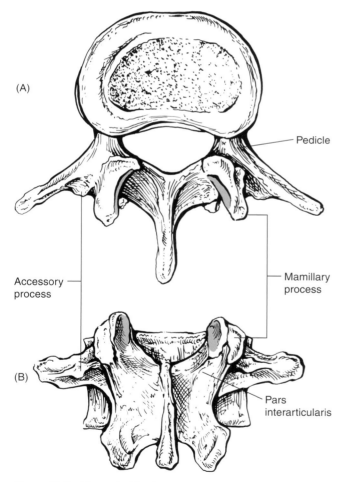

(A)

Pedicle

Accessory process

Mamillary process

(B)

Pars interarticularis

Figure 13.5 The typical lumbar vertebrae. (A) Superior view showing the kidney-shaped body with the transverse dimension (width) being greater than the anteroposterior dimension. (B) Posterior view showing how the superior articular processes face each other to grasp the inferior processes of the segment above. (A, B) From Cramer & Darby (1995), with permission.

The above types apply to bilateral findings and a fourth category is where the facet orientation is not bilaterally symmetrical and there is tropism at that level (Singer 1989).

Movement at T12–L1 is quite restricted due to the form closure and is essentially limited to flexion. Axial rotation is a reasonable movement of the thoracic segments above and becomes limited in the lumbar spine due to the sagittal orientation of the zygapophyseal facets and the resistance of the disk to shear stresses. The transitional change in movement through the thoracolumbar junction varies between being smooth and becoming abrupt (Singer et al 1989). The T12–L1 level consistently demonstrates the least mean range of rotation. There are also large synovial folds which protrude into these zygapophyseal joints, which again emphasize the limitations to rotation (Giles & Singer 1997).

The morphology of the three lumbar segments (L1, L2, and L3) is essentially as described above for a typical lumbar segment. The body has become kidney-shaped in the transverse plane (Fig. 13.5) and is wider from side to side than it is anterior to posterior. The more clinically relevant characteristics of these three segments in this transitional spine are that L3 sits essentially in the horizontal plane while L2 and L1 are each angled anterosuperiorly about the x-axis, reflecting the proximal portion of the lumbar lordosis. The implications are many for reliable assessment and adjustment of the spinal motion units (SMUs) in the thoracolumbar region.

The other significant structural anatomical features of the thoracolumbar region relate to the muscular attachments, which are described in detail under Assessment of muscle change, below. In particular the crura of the diaphragm and the psoas and quadratus lumborum are key functional muscles of clinical importance.

ASSESSMENT OF KINEMATIC CHANGE

Postural assessment

Most forms of scoliosis include the thoracolumbar region; however the practitioner must be careful to differentiate between scoliosis arising due to structural changes within the spine and scoliosis secondary to muscular weakness and subluxation patterns (Schafer 1983). The subject of scoliosis is extensively covered elsewhere and this work will not address this matter other than stating that, as with the mid thoracic spine, a most important component of spinal assessment is observation for scoliosis.

The identification of a rib hump in forward bending (Fig. 12.9) is more an indicator of a scoliosis extending into the mid and upper thoracic spine; however, any such finding will usually be accompanied by scoliosis through the thoracolumbar region. It is thought that a scoliosis suspected in the standing patient which does not produce a rib hump in flexion may be considered as a functional scoliosis. A compensated scoliosis is more difficult to observe than one which is not compensated. In the latter instance, the practitioner may observe lateral head shift, typically with altered levels about the shoulder and a unilateral altered angle of arm carriage. A compensated scoliosis typically has the external occipital protuberance in alignment with the S2 tubercle but may demonstrate altered body contours and unilateral changes in the angle of carriage.

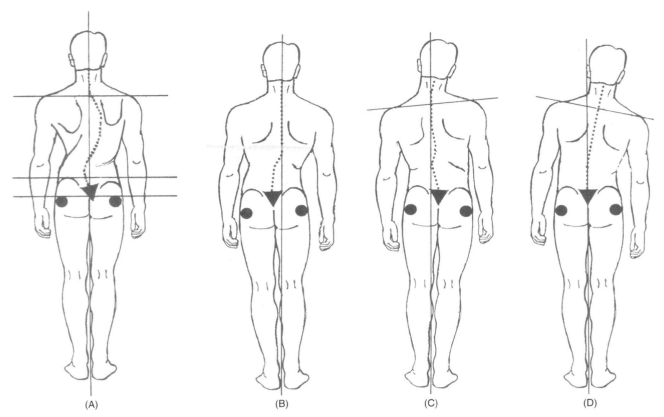

(A) (B) (C) (D)

Figure 13.6 Typical subluxation postures. (A) Probably muscular. Assess rhomboids and splenii on the concave (thoracic) side and the psoas and quadratus lumborum on the side of the low pelvis. (B) Consider a lateral flexion subluxation within the thoracolumbar spine. The shoulders may be high on the side of the lateral pelvic shift in the acute stage. (C) Consider a rotary subluxation within the thoracolumbar spine. The posterior side is usually opposite to the side of the lateral sacral shift. (D) Consider a subluxation complex with rotation and lateral flexion components of some magnitude within the thoracolumbar spine, possibly posterior and superior on the side opposite head shift. From Schafer (1983), with permission of ACA Press and Frank M Painter, DC.

The postural assessment will proceed from global to regional and will attempt to identify postural change secondary to muscle weakness which may present as functional scoliosis. It is not possible to separate the assessment of one particular clinical dimension, such as posture, from another clinical dimension, such as kinematic changes in the form of an SC producing functional scoliosis. The following is to be integrated with the basic principles presented in Chapter 6 and the specific notes which follow in this chapter.

A smooth C-shaped scoliosis through most of the spine suggests that a simple muscular distortion pattern generates where the pelvis is low on the convex side (Fig. 13.6A). The shoulders are level and the head will tilt to the concave side. Weakness may be found in the rhomboids and splenii on the concave side. The psoas and quadratus lumborum will usually be weak, but the side will vary depending on many factors.

This simple C curve usually progresses to a double S-curve scoliosis in which the head and shoulders may be level, having compensated for the upper component of the curve, but the pelvis remains unlevel. It is thought that the majority of these curves are concave to the right in the lumbar spine and to the left in the thoracic spine. The transitional zone lies within the thoracolumbar spine. The shoulders may come to drop on the same

side as the low pelvis and, over time, the overall patterns will become more complex.

When the postural assessment suggests functional scoliosis, the patient should be asked to stand on both toes and attempt equal left–right weight distribution. If a decrease in the distortion pattern is observed, including a shift of the head to become level and in the midline, it is strongly indicative of muscle involvement. Again, the quadratus lumborum and psoas muscles are implicated along with latissimus dorsi and both the lower and upper trapezius fibers.

When scoliotic curves are observed secondary to SC they may be considered as subluxation patterns manifested as scoliosis (Schafer 1983). They largely include the thoracolumbar spine and are considerably more complex to analyze but should be noted on postural observation at rest. They usually remain evident when the patient raises up on to the toes. Typically an isolated SMU with subluxation will lie on the mid sagittal gravity line due to this being the point of least additional stress. Schafer (1983) identifies the key points to include in the postural assessment as follows:

- An unlevel pelvis such as a high ilium, with an ipsilaterally tilted sacrum, is generally associated with a short lumbar curve with a more significant thoracolumbar curve concave on the side of the high ilium and tilted sacrum. The patient will compensate in the upper thoracic and cervicothoracic regions (Fig. 13.6A).

- A lateral shift of the pelvis to one side with a compensation of the head shifting to the opposite side suggests subluxation of a thoracolumbar SMU with segmental superiority on the side of the pelvic shift. This is a lateral flexion fixation with little or no rotation. In time the head compensation may neutralize back to the gravity line but the lateral shift of the pelvis remains (Fig. 13.6B).
- A lateral shift of the pelvis and head to the same side suggests subluxation of a thoracolumbar SMU with body rotation to the opposite side. This is a rotation fixation with little or no lateral flexion. The shoulder on the contralateral side of body rotation is usually high in the acute phase and the patient may also complain of torticollis which will be secondary as compensation to this type of thoracolumbar SC (Fig. 13.6C).
- A tilt of the spine suggests subluxation of a thoracolumbar SMU with both lateral flexion and rotation fixation. In the early phase the tilt is away from the superior side and the spine above may overcompensate with head tilt to the superior side but then stabilize with the head in the gravity line. At this point two relatively shallow spinal curves may be observed (Fig. 13.6D).
- Altered rib alignment suggests lateral flexion and rotation fixation of thoracic segments.

The thoracolumbar region is best palpated with the patient prone to facilitate assessment of posterior to anterior resiliency. Care must be taken with deep palpation and soft-tissue technique to protect the kidneys and ureters. An awareness of tender points, trigger points, and neurolymphatic points is useful to guide palpation. The most common tender areas lie lateral to the T12 and L1 spinous processes and these may refer pain to the ipsilateral iliac crest. Rib 12 may be absent and, if so, usually bilaterally.

Asymmetry may be seen in the musculature about the region and careful assessment should be made of the comparative bulkiness and tone of the paraspinal muscles. Changes in the large, flat muscles (lower trapezius, latissimus dorsi) should also be identified as it is considered that the trapezius is closely associated with the postural distortion patterns given above. Both the upper and lower fibers should be tested for weakness, particularly when the head and neck are involved in the pattern. Specific trigger points in the musculature of the region are discussed in under Assessment of muscle change. Their pain referral patterns include the buttocks, anteriorly to the lower abdomen, and superiorly, paraspinal.

Radiographic analysis

Complete assessment of this region may require analysis of both the thoracic and lumbar anteroposterior (AP) and lateral series, particularly when assessing the nature and extent of any scoliosis or lateral tilt. The region may also be imaged on lateral plain film with functional views such as flexion and extension.

Objective structural change of SMU mechanics

Common anomalies include non-union of the transverse process, particularly at L1. When rib 12 is absent it is typically absent bilaterally. The anomalies discussed in the preceding chapter may also be seen in this region. These include a hemivertebra which is indicative of functional scoliosis, the butterfly vertebra, which is more likely found in the lumbar segments than the thoracic, the Schmorl's node, which is typically painless, except in the acute stage which is indicative of compressive trauma, the giant Schmorl's node, nuclear impression, and endplate irregularities.

Notwithstanding the acceptance that the Schmorl's node is typically asymptomatic or painless in the normal population, a significant correlation has been reported between it and back pain in athletes (Swärd et al 1990). Significant covariation between Schmorl's nodes, reduced disk height, and changes in the configuration of vertebral bodies was also found in that study but it was only the non-apophyseal Schmorl's nodes on their own which maintained a correlation with back pain. It seems these nodes are different to the nodes typically found in the control group of non-athletes in that those in the athletes were more frequently in the anterior part of the endplate and may have involved the anterior part of the ring apophysis (Swärd et al 1990).

The typical fractures of this region involve compression of the vertebral body secondary to either trauma or metabolic change. The transition in sagittal curvature of this region may protect these segments more than those in the mid thoracic spine where compression fractures are more common. The Chance fracture typically occurs in the mid lumbar spine and may be secondary to a motor vehicle accident, particularly when only a lap seat belt has been worn.

The posterior limbus vertebrae may be seen as a fracture secondary to acute or repetitive trauma or as a result of growth disturbance of the ring apophysis (Goldman et al 1990). While L4 is the most common site, it is seen on the plain lateral radiograph as high as T11, appearing as a corticated osseous fragment that may be triangular or circular about the posterior inferior margin of the vertebral body, although it has also been reported as being superior and anterior. The major differential diagnosis of a posterior inferior limbus vertebra is fracture of the posterior cortex of the vertebral body (Goldman et al 1990) and it is important to rule out trauma, especially when the adolescent or young adult patient presents with radiating back pain.

Avulsion may be seen in the tips of the transverse processes of the lumbar segments and needs to be differentiated from benign non-union. A history of trauma would increase the index of suspicion, along with localized pain. Dislocation is secondary to relatively severe trauma and is not commonly seen in manual practice. Hypertrophy of the posterior facets and related elements is seen and may be indicative of altered loads secondary to chronic subluxation and postural changes, while hypertrophy of an individual vertebral body suggests Paget's disease.

Other diagnostic imaging assessment

The axial computed tomography (CT) scan is the axial imaging modality of choice and is commonly used to identify the nature of disk protrusion and disruption to the internal elements of the SMU. Magnetic resonance imaging (MRI) is perhaps more useful to demonstrate soft-tissue relationships about the spine in this region but is not commonly used in manual practice.

Subjective nature of movement

This region must be closely inspected during active global range of motion assessment, particularly in lateral flexion and flexion. During lateral flexion the gutter over the spinous processes formed between the paraspinal muscles is inspected for smooth continuity. The finding of a kink or other deviation in the gutter is an indicator of altered movement at a particular SMU. Active lateral flexion is induced by asking the standing patient to run one hand down the ipsilateral leg, without bending at the hips or knees.

The instruction to the patient for forward flexion while standing should include the request for the patient to curl forward from the head and neck. The Adam's position is reached at about 90° and this is most useful for identifying structural scoliosis about the thoracic spine. Further flexion then involves the thoracolumbar region and levels with restricted flexion may be identified. Rotation is best assessed with the patient seated in order to support the pelvis and maximize rotation to the spine.

Quantification is made of the combined thoracic and lumbar movements such as lateral flexion, and the thoracolumbar region, while naturally included, is not specifically identified or measured.

An assessment of the passive range of motion of the region is made with the patient seated while being guided through the planes of movement, starting with flexion/extension. Palpation of the spine during these movements can quickly identify levels of restriction. The practitioner's indifferent forearm and hand support the patient's folded arms, while the contact hand forms a fist and the dorsal surface of the fingers is used for palpation. The practitioner should be in a fencer stance, posterolateral to the patient, and will combine the movements of raising and lowering the indifferent hand with a posterior–anterior–posterior cycle of the contact hand to induce flexion and extension of the patient's spine over the contact hand. This is the same process explained in detail in Chapter 4.

The initial contact is about the thoracolumbar region and the contact hand is moved up the spine and then down, covering two or three SMUs at a time, with particular attention to identifying any region of restriction and any areas of pain or tenderness. These levels are then assessed for segmental dysfunction.

Palpation is completed with an assessment of the quality of movement in each of the six planes (flexion and extension, left and right lateral flexion, and left and right rotation) within the region. Palpation in the prone patient allows assessment of the quality of end-feel at the elastic barrier and a posterior to anterior springing is used for rotation about the x-axis, or flexion and extension. The assessment then progresses to individual segments.

Assessment of the individual joints

T10–11

The patient may be seated or prone. The T10 spinous process is larger than that of T9; in fact, the T9 spinous is quite small. The seated patient is supported as described above for passive assessment of the region; however the practitioner palpates the individual segment with the fingers and thumb. When the patient is fully flexed at the T10–11 SMU, an assessment is made as to whether there is any restriction in the movement of the spinous process into flexion. The inferior tip of the spinous process is provoked in full flexion to test for tenderness, which may indicate myotendinosis of the interspinous ligament.

As the patient is extended the interspinous space between T10 and T11 is assessed for closure. It is expected that the spinous processes will move apart in flexion and together in extension. An extension fixation is indicated by reduced movement of the T10 spinous process in flexion, while a sensation of closing movement should remain with extension. Some practitioners consider that flexion fixation is not possible at this level; however, there are sufficient structures about the SMU which may alter the nature of movement into flexion. In the case of hypertonicity of the superior muscles attaching to T10 there would be reduced closure of the spinous process in extension and a sensation of increased movement into flexion.

Lateral flexion is induced by the practitioner's arm over the posterior shoulders of the patient producing a force vector which is inferior and medial, directed at the T10–11 SMU. The T10 spinous process is palpated for both the quantity and quality of movement to the contralateral side of lateral flexion, i.e., as the patient is laterally flexed to the right, the spinous is palpated for its movement to the left. In full lateral flexion the end-feel about the spinous is assessed, both in the direction away from the side of lateral flexion and in the direction back to the side of lateral flexion. It is expected that the spinous process will move better into subluxation and be restricted in moving away.

Rotation is induced in the patient by either the practitioner's arm over the shoulders or by using the elbows of the folded arms as a lever. The palpating fingers are initially placed inferior to the spinous process but lightly in touch with it so that the slightest movement may be detected. Given the total range of bilateral rotation is less than 8°, the greater sense of movement will be detected through subtle tissue changes which occur more towards the end of segmental movement than at the beginning.

The spinous is provoked at the end-ranges of rotation to assess for end-feel. The medial border is gently sprung laterally to assess end-feel away from the midline, as if the segment was rotating further, and then with a springing force against the lateral border of the spinous, back towards the midline of the segment. The end-feel away from the midline is normally elastic as the spinous is limited by ligaments while the end-feel towards the midline is normally a little springier and restricted.

Kinematic change may be suspected if there is a perceived asymmetry in the quantity of movement accompanied by tenderness and pain findings. The initial differentiation is between hypomobility, suggestive of restriction or fixation, and hypermobility, suggestive of altered ligamentous integrity.

The nature of any kinematic change is inferred from the quality of the movement during each phase and then from the quality of the end-feel at the end of each phase. It is thought that if a subluxation is visualized as including rotation of the vertebral body to the left (with spinous to the right), then the spinous will move more easily to the right in rotation of the patient to the left and will feel restricted when provoked towards the left. If the subluxation is visualized as including lateral wedging of the body to the right, then it is thought that the movement of the spinous will feel restricted in lateral flexion of the segment to the left, while with lateral flexion to the right, it will not.

Rib 10

The single articulation with the T10 body renders rib 10 more mobile and less likely to subluxate; however, kinematic and positional changes may be associated with muscle hypertonicity about the rib. The anterolateral margins of each rib should also be palpated. The costal cartilage may articulate with that of rib 9 above through a fibrous joint, but this is quite variable.

T11–12

This is assessed in the same manner as described for T10–11, bearing in mind the transition towards lumbar morphology and the dramatic decrease in rotation which will typically be found between T12 and L1 but which may occur at this SMU.

Rib 11

As well as the simpler, single articulation with the T11 body, the distal end of rib 11 does not relate to any costal cartilage and does not articulate with that of rib 10 above. This means rib 11 is a floating rib and is less likely to subluxate.

T12–L1

Typically this is the transitional segment with markedly decreased rotation. It is assessed in a manner similar to that described for T10–11 but with an emphasis on the nature of movement in flexion and extension.

Rib 12

As with rib 11, rib 12 is considered a floating rib. It articulates with T12 and has ligamentous attachments to the L1 transverse processes. Rib 12 is considerably shorter than rib 11 and may be absent.

The diaphragm is convex superiorly and attaches around the entire border about the thoracic outlet. Posteriorly it attaches in broad fashion to the deep surface of the lower six ribs and their costal cartilages (Cramer & Darby 1995). It forms a left and right crux about the spine, each of which attaches to the respective anterolateral surface of L1, L3, and L3 plus the respective disks and the anterior longitudinal ligament. The three splanchnic nerves pierce the posterior aspect of the diaphragm and synapse in one of several prevertebral ganglia. This is discussed under Assessment of neural change, below.

A lateral lumbocostal arch is formed as the lateral arcuate ligament from the thickening of the fascia about the quadratus lumborum. It runs from the L1 transverse process, over the upper portion of the quadratus lumborum, to attach laterally on the lower border of rib 12. The diaphragm, quadratus lumborum, and psoas muscles must be considered with any finding of kinematic change in the spinal segments in this region.

L1–2

The L1 segment is characteristic of the lumbar region and has a total of about 2° or 3° bilateral rotation. In the prone patient it must be remembered that the disk is angled anterosuperiorly to represent the commencement of the lumber lordosis. The SMU is assessed in the typical manner as described above, but with an emphasis on kinematic change in flexion and extension, given the minimal amount of rotation which occurs.

A medial lumbocostal arch is formed as the medial arcuate ligament, also from thickening of the fascia about the quadratus lumborum, and runs from the L1 transverse process to the lateral aspect of the L1 or L2 body by arching medially over the psoas major. The quadratus lumborum and psoas major are key muscles to support the lumbosacral transitional spine and are usually associated with any kinematic change.

L2–3

Bearing in mind the close relationships with the diaphragm, quadratus lumborum, and psoas major, this level is assessed in a manner similar to that described for L1–2. In the prone patient the disk is angled slightly anterosuperiorly.

L3–4

L3 is the midpoint of the lumbar spine. On the lateral radiograph it represents the indicator segment for weight-bearing; a plumb line dropped from its center should pass through the anterior border of S1. As the midpoint, the segment should lie in the horizontal plane when the patient is standing. In the prone patient the L3 disk is typically in the neutral vertical plane. The segment is assessed in a manner similar to that described for L1 and L2.

ASSESSMENT OF CONNECTIVE TISSUE CHANGE

Careful assessment is required of the subcutaneous connective tissue throughout this region as it is also significantly transitional for muscle and its fascia. The erector spinae as a group, and the iliocostalis and longissimus thoracis as distinct muscle bundles, coalesce into broad aponeuroses towards the lower levels of this region.

The intervertebral disk

The morphology of the disk changes to reflect the increasing mechanical demands of this region, from the thinner, smaller thoracic disk to the larger, thicker, more kidney-shaped disks of the lumbar region. Apart from this changing shape, the disks retain the typical characteristics of a nucleus surrounded by the annular fibrosis attached to the longitudinal ligaments. The nerve supply to a normal, healthy disk is to the outer annulus.

The spinal cord transitions to the cauda equina through the thoracolumbar spine and disk lesions manifest themselves variously to include the upper and lower neurons of the spinal cord, cauda equina, and nerve root. Typically, herniations of the T10–11 and T11–12 disk generate upper neuron disorders with lower-extremity weakness and an increased patellar tendon reflex. There may be sensory disturbances of the entire lower extremities and bowel and bladder dysfunction may be reported (Tokuhashi et al 2001).

Lesions of the T12–L1 disk are typically considered lower neuron disorders, presenting with muscle weakness and atrophy below the leg. These include uni- or bilateral foot drop, sensory disturbance in the sole of the foot and around the anus, and absent patellar and Achilles tendon reflexes. Bowel and bladder dysfunction may also be reported (Tokuhashi et al 2001). Disk herniation in this region has previously been considered rare; however, contemporary diagnostic imaging methods suggest they are more prevalent than originally thought (Vernon & Cala 1992).

Lesions of the L1–2 disk are typically considered as mild disorders of the cauda equina; and of the L2–3 disk, as nerve root pain or radiculopathy. Herniation of the L1–2 disk may be associated with severe thigh pain and sensory disturbance on the anterior or lateral aspect of the thigh. Typically there are no clear signs of lower-extremity weakness, muscle atrophy, deep tendon reflex change, or bowel and bladder dysfunction. On the other hand, herniation of the L2–3 disk produces severe thigh pain and sensory disturbance of the anterior or lateral aspect of the thigh, and muscle weakness which may be found in the quadriceps or tibialis anterior. Most of these patients will also demonstrate a decreased or absent patellar tendon reflex. Interestingly, there is no clear pattern of nerve root tension tests for this level, with some patients demonstrating a positive SLR and others a positive femoral nerve tension test (Tokuhashi et al 2001).

These hard neurologic findings are less likely to be seen in the adolescent patient (Kazemi 1999). Disk herniation in this demographic is to be differentiated from apophyseal ring fracture, disk infection, and tumors causing nerve root pain. Trauma, including sports injuries, along with lifting injuries and chronic repetitive strain have been reported as having a causative association (Kazemi 1999).

The porcine model has been used to demonstrate a pathway between the posterolateral annulus fibrosis of the L3–4 disk and the paraspinal musculature (Indahl et al 1997). Stimulation of the nerves in the posterolateral annulus of that disk elicited reactions in the lumbar multifidus and longissimus, bilateral to the L4 spinous process. The action of this pathway was reduced by the introduction of physiologic saline into the zygapophyseal joint, which suggests the joint may have a regulating function in controlling the intricate neuromuscular balance in the lumbar SMU (Indahl et al 1997). This pathway needs to be considered together with that from the supraspinous ligament to the multifidi described below.

Ligaments of the SMU

The anterior longitudinal ligament attaches to the anterior aspect of each body in this region and intermingles with the anterior fibers of the annulus of each disk. The posterior longitudinal ligament continues through this region, largely as previously described.

The ligamentum flavum is paired left and right and each runs between the laminae at each level. As noted by Giles & Singer (1997), it is associated with the intra-articular synovial folds of the zygapophyseal joints. They have a particular function to limit forward flexion and may hypertrophy to compromise the contents of the spinal canal. Ossification of the ligamenta flava is seen in Japanese patients, sometimes in Caucasians, and more rarely in Black people (Rivierez & Vally 2001). When the ligament hypertrophies secondary to ossification in this spinal region, it may cause canal stenosis. A hematoma in the ligamentum flavum of the low thoracic spine has also been reported (Maezawa et al 2001).

The interspinous ligaments become more significant in this region. Herzog (2000 p. 37) observes that they demonstrate a large angle of obliquity as they connect adjacent posterior spinous processes. The obliquity is from the inferior surface of the posterior aspect of the spinous above, to the more anterior aspect of the superior margins of the spinous below, although this orientation is thought to be variable (Behrsin & Briggs 1988). Herzog disagrees that this ligament acts to limit flexion; rather he agrees with Heylings' (1978) suggestion that it acts more like a collateral ligament of the knee. It is thought that it controls the vertebral rotation so it follows an arc throughout the flexion range, which in turn assists the facet joints to remain in contact, gliding with rotation. Its oblique angle also protects against posterior shearing of the superior vertebra (Herzog 2000 p. 37).

The interspinous ligament has been found with fat-suppressed, T2-weighted MRI to be sprained or frankly ruptured at the lumbosacral and higher levels in many patients with low-back pain in one sample (Jinkins 2002). The mechanism is least likely to include flexion, as Gudavalli & Triano (1999) found it to be the ligament least strained during the application of a flexion load to the lumbar SMU, which is evidence against any important role in limiting flexion. A fat-suppressed T2-weighted sagittal sequence of MRIs is recommended for accurate evaluation of posterior ligament complex injury in this region (Lee et al 2000).

The supraspinous ligament is a distinctly different structure to the interspinous ligament, although some class these as the same structure. It is aligned more or less to the compressive axis of the spine and connects the tips of the spinous processes, providing resistance against excessive forward flexion (Herzog 2000 p. 37). Cramer & Darby (1995 p. 208) consider it to be more correctly termed a *lumbar supraspinous restraint* as opposed to *ligament*, to reflect its true nature as a fibrous band of tissue. The "ligament" in this region is a system of dense connective tissue drawn largely of the posterior layer of the thoracolumbar fascia and the spinal attachments of the longissimus thoracis and multifidi (Johnson & Zhang 2002).

Further, there is an intimate functional relationship between the ligament or restraint and the multifidi. Activation of the mechanoreceptors in the supraspinous ligament by deformation or stress has been shown to recruit multifidus muscle forces to stiffen one to three lumbar segments and prevent instability (Solomonow et al 1998). Prolonged flexion of the lumbar spine results in tension–relaxation and laxity of its viscoelastic structures accompanied by altered electromyogram activity in the multifidus and other posterior muscles (Williams et al 2000). Spasms of the multifidi were observed within 2–3 min after the spine was loaded in some cases, and up to 20 min after the load was removed. The clinical result is a loss of reflexive muscular activity, and spasms of the multifidus which may cause pain due to ligamentous (or restraint) overloading which may not fully recover even after 7 h of rest (Jackson et al 2001).

Transforaminal ligaments

A fine network of ligaments was first reported in 1969 (Golub & Silverman) as lying across the exit of the IVC (Fig. 13.7). They are considered to be ligaments of the SMU but are discussed separately here to emphasize their unique relationship to the neurovascular structures which exit through the IVC. They are discussed in some detail in Giles & Singer (1997) and may well provide the mechanism for any compressive effect on the exiting neurovascular structures. It is extremely unlikely that, under normal conditions, the bony elements about the IVC would come to such a position that neurovascular structures would be compromised. However, when it is appreciated that the canal is criss-crossed by a lattice of these fine ligaments and that, as ligamentous tissue, they react to microtrauma with sprain, strain, and edema, a possible mechanism for nerve root compromise can be seen.

Transforaminal ligaments have also been demonstrated in fetal specimens. Their appearance in all specimens shows a smooth, glistening surface covered by loose areolar tissue which separates them from the overlying vessels and muscle. Generally the ligaments are stronger in the upper lumbar region than in the lower levels (Amonoo-Kuofi et al 1988).

The ligaments have been evaluated by MRI and it is now known that they can be subgrouped as thick, medium, and thin, and that they cross the foramen in both vertical and horizontal directions (Cramer at al 2002). The data reported by Cramer et al are represented in Figure 13.7. When identified by a trained radiologist there is an 87% chance one is actually present, and when not seen by a trained radiologist there remains a 51% chance that one is present (Cramer et al 2002).

When present, the ligaments help define a compartment at the foraminal exit zone of the IVC and act to reduce the total area of the opening (Bakkum & Mestan 1994). Horizontally oriented ligaments can reduce the superior to inferior dimension of the foramen by as much as 31.5%. The vertically oriented ligaments have not yet been found to reduce the anterior to posterior dimension (Bakkum & Mestan 1994). The clinical relevance of their existence is that there is less space in the exit zone of the IVC for the spinal nerve, particularly the ventral ramus, and this could account for clinical symptoms after trauma or degenerative changes (Bakkum & Mestan 1994).

The zygapophyseal joints

The zygapophyseal joint capsules undergo a transition through this region to become quite a feature of the lumbar spine. The outer layer of the capsule consists of dense regular connective tissue composed of parallel bundles of collagenous fibers. The fibers run in different directions in the superior and inferior parts of the capsules, while those in the middle layer include large quantities of elastic fibers in the root area of the capsule (Zhang et al 2002). This allows the capsule to withstand loads from various directions.

A common characteristic of the thoracolumbar junction zygapophyseal joints is the presence of small fibrous synovial folds which extend from fat pads adjacent to the ligamentum flavum and fibrous joint capsule. These are located in the superomedial joint recesses. In contrast, the inferomedial aspect of the zygapophyseal joints consistently demonstrates fibroadipose synovial folds, of various lengths, originating from the inferior joint recess between the articular surfaces (Singer et al 1990).

These small intra-articular folds are known as zygapophyseal menisci and they become more clinically significant as they develop into larger structures in the lumbar region, often becoming involved in acute entrapment with flexion and rotation of the patient, typically while lifting. They are pain generators (Giles & Singer 1997) but the extent of their contribution to low-back pain is not yet understood. It is thought they are involved with acute clinical presentations such as the "locked back", which can be classified as an acute facet syndrome.

Ligaments about the ribs

The costovertebral capsules are relevant for ribs 10, 11, and 12 but are typically less complex than those of the ribs above due to the absence of articulation to the transverse process. Ribs 11 and 12 clearly have a single facet on the head of the rib and no neck or tubercle. They articulate directly to the vertebral body and do not spread across the disk, hence the articulation and its ligamentous support are much simpler.

The thoracolumbar fascia

The importance of the thoracolumbar fascia for the mechanics of normal spinal function is now recognized, as is its role in back pain (Vleeming et al 1997b, Chaitow & DeLany 2002). The thoracolumbar fascia acts to transfer load from the latissimus dorsi of one side to the gluteus maximus of the other (Fig. 2.10). The superficial lamina of the fascia is tensed by the contractions of muscles such as the latissimus dorsi, gluteus maximus, and erector spinae, while the deep lamina is tensed by contraction of the biceps femoris (Vleeming et al 1995). These relationships are shown in Figure 13.8.

Apart from the diagonal transmission of forces through the thoracolumbar fascia, it is important to note the chain of communication which arises from the biceps femoris tendon. It

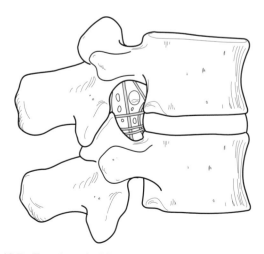

Figure 13.7 Transforaminal ligaments, showing the lattice of transforaminal ligaments in the lumbar spine. Source data from Cramer et al (2002).

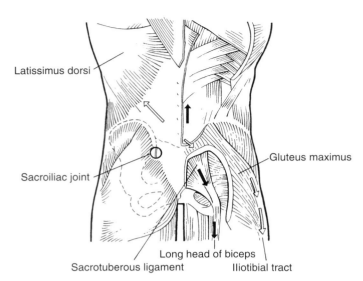

Latissimus dorsi

Sacroiliac joint

Gluteus maximus

Long head of biceps

Sacrotuberous ligament   Iliotibial tract

Figure 13.8 Relationships about the thoracolumbar fascia. The crossover relationship through the thoracolumbar fascia is shown here between the left latissimus dorsi and the right gluteus maximus. The right side of the figure demonstrates the deeper muscle–tendon–fascia sling which is unilateral. There is a continuum between the biceps femoris tendon, the sacrotuberous ligament, and the aponeurosis of the erector spinae. From Vleeming et al (1997a), with permission.

ascends to the spine through the sacrotuberous ligament and into the aponeurosis of the erector spinae. It is also known that the thoracolumbar fascia makes a major contribution to the supraspinous ligament in the lower thoracic spine and that the supraspinous ligaments in the upper thoracic spine form into the deep fascia of the trapezius, rhomboid major, and splenius cervicis (Johnson & Zhang 2002). It is also known that the superficial lamina of the thoracolumbar fascia is continuous with the rhomboids while the deep lamina is continuous with the tendons of splenius cervicis and capitis (Barker & Briggs 1999).

Chapter 9 discussed the formation and importance of the ligamentum nuchae and its connections to the spinal dura at the suboccipital space, and included the trapezius, rhomboid minor, and splenius capitis as three of the four muscles contributing to that ligament. The technique of plastination is now revealing the anatomy of the midline connective tissue and it is becoming apparent that there is a physical continuum between the ligaments about the sacrum and those about the occiput and dura. Both the Logan Basic and Sacro-occipital techniques have empirically addressed these relationships for many years.

The thoracolumbar fascia demonstrates viscoelastic properties, which means there is an increase in stiffness when successively stretched so that strains produced by successive and identical loads decrease, and if a sufficient resting period is allowed between loadings, stiffening is reversed and strains tend to recover initial values (Yahia et al 1993). A third characteristic is that there is ligament contraction in samples which are stretched and isometrically held, suggesting that muscle fibers capable of contracting could be present in the lumbodorsal fascia ligaments (Yahia et al 1993).

Free nerve endings have been identified in the thoracolumbar fascia (Yahia et al 1992), thus it may or may not be a pain generator

in its own right. Yahia et al (1992) also identified two types of encapsulated mechanoreceptors (Ruffini's and Vater–Pacini corpuscles) in their samples and consider that the fascia may play a neurosensory role in the lumbar spinal mechanism. The medial branch of the superior cluneal nerve (cutaneous nerve of the buttock, arising from the lateral branches of dorsal rami of L1–3) is confined within a tunnel formed by the fascia over the superior rim of the iliac crest (Lu et al 1998). Entrapment at this site has been reported as producing low-back pain (Berthelot et al 1996).

An assessment of the status of the thoracolumbar fascia must be a component of the assessment of any of the many muscles which arise from and attach to and about it.

ASSESSMENT OF MUSCLE CHANGE

A number of muscles relevant to the thoracolumbar spine ascend through the mid thoracic and cervicothoracic regions and have been previously discussed. These include the lower trapezius (Fig. 12.15) and the generic back extensors (Ch. 12). The extensors are discussed in more detail below. The most significant spinal muscles are the latissimus dorsi, quadratus lumborum, and psoas major; they are also discussed below. The remaining muscles described here are clinically relevant to the region.

Diaphragm

The diaphragm has been briefly discussed in the earlier parts of this chapter. It is a dome-shaped fibromuscular sheet which attaches around its periphery to the bony structures which form the thoracic outlet. These include the xiphoid process, the internal surfaces of the cartilages and adjacent parts of the lower six ribs, and importantly, to the vertebral column. These tendinous crura blend with the anterior longitudinal ligament and the anterolateral surfaces of the bodies and disks of L1 and L2, with the right crus extending to include L3. There is a lateral arcuate ligament over the quadratus lumborum to join the anterior surface of the L1 transverse process to the lower margin of rib 12 near its midpoint. A medial arcuate ligament arches over the psoas major to attach to the anterior surface of the L1 transverse process and the lateral margins of the L2, and sometimes the L1, body. The phrenic nerve supplies the motor fibers and the lower six or seven intercostal nerves are sensory to the perimeter.

The diaphragm is assessed in cases of respiratory complaint and palpated for nodular myotendinoses around the posteroinferior aspect of the anterior costal margins and the lower ribs at the posterior. The technique of palpation for the anterior aspect is with the patient supine with the knees flexed. A broad contact is taken bilaterally along the long axis of the thumbs and the patient is asked to breathe slowly and deeply. The thumbs lightly ride up in inspiration. During expiration the thumbs roll under the costal margin and apply gentle pressure around the nodular areas.

The other muscles of respiration, the external intercostales, subcostales, and levatores costarum, are included in the observation and palpation of the intercostal space. The more relevant muscle groups around the lower thoracic cage are the rectus abdominis, transversus abdominis, and the internal and external obliques.

The abdominals

The rectus abdominis arises from the symphysis pubis and crest of pubis and attaches to the anterior surface of the xiphoid process and surface of the costal cartilages of ribs 5, 6, and 7. It is innervated by the anterior primary rami of the intercostal nerves from T7 through T12 and acts to support the abdominal viscera, compress the abdomen, maintain the pelvic tilt and limit anterior tilt, and as a muscle of respiration in forced expiration. It is a type 2 phasic muscle with a tendency to inhibition and weakening (Chaitow & DeLany 2002 p. 284) and acts to flex the spinal column.

Chaitow & DeLany (2002) present detailed material on the assessment and treatment of the abdominals (pp. 276–291). As far as assessment of the spine is concerned, the practitioner needs to rule out these muscles firstly, as a source of referred pain from trigger points (Fig. 13.9B, C) and secondly, as a contributor to mechanical dysfunction due to weakness. The first is addressed through palpation of the muscles for trigger points, and the second is assessed through testing the strength and function of the muscles.

The supine patient is asked to bring the trunk up to a seated position, keeping the legs flat, and folding the arms (Fig. 13.9A). The stabilization is across the knees and the test force is in the midline, posteriorly, to extend the patient. It is thought the oblique abdominal muscles may be tested as a variant of this test by varying the contact hand and force direction.

For example, the patient may lean back about 45° from the supine seated position and rotate one shoulder forward. Stabilization remains across the legs and the test force is directed against the shoulder to derotate and extend the patient. The muscles tested are the internal oblique on the side of anterior shoulder and the external oblique on the contralateral side (Fig. 13.9A).

The oblique muscles are thought to form an anterior system of force transmission between the body and the lower limbs (Lee 2000 p. 60), in a manner similar to that of the posterior system between latissimus dorsi and gluteus maximus. It is thought the anterior layers of the oblique abdominal muscles link with the contralateral adductor muscles of the thigh through the intervening anterior abdominal fascia and across the symphysis pubis (Lee 2000). The clinical implication is the need to assess muscles of the thigh, including the adductors, when assessing the abdominal muscles.

Serratus posterior inferior

This small muscle originates in the lumbar fascia and from the spinous processes of T11 through L2 and inserts into the inferior border of the lower ribs, from rib 9, a little distal to the angle. It is innervated by the anterior primary rami of T9 through T12 and acts to counter the pull of the diaphragm by drawing the lower ribs downwards and backwards. It is a type 2 phasic muscle which weakens when stressed (Chaitow & DeLany 2002).

Its role as a muscle of respiration is debatable. As with the serratus posterior superior, Vilensky et al (2001) propose this muscle may act as a spinal proprioceptor. They argue that there is no electromyogram evidence to support any role in respiration and consider that, even though its muscle spindle density is a low 2.97/g, which renders it unlikely to be primarily proprioceptive, its true role is unclear (Vilensky et al 2001).

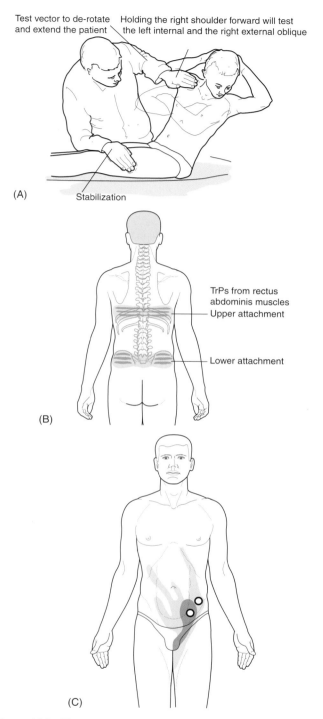

Figure 13.9 The abdominals. (A) Testing positions for the oblique abdominal muscles. The patient's arms may be placed behind the head, in which case the muscles have 100% strength if the patient can hold the position with no test force. If not, patients fold their arms and then, if they can hold with no test force, the muscles are rated as 80% of normal. Resistance testing and "lock-in" testing is then performed, with the arms folded. (B) Dull bilateral back pain in a band either in the mid-back or low back may be referred from trigger points (TrP) in the attachments of rectus abdominis. (C) Trigger points in the lower abdominal wall may refer to the groin and scrotum and need to be differentiated from sacroiliac dysfunction.

However, it is an important muscle to consider with respiratory complaints and its pain is a backache which mimics that of renal dysfunction. When renal disease has been excluded, the trigger point is sought in the prone patient, about the center of the muscle, about the midpoint of rib 11. Its pain is a dull, local pain about the muscle. There is no specific muscle test but dysfunction may be implicated in respiratory disorders and especially when the patient has been coughing excessively.

The back extensors

While the back extensors are quite complex anatomically, clinically they are understood as forming three groups (Fig. 13.10):

- The spinalis, which lie most medial, being long slips which run over several segments, attaching to the lateral borders of the spinous processes. The spinalis blend with the medial longissimus fibers.

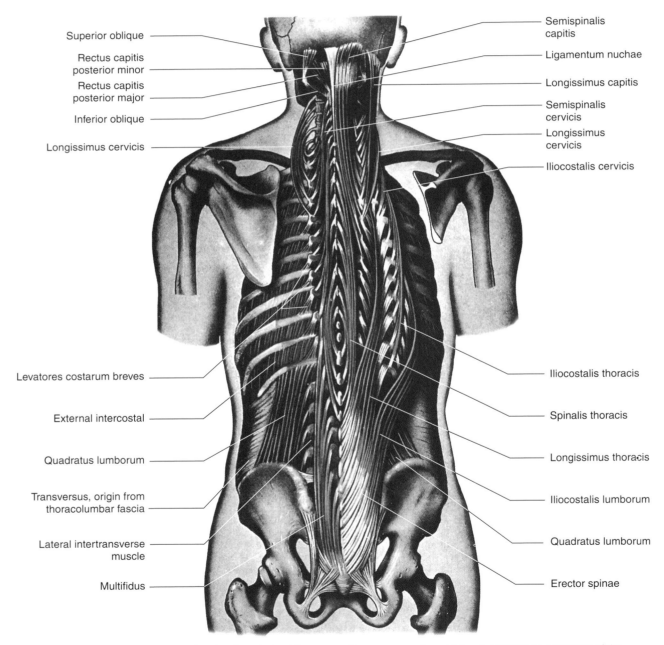

Superior oblique

Rectus capitis posterior minor

Rectus capitis posterior major

Inferior oblique

Longissimus cervicis

Levatores costarum breves

External intercostal

Quadratus lumborum

Transversus, origin from thoracolumbar fascia

Lateral intertransverse muscle

Multifidus

Semispinalis capitis

Ligamentum nuchae

Longissimus capitis

Semispinalis cervicis

Longissimus cervicis

Iliocostalis cervicis

Iliocostalis thoracis

Spinalis thoracis

Longissimus thoracis

Iliocostalis lumborum

Quadratus lumborum

Erector spinae

Figure 13.10 The back extensors, showing the relationships among the many muscles which act primarily as extensors of the back. Note the three bundles which arise out of the thoracolumbar fascia: the spinalis lie most medially, with the longissimus sweeping out almost to the angle of the rib, and the iliocostalis lies most laterally. From Williams & Warwick (1980), with permission.

- The longissimus, which lie medially, over the transverse processes and rib articulations and laterally to about the angle of the rib. Inferiorly the fibers form a broad, thick tendon attaching with the lumbocostal aponeurosis, and superiorly they may be palpated as individual bundles of fibers attaching to the ribs between the tubercle and the angle.
- The iliocostalis, which lie more laterally and attach as individual bundles of muscle fibers about the lower border of the rib, around the angle. Inferiorly the iliocostalis blends into a broad think tendon with the longissimus, attaching to the sacrum, the lumbar spinous processes, and the medial, inner surface of the iliac crest.

The muscles are innervated by the posterior primary rami of the spinal nerves and variously act to extend, laterally flex and rotate the spinal column, and to move the pelvis laterally.

The posterior trunk muscles are grouped together for testing in the prone patient. The general function of all back extensors is tested by the patient extending with the testing force being applied in a posterior to anterior direction in the midline, with stabilization over the gluteals and pelvis. Each side may be tested by the patient extending one shoulder further in posterior rotation, with the testing force applied to that shoulder with stabilization on the contralateral ilium.

An indication of the bilateral tone of the muscles is gained from the "sit and reach" test, where the patient is seated on the bench or floor with both legs extended. Patients are instructed to reach out their arms and fingers and lean as far forward as possible, bringing their fingers to their toes. This is only a general test as reach can be limited by tight hamstrings and calf muscles, as well as by the back extensors. Some differentiation may be gained by asking patients to indicate where they feel restriction or tightness.

Weakness of one side may be indicated in standing patients when they laterally flex to run one hand down the ipsilateral leg. They will be able to reach further towards the floor on the side contralateral to the weak fibers. The distance from the fingertips to the floor may be measured to quantify the assessment and monitor outcomes of intervention.

The trigger points typically refer pain in a vertical band in the ipsilateral side of the spine. The trigger points in the longissimus and iliocostalis about the thoracolumbar spine may refer pain to the iliac crest or as far down as the buttock.

Latissimus dorsi

This muscle arises as a broad aponeurosis from the spinous processes of T7 downwards and across to the posterior crest of the ilium (Fig. 13.11A). It may also attach to the lower three or four ribs and the tip of the scapula. It twists on itself to insert into the floor of the intertubercular groove of the humerus and acts to extend, adduct, and medially rotate the humerus. This action moves the upper limb or raises the entire trunk in brachiation. Its possible contribution to extension of the lumbar spine is trivial, as is its capacity to brace the sacroiliac joint (Bogduk et al 1998).

It is innervated by the thoracodorsal nerve from the brachial plexus (C6, C7, C8) and has the same neurolymphatic point as the mid and lower trapezius fibers. Weakness may allow a high shoulder with a level head, but this pattern may be confused by the upper trapezius.

The muscle is tested with the patient prone or standing (Fig. 13.11B). The ipsilateral arm is held in medial rotation and adduction with slight extension. Stabilization in the standing patient is over the ipsilateral shoulder tip. The test force draws the arm into abduction with some extension to flex the shoulder.

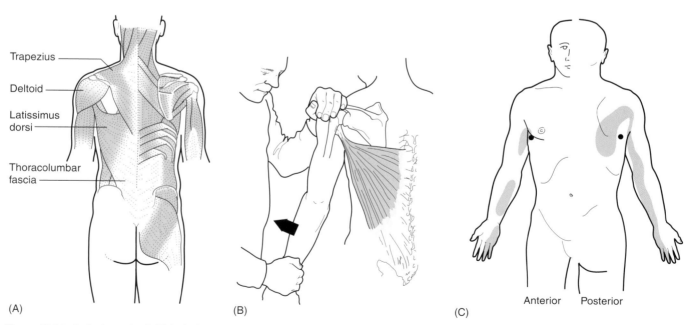

Trapezius

Deltoid

Latissimus dorsi

Thoracolumbar fascia

(A)　　　　　　　　　(B)　　　　　　　　　(C)　　　Anterior　　Posterior

Figure 13.11 Latissimus dorsi. (A) Latissimus dorsi arises from the thoracolumbar fascia and ascends to insert into the floor of the intertubercular groove of the humerus. (B) The muscle is tested in the standing or prone patient who holds the arm in medial rotation with slight extension and adduction. The test force is into abduction and slight flexion. (C) The trigger points are found in the free border and refer pain around the inferior angle of the scapula and into the medial arm, reaching to the fingers. (A) From Chaitow & DeLany (2002), with permission.

The key trigger point is found in the mid portion of the most craniad group of fibers in the region of the posterior axillary fold (Fig. 13.11C). It refers a constant ache to the inferior angle of the scapular and the surrounding mid thoracic region. Pain may also refer about the shoulder and down the medial aspect of the arm, to the ring and little fingers.

Bogduk et al (1998) comment that the latissimus dorsi is of little mechanical importance in the lumbosacral region. They make this observation after conducting a biomechanical analysis of the muscle. Their observation may be valid when considering the muscle on its own; however, contemporary thinking acknowledges its role in a myofascial chain, as discussed above under the Thoracolumbar fascia (Fig. 13.8), and its clinical importance with low-back presentations should not be underestimated, especially when postural assessment implicates shoulder distortions. Further, there is reason to believe that the sacroiliac joint plays a regulatory role involving reflex muscle activation of spinal and gluteal muscles (Indahl et al 1999).

Quadratus lumborum

The quadratus lumborum and psoas major are commonly associated with dysfunction of the thoracolumbar spine and subsequent low-back pain (Fig. 13.6A). Clinically, their role may be understood by considering the quadratus lumborum as lying posterior to the axis of the spine, and the psoas as anterior. The wise practitioner will always assess the four muscles and look for any paired, contralateral involvement, such as left quadratus lumborum and right psoas. Psoas contraction contralaterally rotates the lumbar vertebrae and ipsilaterally laterally flexes the lumbar spine, thus shortening the ipsilateral quadratus lumborum but tightening that on the contralateral side.

The quadratus lumborum is a broad, flat muscle attaching about the iliolumbar ligament and the iliac crest, and arising to the transverse processes of L1 to L4, and the inferior border of the last rib (Fig. 13.12A). It is innervated by the anterior primary divisions of T12 through L3, and based on an assessment of the branching patterns of the intercostal nerves, it is considered to be homologous to the external intercostal muscles (Sakamoto et al 1996).

The structure of the muscle is clinically relevant, especially for the application of soft-tissue technique (Fig. 13.12A). It can be considered as having three layers of bands – the superficial iliolumbar fibers, which run superomedially and act as guy ropes to the thoracolumbar spine; the deep lumbocostal fibers, which run superolaterally and include the last rib and also act as guy ropes, especially in lateral flexion; and the more vertical iliocostal fibers, which form the lateral border, and which interdigitate extensively with the iliolumbar ligament. These fibers lie posterior to the spine and therefore contribute to maintaining the lordosis and extension.

The quadratus lumborum acts as a major stabilizer of the lumbar spine. It is active during flexion-dominant tasks, extensor-dominant tasks, and lateral bending tasks (Herzog 2000 p. 36). The highest activity is observed in ipsilateral trunk flexion in a side-lying position (Andersson et al 1996). The deep lateral erector spinae are also active in this position and this diminishes the clinical usefulness of any test for quadratus lumborum strength or function. The quadratus lumborum is also thought to assist the diaphragm in respiration by depressing the last rib.

It is a difficult muscle to test reliably and the more valuable clinical information is gained from palpation and from careful observation for elevation of the last rib, both during postural assessment and from the AP radiograph. It is thought the lumbar spine may deviate away from a weak muscle (Walther 1981).

The trigger points refer pain locally and to the ipsilateral iliac crest, hip, and buttock (Fig. 13.12B). Typically the trigger points may be found superficially in the lateral fibers about the inferior and superior margins respectively, and deeper about the medial border, at the interspace between the L4 and L5 transverse process, and about the L3 transverse process.

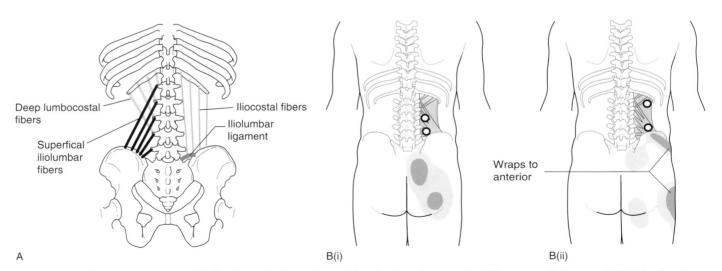

Deep lumbocostal fibers

Iliocostal fibers

Iliolumbar ligament

Superfical iliolumbar fibers

Wraps to anterior

A   B(i)   B(ii)

Figure 13.12 Quadratus lumborum. (A) Quadratus lumborum is considered to have three bands of fibers, namely the superficial iliolumbar fibers, the deep lumbocostal fibers, and the more vertical iliocostal fibers. (B) Four trigger points may be identified. Two are superficial and are found in the lateral fibers about the inferior and superior margins respectively (i). Two are deep and lie medially, one about the interspace between the L4 and L5 transverse process, and the other about the L3 transverse process (ii). Their pain referral is local and to the ipsilateral iliac crest, hip, and buttock.

Psoas major

The psoas major arises from the anterior surface of the transverse processes, the lateral border of the bodies, and the corresponding disks, of T12 through L5, and blends with the iliacus fibers to insert into the lesser trochanter of the femur (Fig. 13.13A). The typical AP lumbar film will show the psoas major and renal outlines.

Innervated by the ventral rami of L2 and L3, it acts as a powerful flexor of the thigh, contributing a little to external (lateral) rotation. Conventional thinking is that, when the thigh is fixed, the psoas acts unilaterally to flex the spine laterally; it may act to extend the spine in the standing patient; it is a powerful flexor of the trunk, especially during sit-ups; and it stabilizes the spine in the seated patient. Recent experiments show that the psoas major probably functions as a stabilizer of the lordotic lumbar spine in an upright stance by adapting the state of contraction of each of its fascicles to the momentary degree of lordosis imposed by factors outside the lumbar spine, such as general posture, general muscle activity, and weight-bearing (Penning

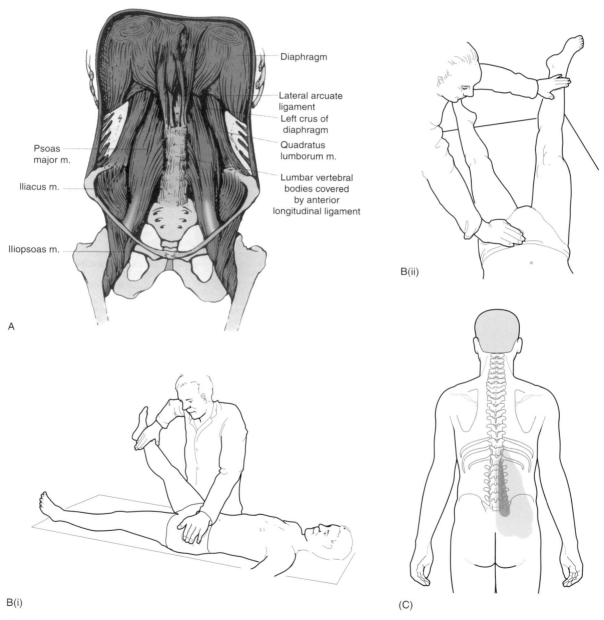

Figure 13.13 Psoas major. (A) The intimate relationship of the psoas to the lumbar spine is shown. The psoas major blends with the iliacus which arises from the anterior surface of the ilium, and together they insert into the lesser trochanter. Given this, the psoas is also termed the iliopsoas muscle. (B) Psoas is tested with the patient supine and the leg raised 45° into flexion and also into abduction. The test vector is into extension and further abduction. (C) The pain referral pattern is paraspinal and may reach into the buttock and about the sacrum. (A) From Cramer & Darby (1995), with permission; (C) from Chaitow & DeLany (2002), with permission.

2000). Its actions are dependent on the degree of hip flexion: it is an erector of the lumbar spine and a stabilizer of the femoral head in the acetabulum at 0–15°; the stabilizing function lessens while the erector function is maintained between 15° and 45°; and it becomes an effective flexor of the lower extremity from 45° to 60° (Yoshio et al 2002).

It is a type I postural muscle prone to shortening under stress (Chaitow & DeLany 2002 p. 231). Dysfunction in the psoas can have a relay effect by distorting posture, which then overloads other muscles in the back and neck (Fig. 13.6A). In particular, when suspecting psoas involvement, the practitioner should also assess the hamstrings, gluteals, the longissimus and iliocostalis, and the posterior cervical muscles.

Bilateral weakness is suspected in patients with a reduced lumbar lordosis. Unilateral weakness allows deviation of the lumbar spine away from the side of weakness, with a low pelvis on that side. The muscle is tested in the supine patient, who is asked to raise the leg 45° off the table and hold it away at about 45° with external rotation of the foot (Fig. 13.13B). This is achieved by flexion at the hip with external rotation and abduction. The knee is kept in extension and the contralateral ilium is stabilized. The test force is applied about the patient's raised knee in a direction to take the leg and thigh into extension and abduction. Weakness may implicate an SC of the L1–2, L2–3 or L3–4 SMU.

The psoas trigger point is in the belly of the muscle and is palpated in appropriate patients with a covered-finger approach which is deep into the abdomen about the level of the umbilicus. Palpation commences lateral to the main bulk of rectus abdominis and is then lateral to medial as well as anterior to posterior. Care must be taken not to aggravate the abdominal viscera. A more accessible tender point lies in the iliacus and is palpated, again with a covered-finger approach, just medial to the anterior superior iliac spine (ASIS). The palpation is anterior to posterior with medial to lateral pressure to palpate the iliacus against the ilium. This point is also the therapeutic point for treating and strengthening the iliopsoas. A third point may be palpated about the insertion into the lesser trochanter. The thigh is flexed and abducted and informed consent is required. The patient is supine in all cases. The general pain distribution is shown in Figure 13.13C.

ASSESSMENT OF NEURAL CHANGE

The spinal nerves

The spinal nerves of the thoracolumbar junctional spine and the levels at which they exit are:

- spinal nerve T10 from the T10–11 SMU
- spinal nerve T11 from the T11–12 SMU
- spinal nerve T12 from the T12–L1 SMU
- spinal nerve L1 from the L1–2 SMU
- spinal nerve L2 from the L2–3 SMU
- spinal nerve L3 from the L3–4 SMU.

While the spinal nerves exit the spinal column as noted above, it must be appreciated that the level of the spinal cord from which they arise becomes progressively higher in relation to the vertebral level, as the number of the spinal nerve increases. The typical relationship between the spinal nerve and the vertebral segment is:

- spinal nerve T10 arises about the level of the T8–9 disk
- spinal nerve T11 arises about the level of the T9 body
- spinal nerve T12 arises about the level of the superior portions of the T10 body
- spinal nerve L1 arises about the level of the T10–11 disk
- spinal nerve L2 arises about the inferior level of the T11 vertebra
- spinal nerve L3 arises about the level of the T11–12 disk.

The subcostal nerve from T12 is sensory to skin of the abdomen inferior to the umbilicus, and is motor to the pyramidalis and quadratus lumborum. The iliohypogastic nerve from L1 is sensory to the gluteal, inguinal, and suprapubic regions and provides some motor to the anterior abdominal wall muscles. The ilioinguinal nerve, also from L1, is motor to the anterior abdominal wall muscles. The genitofemoral nerve is formed from L1 and L2 and is sensory to the femoral triangle. The genital branch has a motor function only in the male, to the dartos and cremaster muscles.

The cutaneous skin reflex for T10, T11, and T12 is elicited by stroking the skin of the abdomen, from superolateral to inferomedial, inferior and lateral to the umbilicus (Fig. 12.19 arrow B).

The lateral femoral cutaneous nerve arises from L2 and L3 and is sensory to the lateral thigh. It is involved in the classic meralgia paresthetica, a loss of sensation about the anterolateral thigh. The femoral nerve arises from L2, L3, and L4, and is motor to the psoas and iliacus before leaving the abdominopelvic cavity and innervating muscles in the lower limb (Cramer & Darby 1995).

The classic meralgia paresthetica is paresthesia along the anterolateral side of the thigh, corresponding to the distribution of the lateral femoral cutaneous nerve (Ebrall 1989, 1990). This nerve arises from the anterior rami of L2 and sometimes L3 levels and may become irritated or entrapped about the inguinal ligament. Meralgia paresthetica is not a rare presentation in clinical practice (Kadel et al 1982, Kadel & Godbey 1983, Ferezy 1989).

The L2 myotome is responsible for hip flexion and this may be assessed in either the supine or seated patient. In the latter, the practitioner places the hand on the anterior thigh about the knee and asks the patient to "lift up". In the supine patient, the hip and knee are flexed and the patient is asked to resist the practitioner extending the hip.

The L3 myotome is involved in knee extension. This function is best tested in the seated patient. The practitioner places the hand about the anterior distal leg and asks the patient to "straighten the leg".

Pain assessment

Local pain may arise either in the surrounding musculature and ligamentous network, secondary to sprain and strain following either acute or chronic overload, or from the structures intrinsic to each SMU. The questions associated with the differential diagnosis of low-back-pain presentations must take into consideration the intimate assessment of the structures forming and attaching to the thoracolumbar spine. This assessment must include the diaphragm, especially its anterior attachments.

Referred pain

Pain may refer about this region due to active trigger points in the paraspinal musculature, particularly the iliocostalis and longissimus. The deeper multifidi may generate local pain referral patterns. Pain and tenderness about the tip of the last rib and around the umbilicus may represent dysfunction about T10 and perhaps referral from the liver, gall bladder, upper colon, kidney, ureter, prostate, testes, ovaries, or uterus (Masarsky & Todres-Masarsky 2001).

Dysfunction about T11–12 typically refers pain to the lower abdominal quadrant, about the level of and medial to the ASIS. Posteriorly, tenderness may be felt about L5–S1. Dysfunction about the specific thoracolumbar junction (T12–L1) typically refers pain to the iliac crest, lateral hip, and into the groin, perhaps with pubic tenderness (Maigne 1996). It is thought these distributions follow the anterior ramus, posterior ramus, and lateral perforating branches of the T12 and L1 spinal nerves. Dysfunction about L2–3 will typically refer pain to the lateral thigh, while dysfunction about L3 will typically refer pain to the medial knee. These pains are emphasized with skin rolling.

Pain which arises from abdominal viscera varies from dull to severe but is poorly localized (Fig. 13.14). It tends to radiate to the part of the body served by the somatic sensory fibers associated with the same segment of the spinal cord which receives visceral sensory fibers from the particular viscus (Moore 1980).

Autonomic effects

The abdominal and pelvic organs receive their motor innervation from both the sympathetic and parasympathetic systems. Sensation from the viscera is conveyed to the spinal cord by nerves running with the autonomic distribution.

The trunks of the sympathetic ganglia with their gray and white rami communicans overlay and are adjacent to the psoas major at the level of T12 and L1 trough L3. The medial branches passing from the lumbar sympathetic ganglia are the lumbar splanchnic nerves and they typically synapse in the mesenteric ganglia. The splanchnic nerves which arise from the thoracic ganglia pierce the crus of the diaphragm, with the greater and lesser ending in the celiac ganglion and the lowest ending in the renal plexus.

The autonomic preganglionic cells in the thoracolumbar region (T10–L3) are sympathetic. The T10 ganglia may contribute to the greater splanchnic nerve. The ganglia about T11 and maybe T10 contribute to the lesser splanchnic nerve. The T12 ganglia give rise to a least or third splanchnic nerve in about 56% of dissections (Cramer & Darby 1995). The splanchnic nerves pierce the diaphragm and, together with the lumbar ganglia, provide sympathetic motor supply to the abdominal viscera.

The parasympathetic supply is from the vagus nerves above, and the pelvic splanchnic nerves below L3.

Traditional concepts

The following notes attempt to present a summary as being suggestive of what may be seen in clinical practice. The references below regarding the stimulation of a spinal center are from Schafer (1983 p. 371). As in previous chapters, the references to the Lovett Brother relationship are from Walther (1981 p. 67).

About T10 – the T10–11 SMU

Traditional chiropractic associates this level with the kidneys. The Lovett Brother relationship to the T10 body is movement in the opposite direction of the T1 body. Adjusting here is considered to produce a sympathetic effect and Gonstead associates this level with systolic hypertension (Plaugher 1993 p. 367).

Osteopathy considers this level is a reference site for abdominal and pelvic viscera (Beal 1989 p. 20). Faridi (1995) associates the T10 vertebral segment with sympathetic neural pathways to the small intestines and relates this level to irritable bowel syndrome. Stimulation of the spinal reflex center is thought to initiate slight visceromotor renal contraction, enhance pancreatic secretion, relax the intestines and colon, and stimulate adrenals when applied bilaterally, and to initiate splenic contraction (and circulatory blood cells) when applied on the left.

The T10 lamina (T8–11) is the location of the posterior neurolymphatic point for the quadriceps muscle (Walther 1981 p. 276). In acupuncture terms, the site for Du 7 Zhongshu is below the spinous process of T10 and is indicated for jaundice, vomiting, abdominal fullness, lumbar stiffness, and pain (Qiu 1993 pp. 154–155).

About T11 – the T11–12 SMU

Traditional chiropractic associates this level with the kidneys and ureters. Adjusting here is considered to produce a sympathetic effect and Gonstead associates this level with systolic hypertension (Plaugher 1993 p. 367). The Lovett Brother relationship to the T11 body is movement in the opposite direction of the C7 body.

Osteopathy considers this level is a reference site for pelvic viscera (Beal 1989 p. 20). Faridi (1995) associates the T11 vertebral segment with sympathetic neural pathways to the kidney and upper urethra. Stimulation of the spinal reflex center is thought to initiate slight visceromotor renal contraction, enhance pancreatic secretion, relax intestines and colon, to stimulate adrenals when applied bilaterally, and to initiate splenic contraction (and circulatory blood cells) when applied on the left.

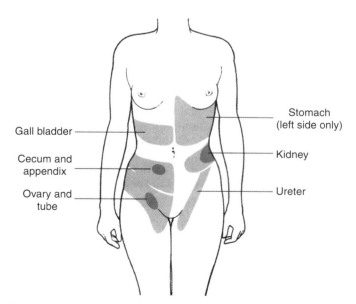

Figure 13.14   Referred pain about the abdomen. From Seidel et al (1999), with permission.

The T11 lamina (T8–11) is the location of the posterior neurolymphatic point for the quadriceps muscle (Walther 1981 p. 276). The posterior point for gastrocnemius, soleus, tibialis posterior, sartorius, and gracilis is bilateral and near the laminae of T11–12 (Walther 1981 pp. 277, 332, 336, 340). There are two posterior neurolymphatic points for quadratus lumborum; one lies over the T11 lamina and the other at the distal superior border of rib 12 (Walther 1981 p. 456). In acupuncture terms, the site for Du 6 Jizhong lies below the spinous process of T11 and is indicated for diarrhea, jaundice, hemorrhoids, epilepsy, infantile malnutrition, and anal prolapse (Qiu 1993 p. 154).

About T12 – the T12–L1 SMU

Traditional chiropractic associates this level with the small intestines and lymph circulation. Adjusting here is considered to produce a sympathetic effect and Gonstead associates this level with systolic hypertension (Plaugher 1993 p. 367). The Lovett Brother relationship to the T12 body is movement in the opposite direction of the C6 body. Maigne (1996 p. 102) suggests dysfunction at T12–L1 may be associated with chronic dysfunction at L4–5 and dysfunction at C2–3 and C6–7.

Osteopathy considers this level is a reference site for pelvic viscera (Beal 1989 p. 20). Faridi (1995) associates the T12 vertebral segment with sympathetic neural pathways to the bladder and urethra and relates this level to bladder infection. Stimulation of the spinal reflex center is thought to initiate prostate contraction and increase tone of the cecum and bladder sphincter. The posterior neurolymphatic point for psoas and iliacus lies between the spinous and transverse processes of T12–L1 and the posterior neurolymphatic point for infraspinatus lies over the T12 lamina (Walther 1981 pp. 304, 404).

About L1 – the L1–2 SMU

Traditional chiropractic associates this level with the large intestines and the inguinal rings. Adjusting here is considered to produce a sympathetic effect (Plaugher 1993 p. 357). The Lovett Brother relationship to the L1 body is movement in the opposite direction of the C5 body.

Faridi (1995) associates the L1 vertebral segment with sympathetic neural pathways to the ileocecal valve and relates this level to the ileocecal valve syndrome. Stimulation of the spinal reflex center is thought to initiate uterine body, round ligament, and bladder contraction, relieve pelvic vasoconstriction, and cause vesicular sphincter relaxation.

In acupuncture terms the site for Du 5 Xuanshu lies below the spinous process of L1 and is indicated for diarrhea, abdominal pain, lumbospinous stiffness, and pain. The site for Extra 21 Pigen lies 3.5 cun lateral to the lower border of the spinous process and is indicated for abdominal masses and lumbar pain (Qiu 1993 pp. 154, 177).

About L2 – the L2–3 SMU

Traditional chiropractic associates this level with the appendix, abdomen, and upper leg. Adjusting here is considered to produce a sympathetic effect (Plaugher 1993 p. 357). The Lovett Brother relationship to the L2 body is movement in the opposite direction of the C4 body. Faridi (1995) associates the L2 vertebral segment with sympathetic neural pathways to the cecum and relates this level to duodenal ulcers.

Stimulation of the spinal reflex center is thought to initiate uterine body, round ligament, and bladder contraction; relieve pelvic vasoconstriction, and cause vesicular sphincter relaxation. The posterior neurolymphatic point for tibialis anterior and the sacrospinalis (as a group) lies over the L2 transverse process (Walther 1981 pp. 339, 447). In acupuncture terms, the site for Du 4 Mingmen lies below the spinous process of L2 and is indicated for impotence, nocturnal emission, leucorrhea, irregular menstruation, diarrhea, lumbar spinal stiffness, and pain (Qiu 1993 p. 154).

About L3 – the L3–4 SMU

Traditional chiropractic associates this level with the sex organs, uterus, bladder, and knees. Adjusting here is considered to produce a sympathetic effect (Plaugher 1993 p. 357). The Lovett Brother relationship to the L3 body is movement in the same direction of the C3 body.

Faridi (1995) associates the L3 vertebral segment with sympathetic neural pathways to the endocrine glands (thyroid, pancreas, adrenals, etc.) and relates this level to endocrine dysfunction. Stimulation of the spinal reflex center is thought to initiate uterine body, round ligament, and bladder contraction, relieve pelvic vasoconstriction, and cause vesicular sphincter relaxation.

ASSESSMENT OF VASCULAR CHANGE

The vascular structures of the abdomen are shown in Figure 13.15A. It is important to assess for signs of an abdominal aortic aneurysm by palpation of the abdomen to the left of and superior to the umbilicus to assess for the pulse width of the aorta (Fig. 13.15B). A normal aortic pulse is projected anteriorly with no lateral expansion; aneurysm is suspected when a lateral, expansile pulse is palpated.

The suspicion of abdominal aortic aneurysm indicates a need for careful consideration of patient positioning and selection of appropriate techniques for spinal adjustment. Both the AP and lateral radiographs of the lumbar spine may also indicate aortic calcification, in which case the cautions associated with aneurysm are elevated to the next level. It is erroneous to associate calcified aortic aneurysms only with aging; a case of idiopathic, isolated infrarenal aortic aneurysm has been reported in a 12-year-old boy (Dittrick et al 2002). Whilst rare, most cases of aneurysm in the young have a clear associated cause, such as connective tissue disorders, infectious processes, inflammatory states, or trauma. The case reported by Dittrick et al (2002) had dense intramural calcification and sterile mesenteric lymphadenopathy.

Edema about the abdomen may be noted as ascites and raises significant diagnostic issues. From a musculoskeletal perspective, the practitioner will inspect and test for signs of edematous swelling about the thoracolumbar region. It is not common. Similarly, inflammation about the thoracolumbar junction and lower ribs is not common.

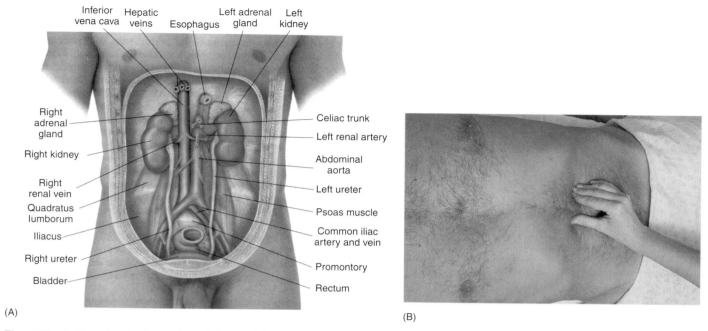

Figure 13.15 Vascular structures of the abdomen. (A) Landmarks for the abdominal aorta; (B) palpation of the abdominal aorta to assess for an indication of aneurysm. (A, B) From Seidel et al (1999), with permission.

CONCLUSION

The architectural change at the thoracolumbar junctional spine is as dramatic as that at the cervicothoracic region, yet the region seems considerably easier to assess. Perhaps this is due to the illusion of greater intersegmental movement, combined with the greater posterior to anterior flexibility.

The area remains intimately involved with the sympathetic nervous system and it is important to include abdominal and pelvic visceral function in the assessment of neural change. The practitioner must also remain alert to referred pain from other visceral structures in every complaint of mid-back pain.

14

The lumbosacral spine and pelvis

KEY CONCEPTS

The L5 vertebral body is the largest in the spine. It is taller at the anterior margin than at the posterior margin and this contributes to the lumbar lordosis. The transverse processes originate from the entire lateral aspect of the pedicle and, while not extending as far laterally as the transverse processes of the other lumbar segments above, they are much wider from anterior to posterior and superior to inferior.

The sacroiliac joint (SIJ) is planar in the child and develops during the teenage years and into the 20s, along with ossification of the sacrum. The joint surfaces become rough and irregular in the adult. Movement and dysfunction are clinically different across age groups.

Movement within the SIJ is small but extremely complex. It can be simply conceptualized as a rotation about the x-axis, allowing the posterior superior iliac spine (PSIS) to move anterior and superior or posterior and inferior, and a rotation about the y-axis, allowing the PSIS to move medially (internally) or laterally (externally).

The ischial tuberosities move apart to widen the support base when sitting. The iliac crests thus approximate and increase the forces of form closure in the SIJ. These simple biomechanical movements reduce the sensitivity of any assessment for kinematic change in the SIJ in the seated patient.

Postural change secondary to subluxation is a process and should not be seen as conclusive. While the body will undergo a series of changes in a chain of cause and effect, there are some patterns which act as indicators of functional lesions in the lumbosacral spine and pelvis. The patterns of gait are similar indicators of certain dysfunctions.

The critical nerve roots to assess are L4, L5, and S1. Sensation may be assessed in identified areas of high probability for each. Motor function and tendon reflexes are also important to identifying levels of dysfunction in the spine.

CLINICAL ANATOMY

The lumbosacral spine and pelvis consist of the two lowest lumbar segments, L4 and L5, and the sacrum in the adult or sacral segments in the developing child, the SIJs, and the symphysis pubis within the complete pelvic girdle. This region is a transitional zone between the entire spine above and the strong, supportive pelvic ring for the transmission of ambulating forces to and from the lower limbs.

The pelvic ring consists of the left and right innominate and the sacrum. Each innominate bone ("without a name") consists of an ilium, ischium, and pubis. The three bones fuse within the

acetabulum and, with respect to discussing the SIJ, "ilium" is interchangeable with "innominate". The commonly used landmarks of the ilium are the anterior superior iliac spine (ASIS) and the PSIS (Fig. 14.1A, B, C). The commonly used landmark of the ischium is the tuberosity and this takes the weight of the body in the seated position. When standing it is covered by the gluteus maximus. The ischium serves as an important attachment site for many of the powerful muscles of the hip and thigh.

The lumbosacral spine and pelvis include the following major articulations:

- L4–5
- L5–S1 (lumbosacral joint)
- left sacroiliac joint (SIJ)
- right sacroiliac joint (SIJ)
- sacrococcygeal joint
- symphysis pubis.

Cramer & Darby (1995 pp. 197–247) provide the appropriate level of anatomy of this region for the student and can be read in

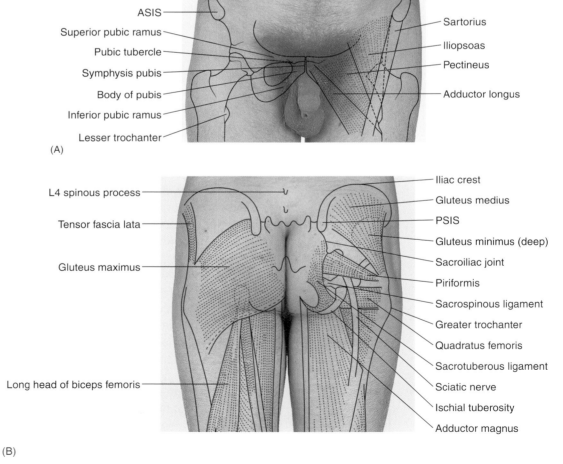

(A)

(B)

Figure 14.1 The lumbosacral spine and pelvis. Landmarks and muscle locations about the pelvis: (A) anterior view; (B) posterior view; (C) lateral view. ASIS, anterior superior iliac spine; PSIS, posterior superior iliac spine. (A–C) From Lumley (2002), with permission.

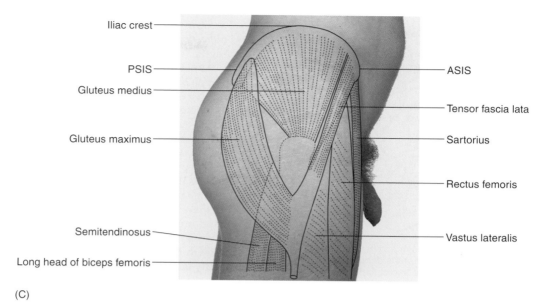

(C)

Figure 14.1 (*Continued*).

conjunction with this chapter. Key landmarks of the lumbosacral spine and pelvis are shown in Figure 14.1 and the following relationships should be noted:

- L4 spinous: usually palpated as being level with the iliac crests
- L5 spinous: usually a smaller, deeper structure palpated in the midline, inferior to the L4 spinous
- S2 tubercle: usually the most prominent and superior tubercle inferior to the L5 spinous, in the midline of the sacrum. The arachnoid mater and dura mater of the spinal canal end at this level
- S4 tubercle: usually the most inferiorly palpable tubercle immediately above the sacral hiatus
- sacral apex: about the sacral hiatus, which is bordered by the sacral cornu
- posterior aspect of the SIJ: immediately medial to the PSIS and at the lateral margin of the sacral alar, lying deep under the posterior and interosseous ligaments
- sacrotuberous ligament: the lateral band attaches about the transverse tubercle of the lateral sacral crest on the lateral margin of the sacrum between the level of the S2 and S4 tubercles
- sacrococcygeal joint: palpated distal to the sacral hiatus
- symphysis pubis: palpated in a superior to inferior direction in the midline of the supine patient.

Given that spinal cord ends in the conus medullaris around L1–2, the contents of the spinal canal in this region are the cauda equina, which includes the nerve roots of L4 through coccygeal. The spinal segments of the cord and the origin of their corresponding spinal nerves lie well above their exit canals and foramina. The S1 nerve root passes completely over the L5 disk as it travels the intervertebral canal (IVC), which is bounded posteriorly by the ligamentum flavum, thereby being exposed to

compression by a number of mechanisms, including disk protrusion, ligamentum flavum hypertrophy or buckling, or hypertrophy of the superior facet of the sacrum.

As the dura mater ends about S2, the nerve roots which exit below this level pierce the arachnoid and continue as individual nerve roots, each in a dural root sleeve. The dorsal and ventral roots unite within their dural sleeve and form a mixed spinal nerve before exiting the sacral canal laterally through a foramen which is continuous with an intervertebral foramen (IVF) on the pelvic surface of the sacrum and an IVF on the dorsal surface. The left and right S5 and coccygeal nerves exit the sacral hiatus medial to the sacral cornua on the respective side. The filum terminale, which originates from the most inferior aspect of the spinal cord and pierces the dura at the level of the S2 bony segment, also exits the sacral hiatus and attaches to the posterior surface of the first coccygeal vertebral segment (Cramer & Darby 1995 p. 225).

The innervation of the SIJ and its ligaments is derived exclusively from the dorsal branches of the sacral spinal nerves (Fig. 14.2) (Kissling & Jacob 1997). All dorsal nerve trunks pass between the layers of the sacrotuberous ligament and, after piercing the origin of the gluteus maximus, reach the skin as the medial cluneal nerve. The ventral rami of L4, L5, S1–3, and part of S4 form the sacral plexus, while those of S4 (part), S5, and the coccygeal nerves pierce the coccygeus muscle and enter the inferior aspect of the pelvis where they are joined by parts of the ventral rami of S4 and form the coccygeal plexus, which provides sensory innervation to the skin adjacent to the sacrotuberous ligament (Cramer & Darby 1995 p. 225). The sacral plexus gives rise to the posterior cutaneous nerve of the thigh, the pudendal nerve, sciatic nerve, superior and inferior gluteal nerves, and the nerves to the obturator internus and quadratus femoris (Cramer & Darby 1995 p. 243). The S2–4 nerves also give rise to the parasympathetic innervation to the pelvic viscera.

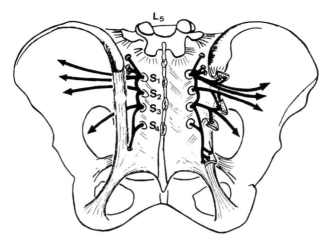

Figure 14.2 Innervation of the sacroiliac joint and its ligaments. The dorsal nerve trunks of S1 through S4 exit the dorsal intervertebral foramen and pass between the layers of the sacrotuberous ligament and, after piercing the origin of the gluteus maximus, reach the skin as the medial cluneal nerves. From Kissling & Jacob (1997), with permission.

The morphology of the L4 vertebrae (Fig. 14.3) is that of a typical lumbar segment and is much as described in the preceding chapter. By comparison, the body of L5 is the largest within the spine and is taller at the anterior than the posterior, contributing to the lumbar lordosis. The L5 spinous process is small and, as it projects inferiorly, it is palpated more deeply than that of L4. The dimensions of the L5 body in Asians are slightly larger compared to Caucasians, with a maximum average difference of +8% for the posterior vertebral body height; however, the spinal canal and pedicle width in Asians are significantly smaller, by an average of 30% and 20% respectively (Tan et al 2002). Notwithstanding these findings, it is also reported that the cross-sectional area, moment arms, and line of action of tissues at the lumbosacral joint in Asian males do not differ from the white population (Lin et al 2001).

The L5 segment articulates with the sacrum through the L5–S1 disk and two zygapophyseal joints which, while the most coronal of the lumbar facets (Fig. 2.5B), are variable in their orientation and commonly demonstrate tropism (Cramer & Darby 1995 p. 203).

The transverse processes of L5 originate from the entire lateral aspect of the pedicle and, while not extending as far laterally as the transverse processes of the other lumbar segments above, they are much wider from anterior to posterior and superior to inferior. The lateral aspects also angle superiorly (Cramer & Darby 1995 p. 203). The iliolumbar ligament is a key ligament of the lumbosacral junction and its attachments include the L5 transverse process. The lumbosacral articulation is a common site of developmental anomalies, described below.

The L5 disk is narrower than the others of the lumbar spine and the IVC between L5 and S1 is also smaller. This results in more than one-third of the area of the L5–S1 IVF being occupied by the mixed spinal nerve. Narrowing of the disk space significantly alters the vertical diameter of the IVC but has no significant effect on its sagittal dimensions (Cinotti et al 2002). Narrowing of the lumbosacral disk space is likely to compromise

the L5 ventral rami and dorsal root ganglia, especially in the presence of a lumbosacral ligament which extends medially across the ventral ramus (Briggs & Chandraraj 1995).

The sagittal dimensions of the IVC are strictly related to the sagittal diameter of the spinal canal and the pedicle length (Cinotti et al 2002). The L5–S1 articulation is also more mobile than the other lumbar spinal motion units (SMUs), allowing up to 5° of unilateral rotation, 3° of lateral flexion, and up to 10° each of flexion and extension (Cramer & Darby 1995 p. 205).

The sacrum consists of five and sometimes six vertebrae (Fig. 14.3). Ossification is a process which continues into adulthood. The disk is represented by a fibrocartilaginous plate about the eighth year as the costal elements unite laterally. These elements start to fuse vertically some time after puberty as the bodies form and these begin to fuse with each other about the 20th year. The central area and greater part of each intervertebral disk remain unossified up to or even after middle life. The coccyx also ossifies during the first 20 years or so of life and its segments are typically united by about the age of 30 years, and may later fuse to the sacrum, especially in females (data from Taylor & Resnick 2000 p. 332).

The sacrum is shorter and wider in the female and is placed at a varying depth between the ilia in both males and females, depending on the overall morphology of the pelvis (Fig. 14.4). The four basic shapes are given in the figure and the classification system centers largely on the characteristics of the pelvic apertures, which have a significant role in the birth process. It is perhaps more relevant within the manual disciplines to consider the depth of placement of the sacrum within the pelvis and the nature of the biomechanical changes which would be associated with such structural change. It has been suggested that low-back pain may arise secondary to altered biomechanics in the lumbosacral area resulting from the depth to which the sacrum is placed by nature within the pelvis (Ebrall 1994). It has also been suggested that, when L5 is deep-seated within the pelvis, the L5–S1 disk is relatively protected and disk protrusion would more likely occur at the L4–5 disk (MacLean et al 1990). This is an area for further investigation.

The base of the sacrum forms the superior border to articulate with L5 and projects anteriorly as the sacral promontory. The sacrum articulates with an auricular surface on each ilium and acts as a keystone in an arch; the shapes of the articular surfaces give the two SIJs a high degree of strength and stability through a degree of form closure. In order for there to be movement within the SIJ, the form closure is not complete and a degree of force closure is required for stability (Vleeming et al 1997a). This is provided by the erector spinae, multifidus, gluteus maximus, latissimus dorsi, and biceps femoris (Lee 1997). Compression of the SIJ occurs when the gluteus maximus and contralateral latissimus dorsi contract.

The articular surface on the ilium is like a gumboot or Wellington which has fallen on its back from facing frontward. The long leg lies anteroposteriorly and tilts inferiorly, and the short foot part runs inferosuperiorly. The boot–shaped surfaces are matched by those on the sacrum (Fig. 14.3) and each SIJ is supported by a strong, complex ligamentous arrangement (see Fig. 14.17, below). In the adult the joint surfaces are rough and irregular; however, during the first decade of life the surfaces are planar (Lee 2000). During the teenage years the SIJ surfaces

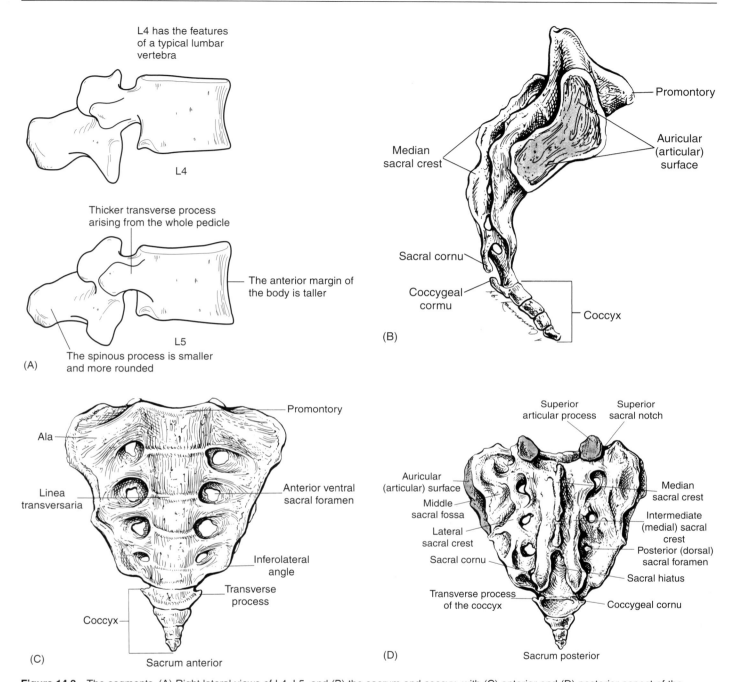

Figure 14.3 The segments. (A) Right lateral views of L4, L5, and (B) the sacrum and coccyx, with (C) anterior and (D) posterior aspect of the sacrum and coccyx.

develop a convex ridge along the entire length of the articular surface on the ilium, matched by a corresponding sacral groove. By the end of the third decade the superficial layers of the articular cartilage are fibrillated with some crevice formation and erosion (Lee 2000). Degenerative changes can appear as early as the third decade but are markedly more frequent from the fifth. Degeneration progresses further in women than men and faster in parous than nulliparous women (Shibata et al 2002).

The changing nature of the articular surfaces of the SIJ has implications in its clinical assessment across age groups. Articular hypomobility is more likely in patients from their late 20s, while movement patterns in the child and adolescent will typically be smoother and not demonstrate the "catching" of the ilium on the sacrum, which is seen in the mature patient as the hip is flexed past 45°. The assessment of kinematic change as described in this chapter is that which is most relevant to the mature patient.

Mechanosensitive receptors have been identified in the SIJ and adjacent tissues. The mechanical thresholds of those within the SIJ (greater than 7 g) suggest they act as nociceptors and the SIJ is confirmed as a source of low-back pain (Sakamoto et al 2001).

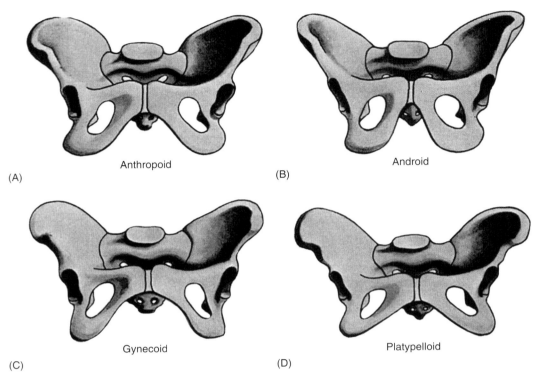

(A) Anthropoid (B) Android

(C) Gynecoid (D) Platypelloid

Figure 14.4 Morphology of the pelvis. (A) The anthropoid pelvis is a common shape in males. (B) The android is also a common pelvis in males and is seen in females. On radiographs it appears with quite tall innominates and the infrapubic angle is sharper than in the anthropoid. (C) The gynecoid pelvis is common in the female and has a large pelvic aperture. (D) The platypelloid pelvis is rare and appears as a flat, low, wide pelvis.

In the porcine model, noxious stimulation of the anterior aspect of the joint under the capsular membrane elicited responses in the multifidus, gluteus maximus, and quadratus lumborum muscles (Indahl et al 1999). This finding suggests a possible regulatory function of the SIJ in locomotion and body posture.

The pelvic ring is completed by the symphysis joint between the medial surfaces of the pubic bones. This is a fibrocartilaginous joint supported by superior and arcuate ligaments and is angled anteroposteriorly (see Fig. 14.17D). Torsional stress about the symphysis pubis creates inflammation as osteitis pubis. Disrelationships across the symphysis are a common clinical finding and typically present as a unilateral superior pubic ramus, usually secondary to dysfunction at the SIJ or muscle imbalance between the abdominals and adductors. Frank dysfunction may occur in the female patient during pregnancy and childbirth and diastasis may follow trauma. It is common for females to have bruising of the parasymphyseal pubic bones postpartum (Wurdinger et al 2002).

ASSESSMENT OF KINEMATIC CHANGE

The terminology for listing the spinal segments is familiar; however, new concepts are required to visualize movement about the SIJ. While the movement is small, it is able to be detected and measured by roentgen stereophotogrammetric analysis (RSA). This process has identified the movements within the SIJ as including rotation about each of the x-axis, y-axis, and z-axis, a rotation about a helical axis, and translation (Sturesson 1997).

The motion of the joint is complex, involving simultaneous rotations of 3° or less, and translations of 2 mm or less, in three dimensions (Harrison et al 1997). The average values for rotation and translation are low, being 1.8°/0.7 mm for males and 1.9°/0.9 mm for females (Kissling & Jacob 1996). These very small values hold true even when an experimental force of 1000 N is applied (Zheng et al 1997). No mobility of the sacrum has been found during stresses in lateral flexion (Barthes et al 1999). For the purposes of clinical assessment the kinematic change within a SIJ may be simplified and described by identifying perceived positional change in either the ilium or the sacrum.

The reference point for describing kinematic change in the ilium is the PSIS. If the ilium rotates into extension about the x-axis the PSIS is considered to move anterior and superior, AS. Extension is the movement which "opens" the anterior plane of the innominate away from the anterior plane of the trunk. This is clockwise rotation about the x-axis when viewing the right lateral perspective.

Conversely, when the ilium flexes and rotates posteriorly about the x-axis, the PSIS is considered to move posterior and inferior, PI. Flexion is the movement which "closes" the anterior plane of the innominate towards the anterior plane of the trunk. This is counterclockwise rotation about the x-axis when viewing the right lateral perspective.

When the ilium rotates about the y-axis the PSIS will either move laterally and open the SIJ or medially and close the SIJ. Lateral movement of the PSIS is considered external rotation (Ex) at the SIJ and medial movement is considered internal rotation (In). By way of a note of clarification, the reference point of the ilium is the PSIS, lying on the posterior aspect, and its movement in rotation about the y-axis is the reverse of the movement of the ilium, i.e., *external rotation of the ilium* (for example, the right ilium rotates to the right about the y-axis) produces *internal rotation of the PSIS* (the PSIS closes on to the sacrum and "closes" the SIJ).

Kinematic change of the ilium about the SIJ is described by listing the PSIS. The paradoxical movements of the sacrum mean that it is not really useful for describing kinematic change about the SIJ. Its preferred role is to describe certain positional changes with relation to L5 above, thus being descriptive of kinematic change at the lumbosacral articulation (Peterson & Bergmann 2002 p. 319). These changes may or may not include an SIJ (see below).

Depending on the paradigm in which the practitioner chooses to practice, the ilium may be listed by one of the following:

- PI: when the ilium is perceived to be fixated in flexion and movement into extension is restricted or limited
- AS: when the ilium is perceived to be fixated in extension and movement into flexion is restricted or limited
- In: when the ilium is perceived to be fixated in external rotation such that the PSIS has internally rotated on to the sacrum and movement of the ilium into internal rotation is limited
- Ex: when the ilium is perceived to be fixated in internal rotation such that the PSIS has externally rotated away from the sacrum and movement of the ilium into external rotation is limited
- PIIn: when the ilium is perceived to be fixated in flexion and external rotation and movement into extension and internal rotation is limited
- PIEx: when the ilium is perceived to be fixated in flexion and internal rotation and movement into extension and external rotation is limited
- ASIn: when the ilium is perceived to be fixated in extension and external rotation and movement into flexion and internal rotation is limited
- ASEx: when the ilium is perceived to be fixated in extension and internal rotation and movement into flexion and external rotation is limited.

The Gonstead system of pelvic analysis attempts to identify the above listings from measurements on the erect anteroposterior (AP) lumbopelvic radiograph and this is described later in this chapter. This method also generates radiographic listings for the sacrum and these may be at variance with listings obtained by palpation.

In essence, the sacrum may rotate about the x-axis in unison, or bilaterally. It may also be perceived to rotate or tilt about the z-axis, and rotate about the y-axis. The movements are actually much more complex than any single movement about one axis and the question of which reference point to use is challenging. The following listings for the sacrum are those which may be perceived by a trained practitioner with a rational consideration of palpatory findings and perhaps of radiographic suggestions:

- Base anterior: when the sacrum has rotated about the x-axis such that the sacral promontory has moved anteroinferior with respect to the anterior margins of L5. In biomechanical and medical terms this movement is nutation. In manual assessment nutation may be palpated and is also observed from lateral radiograph. It needs to be differentiated from retrolisthesis of L5 on S1. The pain findings and tenderness are about the

sacral base if the sacrum is fixed in nutation whereas they are more about L5 with retrolisthesis of that segment.
- Base posterior: when the sacrum has rotated about the x-axis such that the base has moved posteroinferior with respect to L5. In biomechanical and medical terms this movement is counternutation. In manual assessment this may be observed from a lateral radiograph and needs to be differentiated from a spondylolisthesis of L5 on S1. The pain findings and tenderness are usually quite marked about the sacral tubercles when the sacrum is fixed in counternutation or with its base posterior.
- LA or RA: when rotation about the x-axis is combined with rotation about the y-axis such that one alar moves anterior relative to the other.
- LP or RP: as directly above, except the posterior alar is listed.

Herein lies the conundrum; other authors suggest that there is also rotation about the z-axis in these cases, such that the anterior side is also inferior (I). Diversified listings thus consider the sacrum to be listed as either LAIS (left anterior inferior sacrum) or RAIS. On the other hand, Gonstead lists the posterior side and also considers it to be inferior, thus either a left PI (left posterior inferior [sacrum]) or right PI. Quite clearly, if the sacrum is rotating about the y-axis such that one alar becomes anterior whilst the other is posterior, then rotation about the z-axis such that one alar becomes inferior must imply that the other alar is superior. Hence it is not possible to accept that an LAIS is the converse of right PI.

A resolution would seem to be to accept the biomechanical argument of Janse (1976 p. 137) for unilateral anterior-inferior wedging of the sacrum and to consider that its correction would be by contact on the most posterior aspect of the sacrum. Often this is not the opposite alar but is on the contralateral side about the apex.

Postural assessment

The postural changes most relevant to this region are those which affect pelvic leveling and the lower limbs. Schafer (1983) described a number of these patterns which are indicative of lumbopelvic subluxation (Fig. 14.5). There are also a number of distortions indicative of muscle involvement which are discussed later in this chapter.

The golden role of assessment holds true: the patient is assessed in the sequence of global change, regional change, then segmental change. Given that significant regional change generally affects the extent of global movement, it is important for the practitioner to observe global movement with an open mind to the various regional involvements which will be occurring throughout the spine.

Some practitioners look for set patterns of postural change and claim they reflect definitive types of subluxation. It is more likely that postural change secondary to subluxation is an ongoing process as the body undergoes a series of changes in a cumulative chain of cause and effect. As with the upper cervical complex (Fig. 9.7), there are some basic postural changes which act as pointers to dysfunction in the lumbosacral spine and pelvis. Of course, there are a number of other possibilities and these will be discussed later in this chapter; however, from a point of view of observing postural change, it is useful to simplify matters.

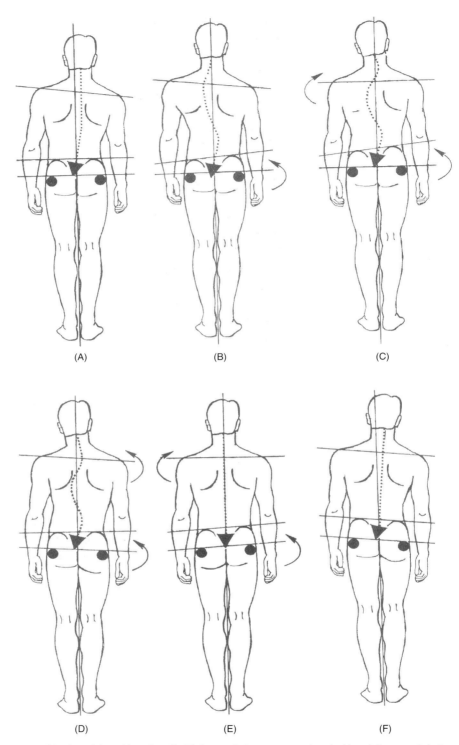

Figure 14.5 Postural indicators of lumbopelvic subluxation. (A–E) Postural changes associated with a right anteroinferior sacrum are shown. The subluxation is minor and in the early stage in (A). Note the sacral apex is left of the midline and the right base is tilted low; however, the iliac crests are level. As it progresses in severity and chronicity, the ipsilateral iliac crest becomes high (B) and a secondary scoliosis develops. The functional curves can become quite established (C) and the pelvis rotates to the left while the high right crest rotates posteriorly. Compensation is provided by the left shoulder rolling forward. This pattern is complicated by a functional short leg on the right (D) which draws the ipsilateral (right) shoulder forward. A paradox occurs with this sacral subluxation when the short leg is on the left (E). The sacrum appears level and the spine is in the midline; however, the pelvis is tilted to the left. (F) Postural changes associated with acute ilia fixation, in this case either left anterior or right posterior. A functional short leg is produced and the entire spine leans to the right of midline. The head is to the right of midline as compensation for left sacroiliac joint (SIJ) pain; if the pain is in the right SIJ, then upper cervical subluxation is also suspected. (A–F) From Schafer (1983), with permission.

The noted chiropractic author Richard Schafer (1983) compiled the following, using a right anteroinferior sacrum (RAIS) as the example (Fig. 14.5A–E). When the subluxation is minor and in the early stage (Fig. 14.5A), it creates a "leaning tower" where the trochanters and iliac crests are level but the sacrum is tilted towards the anteroinferior side. The low lumbar spine follows the sacrum by tilting to the right but corrects from the low or mid thoracic spine. The shoulders may be low on the side of the anteroinferior sacrum and the head and neck will also be laterally shifted to that side. The right SIJ will palpate as tender and the right psoas and erector spinae will be hypertonic.

As the subluxation progresses in severity and chronicity, the ipsilateral iliac crest becomes high (Fig. 14.5B) and a secondary scoliosis develops. The pelvis is noted to have rotated to the left to be "right anterior" (arrow). The occiput has come back to the midline but may be high on the left, depending on cervical compensation. The functional curves can become quite established (Fig. 14.5C) and, as the pelvis has rotated to the left about the y-axis, the high right crest rotates posteriorly about the x-axis. The practitioner will observe a distinct right sacral dimple. The shoulders may be level, depending on the site of thoracic transition, but compensation for the pelvic rotation will be provided by the left shoulder rolling forward.

The patterns associated with an anteroinferior sacrum are complicated by a functional short leg. When the short leg is on the side of the anteroinferior sacrum (Fig. 14.5D), the ipsilateral (right) shoulder tends to lower and roll forward. The occiput may be low on the contralateral (left) side. A paradox occurs with this sacral subluxation when a congenital short leg is present. In the example shown it is on the contralateral side to the anteroinferior tilt of the sacrum (Fig. 14.5E). In this case the sacrum will appear level and the spine will lie on the plumb line; however, the pelvis will tilt to the side of the short leg (left).

It is obvious that the process of relating postural change to a specific subluxation is quite complex. For example, what happens when the anteroinferior tilt of the sacrum is towards the side of a congenital short leg? The practitioner must be thorough and complete with the postural examination and enthusiastic in exploring a dynamic mix of actions and compensatory reactions.

The postural changes thought to be associated with acute ilia fixation, in this case either left anterior or right posterior, are shown in Fig. 14.5F. A functional short leg on the posterior side will be produced and the ipsilateral iliac crest and trochanter will be low. The sacrum will tilt to the low side and the entire spine will thus also lean to that side. The head may tilt to the side of the low pelvis (right of midline in this example) as compensation for left SIJ pain; if the pain is in the right SIJ then upper cervical subluxation is also suspected (Schafer 1983 pp. 476–478). Thorough movement palpation must be undertaken to determine if the fixated SIJ is on the right, listed as RP, or on the left, listed as LA.

It is important for the practitioner to synthesize a three-dimensional understanding of the patient's posture, and to ensure that changes such as anterior shoulder rotation are noted. Other important findings include popliteal fossa and Achilles tendon tension, as well as other palpatory assessments of muscle function. Postural change may not be indicative of lumbopelvic subluxation; rather, it may reflect changes in muscle tension which may be secondary to either subluxation at a higher spinal level or other factors. The practitioner must integrate the postural

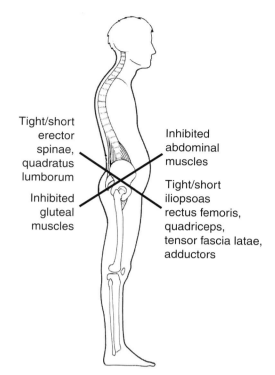

Figure 14.6 Lower crossed syndrome, after Janda and Chaitow. From Chaitow & DeLany (2002), with permission.

findings with the remainder of the assessment procedures and other findings.

In addition to these postural changes, the practitioner should specifically assess for evidence of a lower crossed syndrome (Fig. 14.6). The posture in the sagittal plane will demonstrate tightness and shortening of the iliopsoas, rectus femoris, tensor fascia latae, short adductors of the thigh, and the erector spinae group, in conjunction with weakness and inhibition of the abdominals and gluteal muscles (Chaitow & DeLany 2002 p. 318). The result is anterior tilting of the pelvis with flexion of the hip joints and exaggeration of the lumbar lordosis. The pattern is associated with various degrees of pain and discomfort and leads to cumulative dysfunction throughout the spine and lower extremities.

Radiographic analysis

The two essential radiographs are the AP and lateral lumbopelvic. They must be taken with the patient standing and the radiographer should pay close attention to patient positioning, especially if the practitioner is intending to make measurements of structural dimensions within the pelvis. Other views are taken when indicated, namely a left and right oblique view to demonstrate patency of the IVF and the presence of spondylolisthesis, and flexion/extension views (in the sagittal plane on a lateral radiograph) to demonstrate segmental instability. Some may also find the lateral flexion view (AP projection) useful for identifying segmental movement, particularly rotation, although the clinical application may be questionable.

Vertebral osteophytes are one of the principal radiographic diagnostic criteria for degenerative change in this region.

The prevalence of lumbar osteophytes is greater in men than in women and increases with age. They occur most frequently at L4 in males and at L3 in females (Shao et al 2002). These sites are near the maximal sagittal lumbar curvature. Osteophytes are typically classified as being either a traction spur or a claw spur. The former is thought to be a sign of spinal instability. It has been found that traction and claw spurs frequently coexist on the same vertebral rim, which suggests they may result from the same degenerative processes and not necessarily reflect the results of two distinct pathological processes (Heggeness & Doherty 1998). In this case, both are suggestive of spinal instability.

Objective structural change of lumbopelvic mechanics

The lumbosacral junction is a common site for anomalies. These range from the relatively common facet asymmetry or tropism to the more complex transitional segments at L5–S1. It is academic whether such segments represent sacralization or lumbarization; the clinical relevance is the nature of the resulting segments and their effect on the biomechanics of the region. It is known that in the younger age group without degeneration, there is no difference between subjects with lumbosacral transitional vertebrae and those without, for the dimensions of spinal canal sagittal diameter, interpedicular distance, interfacet distance, and lateral recess diameter (Oguz et al 2002). On the other hand, Santiago et al (2001) report that patients with lumbarization showed smaller diameters of the spinal canal. A description of the full variety of anomalies is beyond the scope of this text and the reader is referred to authoritative sources such as Taylor & Resnick (2000 pp. 218–428) or Yochum & Rowe (1996 pp. 231–239; 282–291).

The patient record should contain notation of anomalies and variants observed on radiograph. The more common findings include agenesis of a lumbar pedicle (to be differentiated from an osteolytic lesion), spina bifida occulta (typically of little or no consequence), transitional segments, facet tropism (not only at L5–S1), and kissing spinous processes (seen on the lateral view). The ossification status of the sacrum should be noted, as it may contraindicate the use of modalities such as ultrasound in the paraspinal region. Some six types of anatomical variants have been determined from computed tomography (CT) images and described for the SIJ (Prassopoulos et al 1999). It is not known how these impact on clinical assessment and treatment.

The ossification status of the iliac crest apophysis must also be noted in the growing patient with scoliosis. The epiphysis first appears at the ASIS between 14 and 16 years and progresses posteromedially towards the PSIS before fusing to the ilium between the ages of 18 and 25. It is graded by the amount of quadrants of the crest which are covered, from 1 through 4, and then grade 5 when ossification is complete (Yochum & Rowe 1996 pp. 321–322). Once the epiphysis becomes visible the progression of a scoliotic curvature slows, and usually ends when ossification of the epiphysis is complete. The Riser grade (1–5) is an accepted sign of skeletal maturity. The normal appearance of the epiphysis of the ilium must be differentiated from traumatic avulsion.

Spondylolysis is non-union of the pars interarticularis (Fig. 14.7C). It may be uni- or bilateral and rarely, at three sites, including the center of the right lamina, in the same vertebra (Ariyoshi et al 1999). While occurring at other levels of the spine, including

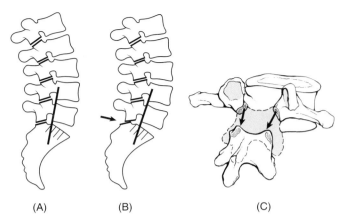

(A)   (B)   (C)

Figure 14.7 Spondylolysis and spondylolisthesis. (A) Normal relationships showing Meyerding's method of measuring spondylolisthesis, where a line along the inferior segment (in this case, the sacral base) is divided into four equal parts. A line projected inferiorly along the posterior aspect of the superior body (in this case, the L5 body) then indicates the grade of anterior slippage. (B) A Meyerding grade 1 spondylolisthesis. (C) The nature of a bilateral pars defect with slippage. (A, B) From Schafer (1983), with permission; (C) from Cramer & Darby (1995), with permission.

cervical, it is a relatively common finding of the L5 segment and is mostly asymptomatic (Standaert & Herring 2000). Non-union infers a congenital or developmental cause, while separation is typically secondary to trauma, most likely repetitive stress imposed by physical activity (Standaert et al 2000). A variant is degenerative spondylosis where there is anterior vertebral displacement of one segment on another secondary to zygapophyseal joint degeneration without a defect of the pars interarticularis (Taylor & Resnick 2000 pp. 242–243).

If the lysis of the pars is such that the vertebral segment displaces itself anteriorly on the segment below, then the condition is spondylolisthesis – a "slippage" (Fig 14.7B). The degree of anterior slippage can be categorized after Myerding, who divided the inferior segment into four equal parts (Taylor & Resnick 2000; Fig. 14.7A). A grade 1 spondylolisthesis exists when a line extending from the posterior border of the superior body falls within the first quarter. Subsequently it is grade 2 when in the second quarter, and so on. A grade 5 exists when the posterior margin of the superior body is beyond the anterior margin of the body below. A spondylolisthesis of grade 2 or above is cause for referral and a slippage of 50% or more will probably be treated with surgical fusion (Seitsalo et al 1990). A grade 1 requires careful assessment and is appropriate for conservative management.

The important differential is whether the spondylolisthesis is congenital or developmental, in which case it may well be stable in the adult patient and not likely to progress, or secondary to trauma, in which case it may well be unstable and require surgical assessment. Once trauma is ruled out as a cause, stability can be assessed from lateral views of the lumbopelvic spine in full flexion and then extension. There should be little, if any, change in position of the anterior segment. It has been reported that the spondylolytic defect in pars interarticularis does not cause permanent instability/hypermobility in the adult patient with low-back pain and low-grade olisthesis (Axelsson et al 2000); however, the incidence of spondylolisthesis has been reported to

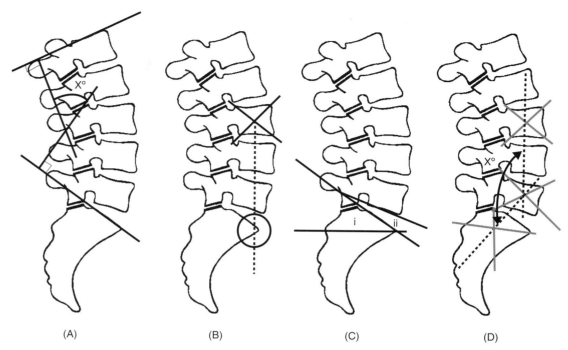

Figure 14.8 Measurements of the lumbar spine. (A) Quantitative measurement of the lumbar lordosis; (B) determination of the lumbar gravity line; (C) quantitative measurement of the sacral base angle (i) and the lumbar disk angle (ii); (D) quantitative measurement of the lumbosacral lordosis angle.

increase from 17% in the second decade to 51% in the sixth when the defect is present (Ishida et al 1999).

By way of a clinical note, a grade 1 spondylolisthesis in the developing spine (mid teenage years) may change the point of inflexion between the lumbar spine and sacrum. In the normal spine it is considered that the base of the sacrum will nutate or move anteroinferiorly when the lumbar spine extends, and vice versa. This point of inflexion may move up the spine, as high as L2 or L3 in the presence of a non-traumatic, bilateral spondylolisthesis at L5–S1.

While much is made of the involvement of spondylolisthesis and anterolisthesis, any finding of retrolisthesis, particularly of the L4 or L3 vertebrae, must be noted. Recent evidence associates retrolisthesis of a lumbar segment with a mild degree of axonal damage in the posterior branch of the lumbar nerve root innervating the medial paraspinal muscles (Sihvonen et al 1997). Clinically this is manifested by radiating sensations (numbness and pain) into the lower limbs with no evidence of nerve root impingement. The tendency to retrolisthesis is seen as a 3–4 mm posterior translation of the vertebral body during extension with no clear anterolisthesis during flexion (Sihvonen et al 1997).

Naturally this region is subjected to degenerative change of the same elements as the spine above and careful assessment should be made of the extent of such change, particularly in the spinal elements. The SIJ may also demonstrate degenerative change and is a common site for identifying pathological processes such as ankylosing spondylitis and other arthritides. The degree of osteoporosis throughout this region in the aging patient should also be noted and must be considered when determining the most appropriate type of manual therapy.

A number of clinically relevant measurements of the lumbosacral spine are taken from the lateral radiograph (Fig. 14.8). The data for the values given are taken from Yochum & Rowe (1996). The measurements include:

- The lumbar lordosis: the superior margins of the L1 body and of S1 are extended posteriorly (Fig. 14.8A). Perpendicular lines then intersect providing an angle which is representative of the lumbar lordosis. The normal angle varies widely but an average of 50–60° is accepted.

- The lumbar gravity line: the center of the L3 body is found by drawing lines which connect the anterosuperior margin with the posteroinferior margin and the anteroinferior margin with the posterosuperior margin (Fig. 14.8B). A vertical line dropped from their intersection indicates the gravity line of the lumbar spine. It is expected to pass through the anterior lip of the sacral base when relationships are within normal limits. It may fall anterior to this point and indicate anterior weight-bearing (rare), or posterior to indicate a posterior shift in weight-bearing (common). A posterior shift is not automatically indicative of an increased lordosis as many factors are involved, including the inclination of the sacrum.

- The sacral base (Ferguson's angle) and the lumbosacral disk angle: these two measurements are important to establish the nature of the lordosis above. Ferguson's angle (Fig. 14.8Ci) is sometimes called the lumbosacral angle; the angle represents the angle of the sacral base against a true horizontal line and this angle is integrated with the lumbar spine above. Normal values lie between 26° and 57° with a mean of 41°. The sacral disk angle (Fig. 14.8Cii) is relevant as an increase has been associated with low-back pain and a decrease is thought to be present with acute herniation of the L5 disk (Yochum & Rowe 1996 p. 161). The normal range appears to lie between 10° and 15°.

• The lumbosacral lordosis angle (Fig. 14.8D): this angle can be considered as the true lumbosacral angle as it reflects the relationship between L5, as (usually) the lowest segment in the lumbar spine, and the sacrum. It is found by taking the angle between lines representing the axis of the lower lumbar spine and the axis of the S1 segment. The former is derived from a line which connects the center of the L3 and L5 bodies. The center of each is found in the manner as described above for L3. The latter is found by finding the center of the S1 segment (in the same manner as for L3), which is dependent on being able to identify the inferior margin of S1 on the radiograph. A line is extended from the center of the S1 segment to meet the center of the L5 body. The angle between this line and the line connecting the centers of L3 and L5 represents the lumbosacral lordosis angle. The range of normal values is given as 124–162°, with a mean of 146°. The significance of this value is not known in the scientific sense; however, from a clinical perspective it is as valuable to the practitioner as it is to separate the upper cervical complex from the cervical lordosis.

It is not appropriate to take any one value as being especially relevant or indicative of a particular presentation; rather, all values should be taken and then considered within the context of the patient's presentation and other clinical findings. As always, it must be expected that some values which may be considered extreme may well be "normal" for a particular patient. The important clinical achievement is the ability to associate changes in the above values with a particular presentation, and then justify the relationship so that it better informs the treatment.

Observation should be made of the disk space height as seen on the lateral radiograph. It is known that the average height of the lumbar disk spaces of males and females in the age range of 20–69 years increases slightly but linearly with increasing age (Shao et al 2002). It declines from the seventh decade and may then contribute to loss of stature. Narrowing of the disk space height is associated with disk disruption. A direct correlation has been reported between the degree of disk space narrowing and the extent of the annular bulge or protrusion (Kambin et al 1988).

There are also important measurements to make about the hip; however, these are considered to be part of the assessment of the lower limb and are not included in this text.

Other diagnostic imaging assessment

The axial CT scan may be particularly useful for quantifying the extent of degenerative bony change, particularly when such change leads to stenosis of the spinal canal and/or the IVC. The CT is also useful for imaging pelvic structures and relationships. The magnetic resonance imaging (MRI) is useful in specialist situations but is not commonly used in general practice. Transvaginal and transrectal ultrasound probes are commonly used in medical diagnosis but these have no relevance in manual healthcare apart from establishing or ruling out any primary source of carcinoma which may metastasize to the bone or spine. Scans of radioisotope distribution are particularly relevant to indicate areas of increased metabolic activity, whether they be due to inflammation or metaplasia.

Subjective nature of movement

The intimate relationship between the lumbosacral spine and pelvis and the lower limbs places a great emphasis on the assessment of dynamic posture. Gait can be considered as the most fundamental form of dynamic posture and is the basis of holistic biomechanical analysis of the patient (Schafer 1983 p. 107).

The protocols for gait analysis have been described in Chapter 4. They are especially applicable to assessing the lumbosacral spine and pelvis as this region is the key locomotor center of the body. Dysfunction in the mechanics of this region is more likely to produce primary gait changes, while dysfunction in the spinal regions above more alters gait as a secondary consideration.

The first observation remains that of the way the patient rises from the chair. This may occur casually as the practitioner greets the patient in the waiting room, or formally as part of the controlled gait analysis. The patient is asked to stand and the practitioner is looking for signs of the patient shifting the body weight to a pain-free, uninvolved side of the body. This is Minor's sign (Evans 2001 pp. 576–577) and is positive when the patient is seen to support the body while sitting by balancing on the uninvolved leg and then using the hands to raise the body from the chair. A positive finding suggests sacroiliac involvement, lumbosacral sprains and strains, disk protrusion with nerve root pain into a leg, and other more worrisome conditions such as lumbopelvic fractures, muscular dystrophy, and dystonia (Evans 2001).

A patient with a positive Minor's sign will obviously demonstrate a significantly altered gait, restrictions to range of motion (ROM), and possibly an antalgic lean, especially with non-central disk protrusion. There is little point in forcing such patients through a series of provocative intermediate tests and it is more appropriate to proceed with a directed examination which focuses on the process of ruling in and ruling out the relevant differential diagnoses.

For those patients who are able to ambulate, the observation aims to assess whether the body is progressing smoothly and fluidly through space with symmetry of movement and elegance of balance. Once a neurologic gait has been excluded, the assessment should determine whether there are asymmetries in the gait cycle which may reflect mechanical dysfunction.

In particular the practitioner must look for symmetry of the stance phase, an even left/right stride length, a smooth vertical excursion, a balanced carriage of the head and trunk, and an arm swing which is free, equal, and alternate to leg swing. The lower limbs are inspected to assess heel strike, knee extension, and any presence of toe-walking.

The pelvis should remain centered over the line of progression while shifting laterally a couple of centimeters to each weight-bearing side during the cycle. Accentuated lateral shifting suggests gluteus medius weakness. It should also rotate and tilt smoothly in the manner described by Greenman (1990; Fig. 4.6B) and restrictions in these movements may indicate SIJ fixation. A forward lurch of the hip suggests a weak gluteus maximus. Significant anterior rotation of the pelvis to provide thrust for the leg suggests weak quadriceps. A pelvis which "waddles" indicates weak or ineffective proximal muscles caused by proximal myopathies. It may also suggest bilateral congenital dislocation of the hip.

Leg swing is assessed to determine whether the adductors are weak and allowing the leg to swing outwards from the hip. Weak medial hamstrings may allow the foot to rotate externally and flare during the swing phase. The foot may appear to turn outwards with a normal piriformis if the contralateral piriformis is weak. An inturned foot may suggest a weak psoas on the same side.

These particular components are evaluated within the context of the overall progress through the gait cycle, as described in Chapter 4, and the findings from the gait analysis must be considered with the postural findings in an attempt to direct the regional and segmental examinations better.

Assessment of the individual joints

The uniqueness of relationships between L4, L5, the sacrum and the ilia, within the lumbosacral triangle (Fig. 14.9), requires the practitioner to develop a specific sequence to the assessment of the individual joints. If the patient has presented with generalized back pain, then the thoracolumbar junctional spine will have been assessed first. It is reasonable to apply these standard SMU assessment protocols for L3 on L4, and, depending on the patient's body type, for L4 on L5. If this has occurred in the seated patient, then it is reasonable to continue to assess L5 on S1, and then the SIJs and, if indicated, the symphysis pubis.

Should the patient present with a specific lumbosacral problem, then the practitioner may elect to assess the lumbosacral region first, starting with L5 on S1 and progressing through each SIJ, before assessing the thoracolumbar spine above. In this case L4–5 may be assessed after L5–S1, or be appended to the thoracolumbar assessment after L3–4. The reason for this approach is to reflect the clinical decision making associated with selecting the contact point for the adjustment in the lumbosacral triangle. The rule of thumb is:

- if L5 is subluxated on S1 and each SIJ is considered normal or free of fixation, then the contact for the adjustment is on L5 so that it is the lumbosacral articulation to which normal movement is restored
- if L5 is considered to have normal movement on S1, and one of the SIJs is considered to be subluxated, then the contact for the adjustment is on the PSIS of the subluxated SIJ
- if L5 is subluxated on S1 and one SIJ (or rarely both) is (are) subluxated, then the adjustive contact is on the sacrum so that normal movement is restored to both the lumbosacral articulation and the SIJ(s).

Knowing this, the practitioner should first assess L5–S1, then each SIJ, the symphysis when indicated, and then the remainder of the spinal segments above. The following description of segmental assessment is sequenced in this manner. The sacrococcygeal joint will only be assessed when specifically indicated by a history of trauma or of a pain history implicating the coccyx.

L5–S1

The patient is seated. Typically, the first movement to be lost with subluxation at L5 is flexion and extension, therefore the patient is asked to bend forward as far as possible, until the L5 segment is maximally flexed. The practitioner may either stand beside the patient with the indifferent hand on the shoulder to guide the patient and the palpating finger of the contact hand in the space under the L5 spinous, or kneel behind the patient and palpate in that space with the thumb. At maximal flexion the spinous is provoked into further flexion. Restricted flexion is quite apparent by reduced movement of the spinous and tenderness on provocation.

The patient is then asked to sit up and lean backwards over the palpatory contact while the practitioner feels for closure of the spinous process on the sacrum. Typically, a small, pain-free movement into extension will be found in association with a painful restriction into flexion. This suggests the L5 segment is subluxated in extension, which gives it a posterior (P) component.

It is reasonable to assess the movement of L5 in lateral flexion in the same manner as previously described for segments above; however, it is difficult to draw a conclusion as to the position of the spinous in relation to the side of open wedge without reference to the AP lumbopelvic radiograph. Typically the side of the open wedge at levels above L5–S1 will be on the side of any convexity associated with scoliotic curvature and the spinous will usually move to the side of open wedge, allowing for side-lying placement of the patient on the concave side of the scoliotic curve and an adjustive contact on the spinous process. In summary, in the side-lying patient for adjustment, the concavity of the scoliosis is down and the side of segmental open disk wedge is up. There are cases in the segments above where the spinous will move to the side of the closed wedge, in which case the patient is still placed in the same manner but the adjustive contact is taken on the mamillary process on the side of convexity so that the adjustive force remains on the side of open wedge and on the side of convexity. These are the principles discussed in Chapter 3.

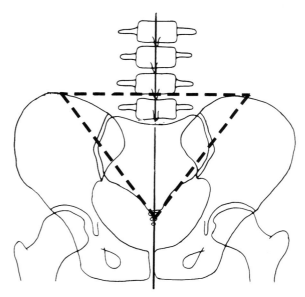

Figure 14.9 The lumbosacral triangle incorporates L4, L5, each ilia, and the sacrum. Assessment must determine the sites of fixation as being L4 on L5, L5 on S1, a sacroiliac joint, or any combination. From Schafer (1983), with permission of ACA Press and Frank M Painter, DC.

The L5–S1 SMU behaves in a more complex manner than those above in that the side of the open wedge may not correlate with the side of convexity of any lumbar scoliosis, while the spinous may still move to either the side of open wedge or the side of closed wedge. This introduces two additional concepts for adjusting L5: namely, while the concave side of any lumbar scoliosis is always placed downwards, the open wedge of the L5–S1 disk may also be down. The adjustive contacts are suitably amended to be the spinous process if it is on the side of the closed wedge (which would also be the side of convexity), or the mamillary process on the side of convexity if the spinous has moved to the concave (down) side (the side of concavity). The end-result is that the adjustive contact is always taken with precedence to the convex side of any scoliosis and on the side of convexity, with secondary consideration of the side of open disk wedge. These additional options seem only to occur at L5 and are extremely difficult to discern from palpation alone.

It is quite difficult to assess movement of the L5 spinous in rotation in the seated patient and the more consistent clinical information seems to be derived from the assessment of this parameter with the patient prone. The practitioner's thumbs are used to induce a left–right movement of the L5 spinous to simulate the minimal amount of rotation which is possible at L5. The findings of movement are integrated with the report of pain and tenderness by the patient to determine any component of "spinous right" or "spinous left".

The sacrum

Positional change in the sacrum is rarely used to infer dysfunction in the SIJ; rather, it reflects unique disrelationships with L5 above. The typical SMU in the regions above is assessed with consideration of the superior segment's perceived relationship on the inferior segment. This convention does not hold at the lumbosacral junction because it is a major point of inflexion, meaning that, while the lumbar spine flexes anteriorly, there are conditions under which the sacrum will break the pattern and counternutate. This produces a palpable movement of the sacral alar to the posterior in the seated patient when he or she flexes fully forward. The movement of the sacrum is variable and it may nutate during the initial stages of trunk flexion (Lee 2000 p. 49). The axis of rotation of the sacrum is within the interosseous ligament.

Conversely, when the seated patient extends the lumbar spine by leaning fully backwards, the sacrum nutates so that the sacral base moves anteroinferiorly and the apex moves posterosuperiorly. These movements are palpated in the seated patient with a bilateral thumb contact over each PSIS on to each sacral alar, while instructing the patient to bend fully forward and then sit up and bend backwards over the thumbs. The fingers rest on the ilia. If it is difficult to ascertain kinematic change then the seated patient can be asked to stand while the sacral alars are palpated. The sacrum moves into nutation when moving from supine lying to standing (Lee 2000 p. 49).

The posterior movement of the sacral base during seated trunk flexion accentuates any fixation of L5 (with reference to the spinous). Importantly, it facilitates determination of whether the sacrum has equal bilateral movement or whether it is unilaterally fixed with reference to L5.

The alar of the sacrum may be listed "posterior" when it is palpated as moving posteriorly while the patient flexes forward, but does not palpate as moving anteriorly when he or she extends backwards over the thumbs. Conversely it is listed "anterior" when it is palpated as moving anteriorly when the patient extends backwards but does not move posteriorly when the patient flexes forward. These listings of anterior or posterior may be a unilateral finding, in which case it is identified as being either left or right, or a bilateral finding, in which case the sacrum is listed as either a base posterior or base anterior.

It is advisable to seek further information from the lateral radiograph before determining a listing of either base anterior or base posterior. The radiograph will demonstrate a parallel L5–S1 disk space and a reduced lumbar lordosis with a base posterior sacrum, and an increased lumbar disk angle with an increased lumbar lordosis with a base anterior sacrum.

There is no real value in attempting to assess the sacrum with rotation of the lumbosacral spine in the seated position for the reason that, when seated, the separation of the ischial tuberosities is accompanied by an approximation of the iliac crests and this increases the form closure about the sacrum and reduces its movement. Also, the concept of tilt about the z-axis is more a postural finding or a radiographic indication and, while not really relevant to determining adjustive technique, may be clinically useful for assessing leg length and considering a heel lift.

The movement of the sacrum is a complex matter and there is considerable difference among authors, largely due to the perspective from which they see the movement and the reference points they elect to use to describe it. Plaugher (1993 p. 153) states: "when sitting or standing, forward flexion of the trunk causes the sacral base to pivot anteriorly and inferiorly, while the apex moves posterior and superiorly". Peterson & Bergmann (2002 p. 319) state: "lumbosacral extension does involve anteroinferior movement of the sacral base". They go on to describe motion palpation tests, such as the sacral push, which reflects that the sacral base moves anteriorly when the seated patient extends.

Lee (2000 p. 49) considers counternutation (the posterior movement of the sacral base) occurs in some patients towards the end of forward bending of the trunk, which is consistent with Peterson & Bergmann. On the other hand, DonTigny (1997) suggests there is a tendency for the sacrum to nutate on the stabilized innominate bones with flexion of the lumbar spine, and to counternutate with extension, probably on a transverse axis.

Snijders et al (1997) describe their "click-clack" phenomenon and state "movement into nutation or counternutation (related to lumbar extension and lumbar flexion respectively) is primarily connected with the inclination of the trunk in the gravity field". This is also inferred by Harrison et al (2002b), who demonstrated that thoracic cage anterior-posterior translations cause significant changes in the lumbar curve and pelvic tilt. It is quite clear that the movement characteristics are not only incompletely known, but that existing descriptions utilize different reference points.

The ilium

The PSIS is the reference point on the ilium for palpatory assessment of the kinematics of the SIJ. Notwithstanding the complexities of movement about the SIJ, the PSIS can be easily assessed for its movement about the *x*-axis and the *y*-axis. The movement of the PSIS is empirically considered to be a good indicator of fixation within the SIJ. Pain alone is a poor indicator, given the complex patterns of referred pain to the area of the SIJ, sacrum, and buttock from other structures in this region (see Assessment of connective tissue change, below). In particular, pain from a hypertonic tensor fascia lata refers about the PSIS and can mimic SIJ pain and dysfunction (see Assessment of muscle change, below).

It must be noted that the SIJ may exhibit dysfunction due to either ligamentous or articular causes, and that the dysfunction may well be hypermobility as opposed to the hypomobility expected with a dysfunctional joint assessed within the "fixation" model. Further, any fixation may be more ligamentous than articular, therefore presenting further challenges to the clinician. These options are depicted in the algorithm given in Figure 14.10. The discussion below assumes that hypermobility has been ruled out and the practitioner is assessing the SIJ for hypomobility or fixation. Hypermobility is suspected when one joint demonstrates greater movement than the other, yet the other demonstrates normal movement with no evidence of ligamentous or articular fixation. Ligamentous laxity, with increased

SIJ mobility, is a normal feature during and after pregnancy and should not be considered pathological.

The difference between ligamentous fixation and articular fixation is quite difficult to discern, and also reflects the individual practitioner's paradigm of practice. Some may categorize most fixation as ligamentous and utilize low-force procedures such as biomechanical wedges or blocking. Others may perceive all fixation as articular and apply high-velocity, low-amplitude (HVLA) adjustive thrusts in every case. There is a middle ground and it probably reflects the severity of the findings and becomes a matter for individual judgment. The point of the following discussion is to apply Pletain's (1997) structured approach in a manner which informs the reader that there are ligamentous contributions to SIJ dysfunction and the better approach is probably one which takes these into account, along with any perception of articular dysfunction.

The SIJ – PI or AS

Movement about the *x*-axis is assessed with the patient standing, preferably beside a bench or chair-back so that the patient may hold it with one hand for support. Prior to making contact, the practitioner demonstrates to the patient the manner in which the leg is raised, namely with the knee straight, and slowly from the floor, through 45°, and then to the point of maximal comfort or ability. The straight leg gives the tests greater sensitivity; however, if patients are unable to do this, then they may raise their leg with the knee bent.

The thumbs are placed as shown in Figure 14.11A. The left thumb contacts the S2 tubercle while the left hand lies gently around the buttock below the iliac crest. The left thumb is the reference point for movement of the right thumb which contacts the right PSIS to assess the right SIJ. The right hand and fingers similarly lie gently around the right buttock.

The patient is asked to raise the right leg. The subsequent sequence of expected events is:

- The instant the right foot comes off the floor, the pelvis will raise on the right side as the left gluteus medius and gluteus minimus contract. The purpose is to allow the right foot to clear the floor as if the patient were to commence walking. This is actually a variant of Trendelenburg's test and failure of the pelvis to raise, or if the pelvis tilts downwards on the right, is a positive finding for weak adductors on the left (Evans 2001 pp. 738–739).
- As the leg is raised to about 45°, the right PSIS moves posterior and inferior (PI) with reference to S2, which remains stable.
- At about 45° the ilium will "catch" on the sacrum at the SIJ and, as the leg is raised higher, both the right PSIS and the S2 tubercle will move downwards (PI) together.

The patient then replaces the leg and is instructed to move it straight backwards. This produces extension at the hip and the expected finding is:

- the PSIS will move anterior and superior (AS) with reference to a stable S2.

The patient replaces the right leg. To continue the assessment for the left SIJ the practitioner changes contacts so the left thumb is on the left PSIS and the right thumb becomes the reference

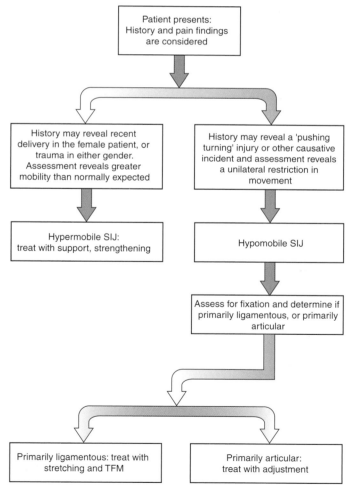

Figure 14.10 A diagnostic approach to the sacroiliac joint (SIJ). TFM, transverse friction massage.

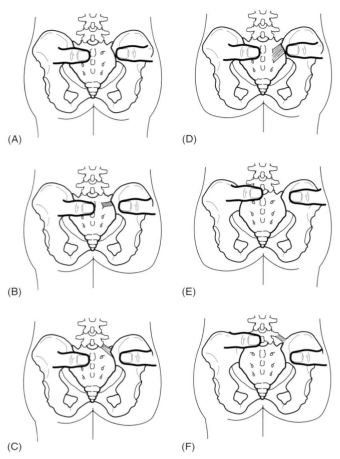

(A)

(B)

(C)

(D)

(E)

(F)

Figure 14.11 Palpation of the sacroiliac joint (SIJ). (A) The basic contacts for standing palpation of the right SIJ. The left thumb palpates the S2 tubercle as the reference point, while the right thumb palpates the right posterior superior iliac spine (PSIS), while the right leg is raised. (B) Findings suggestive of fixation in the horizontal ligament fibers are no movement of the PSIS downwards compared to S2 in the early stage of leg raising. (C) Findings suggestive of fixation in the oblique downwards fibers are downwards movement in the early stage of leg raising for both the S2 tubercle and the PSIS. (D) Findings suggestive of fixation in the oblique upwards fibers are no movement of the S2 tubercle against the PSIS when the contralateral leg is raised past 45°. (E) When both SIJs are functioning normally, raising the contralateral (in this case, left) leg while palpating S2 and the right PSIS will show no movement of S2 in comparison with the right PSIS until the left leg passes through about 45°. At this point the left SIJ will "catch" the sacrum and then draw down S2 in comparison to the right PSIS as the left leg is raised further. (F) The thumb contact is moved to the L5 spinous and findings suggestive of iliolumbar ligament involvement are movement of the spinous to the left as the right left is raised. (A–F) From Pletain (1997), with permission.

point on S2. The patient raises the left leg and the same sequence and findings are expected for the left PSIS.

The listings which may be found are:

- PI: the ilium is considered to be fixed in a PI position when it is palpated as moving into a posterior inferior position but not into an anterior superior position. In other words, the PSIS will move backwards on to the thumb as the leg is raised but will not disappear anteriorly when the leg is extended.

- AS: the ilium is considered to be fixed in an AS position when it is palpated as moving into an anterior superior position but not a posterior inferior position. In other words, the PSIS will move anteriorly away from the thumb when the leg is extended, but will not palpate as moving PI on to the thumb as the leg is raised.

Pletain (1997) identifies a range of subtle changes to the expected sequence described above and associates these with various ligamentous findings. The following discussion is with reference to the right SIJ.

The first variant is that the PSIS fails to move downwards relative to S2 in the early phase of raising the right leg (Fig. 14.11B). This is considered to indicate fixation in the horizontal fibers across the posterior aspect of the SIJ. These are probably the cranial band of the deep layer of the interosseous ligament (Cramer & Darby 1995 p. 228).

The second variant is for S2 to move downwards with the right PSIS in the early phase of raising the right leg (Fig. 14.11C). This is considered to indicate fixation in the oblique downwards fibers across the posterior aspect of the SIJ. These are probably the fibers of the short posterior sacroiliac ligament (Cramer & Darby 1995 p. 237). Contracture of these ligaments would tighten the right SIJ so the right ilium and sacrum would move as one on the left ilium.

A third variant is noted when the left leg is raised while still palpating the right SIJ with the same contacts (Fig. 14.11D). When both SIJs are functioning normally it is expected that there will be no movement of S2 with reference to the right PSIS during the early phase of left-leg raising. When the left leg has passed through 45° and has "caught" the sacrum, it draws it downwards with the left PSIS (Fig. 14.11E) as the left leg is raised higher.

The clinical variant is that the S2 tubercle fails to move downwards relative to the right PSIS after the left leg has passed through 45°. It is thought that this indicates a fixation in the oblique upwards fibers of the right SIJ and these are also probably differently oriented bands of the short posterior sacroiliac ligaments (Chaitow & DeLany 2002 p. 305). Contracture of these fibers would draw the sacrum towards the right PSIS and resist its downwards movement secondary to the raising of the left leg.

A fourth and important variant involves the iliolumbar ligament. The reference point is now the L5 spinous process and the left thumb is moved to that position (Fig. 14.11F). As the right leg is raised, the L5 spinous process may rotate to the left. This is considered to indicate fixation in the right iliolumbar ligament as it connects between the right ilia and the L5 transverse process. As the right PSIS moves PI it draws the L5 transverse process and body to the right, causing the spinous to rotate to the left.

If the findings from the above procedures are equivocal and there is doubt as to whether it is the left or right SIJ which is subluxated, the status of the ischial tuberosity flare can provide an indication.

The patient remains standing and the practitioner changes contacts. The reference point is now the S4 sacral tubercle and the contact point is the ischial tuberosity, firstly of one innominate and then of the other. The right thumb contacts the right ischial tuberosity while the left thumb palpates S4, and vice versa for the left.

The patient is asked to raise the leg again from the ground. As the leg reaches its maximum height the innominate is expected to tilt so the iliac crest moves medially and the ischial tuberosity moves laterally. This is a replication of the movements associated with sitting which require the hip to be flexed towards 90°, which in turn causes the ischial tuberosities to flare to broaden the sitting base.

In the standing patient the ischial tuberosity on the side of a normal SIJ will flare outwards, away from the reference thumb, towards the end of leg raising. Failure of the ischial tuberosity to flare in this manner is indicative of dysfunction within the SIJ of that side, probably in the inferior aspect of the joint.

The SIJ – In or Ex

The final component of the SIJ listing is an indication of whether the ilium is fixated in a closed position on to the SIJ, representing internal rotation (In) of the PSIS (and external rotation of the ilium about the y-axis as discussed earlier), or whether it is fixated in an open position, representing external rotation (Ex) of the PSIS. The characteristics of the two listings are:

- In: the PSIS is considered to have rotated medially or internally to close the SIJ when it is palpated as moving easier in a medial direction than in a lateral direction at the SIJ.
- Ex: the PSIS is considered to have rotated laterally or externally to open the SIJ when it is palpated as moving easier in a lateral direction than in a medial direction at the SIJ.

The patient is placed prone and the practitioner takes a square stance at the level of the pelvis. The following description is for the right SIJ with the practitioner standing on the right.

The practitioner's right or cephalad hand palpates the right SIJ. The first and second fingers lie over the PSIS and on to the right alar of the sacrum, with a slight pressure laterally against the medial border of the PSIS. The left or caudad hand takes the patient's ankle and flexes the knee to 90°. It then moves the leg away from the practitioner so that it crosses the midline of the patient and externally rotates the femur, drawing the right ilium after it, thus emphasizing a medial or internal rotation of the PSIS on to the right SIJ.

The leg is then drawn towards the practitioner and pressed outwards so as to rotate the femur internally and draw the right PSIS laterally into external rotation at the right SIJ. The end-feel movement of the PSIS is important in both cases to give the better indication of the state of any rotation of the ilium about the y-axis as it may affect the SIJ.

In the case of an Ex listing, the PSIS will appear to move laterally or externally as the leg is drawn towards the practitioner but will not appear to close or move medially and internally as the leg is taken over the midline. The findings are reversed for an In listing.

It is also possible that there may be no component of In or Ex and that the listing is simply PI or AS. It should be remembered that the concept of rotation about the y-axis is paradigm-dependent and some practitioners ignore it with respect to listing the SIJ. On the other hand, the findings are clearly palpable and should be considered to complete the assessment of the lumbosacral spine and pelvis.

The SIJ – Lewit's test

Fixation of the SIJ may subtly affect movement of the overlying connective tissues. Lewit & Rosina (1999) have described a test where the practitioner is behind the standing patient and lightly rests the lateral borders of the first finger of each hand on each iliac crest. The hands are deviated to the ulnar side to allow the proximal fingers almost to meet in the midline. The patient is asked to turn the head to one side and the palpating fingers on that side should rise above those opposite. This palpable change in tissue tension is absent when there is restriction in one SIJ (Lewit & Rosina 1999).

The mechanism for the movement is probably the extensive links in the connective tissues between laminae of the thoracolumbar fascia and the ligamentum nuchae. The lack of movement in the presence of SIJ restriction may reflect tension about the long posterior ligament and its connections.

The coccyx

Subluxation of the coccyx is usually secondary to trauma and this should be revealed in the patient history. The coccyx typically subluxates anteriorly with reference to the sacral apex and the findings are pain and tenderness about the sacrococcygeal joint consistent with the history.

The joint may suffer ligamentous strain, in which case external palpation and adjustment are normally sufficient, together with assessment of the surrounding musculature. However, if there is traumatic separation of the joint then internal palpation and adjustment may be indicated. This is an advanced technique which is beyond the scope of this text and it may require lateral radiographs to guide the practitioner better.

The symphysis pubis

The symphysis is the anterior articulation of the pelvic ring and may suffer frank trauma, such as with a fall with spread legs on a gym beam, or more subtle dysfunction secondary to torsional forces generated by dysfunction in the posterior elements. Trauma will be revealed by the history and assessment and treatment will be guided by radiographs. The following discussion relates to identifying the kinematic change present as a secondary effect of lumbopelvic dysfunction.

The symphysis pubis is assessed in the supine patient with express, informed consent. The practitioner should have a chaperone in the room during the procedure regardless of the gender of the patient. The practitioner stands square to the supine patient about the level of the thorax and turns caudad to conduct the examination. The patient should be gowned and wearing underwear, and draped using a towel for modesty.

The palpating contacts are the finger pads of the first and second fingers of each hand. The patient is asked to place their hand in the middle of their pubic bone and keep it there as a reference point. The practitioner's fingers are placed towards the pubic rami, flat on the abdomen, and then gently palpate inferiorly until each pubic tubercle (Fig. 14.1A) is located. When bony contact is made the superior margin of each pubic ramus is palpated to identify zones of pain and tenderness which may indicate myotendinoses at muscle insertions.

The important finding is whether one ramus appears superior to the other. Gentle superior to inferior springing may help discern whether one ramus appears to have rotated superiorly with reference to the other. In other patients an obvious step defect will be palpated across the symphysis itself. Typically, the superior ramus will be reported as tender, and will exhibit a blocked feel to palpation in an inferior direction.

Such a finding would be reported as left (or right) superior pubic ramus. Minor dysfunction at the symphysis pubis typically resolves following adjustment through the lumbopelvic region and/or with the application of various treatment techniques to involved muscles. The joint is assessed after such treatment and, if palpable findings are again found, consideration is given to specific adjustive treatment aimed at the symphysis dysfunction.

Sequencing the assessment

While a full sequence has been described above for the segments in this region, an efficient clinical approach is to:

- start with the patient standing and assess ROM and then each SIJ for flexion/extension fixation
- assess L5 for restriction in flexion and extension in the seated patient
- assess the sacrum by contact on each ala for restriction in flexion and extension in the seated patient
- assess L5 for restriction in lateral flexion in the seated patient
- assess the segments of the spine above if indicated
- place the patient prone and assess for fixation in rotation at L5
- assess the sacrum for posterior to anterior springiness
- assess each SIJ for internal/external fixation
- assess the sacrococcygeal junction if indicated
- place the patient supine and assess the symphysis pubis if indicated.

This is a smooth sequence of assessment with structured patient placement from standing to seated, prone, then supine. Other assessments may be included as appropriate with each patient position. An ordered approach in this manner prevents patients feeling as if they are on a rotisserie.

ASSESSMENT OF CONNECTIVE TISSUE CHANGE

The L5–S1 and then L4–5 disks generate the most obvious connective tissue involvement in this region and their assessment is inseparable from that for neural and muscle change. This section will provide a basic discussion on the disk for integration with the following explanation of clinical procedures. The iliolumbar ligament is unique to this region, while many of the other ligaments about the SMU have been previously discussed, so only a brief summary will appear here. The ligaments about the SIJ have been introduced above during the assessment for kinematic change, and the thoracolumbar fascia, discussed in the previous chapter, remains particularly important.

The intervertebral disk

Kirkaldy-Willis developed a schema of the phases of degenerative change associated with altered biomechanics and ordered these as dysfunction, the unstable phase, and the stabilization phase (Kirkaldy-Willis 1992b). The contemporary work of Adams et al (2002) formalizes a four-point grading system for disk degeneration (Box 2.1) and this is particularly relevant to the L5–S1 and L4–5 disks.

The grade 2 disks do not distribute loading evenly on to the vertebral body and nearly always concentrate stress in certain regions, usually posterior to the nucleus. The grade 3 disk demonstrates moderate degenerative change, including the annulus bulging into the nucleus and structural disruption to the endplates. It is in this stage that disk protrusion and extrusion occur. It must be appreciated that herniation does not always involve the nucleus, and may consist only of annular fibers (Lebkowski & Dzieciol 2002). The fourth stage is severe degeneration and Kirkaldy-Willis sees this as a stabilization phase.

It is clearly not possible to reverse severe degenerative change; however, treatment may well be directed at restoring movement to some degree, along with normalizing the supporting musculature. It appears likely that the assessment and intervention of the manual physician is most effective in both the grade 2 and 3 stages and it could be argued that greater efficiency and benefits would be derived from early detection of grade 2 change which may be associated with small degrees of kinematic change.

The process of disk degeneration includes disruption to the annular fibers (Fig. 14.12) as well as the nucleus (Fig. 14.13). If the nucleus is contained by the fibers of the disk or the posterior longitudinal ligament, the bulge is termed a protrusion. It may be focal or broad-based and is described by location (Fig. 14.14). The posteromedial (Fig. 14.14B) and posterolateral (Fig. 14.14D)

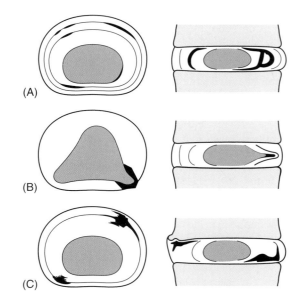

(A)

(B)

(C)

Figure 14.12 Types of annular damage. The disrupted annular tissue is shown in black and the nucleus in gray. The sagittal sections (right) show the anterior of the disk on the left. (A) Concentric clefts; (B) radial fissures with distortion of the nucleus; (C) peripheral rim tears. (A–C) From Adams et al (2002), with permission.

protrusions are most common. When the nuclear material penetrates through damaged fibers it is termed an extrusion, and if a piece of material separates, it is a sequestration (Fig. 14.13). Once disk material comes into contact with epidural tissue, it is considered to be uncontained (Ito et al 2001).

The locators "medial" and "lateral" are with respect to the affected nerve root: if the protrusion is medial to the nerve root it will press on the nerve from medial to lateral and the patient will

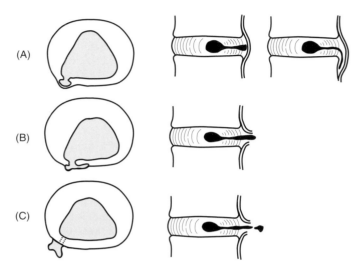

Figure 14.13 Categories of disk prolapse. (A) The prolapsed nucleus may be contained under the annular fibers and posterior longitudinal ligament, in which case it is a protrusion. It may be focal, as shown, or broad-based. The sagittal sections show it may be contained at the level of the disk or travel either superiorly or inferiorly (shown) beneath the ligament. (B) The annular fibers may rupture and nuclear material may extrude into the spinal canal. It may do this through ruptured posterior longitudinal ligament fibers, or around the margins of the ligament. (C) When displaced nuclear material loses contact with the remaining nucleus, it is termed a sequestration. The sequestered fragment may be mobile within the spinal canal. (A–C) Modified from Adams et al (2002), with permission.

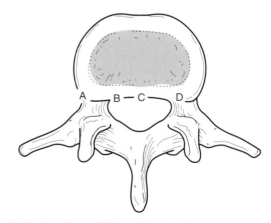

Figure 14.14 Locations of disk prolapse. (A) The far lateral or extraforaminal protrusion is not common. (B) The posteromedial protrusion (left or right) is relatively common. (C) The posterocentral protrusion may be quite focal or diffuse and broad-based across the entire posterior margin of the disk. (D) The posterolateral protrusion may extend into the contained area of the intervertebral canal, in which case it becomes a foraminal protrusion.

lean laterally in an attempt to move the nerve root laterally, away from the protrusion. On postural assessment the patient will be seen with an antalgic lean towards the side of the painful leg (Fig. 14.15A). The leg pain will increase if the patient attempts to straighten (Fig. 14.15B), as this action will move the nerve root medially back on to the protrusion.

The converse is found with a posterolateral protrusion. The patient will adopt an antalgic lean away from the involved leg (Fig. 14.15C) in an attempt to draw the nerve root medially away from the posterolateral protrusion. When the patient leans towards the involved leg (Fig. 14.15D), the nerve root shifts laterally on to the protrusion and replicates the pain. Clinically, the first step is to identify the involved leg and the second is to determine whether the pain increases by leaning more towards the involved leg (posterolateral protrusion) or decreases (posteromedial).

The disk is therefore implicated as a cause of nerve root pain by physically and chemically altering the environment within the spinal canal or IVC and directly irritating the spinal nerve. The resultant pain is typically unilateral nerve root pain and, in this region, the low lumbar and upper sacral nerve roots are affected. The pain may be sudden-onset, as in the case of significant disk damage secondary to traumatic overload, gradual-onset with repetitive injury, or insidious, as with degenerative change. Given that the nerve root pain is felt into the thigh and leg, the presence or absence of leg pain in the patient with low-back pain is an important clinical clue.

The disk itself may be a source of pain, in which case the patient should report a localized low-back pain. This may be acute from traumatic injury to the disk, in which case it will either have the characteristics of a strain/sprain pain or of significant disk injury, such as endplate fracture. The onset of strain/sprain pain will be worsening several hours after the injury to reflect the

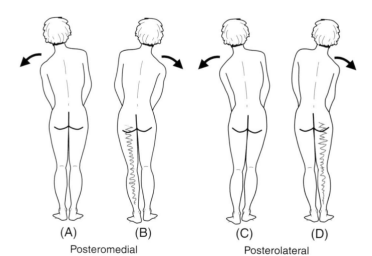

(A)	(B)	(C)	(D)
Posteromedial		Posterolateral	

Figure 14.15 Antalgic posture with discogenic nerve root pain. (A) With a posteromedial disk protrusion the patient adopts an antalgic lean towards the involved leg (in this case, left). (B) When the patient with a posteromedial protrusion leans away from the involved leg, the leg pain is worsened as the involved nerve root is drawn on to the posteromedial protrusion. (C) With a posterolateral disk protrusion the patient adopts an antalgic lean away from the involved leg (in this case, right). (D) When the patient with a posterolateral protrusion leans towards the involved leg, the leg pain is worsened as the involved nerve root is drawn on to the posterolateral protrusion.

inflammation and swelling, whereas the pain of significant disk injury will be immediate and disabling and usually with neurologic signs. Internal disk disruption includes inflammatory degradation of the disk matrix and may follow repetitive trauma such as axial compression and torque, as is common in many sports (Cooke & Lutz 2000).

The disk may also give rise to chronic pain from the slow processes of degenerative change. Internal disruption of the disk is accompanied by nociceptive nerve growth and the resultant pain is dull and vague about the low back. This pain is complicated by associated changes in the supportive tissues which in themselves may then become pain generators.

The zygapophyseal joints

The zygapophyseal joints have been adequately described in preceding chapters. Their role in this region is important, especially within the transitional lumbosacral articulation. In essence they block axial rotation and forward sliding of the vertebrae, thus protecting the disk. Cramer & Darby (1995 pp. 26–28) identify them as pain generators and they are implicated with spinal pain which worsens on extension.

Pain will be local about the involved joint and may refer into the ipsilateral buttock and thigh. Kirkaldy-Willis et al (1992) suggest the pain may also refer below the knee to the calf, ankle, foot, and even toes. Cox (1999) considers it is unusual for the pain to reach below the knee and rare for it to reach the foot. The mechanism is probably scleratogenous and the characteristic of the referred pain is that it is dull, diffuse, and poorly localized. It has been suggested that the distance the pain radiates down the leg depends on the amount of facet irritation and the period of time irritation has been present (Mooney & Robertson 1976).

Pain arising from the zygapophyseal joints is termed "facet syndrome" and is of two distinctly different types and mechanisms. The first is acute, which involves entrapment of the meniscus between the facets. The patient will report a sudden onset of intense pain, usually when straightening up from forward bending, with or without loading. The pain is unilateral and the patient will be antalgic away from the involved side. There is no neurological involvement and the pain is typically localized around the facet and into the buttock, with perhaps a radiation to the groin. This presentation responds well to HVLA adjustment which opens the facets to allow the release of the trapped meniscoid fold.

The second presentation is chronic in nature and develops secondary to degeneration. It may be hastened by the transfer of weight to the posterior column with increased lordosis and typically demonstrates facet hypertrophy with other changes on radiograph. Neurologic signs may be present, depending on the degree of bony remodeling and subsequent compromise of neural structures.

Kemp's test is an appropriate diagnostic test to help implicate a facet syndrome, although care must be taken with this procedure in the acute patient. The patient is seated and the practitioner's fingers form a fulcrum at the level and side of the suspected facet. The indifferent hand stabilizes the patient's shoulder and controls the movement. Given that the aim is to increase axial compression in the spine through extension, the test will also be positive for disk disruption.

As the patient is extended and laterally flexed over the fulcrum, the reported pain must be considered as to whether it is dermatomal or diffuse. If dermatomal, then the cause is probably disk; if diffuse, then the cause may be facet. The onset of diffuse pain early in extension is more suggestive of facet involvement (Brier 1999).

Ligaments of the SMU

The discussion in the previous chapter is generally applicable to the ligaments of the SMU in this region. The anterior longitudinal ligament becomes widest in this region, attaching across the anterior aspects of the vertebral bodies and disks to attach inferiorly to the sacrum. The posterior longitudinal ligament is highly sensitive to pain and flares laterally at the level of each disk where it attaches to the posterior aspect of the annulus. In some cases the dura mater attaches firmly to the posterior longitudinal ligament in this region (Iwamura et al 2001).

The ligamentum flavum forms the anterior capsule of the zygapophyseal joint and attaches to the articular processes. The nerve roots are in direct contact with the anterior surface of these ligaments as they exit the IVC. The L5 nerve roots are particularly susceptible to compromise from hypertrophied ligamenta flava (Cramer & Darby 1995). The ligaments may undergo myxomatous degeneration, producing a mass which has been reported as acutely compressing the lumbar nerve root (Yoshii et al 2001).

There is a small ligament running between the mamillary and accessory processes, forming an open groove through which the medial branch of the lumbar dorsal root passes. Ossification of this ligament was first reported by Chinese investigators in 1978 and a 1991 study of Europeans reported a frequency of 26.4% on the left and 13.5% on the right at L5 (Maigne et al 1991). Such changes introduce the possibility of mechanical interference with the nerve at this point.

The supraspinous ligament typically ends at L5, although Cramer & Darby (1995 p. 208) cite authors who variously report that it ends at L4 or the sacrum. In this region it is a strong condensation of the thoracolumbar fascia and is probably better thought of as being a restraint to flexion more than a ligament. It is thought the posterior border of the ligamentum flavum becomes the supraspinous ligament which in turn is anchored to the thoracolumbar fascia (Lee 2000 p. 28). The thoracolumbar fascia has been discussed in the preceding chapter. The interplay between the fascia and the ligaments in this region is shown in Figure 14.16.

The interspinous ligament has been shown to demonstrate sprain or frank rupture on T-weighted, fat-suppressed MRI studies at the lumbosacral junction (Jinkins 2002) and this has an observational incidence in patients with low-back pain. The transforaminal ligaments, discussed in the preceding chapter, are generally stronger in the upper lumbar region than in the lower levels (Amonoo-Kuofi et al 1988).

The iliolumbar ligament

This important ligament arises from the transverse processes of L5 and sometimes L4, and attaches to the sacrum and iliac crests of the same side. It exists as a series of bands, one of which attaches between the body of L5 and the sacral ala, and another of which attaches to the iliac crest in front of the SIJ (Fig. 14.17A).

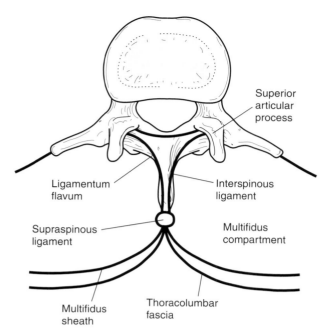

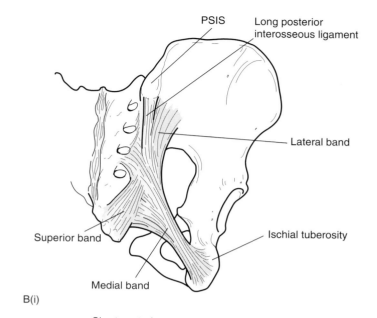

B(i)

Figure 14.16 Transverse view of the interplay among ligaments. A transverse view through a lumbar vertebra illustrating the interspinous–supraspinous–thoracolumbar ligamentous complex. By anchoring the thoracolumbar fascia and multifidus sheath to the facet joint capsules, the complex becomes the central support system for the lumbar spine. Modified from Vleeming et al (1997a), with permission.

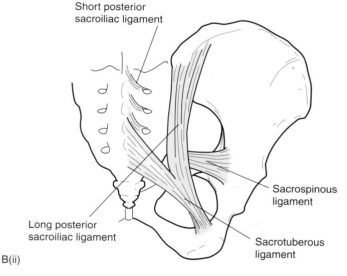

B(ii)

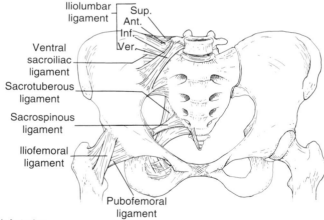

(A) Anterior

Figure 14.17 Ligaments of the pelvic girdle. (A) The anterior of the sacroiliac joint is covered by the anterior or ventral sacroiliac ligament and by the lower bands of the iliolumbar ligament. (B) The sacrotuberous ligament consists of three bands which come to lie over the long posterior interosseous ligament (posterior i). It acts to restrict nutation of the sacrum. The long dorsal ligament (posterior ii) runs between the inferolateral margins of the posterior superior iliac spine (PSIS) and the lower transverse tubercle of the lateral sacral crest. It acts to oppose the sacrotuberous ligament and restrict counternutation of the sacrum. (C) A transverse section of the sacroiliac joint (SIJ) shows the relationships of the articular capsule and the supportive ligaments. (D) The ligaments of the symphysis pubis. (A) From Lee (2000), with permission; (B) from Vleeming et al (1997a), with permission; (C) from Cramer & Darby (1995), with permission. (D) From Lee (2000), with permission.

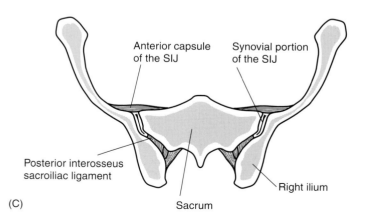

(C)

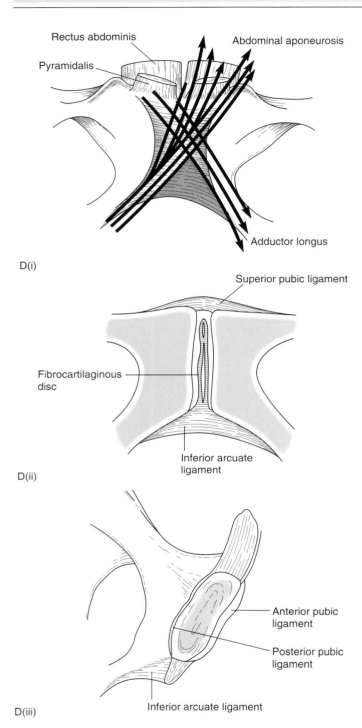

D(i)

D(ii)

D(iii)

Figure 14.17 (*Continued*).

Fibers arise along the entire anteroinferior aspect and the tip of the L5 transverse process.

The structure of the ligament in the newborn was claimed to be muscular by Luk et al (1986), who also reported it was formed by metaplasia of the fibers of the quadratus lumborum and became ligamentous from the second decade. More recent findings suggest it exists in the fetus as a true ligament (Lee 2000 p. 29). Uhtoff (1993) has shown it is always present at the gestational age of 11–15 weeks.

There are conflicting reports of its structure. A 1994 report by Hanson & Sonesson could only find two parts or bands from the L5 transverse process. Hanson et al also reported (1998) that the ligament is a single, markedly longer and wider band in Black people and a shorter, two-band structure in whites. The horizontal and vertical angles also varied greatly between white and Black subjects; however, Rucco et al (1996) suggest the spatial disposition of the ligament is a normal variant depending on the depth to which L5 sits in the pelvis.

It functions as a strong stabilizer of the lumbosacral junction in both the frontal and sagittal planes, limiting rotation and becoming more important as the L5–S1 disk degenerates and the disk space narrows. Flexion of L5 on S1 is mainly controlled by the posterior band, and lateral bending by the anterior band (Leong et al 1987). A sacroiliac part has been identified which arises on the sacrum and blends with the interosseous sacroiliac ligaments (Pool-Goudzwaard et al 2001). These fibers also contribute to the direct restraining effect the ligament has on movement in the SIJ.

Cramer & Darby (1995 pp. 208–209) identify it as a probable primary pain generator due to its innervation by the posterior primary division of the spinal nerves. Its pain referral pattern is about the ipsilateral iliac crest, the lateral hip, and wrapping to the medial thigh and groin (Fig. 14.18A). A trigger point has been thought to exist as a painful insertion of the iliolumbar ligament some 7–8 cm from the midline; however, Maigne & Maigne (1991) have shown that the ligament is not palpable at this location and that the trigger point likely corresponds to pain elicited from a cutaneous dorsal ramus from the thoracolumbar junction which crosses the iliac crest at this point.

Ligaments about the sacroiliac joint

The SIJ only has a joint capsule at the anterior margins. It is lined with a synovial membrane and innervated by nociceptive and proprioceptive nerve endings (Cramer & Darby 1995 p. 228). The anterior sacroiliac ligament is little more than a thickening of the joint capsule and cannot be distinguished from it on imaging (Jaovisidha et al 1996). There are horizontal fibers crossing the joint and intermingling with the capsule. It is the weakest of the ligaments about the SIJ (Fig. 14.17C), although it does function to limit rotation about the x-axis (Wang & Dumas 1998).

The ligament is a pain generator and will reproduce the pain when palpated or stressed. It is palpated deeply about 2.5 cm medially to the ASIS. Care is taken as it may be quite tender. The ligament is stressed in the supine patient as the practitioner presses laterally on each ASIS to open the anterior aspect of the SIJ.

The interosseous ligament is the strongest ligament of the SIJ and runs between three fossae on the sacrum, and the ilium. It has a deep cranial band which lies horizontally and a deep caudal band which lies more vertically. The superficial bands are membranous and lie under the long and short posterior (dorsal) sacroiliac ligaments. A small band is commonly found to run between the superior aspects of the sacral and iliac articular surfaces as the superior intracapsular ligament or Illi's ligament (Freeman et al 1990).

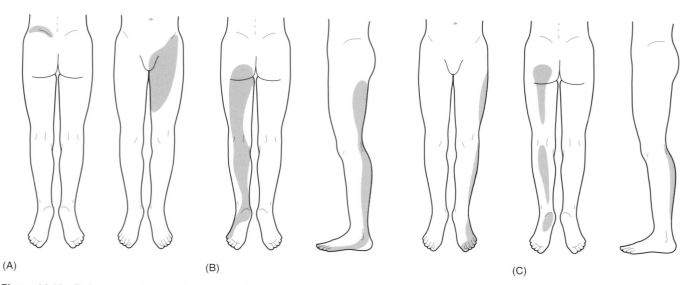

Figure 14.18 Referred pain from pelvic ligaments. The pattern of referred pain from: (A) the iliolumbar ligament; (B) the sacrotuberous ligament; (C) sacrospinous ligament. (A–C) From Dorman (1997), with permission.

Two distinct bands form the posterior sacroiliac ligament (Fig. 14.17 B(i), (ii)). The short band runs in a horizontal plane between the sacral tubercles of S1 and S2 and the medial aspect of the posterior surface of the iliac crest and iliac tuberosity.

The long band, known as the long posterior (or dorsal) sacroiliac ligament, runs vertically downwards from the PSIS to intermingle with the sacrotuberous ligament. It plays an essential role in limiting counternutation of the sacrum. Medially the fibers attach to the deep lamina of the posterior layer of the thoracolumbar fascia and the aponeurosis of the erector spinae (Lee 2000).

It has close anatomical relations with the erector spinae muscle, the posterior layer of the thoracolumbar fascia, and the tuberoiliac part of the sacrotuberous ligament. It is an important functional link between the legs, spine, and arms and it is tensed by hypertonic erector spinae and with sacral counternutation (Vleeming et al 1996). It is reported that women with peripartum pelvic pain frequently experience pain and tenderness within the boundaries of this ligament (Vleeming et al 2002).

Ligaments about the sacral apex

The sacrotuberous ligament has three large fibrous bands. A lateral band runs between the ischial tuberosity and the posterior inferior iliac spine and receives some fibers from the piriformis as it crosses that muscle. A medial band runs between the transverse tubercles of S4–5 and the lateral margins of the sacrum and coccyx and the ischial tuberosity. A superior band runs between the coccyx and the PSIS (Lee 2000). It merges with the long posterior ligament above and often with the fibers of the biceps femoris below (Fig. 14.17B). The sacrotuberous ligament is considered a generator of pain down the posterolateral thigh and leg, into the lateral foot (Fig. 14.18B).

The sacrospinous ligament runs between the anterior surface of the sacrum about the level of S2–4, to the ischial spine. The superior fibers blend about the SIJ. The ligament is thought to represent a degenerated part of the coccygeus muscle and may be responsible for the secondary coccygodynia experienced by patients with dysfunction of the pelvic ring (Lee 2000). It is also considered a pain generator and its pattern of referral is in a narrow strip down the posterior thigh and leg and perhaps into the heel (Fig. 14.18C).

The sacrococcygeal articulation has a small disk and is supported by a number of ligaments. Posteriorly these run between the cornua of the sacrum and the cornua of the coccyx, and on the dorsal aspect about the filum terminale externum; anteriorly the ventral sacrococcygeal ligament is analogous to the anterior longitudinal ligament; and laterally the ligaments run between the transverse processes of the coccyx to the inferolateral angle of the sacrum (Cramer & Darby 1995). A number of muscles also attach to the coccyx.

Ligaments about the symphysis pubis

The symphysis includes a fibrocartilaginous disk and is supported by a superior pubic ligament which connects the superior borders of the pubic rami, and an inferior arcuate ligament below, which blends with the fibrocartilaginous disk (Fig. 14.17D). The pelvic surface is covered by the posterior pubic ligament which blends with the adjacent periosteum and the anterior aspect is covered by the anterior pubic ligament which is a thick, fibrous band which receives fibers from the aponeurotic expansion of the abdominal musculature as well as the adductor longus muscle (Lee 2000 p. 31).

The fibers in the anterior ligament run both horizontally and obliquely and facilitate the transfer of anterior forces diagonally across the joint between the abdominal muscles and the adductors. These muscle groups must be assessed when examining for any dysfunction about the symphysis.

ASSESSMENT OF MUSCLE CHANGE

Postural changes are an important indicator of muscle involvement through this region and have been discussed earlier, along with gait analysis, which is really the dynamic application of muscle function. An important static finding is that of a lower crossed syndrome (Fig. 14.6) where the posture in the sagittal plane will demonstrate anterior tilting of the pelvis with flexion of the hip joints and exaggeration of the lumbar lordosis. This is due to the tightness and shortening of the iliopsoas, rectus femoris, tensor foscia latae, short adductors of the thigh, and the erector spinae group, in conjunction with weakness and inhibition of the abdominals and gluteal muscles (Chaitow & DeLany 2002 p. 318).

A second important assessment in the patient with low-back pain is the recruitment pattern of hip extension. This is a dynamic assessment of muscle sequencing for the crucial postural and gait tasks of pelvic stabilization and provides important clues as to which muscles should be targeted for further assessment and perhaps strengthening.

The patient is placed prone and the practitioner takes a square stance at the level of the pelvis. The thumb and first finger of the cephalad hand palpate the ipsilateral erector spinae and the contralateral erector spinae respectively, about the level of L3-4. The thumb and first finger of the caudad hand palpate the ipsilateral gluteus maximus and hamstrings respectively. The patient is asked to raise the leg off the table. This induces extension in the ipsilateral hip and the palpating digits attempt to identify the order in which the muscles fire to perform this task.

Chaitow & DeLany argue that the correct recruitment sequence is gluteus maximus, hamstrings, contralateral erector spinae, and then ipsilateral erector spinae (Chaitow & DeLany 2002 p. 322) but acknowledge that practitioners differ in their view of this. They cite Janda as suggesting the poorest recruitment pattern is one which commences with contraction of the ipsilateral erector spinae. On the other hand, clinical scientists Vogt & Banzer (1997) have researched the question and identify the recruitment order of muscles during prone hip extension as ipsilateral erector spinae, semitendinosus, contralateral erector spinae, TFL, then gluteus maximus.

These evidence-based findings obviously pose a problem for the clinical observations, especially that which suggests that delayed activation of the gluteus maximus stresses the region during this activity. There is even greater difficulty in determining the most relevant corrective and rehabilitative actions in the face of what is considered "an altered activation sequence during hip extension" (Liebenson 1996 p. 363) when the found sequence in the patient may well be in accord with the reported normal sequence, yet considered by some to represent dysfunction.

Clearly there are other factors involved and these may be as simple as the finding that exercise intensity and multiple sets alter muscle recruitment patterns of the lumbar and hip extensor muscles (Clark et al 2002). When a prescribed exercise activity was performed, the electromyogram (EMG) activity of biceps femoris was significantly greater than that of the paraspinal muscles at 50% exercise intensity. When the intensity increased to 70% there was no difference between the muscles. Further, gluteus maximus activity increased as the number of sets of exercise increased, while there were decrements in the activity of the paraspinal muscles. Other confounders could be the reduced activity of the gluteus maximus in patients with chronic low-back pain (Leinonen et al 2000) and the differences in time-to-fatigue between male and female subjects (Kankaanpaa et al 1998). Admittedly, EMG activity is a different parameter to initial firing; however, the finding that activity levels are variable suggests that different patterns could be found in recruitment sequencing.

In clinical terms it is appropriate to assess recruitment order during prone hip extension but the interpretation of the findings should be made in conjunction with strength and function assessment of each muscle group as well as other clinical findings such as postural imbalance in an attempt to identify pathologic involvement.

Prior to proceeding to assess the following specific muscles, the practitioner should review the longissimus and iliocostalis, along with the smaller back extensors and the quadratus lumborum, for function, strength, and trigger point pain referral.

Piriformis

The piriformis generates leg pain in a number of ways, commonly including entrapment of the sciatic nerve and, rarely, the superior gluteal nerve (Diop et al 2002), both of which give rise to nerve root pain signs and symptoms. There is also dull buttock and thigh pain secondary to dysfunction, including trigger point development, within the muscle itself. The variable collection of signs and symptoms has been termed piriformis syndrome since 1928, yet there is little consensus on its diagnosis and treatment (Silver & Leadbetter 1998).

Some even consider piriformis syndrome a myth (McCrory 2001, Rend 2002), yet informed practitioners have long identified its mechanical dimensions (Kirkaldy-Willis & Hill 1979), described a rational approach to its management (Barton 1991), and developed specific diagnostic tests and outcomes measures (Fishman et al 2002a). A role is being identified for MRI in the diagnosis of the syndrome (Rossi et al 2001) and contemporary invasive treatment includes injection of botulinum toxin A (Fishman et al 2002b).

It has been said it is a diagnosis reached by exclusion (Rodrigue & Hardy 2001), yet the conservative diagnostic approach is no different for the piriformis than it is for any other problem; the history and initial examination allow it to be included as a probable diagnosis, which is then either ruled in or ruled out by specific examination. Practitioners with access to neurophysiologic equipment may find the H-reflex prolonged with hip flexion, adduction, and internal rotation (Fishman et al 2002a). Conservatively, a good indication of piriformis involvement can be found in the side-lying patient where the painful side is up with the leg flexed and the knee resting on the table. This is the standard position for palpating the piriformis. The patient is asked to raise and hold the knee several centimeters off the table and the piriformis is implicated by deep buttock pain with this maneuver (Beatty 1994).

There is no doubt in the mind of experienced practitioners of manual healthcare that the piriformis is frequently involved in various presentations of back pain, not always as an individual muscle syndrome, but more often as an adjunct or associate. It is an important muscle to include in the assessment of all patients with low-back pain.

Piriformis literally means "pear-shaped" and the muscle has broad, muscular attachment along the anterior surface of the sacrum and the gluteal surface of the ilium near the posterior inferior iliac spine, and tapers laterally to a narrow tendinous part which inserts to the upper border of the greater trochanter (Fig. 14.19A; see Fig. 14.21A, below). It has muscular slips arising from the capsule of the SIJ and sometimes from the sacrotuberous ligament. It passes through the sciatic foramen and is innervated by the ventral rami of L5, S1, and S2.

The piriformis acts as an external (lateral) rotator of the neutral-to-extended thigh but its moment arm changes when the thigh is flexed so it becomes an abductor and, more importantly for clinical assessment, an internal rotator (Delp et al 1999). The moment arm only changes for the piriformis; the remaininig lateral hip rotators (quadratus femoris, obturator internus, obturator externus) retain similar actions in flexion as in neutral (Delp et al 1999).

The clinical implication is that the preferred testing position for the muscle is with the hip in neutral. This is achieved with the patient prone, and a testing force is directed by the practitioner's hand against the distal medial tibia while the knee is flexed to 90° (Fig. 14.19B). Stabilization is important to ensure the effect of the test force on the femur is internal rotation and not abduction. The indifferent hand is placed about the distal lateral femur with the fingers in line with the long axis of the femur. Walther (1981 pp. 294–297) describes tests with the patient seated or supine, and even on hands and knees, but as these each require 90° of hip flexion, it is the other lateral rotators which are tested and not the piriformis. When the knee is flexed the piriformis becomes an internal rotator and any test force with a flexed hip would need to account for this.

The piriformis is a postural (type II) muscle and shortens when stressed (Chaitow & DeLany 2002 p. 374). Postural signs therefore include external foot flare on the involved side. A shortened muscle may be accompanied by weakness in its opposite. The assessment for trigger points is conducted with the patient lying with the involved side up. The hip and knee are flexed to about 45° and the knee of the involved side rests on the table.

The practitioner takes a square stance anterior to the patient at the level of the pelvis and constructs an imaginary line between the greater trochanter of the involved leg (up) and the S2 tubercle. This approximates the midline of the muscle. The first trigger point lies about one-third of the distance medially along the line from the greater trochanter. This location is in the myotendinous junction of the muscle and the trigger point is best palpated with a transverse motion across the fibers. The second trigger point lies a further third along the line towards the sacrum. This is within the muscular belly of the piriformis and is palpated with deep but gentle digital pressure.

The pain referral patterns are about the buttock and the posterior thigh (Fig. 14.19C). The common practice of digging into the buttock in the prone patient is a crude and non-specific provocation of many painful structures in the area and is far from an acceptable approach to the piriformis.

Gluteus maximus

A benefit of assessing the piriformis with the patient side-lying is the ease of progression to palpating for trigger points in the gluteus maximus. As the hip is flexed through 45°, the gluteus

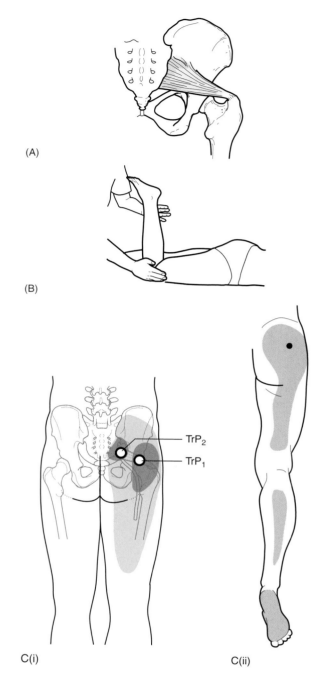

(A)

(B)

TrP₂

TrP₁

C(i)   C(ii)

Figure 14.19 The piriformis. (A) The piriformis arises largely from the ventral surface of the sacrum and inserts into the upper border of the greater trochanter. (B) The muscle is tested with the patient prone. The knee is flexed to 90° and the test force is applied against the medial distal tibia to rotate the femur internally as the piriformis acts to rotate it externally. (C) The two trigger points (TrP) refer pain about the buttock and posterior thigh. Pain from piriformis syndrome may extend well down the leg (right).

maximus fibers move laterally and uncover the ischial tuberosity. The purpose is to remove the muscle from under the tuberosity while sitting so that muscle fibers are not compressed.

Gluteus maximus trigger points are found in the loose medial border of the muscle in the side-lying patient and are best located by a pincer palpation between thumb and finger. The muscle fibers about the ischial tuberosity are gripped while seeking the painful, nodular trigger points. Another trigger point may be palpated inferolateral to the PSIS. The pain referral patterns are generally about the ipsilateral buttock and give the sensation of very-low-back pain and perhaps coccygodynia (Fig. 14.20C).

The broad, thick muscle arises in a sweeping arc from the posterolateral sacrum and along the gluteal line of the ilium to beyond the PSIS (Fig. 14.20A). Superficial fascial tissue lies over the muscle and gives the characteristic shape of the buttock. The muscle fibers intermingle with the thoracolumbar fascia, the posterior sacroiliac ligaments, the sacrotuberous ligament, and the coccyx. They sweep down laterally to merge into the iliotibial band which extends to the knee, with about a third of the muscle inserting into the gluteal tuberosity of the femur. There are up to three bursae under the muscle (over the greater trochanter,

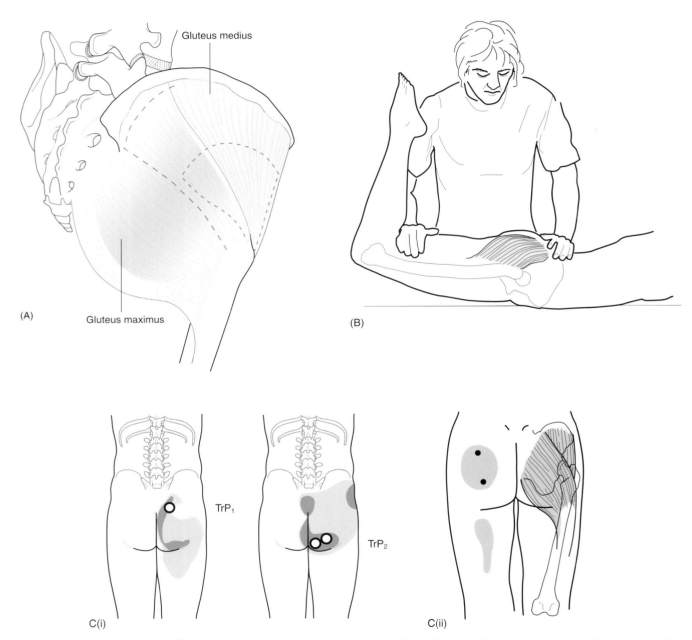

Figure 14.20 The gluteus maximus. (A) The gluteus maximus arises from the gluteal line of the ilium, the posterior surface of the sacrum and coccyx, and the sacrotuberous ligament, and attaches to the greater trochanter and the iliotibial band. (B) The muscle is tested with the patient prone. The knee is flexed to 90° and the patient is asked to raise the leg from the table. The test force is applied at the distal posterior thigh to force the hip into flexion while stabilization is provided over the iliac crest. (C) The trigger points (TrPs) refer pain about the buttock (left and center). There may be two in the medial border about the ischial tuberosity, and a third inferolateral to the posterior superior iliac spine. Isolated pain may refer to the posterior thigh (right). (A, C) From Chaitow & DeLany (2002), with permission.

between the muscle's tendon and the vastus lateralis, and about the ischial tuberosity) which may contribute to localized pain and discomfort.

Innervated by the inferior gluteal nerve from L5, S1, and S2, it acts to extend the hip and laterally rotate the thigh. It is an important stabilizer of the knee through its integration into the iliotibial band and a key symptom of weakness is difficulty in walking uphill or the feeling that the knee will give way, especially when climbing stairs. It is also a stabilizer of the pelvis during gait.

The gluteus maximus is a phasic (type II) muscle with a tendency to weakness and lengthening (Chaitow & DeLany 2002 p. 363). The side of a weak gluteus maximus will show a high iliac crest on postural assessment with perhaps internal rotation of the leg and foot. The popliteal fossa tension may be decreased. The lateral assessment will show anterior pelvic tilt with increased lumbar lordosis. A unilateral weakness will result in anterior pelvic rotation as a combination of anterior tilt with a higher crest.

The muscle has a biomechanical relationship with the contralateral latissimus dorsi (Fig. 2.10C) which transmits forces diagonally across the lower spine between the upper and lower extremities. That muscle must be included in any assessment of gluteus maximus, which is tested with the patient prone (Fig. 14.20B). The knee should be flexed to no more than 90° for consistency, as increased knee flexion restricts hip extension. The indifferent hand provides stabilization over the iliac crest, avoiding the actual muscle itself, and the patient is asked to extend the leg off the table. The test force is applied at the distal posterior thigh to force the hip into flexion.

Gluteus medius and minimus

The gluteus medius arises from the outer surface of the ilium from the iliac crest to the posterior gluteal line, and attaches into the lateral surface of the greater trochanter (Fig. 14.21A). Its posterior third is covered by the gluteus maximus while the anterior two-thirds are superficial. A bursa separates the tendon from the greater trochanter. The gluteus minimus is a smaller muscle lying deep to the medius, attaching to the outer surface of the ilium. It inserts to the anterior surface of the greater trochanter and contributes to the hip joint capsule. There is also a bursa between the tendon and the greater trochanter.

Both muscles are innervated from L5 and S1 by the superior gluteal nerve and act as hip abductors. Their anterior fibers can medially rotate the hip. Their key role is to hold the pelvis level and keep the trunk upright when the contralateral foot is raised from the ground. As phasic (type II) muscles they have a tendency to weakening and lengthening (Chaitow & DeLany 2002 pp. 365–366) and are associated with hip pain which may result in a limp and difficulty in getting up from a chair.

The gluteus medius has trigger points and multiple sites of myotendinoses around the iliac crest and these refer pain into the buttock to and about the sacrum (Fig. 14.21C). The trigger points may be secondary to those in the quadratus lumborum and both muscles should be assessed together. The trigger points in gluteus minimus lie deeper and distal to the crest and can refer severe pain down the posterolateral thigh and into the leg, mimicking sciatic nerve root pain (Fig. 14.21C). The assessment for tender and trigger points is made with the patient lying on the side with the involved leg up, as a continuation from piriformis and gluteus maximus.

The muscles are tested in the side-lying patient with the involved muscles up, and the leg straight at the hip and knee (Fig. 14.21B). Stabilization is provided proximal to and over the iliac crest without compressing the involved muscle fibers. The patient abducts (raises) the leg off the table. If the patient is able to hold this position, a light testing force is applied to the

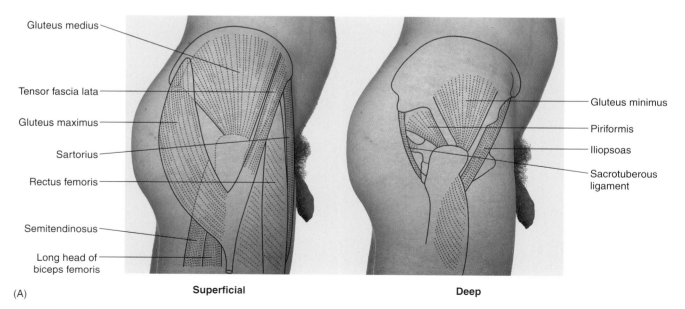

Figure 14.21 Muscles about the lateral hip. (A) The gluteus minimus lies deep to gluteus medius. (B) The gluteus medius and minimus are tested with the patient lying on the side with the involved muscles up. The neutral position accentuates gluteus minimus while a small amount of extension and external rotation accentuates gluteus medius. (C) Pain referral patterns from gluteus medius, gluteus minimus, and tensor fascia latae. (A) From Lumley (2002), with permission; (C) from Chaitow & DeLany (2002), with permission.

distal lateral leg to adduct and slightly extend the limb. When the leg is held in neutral and is in line with the trunk, the test accentuates gluteus minimus. A small amount of extension and external rotation of the leg will accentuate the gluteus medius. The postural findings with a weak gluteus medius include a high pelvis, shoulder, and mastoid on the ipsilateral side.

The pain patterns from the three gluteal muscles are quite easily confused for pain arising from SIJ dysfunction, trigger points in the back extensors, and even nerve root pain. As much as some like to think the trigger point manuals are definitive, it must be remembered that referred pain is both variable and individual. Further, it is unusual for any one mechanical problem to exist on

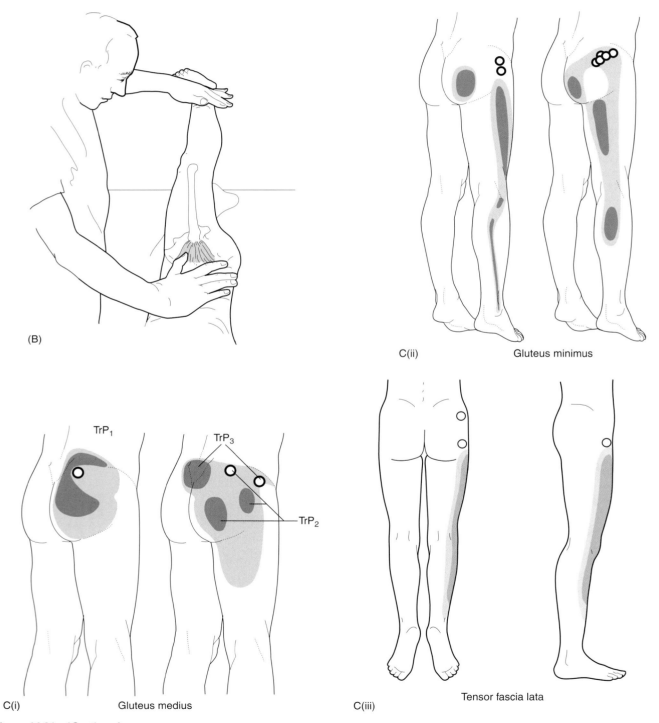

(B)

C(ii)   Gluteus minimus

C(i)   Gluteus medius

C(iii)   Tensor fascia lata

Figure 14.21 (*Continued*).

its own; mostly there are several problems which each need to be addressed in the working diagnosis and treatment plan.

Tensor fascia latae

The tensor fascia latae is the muscular component of the iliotibial band and is commonly overlooked when the lumbosacral spine and pelvis are assessed. It arises from the anterior aspect of the outer lip of the iliac crest and the lateral surface of the ASIS and descends into the iliotibial tract of the fascia latae which in turn descends to attach about the lateral condyle of the tibia (Fig. 14.21A). The greater part of the tendon of gluteus maximus sweeps to join the iliotibial band at about the same level as the tensor fascia latae.

Innervated from L4 and L5 by the superior gluteal nerve, it acts as a stabilizer of the knee through the iliotibial band and assists knee extension. It also participates in flexing, abducting, and medially rotating the thigh at the hip. It is a postural (type I) muscle which shortens when chronically stressed (Chaitow & DeLany 2002 p. 357).

Hypertonicity of the tensor fascia latae can mimic the pain and symptoms of SIJ dysfunction and its pain tends to localize about the PSIS. Kirkaldy-Willis et al (1992) also show that pain from the tensor fascia latae will refer in a narrow band down the lateral thigh and leg, to about mid-calf (Fig. 14.21C(iii)). It is important to include assessment of this muscle with assessment of the SIJ.

The muscle may be tested in the side-lying patient with a variant of the tests used for gluteus medius and minimus. The patient brings the abducted, straight leg into a small degree of flexion at the hip and resists a test force into adduction and extension. The postural findings suggestive of a weak tensor fascia latae include an ipsilateral high pelvis and genu varus of the ipsilateral knee.

Hamstring attachments

The hamstrings are considered muscles of the lower limb; however, their attachments to the pelvis are important to include in the assessment of this region, and their effect on postural change and gait may be seen about the pelvis. The biceps femoris (Fig. 14.21A) is the lateral hamstring and its long head attaches to a medial fossa on the upper half of the ischial tuberosity, with the semitendinosus. Its tendon is common with the sacrotuberous ligament and forms an important longitudinal muscle–tendon–fascia sling (Vleeming et al 1997b) which connects the lower extremity with the contralateral upper extremity (Fig. 13.8).

The biceps femoris has been shown to tighten the sacrotuberous ligament (Dorman 1997) and its attachment to the ischium is minimal in some individuals. The muscle is affected by the degree of nutation of the sacrum, through the sacrotuberous ligament, and by an AS subluxation of the ilium, which draws the ischium superiorly, increasing the tension in the muscle.

The medial hamstrings are the semitendinosus (Fig. 14.21A), which has a common origin with the biceps femoris tendon, and the semimembranosus, which arises from the ischial tuberosity lateral to semitendinosus and biceps femoris. All are postural (type I) muscles which tend to shorten when stressed (Chaitow & DeLany 2002 pp. 432–441). They are innervated by the tibial branch of the sciatic nerve from spinal levels L5 to S2. The long head of the biceps femoris acts to extend, laterally rotate, and

adduct the thigh at the hip and to tilt the pelvis on the hip posteriorly. The other muscles contribute to these actions and also flex and medially rotate the knee.

They are tested with the patient prone and with the knee flexed to about 60°. The test force is applied at the posterior distal leg to take the knee into extension. The pain patterns from trigger points lie about the posterior thigh and proximal posterior leg. Postural findings associated with weak hamstrings include an anterior pelvic tilt and increased lumbar lordosis. External rotation of the foot may suggest weakness of the medial hamstrings, while internal foot rotation may suggest weakness of the lateral hamstrings.

Adductor attachments

The adductors of the thigh are considered muscles of the lower limb; however, their attachments to the pelvis are important to include in the assessment of this region, and their effect on postural change and gait may be seen about the pelvis. Inappropriate assessment and treatment of the adductors, in the absence of informed patient consent and a chaperone, is a cause of formal complaint against practitioners.

The adductors include the gracilis, pectineus, adductor longus, adductor brevis, and adductor magnus (Fig. 14.22). They are postural (type I) muscles which shorten and tighten when chronically stressed (Chaitow & DeLany 2002 pp. 351–358; 416–420). The gracilis arises from near the symphysis on the inferior pubic ramus. The pectineus has a broad attachment along the pecten of the pubis which runs medial to lateral along the anterior margin of the pubic ramus. Adductor longus arises from the front of the pubis between the crest and the symphysis and the adductor brevis arises from the inferior ramus of the pubis. The adductor magnus arises from the inferior ramus of the ischium and pubis. They variously attach about the femur and essentially act to adduct the thigh.

Unilateral weakness of the adductors allows genu varus of the knee and a possible high pelvis on the contralateral side. They may also be implicated with lateral pelvic shift away from the side of weak adductors or towards the side of hypertonic adductors. The thigh abductors need to be assessed in this case to determine if they are unilaterally weak, which may allow the adductors to

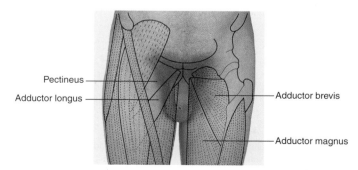

Pectineus
Adductor longus
Adductor brevis
Adductor magnus

Figure 14.22 Pelvic attachments of the adductors. The gracilis (not shown) is the most superficial muscle of the group. From Lumley (2002), with permission.

appear strong, or vice versa. Lateral pelvic shift is accompanied by weight transfer to one leg. Gait analysis may point to weak adductors when the leg is late in returning to the midline during the swing phase.

The adductors tend to generate pain about the groin and medial thigh and may refer pain to the knee. They are commonly strained in sports requiring strong leg action such as horse riding and football and are usually associated with osteitis pubis. They should also be assessed when the patient complains of hip or intrapelvic pain. Naturally they are included with the assessment of the SIJ and particularly of the symphysis pubis.

ASSESSMENT OF NEURAL CHANGE

The spinal nerves

The spinal nerves of the lumbosacral spine and pelvis and the levels at which they exit are:

- spinal nerve L4 from the L4–5 SMU
- spinal nerve L5 from the L5–S1 SMU
- spinal nerve S1 from the S1 foramina
- spinal nerve S2 from the S2 foramina
- spinal nerve S3 from the S3 foramina
- spinal nerve S4 from the S4 foramina
- spinal nerve S5 from the sacral hiatus
- coccygeal nerve from the sacral hiatus.

The course of the nerve roots and their normal relationships are given in Figure 14.23, however, there are many anomalies in this region, categorized as follows:

- Type 1: conjoined roots, where a common dural sheath gives rise to two separate nerve roots, each of which exits the spinal canal through different IVCs.

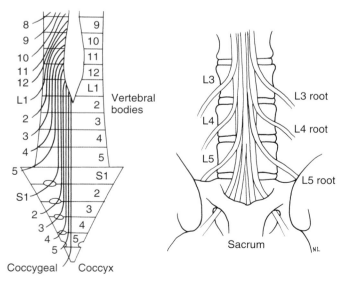

Figure 14.23 Course of the lumbar spinal nerve roots. The low lumbar spinal nerves exit under the pedicle which is placed relatively high on the body. The nerve thus exits the intervertebral canal above its corresponding disk. A disk protrusion of, for example, L4, is more likely to compromise the L5 nerve root than the L4 nerve root. From Peterson & Bergmann (2002), with permission.

- Type 2: where two nerve roots exit through the one IVC, either leaving one IVC unoccupied or representing an additional nerve root (see below).
- Type 3: where adjacent nerve roots are connected within the spinal canal by a connecting root in the form of an anastomosis. This may connect two roots before each exits its respective IVC, or connect two roots which then exit the one IVC.

This classification system was developed from a relatively small sample of 16 anomalies found at surgery (Neidre & MacNab 1983). A recent study using MRI found an anomaly incidence of 17.3% ($n = 65$) in a sample of 376 patients (Haijiao et al 2001). Their classification system was more complex but essentially reflected the categories of Neidre & MacNab (1983). More important was the relatively high incidence (15.1%) of the furcal nerve.

The furcal nerve usually arises at the L4 root level (93% of dissections) and gives branches to the lumbosacral trunk, femoral, and obturator nerves. It usually lies superior and anterior to the L4 root in the L4–5 IVC. It has its own anterior and posterior root fibers and its own dorsal root ganglion (Kikuchi et al 1984). The clinical significance is that the furcal nerve may be involved in presentations with unusual findings, such as sensory impairment in the S1 dermatome with motor weakness in the L4 area (Kikuchi et al 1986).

Neurologic symptoms with two roots involved may be due to four causes:

- two roots may be compromised by a single lesion
- two lesions may be present
- an anomaly of root emergence may be present with two roots emerging through the same IVC
- the furcal nerve may be involved (Kikuchi et al 1986).

The furcal nerve may arise from the common dural sheath either before or within the IVC, or after the bundle has exited the IVC, beyond the pedicle (Haijiao et al 2001). The peripheral nerves also demonstrate anomalies, usually secondary to variations in muscles such as the gluteus maximus (Kirici & Ozan 1999) and piriformis (Saadeh 1988), and the potential for nerve compromise away from the spinal column should always be considered.

The assessment of neural change in this region must be built on a thorough pain history (Ch. 16) which should then direct the examination and assessment. The following should be explored:

- Is there change to cutaneous sensation? If so, is it by dermatome or cutaneous nerve distribution (Fig. 14.28) or is it unusual?
- Is there any change in motor function? Is it myogenic or neurogenic? If neurogenic, is it by nerve root level or peripheral nerve? Does the suspected nerve match other findings?
- Is there any change to the muscle stretch reflexes? If so, how does it fit with other findings?
- Are there any other neurological signs or symptoms? Is there any atrophy of limbs (measure the circumference) with absent reflexes suggestive of a lower motor neuron lesion? Do the findings suggest an upper motor neuron lesion with increased tone and increased reflexes with weak leg flexors? An upper motor neuron lesion may be confirmed by a positive Babinski's sign in which the big toe extends and the other toes spread when the end of the plessor is drawn up the lateral border of the foot and across the foot pad.

- Are the findings suggestive of a cord lesion? A one-sided lesion will give upper motor neuron signs in the ipsilateral leg with loss of position and vibration sense, and spinothalamic signs in the contralateral leg with pain and temperature sensation loss. A posterior column lesion gives bilateral loss of position and vibration sense, and an anterolateral column lesion gives either upper motor neuron and/or spinothalamic tract symptoms in both legs and may be associated with incontinence (Wilkinson 1993 p. 123).

Are the signs and symptoms adding up? If the pain drawings are equal left and right, or bizarre in their marking and distribution, then consider a functional overlay. If the dermatomes are not matched as tightly as expected, then consider a nerve root anomaly or sclerotomal involvement. The sclerotomes of this region are somewhat close to the dermatomal distribution but do demonstrate sufficient lack of congruity to confound the dermatomal findings.

The variability in dermatome maps may be compounded by anomalies in nerve root origin. Practitioners can enhance their intraexaminer reliability by assessing the three key dermatomes in the area where the highest probability of identifying an individual dermatome is known. Nitta et al (1993) (see Fig. 14.29, below) applied selective lumbar spinal nerve block to determine the following:

- the probability that the medial side of the lower leg is subserved by the L4 nerve root is 88%
- the probability that the side of the first dorsal digit is subserved by the L5 nerve root is 82%

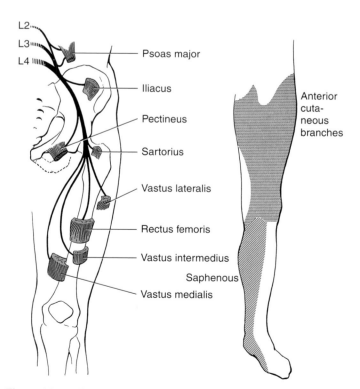

Figure 14.24 Distribution of the femoral nerve, showing motor and cutaneous innervation. From Jenkins (1998), with permission.

- the probability that the side of the fifth digit is subserved by the S1 nerve root is 83%.

The areas given above are those where, within Nitta's sample of 71 patients, there was firstly, the most superimposition of sensory impairment amongst the sample for that particular nerve root and, secondly, the least sensory impairment within the sample after the blockage of adjacent nerve roots. The probability values represent the percentage of patients in various subsets where the specific nerve root block achieved sensory loss. There is considerable clinical value in consistently assessing these three dermatomes in these high-probability areas.

L4 spinal nerve

The L4 spinal nerve is typical in that it has the same anatomical characteristics and relations of the lumbar spinal nerves above and as previously described. The dorsal and ventral roots travel inferiorly as the cauda equina and before exiting the IVF form a mixed spinal nerve which emerges and then divides into the anterior primary division or ventral ramus, and posterior primary division or dorsal ramus (Cramer & Darby 1995 p. 215).

The L4 dorsal ramus tends to form three branches – medial, lateral, and intermediate – which are distributed, respectively, to multifidus, iliocostalis, and longissimus (Bogduk et al 1982). The medial branch innervates two adjacent zygapophyseal joints and ramifies within multifidus, supplying only those fascicles which arise from the spinous process with the same segmental number as the nerve (Bogduk et al 1982).

The structures innervated by the dorsal ramus are all pain generators and include the zygapophyseal joint, interspinous ligament, supraspinous restraint, possibly the ligamentum flavum, the periosteum of the posterior arch and posterior aspect of the spinous process, and muscles including the multifidi and rotatores (Cramer & Darby 1995 p. 216).

The recurrent meningeal nerve innervates many structures within the spinal canal and IVC which are capable of producing pain. The anterior structures about the L4–5 SMU are innervated by gray communicating rami of the sympathetic trunk. These structures include the anterior longitudinal ligament, the periosteum of the anterior and lateral vertebral bodies, and the anterior and lateral annular fibers.

The ventral ramus immediately enters the psoas muscle, which serves to protect the dorsal and ventral roots, and branches to form the lumbar plexus with the ventral rami of L1 through L3 above. Fibers from L4 contribute to the femoral nerve (with L2 and L3) which is motor to the psoas, iliacus, quadratus femoris, and pectineus muscles, and sensory to the anterior thigh and lateral leg (Fig. 14.24). These three anterior rami also form the obturator nerve which is motor to the adductors and sensory to the medial aspect of the thigh (Fig. 14.25).

The clinical evidence of L4 involvement is pain and/or sensory change in a region extending from the midline of the trunk posteriorly, across the buttock, through the lateral and anterior side of the thigh, and the medial side of the leg to the first digit of the foot (Nitta et al 1993).

Weakness may be seen in foot dorsiflexion by the deep peroneal nerve to the tibialis anterior. Foot dorsiflexion is shared by

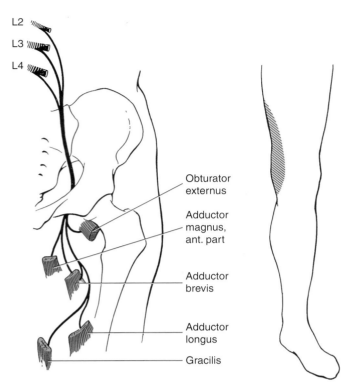

Figure 14.25 Distribution of the obturator nerve, showing motor and cutaneous innervation. From Jenkins (1998), with permission.

L4 and L5 and weakness is demonstrated by difficulty in walking on the heel or in resisting a test force of the foot into plantar flexion. L4 is emphasized through tibialis anterior by inversion of the foot and the specific motor test is to resist foot eversion.

The reflex response is elicited at the infrapatellar tendon which represents the femoral nerve and includes L3.

L5 spinal nerve

The L5–S1 IVC is smaller than those above due to the L5 disk being narrower. This results in more than one-third of the area of the L5–S1 IVF being occupied by the mixed spinal nerve, which in turn increases its susceptibility to compromise. The L5 dorsal ramus is much longer than the others in this region and forms only a medial and an intermediate branch (Bogduk et al 1982). As with L4, the medial branch innervates two adjacent zygapophyseal joints. The ventral ramus unites with a branch of the ventral ramus of L4 to form the lumbosacral trunk which enters the pelvis to unite with the ventral rami of the sacral spinal nerves to help form the sacral plexus (Cramer & Darby 1995 p. 217).

The L5 component of the lumbosacral trunk lies ventral to the iliolumbar ligament, which has a range of variations in its attachment. Connective tissue may form a ligamentous link between the sacrum and the L5 body on the caudal margin of the iliolumbar ligament. This courses ventral to the L5 root which, in one-fifth of specimens examined, adhered to the periosteum of the sacrum distal to the ligamentous link (Kleihues et al 2001). The ligamentous

connection was found to exert pressure on the nerve root during distraction and translation of the root. Clinically this may implicate sacral subluxation with L5 symptoms.

The clinical evidence of L5 involvement is pain and/or sensory change in a region extending from the midline of the trunk posteriorly, across the buttock, through the lateral side of the thigh, the lateral side of the leg and the medial side of the dorsum of the foot, to the first digit (Nitta et al 1993).

Weakness with foot dorsiflexion by the deep peroneal nerve to the tibialis anterior includes L4 and is tested as described above. Specific weakness of L5 may be assessed by asking the patient to dorsiflex the big toe while the practitioner attempts to draw it into plantar flexion. The reflex response for L5 is difficult to elicit. Some consider it may be indicated by the response of the tendon of semimembranosus, while Hoppenfeld (1997 p. 59) suggests tapping the tendon of tibialis posterior. The patient is seated and the foot is taken slightly into eversion and dorsiflexion. The tendon is located on the medial side of the foot as it inserts into the navicular tuberosity. A normal response is a slight jerk into plantar inversion.

S1 spinal nerve

The S1 nerve root is shorter than those of L4 and L5 and lies more vertically in the spinal canal than the others. Its dorsal root ganglion is unique in that it is the largest of the region and is more frequently located intraspinally (Hasegawa et al 1996). It is located more medially and clinically and this means that S1 nerve root pain may arise from both the nerve root and the dorsal root ganglion as a result of either L5 disk protrusion or degenerative L5–S1 facet changes (Hasegawa et al 1996).

The ventral rami of S1, together with those of S2 and S3, part of S4, combine with those that form L4 and L5 to form the sacral plexus which lies on the posterior pelvic wall anterior to the piriformis. The sacral plexus gives rise to the sciatic nerve which has contribution from L4 through S3, and other nerves, including the posterior cutaneous nerves of the thigh, the pudendal nerve, superior and inferior gluteal nerves, and the nerves to the obturator internus and quadratus femoris (Cramer & Darby 1995 p. 243). The anteromedial compartment of the sciatic nerve is the tibial nerve (Fig. 14.26) and the posterolateral compartment is the common peroneal nerve (Fig. 14.27).

The clinical evidence of S1 involvement is pain and/or sensory change in a region extending from the midline of the trunk posteriorly, across the buttock, through the posterior, lateral aspect of the thigh and leg to the fifth digit of the foot (Nitta et al 1993). Sciatic nerve root pain is typically reported as a narrow band of "electric-type" pain down a clearly identified band on the posterior thigh and leg.

The involvement of the S1 level may be suspected with weakness of foot plantar flexion by the posterior tibial nerve to the gastrocnemius. Foot plantar flexion is shared by S1 and S2 and weakness is demonstrated by difficulty in walking on the toes or in resisting a test force of the foot into dorsiflexion. S1 may be emphasized through peroneus longus and brevis by asking the patient to plantar flex and evert the foot while the practitioner attempts to dorsiflex and invert it.

The reflex response is elicited at the Achilles tendon, which represents the tibial nerve and includes S2.

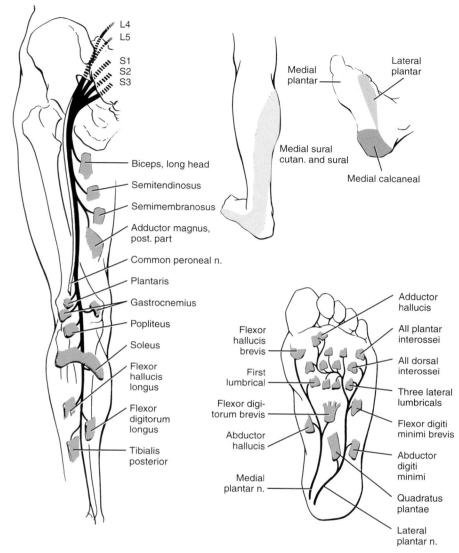

Figure 14.26   Distribution of the tibial nerve, showing motor and cutaneous innervation. From Jenkins (1998), with permission.

Nerve tension tests

There are two clinically relevant nerve tension tests for this region and they traction either the femoral nerve to implicate nerve root involvement at the L2, L3, and L4 levels, or the sciatic nerve complex, to implicate nerve root involvement at the L5 and S1 levels.

The femoral nerve tension test is performed with the patient prone. As with all provocative tests, the unaffected leg is tested first, and then the involved leg. The test is passive for the patient, and the practitioner brings the heel upright to flex the knee to 90°. The leg is then flexed further, within patient tolerance, to bring the heel towards the buttock.

A positive finding is anterior thigh pain which replicates the complaint of the patient. A false-positive finding may arise from stretching a tight quadriceps but this would usually be bilateral. Unilateral anterior thigh pain is suggestive of involvement of the femoral nerve at either the L3–4 or L4–5 level. It is suggested

that radiating pain to the groin is more suggestive of L3 while leg pain to the mid-tibia is more suggestive of L4 (Evans 2001 p. 524); however, as this test also stresses the lumbosacral junction and SIJ, groin pain may implicate these structures.

The sciatic nerve tension test is preferably performed with the patient supine, but may also be applied in the seated patient. The test is also passive, with the leg being raised and controlled by the practitioner, and while correctly known as the passive straight leg raising (PSLR) test, is also termed the Lasègue test. The problem with the PSLR test is that there is no standard procedure and no consensus on the interpretation of results (Rebain et al 2002).

The diagnostic accuracy of the PSLR in detecting disk herniation seems to be limited by its low specificity (Devillè et al 2000). This is because mechanical pain may arise from the knee, hip, SIJ, or lumbosacral junction during the performance of the test,

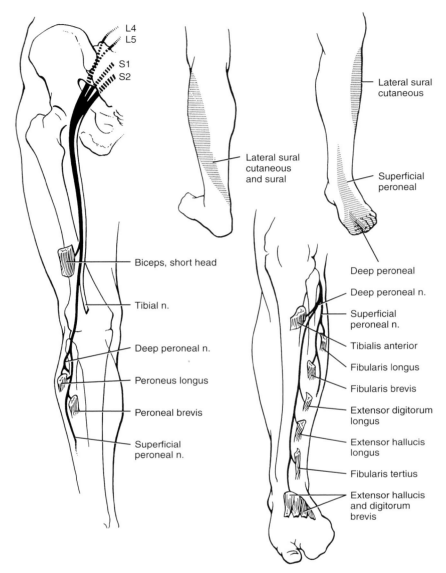

Figure 14.27 Distribution of the common peroneal nerve, showing motor and cutaneous innervation. From Jenkins (1998), with permission.

as well as from disk irritation of a nerve root; however the astute practitioner should be able to apply variations of the test to rule in and rule out various causes of pain. The sensitivity of the test is high, however, in the presence of disk protrusion causing nerve root pain. It has also been suggested that there is greater diagnostic value with a negative finding than with a positive finding (Rebain et al 2002).

The mechanism for detecting discogenic nerve root irritation is the physical traction of the nerve root, which occurs when the straight leg is raised from the bench with the patient supine. The PSLR initially tractions the sciatic nerve as it leaves the pelvis and the leg needs to be raised about 20–30° from the bench before the sciatic nerve is tractioned at the IVF. Traction is greatest at the L5–S2 levels with 60–80° of leg raise and movement is rarely seen at the L3 level or above (Rebain et al 2002).

The test is performed with the practitioner in a square stance to the supine patient at the level of the knee. The patient is instructed to report the onset of pain, at which point the test will stop and the nature of the pain will be explored. The practitioner's cephalad hand is placed lightly over the knee in order to detect any early attempt to ease pain by the patient flexing the knee. If the patient does this, it represents the "buckling" sign. The caudad hand is placed under the heel and the straight leg is slowly raised from the table.

The procedure is first performed on the non-involved leg, in which case it is termed the "well leg raise". If raising the well leg causes pain in the involved leg, then the test is considered a positive "crossed straight leg raise". When the involved leg is raised the practitioner stops at the point of reported pain and eases the leg down a little. The nature of the pain is explored and, if its description is that of nerve root pain familiar to the patient, then the nerve root is provoked by a series of other maneuvers such as dorsiflexion of the foot and then big toe, and internal rotation of the leg.

The variants attempt to isolate nerve root pain from other mechanical pain and this is achieved by stopping the leg raise when the patient reports pain, and then flexing the knee while flexing the hip. Knee flexion significantly reduces the traction force on the sciatic nerve and should allow movement at the hip which, if limited by pain, is probably due to hip or SIJ involvement. If the thigh can be reasonably flexed at the hip without pain, the knee can then be gently extended to introduce nerve tension, which should again produce radiating leg pain in the presence of disk involvement.

Local vs referred pain

The common, painful syndromes of the low back can be summarized as:

- myofascial pain syndromes
- the sacroiliac syndrome
- the lumbosacral subluxation syndrome
- the lumbar facet syndrome
- the lumbar disk syndrome.

The patient is usually driven to the consultation by pain and discomfort and does not conveniently present with one or more of the above labels. The practitioner must therefore learn to discern the subtle characteristics of each syndrome and to conduct the assessment at a high enough level to ensure the resulting working diagnosis is one which bests integrates the history and clinical findings.

A key finding is differentiation between local and referred pain. Local pain will result from direct damage to tissues, be it a strain/sprain of the annulus, or of the posterior SIJ ligaments, or other such structures. The pain will worsen locally with tests which provoke the structures and should be able to be identified by the patient, using one finger to locate the area. Such pain is typically acute and the diagnostic challenges begin when the pain is chronic, or is an acute overlay on chronic pain and dysfunction.

Aside from a disk injury which immediately impinges on a nerve root, most referred pain falls in the insidious or subacute to chronic category. This is simply because mechanisms such as trigger points in muscles need time to develop. The most important ingredient for working back to a source problem from a reported pain pattern is an intimate knowledge of the nature of referred pain patterns in this region and a strong index of suspicion, based on a thorough history, for the causative element.

It is clearly impossible to construct a simple grid which distinguishes between the five syndromes above, or other causes of pain, but there are some basic principles to be applied. These include:

- Dull, vaguely localized pain which wakes the patient at night is ominous and is most likely not of mechanical origin. Patients reporting these findings should be investigated for organic dysfunction and neoplasia.
- Sharp, well-defined pain in known patterns such as a strip down the back of the thigh is typically nerve root pain. In this region these are usually either sciatic nerve root pain on the posterior leg or femoral nerve pain on the lateral and anterior thigh.
- Ill-defined pains radiating into the buttocks, thigh, and legs are more likely due to muscle, ligament, or SIJ. There is no substitute for a systematic evaluation of all likely pain generators.
- Localized pain about the hip worsened by movement implicates the hip joint complex, including the capsular ligaments and bursae.
- Reflex changes typically suggest a nerve root lesion in the presence of supportive signs and symptoms, most notably dermatomal pain and weakness, or central nervous system lesions in the presence of more complex problems.
- Any combination of the above is to be expected, in particular, local low-back pain (secondary to disk injury) with leg pain (secondary to nerve root involvement), complicated by myofascial pain overlays.

Sensory change

Basic assessment includes recording the bilaterally comparative responses to crude touch. Further assessment can include pain or sharp touch, temperature, and vibration. Sensory changes with or without pain can arise from both nerve root irritation and peripheral nerve entrapment. The latter are likely to be either meralgia paresthetica (entrapment of the lateral femoral cutaneous nerve of the thigh) with sensory change on the anterolateral thigh, or common peroneal palsy (entrapment of the common peroneal nerve about the head of the fibula) with sensory change on the lateral leg and foot.

The dermatomes by nerve root and cutaneous nerve are given in Figure 14.28 and the probability areas for the L4, L5, and S1, 2 dermatomes are given in Figure 14.29.

Motor function

Basic assessment includes recording muscle weakness, absent or diminished tone, fasciculations, neurogenic atrophy, and altered deep tendon reflexes. The nerve roots may be assessed as L4, L5, or S1, or the peripheral nerves may be assessed with inference back to the root. The muscles to test for motor function of individual spinal nerve roots are:

- L4: foot inversion
- L4 and L5: foot dorsiflexion
- L5: big toe dorsiflexion
- S1: foot eversion
- S1 and S2: plantar flexion.

Figures 14.24–14.27 identify the motor distribution of these nerve roots and their resultant peripheral nerves in the lower limbs.

Autonomic effects

The preganglionic sympathetic fibers exit the spinal cord in the ventral roots of cord segments T1 to L2 or L3, hence there is no direct sympathetic outflow from this spinal region, although the sympathetic trunk does innervate effectors in the lower extremities, abdominal cavity, and pelvic cavity. The lumbar sympathetic

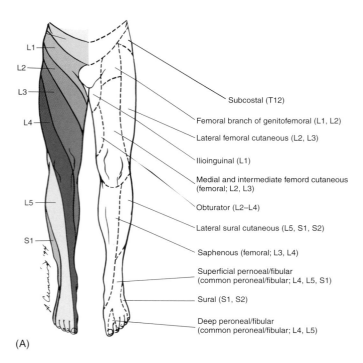

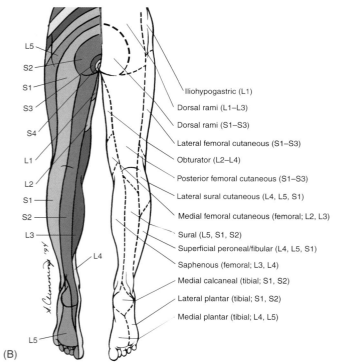

Figure 14.28 Cutaneous innervation. The cutaneous innervation of the lower body is shown by dermatome (left of each image) and cutaneous peripheral nerve (right of each image) for the anterior (A) and posterior (B). From Cramer & Darby (1995), with permission.

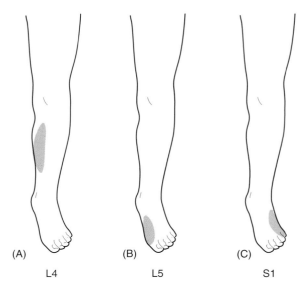

Figure 14.29 Highest-probability dermatome zones. (A) There is an 88% probability that the dermatome for the L4 nerve root will be found on the medial side of the leg. (B) There is an 82% probability that the dermatome for the L5 nerve root will be found on the side of the first digit on the dorsum of the foot. (C) There is an 83% probability that the dermatome for the S1 nerve root will be found on the side of the fifth digit of the foot. After data from Nitta et al (1993).

leg and foot, primarily by traveling with the tibial nerve (Cramer & Darby 1995).

The parasympathetic fibers arise from S2 to S4 and provide innervation to the pelvic viscera through the sacral plexus. The efferents course within the ventral roots and subsequently form pelvic splanchnic nerves. They innervate smooth muscle and glands within the pelvis in those areas not innervated through the vagus. These include part of the transverse colon, the descending colon, sigmoid colon, rectum, bladder, and reproductive organs. This system also conveys important sensory information that provides reflex control of normal bladder, colon, and sexual organ function (Cramer & Darby 1995 p. 327).

While there is ample empirical evidence supportive of achieving positive change in bowel, bladder, and sexual function following manual intervention, including spinal adjustment, there are no specific signs and symptoms of autonomic disturbance yet related in an evidence-based manner to segmental dysfunction of the spine. Notwithstanding the lack of evidence, the astute practitioner will explore these matters as appropriate and monitor the patient for outcomes. Hopefully practitioners will also document and publish their findings and outcomes in case reports to add to the literature.

It is becoming known that pediatric bladder dysfunction and nocturnal enuresis may respond to chiropractic adjustment (Todres-Masarsky et al 2001). Further, many cases of constipation have been described in the literature, usually with lower sacral nerve root irritation. This has given rise to the development of the mechanically induced pelvic pain and organic dysfunction (PPOD) syndrome which includes urologic dysfunction, enterologic dysfunction, and gynecologic and sexual dysfunction. In many cases there is lower sacral neurology which resolves with manipulation, exercises, and home instructions, together with

trunk lies adjacent to the anterolateral aspect of the vertebral bodies and the medial margin of the psoas major. The pelvic sympathetic trunk has four or five ganglia which lie against the pelvic surface of the sacrum. Fibers from here reach blood vessels in the resolution of the symptoms of PPOD (Browning 2001). Clearly the autonomic effect of subluxation in the lumbosacral spine and pelvis is an emerging area of great clinical interest.

Traditional concepts

The following notes attempt to present a summary as being suggestive of what may be seen in clinical practice. The references below regarding the stimulation of a spinal centre are from Schafer (1983 p. 371). As in previous chapters, the references to the Lovett Brother relationship are from Walther (1981 p. 67).

About L4 – the L4–5 SMU

Traditional chiropractic associates this level with the prostate gland, muscles of the lower back, and the sciatic nerve. The Lovett Brother relationship to the L4 body is movement in the same direction of the C2 body. Maigne suggests chronic dysfunction at L4–5 may be reflected in dysfunction at C2–3, C6–7, and T12–L1 (Maigne 1996 p. 102). Adjusting here is considered to have a sympathetic effect (Plaugher 1993 p. 357). Faridi (1995) associates the L4 vertebral segment with sympathetic neural pathways to the large intestine and relates this level to ulcerative colitis and toxic bowel syndrome.

Stimulation of the spinal reflex center is thought to initiate sigmoidal and rectal contraction and to increase the tone of the lower bowel. In acupuncture terms the site for Du 3 Yaoyangguan lies below the spinous process of L4 and is indicated for irregular menstruation, nocturnal emission, impotence, lumbosacral pain, and motor impairment of the lower limbs (Qiu 1993 pp. 153–154). There is also the Extra 22 Yaoyan point in the depression 3–4 cun lateral to the lower border of the L4 spinous process, which is thought to affect the posterior branch of the third lumbar nerve and is indicated with irregular menstruation and leucorrhea (Qiu 1993 p. 177).

About L5 – the L5–S1 SMU

Traditional chiropractic associates this level with the lower legs, ankles, and feet. The Lovett Brother relationship to the L5 body is movement in the same direction of the C1 body. Adjusting here may or may not have a parasympathetic effect (Plaugher 1993 p. 367). Faridi (1995) associates the L5 vertebral segment with sympathetic neural pathways to the ovaries, fallopian tubes, uterus, and vagina and relates this level to dysmenorrhea.

The posterior neurolymphatic point for the abdominal muscles, piriformis, gluteus maximus, gluteus medius, gluteus minimus, peroneus longus, peroneus brevis, flexor hallucis longus, and the intrinsic muscles of the foot lies between the L5 spinous process and the PSIS (Walther 1981 pp. 293, 300, 346, 347, 352). This point may also have a provisional relationship with opponens pollicis and opponens digiti minimi (Walther 1981 pp. 425, 429). The posterior neurolymphatic point for peroneus tertius lies between the L5 transverse process and the sacrum (Walther 1981 p. 342). The significance of the neurolymphatic point lies not only in its possible diagnostic and therapeutic relationship to specific muscles, but to the fact that tenderness to palpation of a certain structure does not automatically infer a local tissue response to kinematic change or subluxation complex.

In acupuncture terms the site for Extra 23 Shiqizhui lies below the spinous process of L5 and is indicated with paralysis of the lower limbs, massive uterine bleeding, and irregular menstruation (Qiu 1993 p. 177). The site for Extra 19 Jiaji (Huatuojiaji) points lies 0.5 cun lateral to the lower border of the spinous process and is used to stimulate the posterior ramus and their arterial and venous plexuses at this level (Qiu 1993 pp. 176–177).

About the sacrum – the S1–2 sacral segments and coccyx

Traditional chiropractic associates the sacrum with the hips and buttocks, and the coccyx with the rectum and anus. Faridi (1995) associates the SIJ with the bladder and urethra, ileocecal valve, and the reproductive system in both males and females. In acupuncture terms the site for Du 2 Yaoshu lies at the sacral hiatus and sacrococcygeal ligament and is indicated for irregular menstruation, hemorrhoids, lumbar spinal stiffness and pain, motor impairment of the lower limbs, and epilepsy (Qiu 1993 p. 153).

ASSESSMENT OF VASCULAR CHANGE

There are several ways in which vascular change can be implicated in pain and dysfunction about the lumbosacral spine and pelvis, including the sequelae of vasoconstriction in muscle, ischemia about the nerve root, and venous hypertension. These have been discussed in general terms in Chapter 8 and are applicable to this region.

Regrettably, there are few, if any, clinical tests specific to vascular change of this nature, but its involvement must be considered when developing the treatment plan and prognosis. The most relevant overt expressions of vascular change are the signs seen on infrared thermography. For some reason, perhaps capital cost and the lack of third-party reimbursement, infrared thermographic imaging is not commonly used in manual healthcare practices.

There is little doubt that quality infrared images can demonstrate sensory neuropathies, thermal changes in the legs secondary to lumbar disk herniation, reflex sympathetic dystrophy, and some myofascial pain syndromes (Christiansen & Gerow 1990). Its current lack of use is regrettable; however the Nervoscope, as used within the Gonstead paradigm of chiropractic practice, does seem able to identify paraspinal levels of thermal asymmetry secondary to changes in the microcirculation (Ebrall et al 1994a).

Vascular claudication is one clinical presentation which has tangible dimensions. Claudication is a descriptive term for the clinical symptom of activity-induced leg pain relieved by rest (Cox 1999 p. 180). Vascular or ischemic claudication is characterized by pain, dysesthesia, and paresthesia which occur with ambulation but are relieved by rest or lying prone. Absent pulses and distal pallor are classic signs and help distinguish vascular claudication from neurogenic claudication. Typically, neurogenic claudication is vague leg pain over the thighs and calves relieved by postural change. If vascular compromise is suspected of the lower-limb circulation, the practitioner must assess the bilateral pulses in the femoral, popliteal, and dorsalis pedis arteries.

CONCLUSION

Dysfunction about the lumbosacral spine and pelvis is the most common presentation in chiropractic practice. Low-back pain in particular is perhaps the most researched entity in manual medicine and has an extensive and strong evidence-base in the literature.

While the majority of low-back pain is termed "mechanical", it must be remembered that, in the context of the subluxation complex, mechanical dysfunction rarely, if ever, exists on its own. It is imperative to master the complete assessment of this region, including the identification of changes to neural function, muscle, and connective tissues, with consideration of the vascular changes, which may range from abdominal aortic aneurysm to venous congestion within the SMU.

A high level of evidence is needed in order best to direct the therapeutic intervention and outcomes measurements.

PART 3

Documentation, patient history, and the diagnosis

You write with ease, to show your breeding,
But easy writing's curst hard reading

Source: Sheridan Richard Brinsley *Clio's Protest*. English dramatist and politician. 1751–1816

15

The clinical record

KEY CONCEPTS

The purpose of the clinical record is to collect all relevant data concerning one individual patient so as to provide an information resource to drive clinical decision making for that patient.

Four dimensions are evident in the process of clinical thinking: (1) the physical dimension of the source data; (2) the temporal dimension of the patient; (3) the interventional dimension which flows from the clinical interaction; and (4) the spiritual dimension or biopsychosocial status and embodied experiences.

The clinical record is to integrate the source data to allow the synthesis of a working diagnosis which will drive the management plan and determine the outcomes measurements. All elements are to be recorded, dated, and structured into one record of the patient.

The clinical record must include progress notes which are a contemporaneous record of every interaction of the patient and include subjective information and objective data, an assessment of that data and its clinical implications, including treatment options and changes, and a plan for the delivery and monitoring of that care.

All entries in the clinical record must be dated and no entry may be removed, deleted, or otherwise rendered illegible, although corrections, additions, and clarifications may be made. The patient has the right to access the clinical record and make alterations and amendments.

The types of care which may be rendered to a patient may be based on signs and symptoms associated with an identifiable event (type 1), signs and symptoms not related to a precipitating event (type 2), provided in order to prevent the return of signs and symptoms as maintenance care (type 3), or provided in the absence of quantifiable signs and symptoms to improve quality of life as preventive care (type 4).

Privacy legislation may require patients to consent to the establishment and maintenance of a clinical record of their interaction with a particular provider and impose strict obligations on the provider to maintain the privacy of the patient.

Treatment may only be provided after patients have authorized by signature their informed consent to specific treatment. Patients must be informed of options to treatment, including no treatment, and of the material risk, which is risk which they consider would influence their decision to agree to specific treatment.

INTRODUCTION

The purpose of the clinical record is to collect all relevant data concerning one individual patient so as to provide an information resource to drive clinical decision making for that patient. In broad terms, this includes the working diagnosis and the

reasons why it was reached, the subsequent management plan, including intervention, and the outcomes of that intervention. The financial relationship of the patient with the provider is a separate issue and the clinical record excludes financial and insurance information except where it may pertain to the clinical presentation, for example, a work-related injury for which compensation is paid.

The steps in the assessment process have been discussed (Fig. 1.3) and the three basic principles of assessment identified (Fig. 1.5). The intent of this chapter is to integrate these theoretical positions with the practical reality of creating the clinical record (Fig. 15.1). The record is discussed in terms of it being a paper-based, hard-copy entity; however, the principles are applicable to electronic records, given that the e-record must be able to be printed out at some stage for access by and provision to the patient, on request.

There are a number of ethical and professional principles which underpin professional practice. Readers must also appreciate the potential for the jurisdiction in which they practice to enact legislation which will impact on the clinical record in a variety of ways. While it is not possible for any one text to provide current information on the requirements of every jurisdiction, Ladenheim et al (2001) is especially relevant to the North American reader and provides an understanding of universal principles from the point of view of developing sound risk management strategies.

This chapter describes the practical application of a range of principles which underpin responsible practice; however, readers are responsible for customizing these to their individual practice jurisdiction. The matter of establishing and maintaining the clinical record is crucial to successful practice where success is defined as a safe and effective environment for both the patient and the practitioner.

A properly constructed and well-maintained clinical record provides protection to the practitioner in the medicolegal sense; however, this should be seen as the byproduct of a record which is established for the express purpose of ensuring the safest and best possible management plan for patients given their clinical circumstances. The intent of clinical practice is to accept, diagnose, and treat individuals to restore or attain their optimal level of health. The clinical record is, as its name implies, the compilation of all relevant data, information, and opinion related to this purpose.

The ideal clinical record will both enhance and reflect the clinical decision-making skills of the practitioner. In order to appreciate how the content and structure may complement each other it is valuable to overview briefly a contemporary approach to clinical thinking in the practice of manual healthcare.

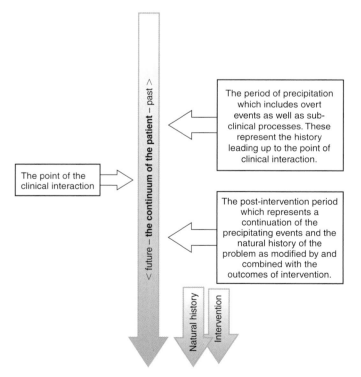

Figure 15.1 Relationships of history on the patient continuum. The continuum of the patient is the temporal dimensions of the clinical interaction, to which the physical, interventional, and spiritual dimensions attach.

A FOUR-DIMENSIONAL MODEL OF CLINICAL THINKING

The process of clinical thinking in chiropractic, osteopathy, and physical therapy can be described as having four dimensions:

1. physical
2. temporal
3. interventional
4. spiritual.

The physical dimension represents the patient as the entity with the potential need for intervention, and includes all his or her physical characteristics which will be recorded as source data. It is these data which are relatively easy to elicit and document in the clinical record. They include the demographics, vital signs, case and pain history and are discussed in detail shortly.

This source data is one-dimensional. It is the physical description and story of the patient at one point in time, the point of initial interaction with the practitioner. The remaining three dimensions represent more of a way of thinking and acting within the clinical environment to allow for a more complete and productive interaction.

The temporal dimension represents a continuum which both leads up to the time of the clinical interaction, and then runs forwards from it (Fig. 15.1). The past elements of the temporal continuum represent the period of precipitation and are explored within the case and pain histories. They include:

- the nature of the clinical situation at the present time
- the nature of any precipitating event, such as external mechanical forces or internal mechanical forces, such as strain/sprain and overuse injuries
- the nature of clinical and subclinical events leading up to this time, including pathological and infective processes.

The future elements of the continuum are postintervention and help determine the preferred outcomes measurements, the likely frequency and duration of care, the "return-to-work" processes where needed. They include:

- the likely natural history leading from the point of clinical interaction
- the variation to natural history which may result from therapeutic intervention
- the supportive processes which may be required in the future
- the outcomes which may be measured at that time.

The interventional dimension describes the full range of therapeutic processes available to practitioners that are included within their training and permitted within their scope of practice. The preferred intervention is determined with consideration of the other three dimensions:

- The physical dimension is a strong determinant of the type of therapy in manual healthcare. The practitioner must, among many things, consider patient age, body type, muscle mass, skin status, and the likely tissue response.
- The temporal dimension is a determinant of the frequency and duration of care and is closely associated with the spiritual dimension, which reflects the patient's locus of health control. In clinical terms, this means the patient may simply want a "quick fix" at one end of the spectrum or may commit to a long-term health and wellness program at the other.

The spiritual dimension represents the biopsychosocial status and the embodied experiences of the patient and can be described in terms of the patient's locus of health control and level of acceptance of his or her role in self-care. Conservative, manual healthcare seems to achieve its best outcomes when the patient is an active participant in the therapeutic process.

These four dimensions represent a way of thinking about the patient in a holistic clinical manner. They also guide the process of record keeping in the sense that they identify and categorize elements of the intellectual property which the practitioner brings to the record.

PRINCIPLES OF CLINICAL RECORD KEEPING

The style and contents of the clinical record will vary in accord with the nature of the clinical discipline. It is obvious that the dental record of a patient will have different content to the record kept by the podiatrist. The only commonality will be the identification of risk factors and informed consent with regard to material risk. The clinical information will be that which is within the scope of practice of the provider.

There are broader areas of commonality among members of a discipline grouping, such as manual healthcare, which includes practitioners from professions such as chiropractic and osteopathy. The basic principles of assessment as discussed in Chapter 1 provide the basis for the principles of record keeping (Fig. 15.2), and these should be common among all members of one discipline grouping.

For chiropractors and osteopaths the first commonality is their role as a primary-contact health provider. This means that patients may attend and consult at their own volition and without referral from another provider. Primary-contact practitioners have express societal obligations to ensure the patient is triaged to the most appropriate provider. Most of the time the patient will have self-selected the appropriate provider but the obligation remains and triage is an important step in the clinical record.

Source data

The source data for the clinical record are obtained from each step in the process of assessment. The key steps are patient presentation and triage, then the contextualization and socioculturalization of the patient which follow the acceptance of the patient into the practice. The aim is to establish a clinical record which will facilitate competent management of the patient.

The source data for triage include the nature of the patient presentation and the vital signs of the patient. Presentations in which the patient is not ambulatory or progresses only with a high degree of assistance provide sufficient red flags to warn of a condition which may well require emergency care, such as significant disk herniation with extrusion.

There are also red flags with headache, including fever and neck stiffness with a new headache, which suggests meningitis, for which prompt referral is the appropriate management at primary-contact level. Similarly, there are numerous cardiac events which in their extreme are obvious but while emergent may mimic musculoskeletal disorders.

The initial source data are thus somewhat subjective and reliant on the receiving practitioner's impression of the presentation of the patient. The vital signs provide objective data which may further inform the practitioner's impression and direct the subsequent clinical actions. No matter the duration of the initial presentation, it must be documented in a clinical record for that patient.

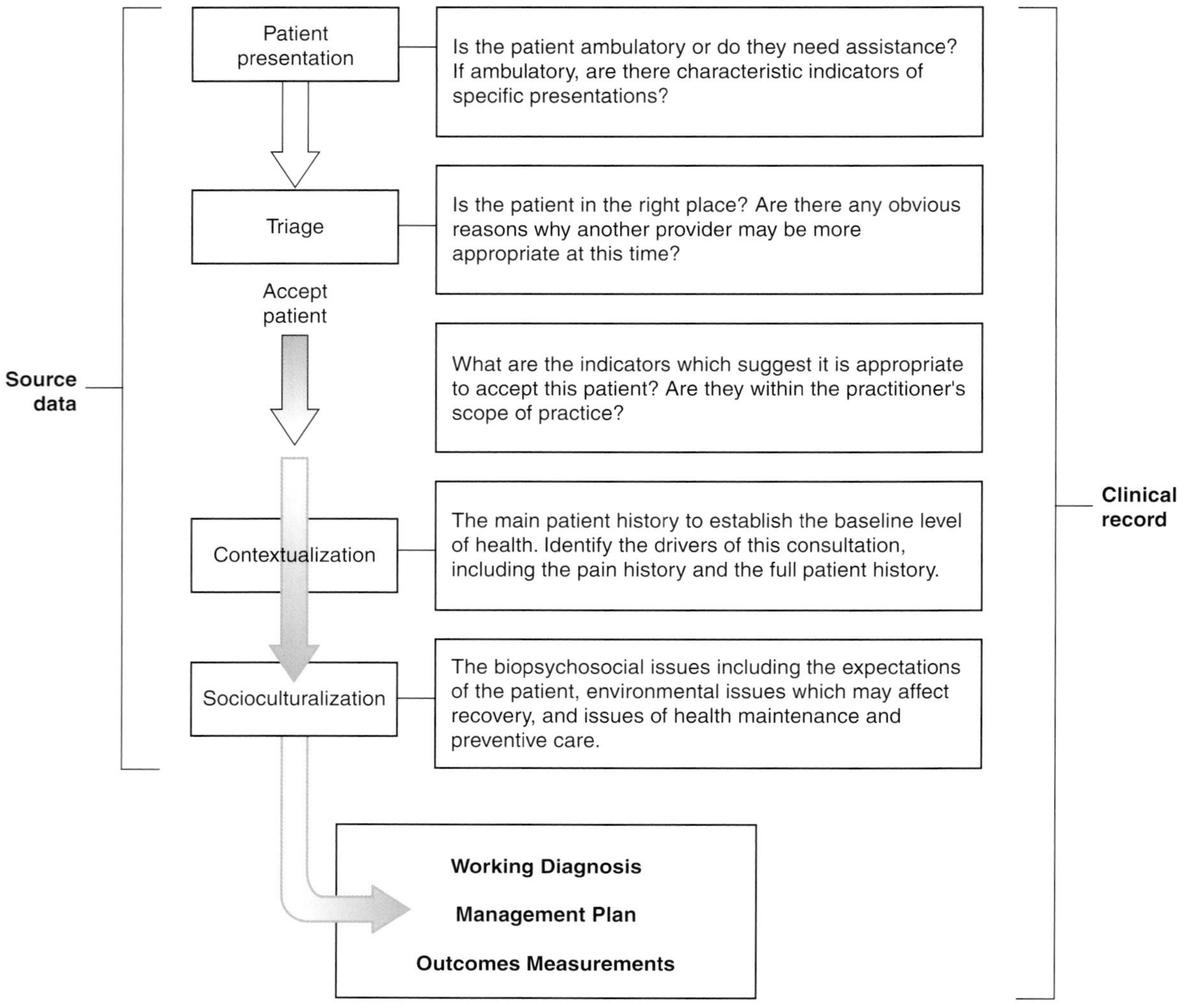

Figure 15.2 Schema of the clinical record. The basic principles of assessment (Fig. 1.5) form the basis for the content of the clinical record.

Once the patient is accepted into the practice of the practitioner, the source data are generated through a wide variety of means and processes. As with the initial data, these include subjective and objective as well as qualitative and quantitative information. They also include information gathered outside the practitioner's clinic and this must be integrated into the clinical record along with the internally generated data. Examples of external data include diagnostic imaging reports, laboratory tests, and audiometry reports. Of course some clinics may generate some or all of these data on-site; however, the principle is that all relevant data and information must be gathered in an ordered manner into the clinical record.

Contextualization

The second commonality among manual healthcare physicians is the provision of primary care, where primary care in this context is that level of care delivered on-site by the individual practitioner. The World Health Organization (WHO) concept of primary care has three levels of meaning, one of which is the primary level of service delivery within the healthcare system. The other meanings relate more to health policy. The characteristic features of primary healthcare as a level of service delivery include accessibility (primary contact), a generalist orientation, continuity of care, and a recognition of the family and social context of health and illness (National Better Health Secretariat 1991 p. 22).

An important component of the clinical record is therefore information which contextualizes the patient. This will ensure that the baseline level of health which is established for the patient incorporates relevant information from a variety of sources, including prior or current medical management. Providers of manual healthcare often function in the insular environment of a sole-practitioner clinic, but this must not be considered isolated. The primary care model of health service delivery incorporates horizontal networking amongst all practitioners who may be associated in some way with an individual patient.

The purpose of contextualizing the patient is to synthesize and generate a working diagnosis. Contextualization therefore represents the main patient history. This will be extensive on the initial visit and will allow the practitioner to reach a working diagnosis which takes into account the presenting demeanor of the patient, the history, which includes health history, family history, and the history of the presenting complaint, physical examination findings, a review of body systems, and any other information which could have a direct bearing on the patient's health status at that moment in time.

Socioculturalization

The third commonality among manual healthcare physicians is a growing recognition that care is best delivered within a wellness model which is holistic, interactive, and uncertain (Jamison 2001). Waddell (1998) recognized this trend when he introduced the biopsychosocial model (Fig. 4.1) and Jamison (2001) has developed a mindset for promoting patient self-care. The process of socioculturalization explores the biopsychosocial dimensions of the patient and integrates them with their capacity, both physical and mental, for self-care.

Socioculturalization incorporates issues of maintenance care and preventive care and allows these to become a legitimate component of clinical practice by documenting both the patient's desire and capacity to participate in care which may not be symptom-based, and their response to that care as it is provided. While pain remains the main driver for the patient to seek treatment, a subset of patients will want to move beyond symptom-based presentation and into a wellness paradigm, especially when this approach to practice is espoused by a competent provider.

The process of socioculturalization integrates and respects the subjective and abstract dimensions of neural change (Fig. 7.1) and brings clinical credibility to the neurocognitive dimensions of health and wellness. It also recognizes the felt experience of dysfunction in the patient's body which allows the lived kinesthetic experience to become part of the doctor–patient interaction. Patients' embodied representation of their pain not only shapes their understanding of the clinical interaction, it influences their understanding of the practitioner's actions and gives rise to their own metaphorical structuring of the abstract concept of health and wellness in general and the subluxation complex in particular.

Patients construct an embodied representation of their health to the extent that inferences enable them to respond to the practitioner's questioning and understand the clinical interaction. This becomes increasingly important the further the encounter moves away from drivers such as pain and dysfunction and towards health maintenance and further towards prevention. The embodied representation is a limiting behavior and is capable of being exploited as patient education. Such education is often an inappropriate training of the individual to respond to the practitioner with modulated words and behaviors nominated by the practitioner as equating to an idealized existence.

The clinical interaction is bidirectional in that it must include the embodied experiences of the patient and the abstract mental models of the practitioner. It places an emphasis on the integrity of the provider to remain as grounded in evidence as possible and not to extend unreasonable ideals which may develop false expectations in the patient. Each statement made about health and wellness should in itself hold true to fundamental laws as

> **Box 15.1** A scheme of types of care
>
> **Type 1**
> A precipitating or causative event can be identified, such as a fall, or a lifting injury, and the pain and dysfunction are associated with that event. This is an expression of evidence-based care with quantifiable parameters.
>
> **Type 2**
> Pain and dysfunction are present but no specific precipitating or causative event can be identified, although the practitioner is able to identify indicators for treatment. This is a transition between evidence-based care and maintenance care.
>
> **Type 3**
> No specific precipitating or causative event can be identified and the patient may not report pain or demonstrate dysfunction, but the practitioner is able to identify indicators for treatment. This is the essence of maintenance care and is validated when the patient returns to a state of pain and/or dysfunction in the absence of treatment.
>
> **Type 4**
> No specific precipitating or causative event can be identified and the patient does not report or demonstrate dysfunction but the practitioner is able to perceive indicators for treatment. This is the essence of preventive care and is yet to be tested in a longitudinal study where the quality of life of those so treated is compared against that of matched samples from the general population.

they are currently known, so then each statement itself will be testable and repeatable.

These statements and the patient's responses to them should be included in the clinical record. A scheme of types of care is given in Box 15.1. These move from the most evidence-based to the least, and provide a useful means of broadly categorizing the stage of the patient encounter as the patient moves from pain drivers to wellness and self-care. Each of these four levels is a valid component of manual healthcare in the contemporary environment and the typical practice will have a spread of patients across all levels.

No matter the level of care determined for the patient, the clinical record must establish an informed starting point common to all patients received by the clinic. This obligation extends from the legal status of chiropractors and osteopaths as primary contact providers of primary care with the responsibility to triage and then either refer or accept the patient.

THE CONTENT OF THE CLINICAL RECORD

The processes of triage, contextualization, and socioculturalization generate a wide range of source data which must be collected and collated in a manner which informs the practitioner in the development and initiation of a management plan and subsequently in the progress of the patient within that plan. The golden rule of the clinical record is for its content to be structured in an organized manner. It is usual for the most recent records to be placed so they are seen when the file is opened, and for the progress notes then to be in an ascending chronological order. This will place the oldest notes towards the back of the file.

There are two exceptions to this. The first is the gathering of like reports under a specific tab, so that all diagnostic imaging reports, for example, are grouped together with the most recent being the first seen under the tab. The second exception is for an overview of the patient also to appear when the file is opened. If a paper-based clinical record is kept within a folder, the progress notes and other source data may be filed on the right side and the overview of the patient, perhaps with contraindications and other critical clinical information such as red flags, on the left. The overview of the patient should be updated from time to time, perhaps to reflect new presentations or the movement from one level of care to another. It should also include the management plan and outcomes measurements, with a record of the patient's progress against those objectives.

The reader will note the absence of recommended forms from this text. This is in recognition of the different emphases, approaches, and clinical languages of the various manual healthcare disciplines. It also reflects the reader's own approach to documenting clinical information. Some are visually oriented and relate easily to clinical drawings and illustrations while others prefer lists, blocks of text, and perhaps algorithms. There are a number of professional associations and some insurers who provide recommended forms to their members.

The clinical record is therefore not a universal, homogeneous document. It is a highly individualized work-in-progress which has a degree of flexibility to accommodate professional sensibilities and practitioner preference. Notwithstanding this flexibility, there are essential categories of data which must be included (Box 15.2). The following may be seen as aspirational yet they reflect not only the opinions of those who defend practitioners from time to time, but also those bodies such as registration boards which determine precedence from time to time.

Patient demographics

The relevant demographics are age, gender, height, weight, body mass index (BMI), somatotype, gene pool, and occupation. These data allow the synthesis of contextualizing statements such as "a 39-year-old female accountant..." which in turn facilitate the association of the patient with disorders common to that demographic. BMI is a function of height and weight (BMI = weight in kilograms/[height in meters]^2) and is a determination of caloric nutritional status. The lowest health risk category occurs for individuals whose BMIs range from 20 to 25, and the highest risk category includes individuals whose BMIs exceed 40. An increased incidence of hypertension, diabetes, and coronary heart disease occurs when BMI values exceed 27.8 for men and 27.3 for women. A BMI between 25 and 30 is considered overweight, and in excess of 30, is obese (McArdle et al 1999).

Notation of the gene pool is relevant as it may alert the practitioner to disorders which have a racially dependent prevalence, such as ossification of the posterior longitudinal ligament which is common in Japan, and neurological disorders such as multiple sclerosis. Occupation is relevant in that it may suggest the mechanism of injury and is usually a factor in the management plan.

Vital signs

The vital signs of the patient, along with other initial observations, effectively provide the data for the triage decision. The vital signs are the patient's temperature, pulse, respiration rate, and blood pressure. Modern instruments may be used as an initial screen; for example, tympanic temperature may be taken within a couple of seconds by a hand-held, infrared thermometer, and indicative blood pressure may be taken by an automated cuff about the finger. If either of these parameters is outside normal limits then more reliable instrumentation should be used to obtain the quantitative data.

The timing of the taking of vital signs must be flexible. Where the practitioner has an early clinical impression that the presentation may require referral, the vital signs should be taken promptly. Where the impression is less obvious, the vital signs may be taken at a relevant point in the history or physical examination process. Vital signs are mandatory at the initial presentation and are then taken as indicated on subsequent visits.

Temperature is indicated with any suspicion of fever or systemic disease process, and in the presence of headache with neck pain and stiffness. Blood pressure is indicated when the initial reading suggests either hyper- or hypotension and the patient is to be monitored, and generally when the patient reports headaches, dizziness, or unsteadiness when standing up. Blood pressure must be recorded in any presentation which suggests cardiovascular change, ranging from micturition syncope to weight gain. Respiration rate is an indicator of respiratory function and should be recorded in any complaint about the thorax, chest, nose, and throat. It may also be elevated when the patient is in pain, along with pulse.

Case history

The case history is a record of the patient and their relationship to the presenting complaint. It is separated into the wide-ranging case history and the specific pain history, when the patient presents with a complaint of pain and/or dysfunction. When the patient presents for maintenance or preventive care, the pain history becomes less relevant but the case history remains important (Ch. 16).

Box 15.2   The essential contents of the clinical record

The clinical record for an individual patient is expected to contain:

- the demographics of the patient
- the vital signs of the patient at initial presentation and then as needed
- a history of the patient and his or her health and disease experiences
- a history of the pain experience of the patient
- details of all relevant physical examination findings, whether positive or negative
- a review of the body systems of the patient
- notation of the family history
- a working diagnosis
- a management plan relevant to the working diagnosis, to include treatment options
- a record of advice given to the patient such as recommended exercises
- progress notes which are a contemporaneous record of what has taken place on each visit
- identification of outcomes measurements relevant to the working diagnosis and management plan and the recording of the patient's progress
- a record of informed consent signed and dated by the patient.

Pain history

The pain history is a specific exploration of the patient's current pain experience and must explore the three essential dimensions of intensity, frequency, and duration. No matter how quantifiable the pain history may appear to be, it remains an embodied kinesthetic experience of the patient, therefore it really cannot be separated from the overall case history and experiences of the patient. Notwithstanding this, the pain experience of the patient is explored and recorded in concise terms (Ch. 16).

The history is neither a simple set of pain measurements nor a collection of unrelated statements; it is a complex, interwoven tapestry of the patient's lived experiences which should be explored broadly but then succinctly documented in the general terms of the overall history of the patient, and in the specific terms of the presenting complaint. These statements are then to be supported by the subsequent steps in the assessment process.

When the patient file is reviewed, the history section should allow an understanding of the experience of the presenting complaint within the overall context of the patient. These self-reported historical data are then supplemented with findings from the physical assessment, review of systems, family history, and assessment of the spine.

Physical examination findings

The primary contact provider of manual healthcare is responsible for the physical examination of the patient to identify conditions which may contraindicate or modify manual intervention. The provider is not expected to reach a definitive diagnosis of any of the systems examined, but must have sufficient diagnostic acumen to raise an index of suspicion about a system which may have findings which fall outside normal limits.

A review of the following body systems of the patient should provide an indication for physical examination where such examination is warranted and may inform the clinical interaction. To this end the practitioner is expected to undertake a physical examination of the following systems when indicated and record the findings, whether they be positive or negative:

- Eyes, ears, nose, and throat, using the otoscope, ophthalmoscope, torch, sinus illuminator, and tongue depressor to inspect and assess all structures visually. Indicated by any reported problems with these special senses, and the wearing of glasses or contact lenses.
- The cardiovascular system, including auscultation of the heart and valves and carotid arteries, palpation of the peripheral pulses and abdominal aorta, and measurement of jugular venous pressure. Indicated when patients do not know their blood pressure, report a blood pressure outside normal limits, report chest pain or that they feel their heart beating, or other indicators of cardiovascular change such as light-headedness or tingling in an extremity.
- The respiratory system, including auscultation and percussion of the lungs and bronchi. Indicated when the patient reports breathing difficulties, chest pain or chest infections, or asthma.
- The gastrointestinal tract, to include auscultation, percussion, and palpation of the abdomen, to include the liver and gall bladder. Indicated when the patient reports problems with

eating or with defecation or urination, including irregular bowel movements and/or urinary incontinence or retention.
- The musculoskeletal system in general terms as well as specifically with the assessment of the spine. Indications are generalized weakness or global muscle dysfunction.
- The nervous system in general terms including the status of the central nervous system, as well as specifically with the assessment of the spine. Indications are global dysfunctions which appear to be unrelated to spinal dysfunction.

The hematological and endocrinological systems are implicated by clinical suspicion and informed by palpation of the spleen and thyroid and the patient is typically referred for laboratory investigation and specialist assessment. Other indications include patients reporting they are taking medication to thin their blood, or that they bruise or tire easily. Patients should be asked if they have been tested for diabetes, and, if female of menopausal age, whether they are taking hormone replacement therapy (HRT).

The genitourinary and reproductive systems are typically assessed through directed questioning with any physical examination being conducted with a chaperone present or, more commonly, by referral to a practitioner specializing in these systems. Males should be asked if they have two testicles and, after puberty, whether they perform testicular self-examination. Females from about the age of 20 should be asked whether they perform breast self-examination, and from the onset of sexual activity, whether or not their Pap smear is current. A menstrual history should also be taken of females of reproductive age, and a birth history should be recorded for females who have previously conceived.

Family history

The history of other members of the individual's family is relevant, particularly with genetic disorders. A scheme for recording the family history is given in Figure 15.3. The family tree was originally developed to track autosomal dominant or recessive genes to determine the individuals in whom certain diseases and disorders may be expressed.

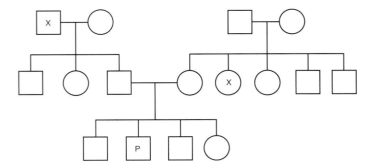

Figure 15.3 The family history tree. Male gender is represented by a square and female by a circle. An X indicates the family member is deceased; a P identifies the patient. Notation should be made of the cause of death. Notation of serious disorders and illnesses should also be made against relevant members. The horizontal line between two individuals represents a productive sexual relationship, with the vertical line linking the offspring.

A further clinical use is to identify clusters of death due to potentially preventable causes and thus allow the identification of individuals who may benefit greatly from medical screening procedures. An example is bowel cancer, where the offspring of an individual who has suffered or died from the disease should be entered into a screening program at an appropriate age (usually in the fifth decade for males). If two generations of antecedents have suffered the same disease, then the screening should begin earlier.

While familial relationships have been noted in various pain syndromes, such as fibromyalgia and compensable low-back pain, these relationships may be more psychosocial than genetic or hereditary and the tree, while suggesting familial disposition, may not be clinically useful.

Assessment of the spine

Given the title of this text and its orientation towards the identification of spinal dysfunction through careful and thorough assessment, it must be expected that the findings from the specific assessment of the spine are recorded in the clinical record.

These findings will be recorded following the initial visit and will set the specific direction for subsequent intervention. The challenge with mechanical findings about the spine is that they are inherently dynamic, in that they may respond totally to one intervention and be absent on subsequent assessment. They may also demonstrate an unpredictable response to intervention, in that they may return as originally identified from time to time, or may stimulate other patterns of findings.

Assessment of the spine is a major clinical task which must be undertaken at each visit. Naturally the subsequent assessments are not as time-consuming as the initial assessment, but this is not an invitation for the subsequent assessments to be unreasonably abbreviated. At all times the findings from subsequent assessment must be considered in the context of the original findings and the patient's response to the previous treatment episode.

Clinical impression

The clinical impression is a mandatory inclusion for return or continuing visits as it represents the subjective opinion of the practitioner as to the status of the patient, including progress or regression. This is discussed shortly under Progress notes.

The inclusion of a clinical impression at the initial visit is optional but may have benefit in that it is capable of capturing the clinical instinct of the practitioner. Instinct is an abstract dimension and, in the same manner in which there is strong clinical justification for recording the abstract dimensions of the patient's presentation, there is justification for recording those of the practitioner.

Care must be taken with the words used to express what is essentially an opinion of the practitioner and the clinical impression should never be a blatant accusation of malingering or mental instability or other functional disorder. Instead, the suspicion of such disorders could be recorded as "query functional overlay" which is a justifiable clinical impression that, in the opinion of the practitioner, there may be value and relevance in making clinical investigation into the possibility of a potentially

unfavorable patient reaction which may well be secondary to the presenting complaint and a valid warp of the biopsychosocial dimensions.

As the practitioner gains experience, the clinical impression sharpens; however, care must always be taken to avoid presumptuous pattern recognition. Notwithstanding this caveat, the clinical impression is an opportunity to capture the gut feel of the practitioner and may be a useful item to revisit in cases where the patient fails to progress as expected.

Working diagnosis

The working diagnosis is the engine built by all the elements discussed above (history, examination, spinal assessment) for the purpose of driving the management plan. It encapsulates the entire purpose of the process of assessment subsequent to the patient presentation, and exists as a succinct, linked series of statements which incorporate the diverse elements identified during the assessment process.

The working diagnosis is descriptive statements which integrate the believed cause with the many elements which are manifested in various forms. The truthfulness of the working diagnosis reflects the comprehensiveness of the assessment yet can only remain a best guess of what is happening to the patient.

The content and structure of the working diagnosis are complex and must integrate all elements of the assessment process (Ch. 17).

Management plan

The management plan is the vehicle built to accommodate the working diagnosis as its engine and incorporates a variety of elements to ensure the safe and successful transport of patients from their presenting condition to the mutually agreed destination. It is, quite simply, a synthesis of what the practitioner conceives to be the most effective way forward given the found data and working diagnosis, but can only ever reflect a direction approved and complied with by the patient.

This is the reason why the question of prognosis is really a quite useless inclusion in the clinical record. Any prognosis must rely upon the precision of the practitioner to reach a working diagnosis and then to select the most appropriate treatment plan, both being acts which are subsequently modified to a significant extent by the patient's elected level of cooperation. Any statement of prognosis thus has the validity of an astrological reading and is better replaced by a reasoned management plan which allows for the various "ifs" and "buts" of normal clinical reality. This is not to deny patients the benefit of a best guess as to how their condition may develop or remit, but this can only be answered in terms of the known natural history of that condition and should attempt to incorporate known modifying factors, such as the patient's lifestyle.

The management plan is driven by the working diagnosis and must include various treatment options. The word "options" is the keyword in this context; it demands that the practitioner be sufficiently informed to be able to recommend valid treatment options to patients, thus allowing them to make an informed decision to accept or reject those treatment options offered by the practitioner. The options will range across the different conservative techniques which can be offered by the practitioner, to the different techniques of related disciplines outside the practitioner's scope of practice.

Practitioners must act as an informed but not authoritative source of information regarding clinical procedures outside their immediate discipline. In the case of manual healthcare, these range from the innocuous but powerful tai chi to the also powerful but irreversible effects of surgical intervention. In order to maintain an appropriate level of knowledge in these matters, participation in multidisciplinary continuing professional education is useful.

The clinical implication is the two levels of options which are to be presented to the patient. The first incorporates those outside the practitioner's scope and the second informs the patient of those within the practitioner's scope. In the case of an overweight 45-year-old male shoe sales assistant with recurrent low-back and left-sided buttock pain without leg radiation, the external options could include medical consultation and analgesics, chiropractic consultation with spinal adjustment, osteopathic consultation with muscle energy techniques, and physical therapy consultation with exercises. Each may also recommend weight management and nutritional advice, workplace assessment, psychological counseling or other adjunctive therapeutic activities.

The internal options are dependent on the practitioner's therapeutic armamentarium and the specific clinical indicators, but could include flexion-distraction traction, prone drop-piece adjustment, prone spinal treatment with the Activator™ adjusting instrument, supine blocking with biomechanical wedges, side-lying high-velocity, low-amplitude spinal adjustment, side-lying spinal mobilization, with or without impulse, or muscle energy techniques. Each of these options may be combined with soft-tissue treatment, trigger point therapy, and adjunctive therapeutics like ultrasound, laser, or interferential. It is quite apparent that a broad-scope practitioner is able to offer a wider selection of options than one who has narrowed his or her scope into a singular paradigm of practice or is limited to only one technique system.

The options must take patients into account, particularly their age. The clinically significant age groupings are neonate, preschool, school-age, adolescent, young adult, and aging. The gravid patient represents an additional grouping.

The management plan must be determined, documented, and defendable. The process of determining the plan leads to the question of informed consent, discussed below.

Progress notes

The progress notes are the most active part of the clinical record and are a contemporaneous record of what has taken place on each interaction with the patient. They are more than a record of treatment, as treatment per se may not be given on certain visits and interaction with the patient may occur by telephone, as with the patient calling for advice. The progress notes must document each such interaction as an entry written at the time the interaction occurred, and dated accordingly. They are generated in an ascending chronological order so that the oldest notes or pages of notes are towards the back of the file and the most recent are on top.

There will be occasions when it is appropriate to clarify a pre-existing progress note or add further information. Any such additions must be initialled by the person who makes them and be dated for the day they were entered. There are no circumstances under which pre-existing information may be erased, blanked out, or otherwise made illegible. Where information needs to be de-emphasized, a single line may be drawn through it; this change must also be initialled and dated.

The degree of comprehensiveness of the progress notes is, to some extent, a preference of individual practitioners. They must, as a minimum, document the care given, comments by the patient, and the responses of the patient following treatment. The common acronym for the progress note is SOAP:

- Subjective: the comments by patients on how they feel they are progressing or regressing, and the clinical impression and any subjective observations of the practitioner.
- Objective: the clinical findings evident at that interaction, including those derived from physical examination and spinal assessment.
- Assessment: the interpretation of the objective findings within the subjective context. This is a crucial step in the management plan of the patient. It provides the opportunity to appraise the intervention to date and forces the clinical judgment of whether the management plan should continue, be altered, or end.
- Plan: the proposed actions in response to the assessment. It includes a description of the spinal segments to be adjusted, the types of technique used, and the patient's response to those interventions after they have been performed. It also includes a directive as to when the patient is next to attend.

A record of advice given

The participation of patients in their journey out of injury and dysfunction and into health and wellness is guided by advice from the practitioner. A record of that advice, as it is given from time to time, must be included in the clinical record.

When printed advice is passed to the patient – for example, an exercise sheet – a copy of that sheet should be entered into the clinical record with specific notation of which exercises were recommended, along with cautions and guidance. This forms a valuable guide for subsequent visits when the exercise routine needs revision.

Outcomes measurement

Outcomes measurement is an integral component of the clinical interaction. It is not enough for patients to think they are improving and for practitioners to continue providing care in the belief they are having a positive effect. Evidence of the outcome of the intervention is needed. The very minimum is a visual analog scale (VAS) marked by patients to record one or more dimensions of their perceived clinical status, and a simple test by the practitioner of patient function, such as range of motion of a joint which may have been previously limited.

It is far better to select specific outcomes measurements which are relevant to the working diagnosis and management plan. Yeomans (2000) discusses the selection and clinical application of outcomes measurements and provides a variety of instruments suitable for use. The completed instruments are dated and collected within the patient record.

ABBREVIATIONS

There are very few abbreviations common to all clinical disciplines. Manual healthcare is practiced by several disciplines which, regrettably, have little congruence in their paradigms and even less standardization among their teaching institutions. Once within a discipline, a degree of common usage of basic abbreviations is found, but there will always remain a range of terms for which individual practitioners have developed their own shorthand or abbreviation.

A fundamental reason for clinical record keeping is that any practitioner in the same discipline group and with a registration or license to practice under the same Act or Bill must be able to read, interpret, and understand the clinical records which are kept by others of that discipline group. This is for the protection of the patient in the event the practitioner is disabled. If the osteopath falls ill, another osteopath should be able to step in and continue care. If the chiropractor dies suddenly, another chiropractor must be able to step in and continue care.

The matter is simply resolved by individual practitioners having a list of abbreviations they use available for reference at the point where the clinical record is accessed.

THE CLINICAL RECORD AND THE LAW

The following principles are drawn from the Health Records Act 2001 of the State of Victoria, Australia and other sources (Ladenheim et al 2001, Risk Management Seminar 2002).

The clinical record is considered to be information or an opinion about the physical, mental, or psychological health (at any time) of an individual, including any disability and any expressed wishes about the future provision of health services to the individual. It includes details of any health service provided, or to be provided, to an individual, and the personal information of the patient which is collected to provide the health service, such as address, phone numbers, and employer and insurance details.

It is important for the clinical record to be handled responsibly in order to maintain the privacy of the patient. In the most simple of terms, the practitioner or clinic owns the physical record (the paper it is written on) while the patient owns the general content. Specific content in the form of a confidential opinion of patients or their condition which is provided to one practitioner from another, may remain confidential from the patient. Apart from this, patients have the right of full access to their clinical record and to control the use of that information.

The health information collected by a clinic about an individual should only be collected from that individual. Exceptions to this are when the individual is unable to offer reliable clinical information, as with a young child or an older senile person, where the parent, guardian, or nominated family member may provide relevant information. Information in the form of data from another practitioner or an external laboratory or imaging center may also be provided and forms part of the clinical record available to the patient.

Box 15.3 Consent to establish a clinical record

I, being the person whose name and signature appear below, consent to the [name of clinic or health service] creating and maintaining a health record of me as an individual for the purpose of recording my health status to determine and manage therapeutic interventions. This record will include details of any health service provided or to be provided to me, and my personal information which is collected in order to provide the health service, such as address, phone numbers, and employer and insurance details.

I understand that the information in this record is private and will not be released to any person or organization except as required by law without my written permission. I also understand that I have access to the information contained within my health record and that, while not deleting information, I may change or correct that information should I consider it appropriate to do so.

Include this statement if there is an intent to use clinical information for research purposes:

I consent to the use of information from my health record for the purpose of research and education on the understanding my identity is removed from my information and its use will not identify me in any way.

Name: Signed: Date:

Witnessed by:

Name: Signed: Date:

An important point is that legislation may require the health service to obtain consent from the individual to create and hold a clinical record. While the intent of such legislation is to protect the interests of the patient in large organizations, the implication is that the clinic should inform the patient that a health record will be created, the purpose of that record, and the uses of the information which will be gathered and recorded. It is noted that information in the health record should not be used for research purposes without the consent of the individual except in certain cases, which may be deemed to be in the public interest, when the data must be de-identified. If the practitioner wishes to use an individual's data for research then consent should be obtained. Statements which may satisfy these requirements are given in Box 15.3.

The clinic must take reasonable steps to protect the health information it holds from misuse and loss and from unauthorized access, modification, or disclosure. All staff who work within the clinic must be aware of this and care must be taken to ensure the clinical record is not accessible by cleaners, tradespeople, or other patients.

An underlying principle is that, once an entry is made into a clinical record it must remain, even if it is later found or claimed to be inaccurate. Any subsequent entry to correct or clarify such information may be entered and, while notation of the new entry may be made adjacent to the original entry, the original entry must remain legible. In the case when an inactive clinical record is destroyed, or an electronic record is deleted from a current file, a written note must be made and retained of the name of the individual to whom the health information related, the period covered by it, and the date on which it was destroyed or deleted. A health service provider who transfers health information to another individual or organization and does not continue to hold a record of that information must make a written note of the name and address of the individual or organization to whom it was transferred.

Information from the patient's clinical record may be made available to another health service provider on request of the patient or request of the other provider when authorized by the patient.

THE RECORDING OF CONSENT TO TREATMENT

Implied consent is not informed consent. Patients must be informed of what the practitioner intends to do. They must be informed of the alternatives to the proposed treatment and techniques and the possible consequences of them not undertaking the treatment which is recommended.

Most importantly, the patient must be informed as to the material risk associated with the treatment and techniques which are proposed. A material risk is a risk the patient would place emphasis on in considering whether to proceed with treatment. With regard to manipulation of the neck by an experienced practitioner, while the risk of an adverse outcome is exceedingly small, the outcome may be devastating and the risk may be considered material by the patient.

The patient should be informed there is a risk of injury or death, and this should be conveyed in language which the patient, a lay person, can understand. A statistical expression of the risks associated with manipulation of the cervical spine is about one in two million. The patient will understand this better if it is explained that the "risk of stroke following neck manipulation has been described as roughly equivalent to the odds a person has of being struck by lightening" (Ladenheim et al 2001).

The consequential risk potential varies with the technique and procedure as well as with the age of the patient and the region being treated. For example, the risk outcome of low-back manipulation is less for an older patient with no evidence of a disk bulge than it is for a younger patient with evidence of a disk bulge. The patient must have the opportunity to discuss the risk potential with the practitioner who will be delivering the care. The wise practitioner will ensure the patient's inquiries are well answered and exhausted.

Informed consent is acknowledged by patients signing and dating a printed informed consent form which they have read and then discussed to their satisfaction. The wording used for such forms differs according to discipline, jurisdiction, and the demands of the professional indemnity insurer. Current forms with appropriate wording should be available from the relevant professional association. The signed and dated form is retained in the patient's clinical record.

CONCLUSION

Clinical practice is richly rewarding but comes with specific responsibilities which are intended to protect both the patient and the practitioner. A thorough clinical record which is well structured and adequately maintained is essential to safe and successful practice.

16

The patient history

KEY CONCEPTS

There is a well-respected understanding among experienced practitioners that the patient will tell the practitioner what is wrong as long as the practitioner is smart enough to give the patient the opportunity and intelligent enough to be listening for the answer.

The importance of the case and pain histories cannot be overestimated for their role in adding to the source data to drive the determination of the most appropriate working diagnosis, management plan, and outcomes assessment.

The responsibilities of the case and pain histories include determination of the nature and extent of the physical examination and the essential inclusions of the examination directly related to the presenting complaint.

The case history is a record of the patient and his or her relationship to the presenting complaint. It is supplemented by the specific pain history when the patient presents with a complaint of pain and/or dysfunction.

The pain history is a specific exploration of the patient's current pain experience and must explore the three essential dimensions of duration, intensity, and frequency in concise terms.

Specific words have specific meanings when used as descriptors of the pain experience of the patient and it is wise to standardize the words used for writing the patient history with those found to be valid and reliable in the worldwide clinical experience.

The history of the pain experience has dimensions of duration, intensity, and frequency which provide valuable elements for the practitioner to explore and document.

The practitioner is responsible for all of the content within the clinical record and any prehistory forms completed by the patient alone must be discussed in detail with the patient by the practitioner.

INTRODUCTION

Many of the steps required to build the clinical record are relatively one-sided in that they involve the practitioner actively performing a test on a passive patient. The establishment of the patient history requires an interactive, bidirectional relationship in which the patient feels sufficiently confident to respond truthfully to the practitioner's questions. The practitioner also has a responsibility to ensure the flow of questions considers and reflects the incoming data from the patient to ensure they are modified to elicit the most comprehensive and relevant patient response.

There is a well-respected adage among experienced practitioners that the patient will tell the practitioner what is wrong as long as the practitioner is smart enough to give the patient the opportunity and intelligent enough to be listening for the answer.

COMMUNICATION WITH THE PATIENT

There is an imbalance of power in every doctor–patient relationship. This is due to the doctor having a professional level of education in a field not shared by the patient, which puts patients at the disadvantage of receiving information about themselves which they do not have the power or ability to test. There is a significant element of trust and a responsibility on the doctor not to abuse or misuse that trust.

Patients are also placing themselves in a relationship which they expect will recommend and then deliver certain therapeutic interventions to them for their benefit. This relationship between the doctor and the patient imposes an obligation of a duty of care on the doctor to ensure benefit for the patient.

The imbalance of power does not mean practitioners should use words of one syllable in short sentences; rather, they should aim to establish a common level of language with the patient in which both feel comfortable. Once it is established that the two are speaking the same language, the art of communication

---

Box 16.1 Ways to improve communication with the patient

- Sit across the corner of the desk – avoid placing a physical barrier.
- Maintain eye contact with the patient while talking – demonstrate you are interested in what the patient has to tell you.
- Use the language of the patient – if the language of the practitioner is the patient's second language, then an interpreter may be needed.
- Use words the patient can understand – consider the patient's age, linguistic capability, education level.
- Demonstrate the boundaries of confidentiality – accept whatever the patient says as "normal" and do not react to or highlight confidential information.
- Be directed and focused on the patient – do not ramble or talk about yourself.

---

moves more to how things are said (Box 16.1) rather than what is actually said.

The words used and the way they are delivered by the practitioner should work together to minimize the discomfort of the patient and thus maximize the quality of the data obtained. Every patient wants to know "how bad is it?" and responses from the practitioner such as "oh dear" or "that is the worst I've ever seen" do little to inspire trust and confidence. When the patient has a significant problem the practitioner should seek to reassure the patient without trivializing the matter: "yes, there is a disk protrusion which seems to be interfering with some nerves in that area and this is causing your pain and preventing you from working, but you've done the right thing by coming here and there are things we can do to help".

Note the use of the plural "we" when the practitioner is speaking. Practitioners should not aim to emphasize themselves as healers. The use of a plural tense infers there is a broader range of expertise available should the practitioner find the problem does not respond to their care and the patient needs referral. Also, it is unlikely that the patient will always see that one practitioner given that at times he or she will be absent and a locum or assistant will continue the care. Finally, "we" includes the patient and it is a central premise of manual healthcare that the patient is a partner in the healing journey.

The subtle and thoughtful use of inclusive words when communicating with the patient may be reinforced by metaphors and models. As dreadfully unrealistic as it may be, describing the effect of the subluxation complex as like "a foot on the hosepipe" effectively conveys an idea which patients can understand. Difficulties seem to arise, however, when the patient conveys this simple understanding to another person or practitioner who does not appreciate the use of the metaphor.

How to structure questions

The asking of a question is an invitation for a response. There are three types of response in the clinical setting: inadequate, useful, and overwhelming. Most patients are cooperative in that they want the practitioner to have the information needed to help them and the type of response will vary between being inadequate and useful, depending on how the practitioner asks the question. The type of response reflects the type of question, and in the clinical setting the question can be either open-ended or closed.

A closed question is one which can be answered with a limited response. An example is "does it hurt when I press here?" to which the response can be "yes", "no", or "sort of". Any one of these answers closes the question and the practitioner must ask another. For example, if the response is "yes" then the practitioner needs to explore that response with a question such as "is this the pain which is your problem?" and so on.

An open-ended question is one which facilitates a descriptive response from the patient. For example, "tell me about any pain you might feel as I touch you here" is an invitation which can't be answered "yes" or "no". The dialogue is thus forced to become interactive and the value of the patient's responses increases.

There are certain patients who will take every opportunity to inform the practitioner of every minute detail of their life story, colored by similar trivia of the lives of their family members and even neighbors. These patients present a challenge and the practitioner should resort to simple, directed questions which can be asked in quick succession, thus limiting the opportunity for the patient to overrespond. The practitioner may have to resort to closed questions to bring the interaction back on track.

The open-ended approach carries into instructions given to the patient during the assessment. For example, the closed instruction "bend down and touch your toes" does not give an opportunity for the person who can reach beyond their toes to demonstrate this. An open-ended instruction is better: "bend down and see if you can touch your toes or go further".

Other examples of open-ended instructions and questions include:

- "show me where you are feeling these pains" to engage the patient in an act of completeness which the practitioner can summarize
- "tell me about any time that you might have had this problem before" will engage the patient in telling a story and this again allows the practitioner to distill the relevant data
- "what do you think the problem is?" is a wonderful question to engage patients in their health interaction. Remember to be listening for the answer!

THE PATIENT HISTORY

There are two components of the patient history. The first is the case history, which is a global overview of the patient as they experience the specific problem of their presenting complaint. The second is the pain history, which is a concise exploration of the pain where the patient has presented with a complaint of pain and/or dysfunction.

Practitioners who function more with type 3 (maintenance care) and type 4 (preventive care) patients (Ch. 15) will place less emphasis on the pain history but must still elicit a complete and comprehensive case history. It may be said that in these circumstances there is a greater responsibility on such practitioners to observe and document the case history in order to develop a justifiable management plan which incorporates the patient's expectations. Practitioners who deal largely with a patient-base driven by pain perhaps have the easier task; pain can be described in a number of ways to justify care and its fluctuation and (hopefully) eventual cessation over time provides ready evidence of a cause-and-effect relationship with the management plan and treatment delivery.

This is not quite so for practitioners delivering preventive care as the markers of the success or otherwise of such care have yet to be identified and tested. Patients receiving maintenance care are usually able to associate the return of familiar pain and dysfunction with withdrawal of care and this in itself provides a certain level of evidence for the need and value of type 3 care.

Practitioners who limit their practice to accept only those presentations for which evidence exists in the literature, preferably in the form of controlled clinical trials, are effectively denying a large number of potential patients the right to a form of care the patient elects to seek out and purchase.

The importance of the case and pain histories cannot be underestimated for their role in adding to the source data to drive the determination of the most appropriate working diagnosis, management plan, and outcomes assessment. Indeed, the case and pain histories play an important role in determining the direction of some other components of the source data, most notably the physical examination.

It is important, and in some jurisdictions mandatory, for the clinical record to include a review of systems. The value of a thorough case and pain history is that, in conjunction with the systems review, it allows the practitioner to reach a decision to conduct a directed physical examination as opposed to routinely completing a full physical examination on every patient.

A directed physical examination is a subset of the full physical examination where that subset is indicated by findings within the histories and systems review. As a subset of the full physical, the directed physical examination is conducted at the same level of thoroughness and competence as it would be if it were performed within the routines of a full physical. Perhaps, in some respects, the directed examination is more thorough in that it is initiated by indicators from the histories, whereas a full physical examination is often conducted in the hope of finding something which may relate back to the presenting problem.

The responsibilities of the case and pain histories are to contribute to the source data and better inform the subsequent steps in the clinical interaction. These include determination of the nature and extent of the physical examination and the essential inclusions of the examination directly related to the presenting complaint. Once again, decent histories can efficiently direct the examination of the presenting complaint and avoid the need to subject the patient to a barrage of tests in the hope that one or two may uncover something.

THE CASE HISTORY

The case history is a wide-ranging record of the patient and his or her relationship to the presenting complaint. It is supplemented by a specific pain history when the patient presents with a complaint of pain and/or dysfunction. When the patient presents for maintenance or preventive care, the pain history becomes less relevant but the case history remains critically important.

There are classic approaches, commonly termed "the eight-point history". The inherent problem is that they generally focus on the presenting complaint and thus become an abbreviated pain history. A more comprehensive history can be built about the patient when the pain history is explored separately. A second benefit is that the pain history can be expanded beyond the usual "what, where, when, how" approach.

The case history seeks to inform practitioners about the patient at the particular moment in time of their interaction with the patient. As such, it should explore why the patient has selected a particular practitioner and try to identify expectations and concerns. This is a combination of contextualization and socioculturalization.

The case history will record:

- The *location* of the problem. A useful generalization is that mechanical problems can usually be pointed to quite specifically by the patient, while a problem which is described as vague and diffuse in nature may be either muscular or non-mechanical. Associated findings, such as weakness or sensation changes, are also documented. The location can also be explored as to whether or not there have been any preceding, seemingly unrelated injuries to the current area of pain.

- The *onset* of the problem. This is explored in terms of when and how, and particularly whether or not the patient associates onset with any event. There are medicolegal implications and the practitioner should retain a clinical detachment which allows an informed judgment of any claims of causation by the patient.
- The *course* of the problem since it became apparent to the patient. Some presentations progressively worsen while others are intermittent or refractory in nature. This information is useful for identifying possible diagnoses and may even point to probable diagnoses. An exploration of the *aggravating and relieving factors* is warranted as it will also help extract the probable diagnoses from the possible.
- Information about any *previous occurrences* and the patient's *response* to those occurrences and the current presentation, including self-medication and consultations for other advice and any treatment.
- A description of *other problems* which may be afflicting the patient and whether or not the patient offers any association between those problems and the presenting complaint.

Each of these dimensions allows the practitioner to explore the point further in relation to the patient's experience. This process may not be completed on the initial visit as more information may be revealed during a course of treatment. The case history is a vital, ongoing document and it is appropriate to return to the initial history to add information and make clarification as long as the date of those entries is shown to differentiate them from the date the initial history was recorded. The entries which are made from time to time to document the changing status of the patient are recorded separately, in ascending chronological order, as progress notes.

THE PAIN HISTORY

The pain history is a specific exploration of the patient's current pain experience and must explore the three essential dimensions of duration, intensity, and frequency. No matter how "quantifiable" the pain history may appear to be, pain remains an embodied kinesthetic experience of the patient and it really cannot be separated from the overall case history and experiences of the patient. Notwithstanding this, the pain experience of the patient is explored and recorded in concise terms.

Characteristics

A variety of verbal descriptors have been tested and found to be reliable and useful for describing the pain experience. Melzack (1975, 1982) collected these into an instrument now known as the McGill pain questionnaire (MPQ), which can be considered the gold-standard instrument for measuring pain outcomes with respect to pain quality (Yeomans 2000 p. 64). Fernandez & Towery (1996) extracted what they consider to be a reliable vocabulary of pain (see also Ch. 7). These terms can be used to

describe the pain experience of the patient during the process of history taking. They are grouped in sensory subcategories:

- temporal: pulsing, throbbing, pounding, beating
- spatial: radiating, spreading
- punctate pressure: drilling, penetrating, stabbing, piercing, pricking
- incisive pressure: cutting, lacerating
- constrictive pressure: pressing, crushing, squeezing, tight
- traction: tugging, pulling, drawing
- hotness: burning, hot, scalding, searing
- coldness: cool, freezing, cold
- brightness: smarting, blinding
- dullness: aching, dull, sore.

The clinical application is for the practitioner to hear the type of pain the patient is attempting to describe, and then to offer relevant words from the list above and record those with which the patient agrees. The use of terms such as these is important for the standardization of pain descriptions among practitioners and across disciplines.

Duration

Pain has a duration which can be described as acute, subacute, or chronic (Box 16.2). These terms reflect the duration of the pain episode and not its frequency or its intensity. A representation of these time periods is given in Figure 16.1 as they relate to the common syndrome of low-back pain. The period of 13 weeks as the delimiter between subacute and chronic pain is commonly used in the clinical context.

Less complex pain experiences, such as those associated with local tissue injury, may have a shortened scale to differentiate between acute and subacute. The delimitation here relates to the pathological processes associated with tissue healing, and an acute condition typically exists for about 72 h before the healing phase sets in and the injury can be considered subacute. The

---

Box 16.2 Questions about the duration of a pain episode

A short-term pain experience may be continuous; however, as the duration lengthens, the pain experience reflects changes in frequency and intensity. The following questions explore a typical pain episode which has been present for a period of time:

- When did the problem start? (to classify it as acute, subacute, or chronic)
- How do you think it started? (the patient should have an opinion about this)
- What were you doing at the time it started? (to identify a likely mechanism of injury)
- What have you done about it since it started? (to identify any medication or other treatment)
- What actions or movements make the pain worse? (mechanical pain is often worsened by specific movement)
- What can you do to ease the pain? (body position to ease pain is an important clinical clue)
- Are there times when the pain has gone away? If so, what makes it return? (clues may be given to understand better the frequency and intensity of the experience)
- Does the pain wake you at night? (mechanical pain typically eases with rest; sinister pain may wake the sleeping patient).

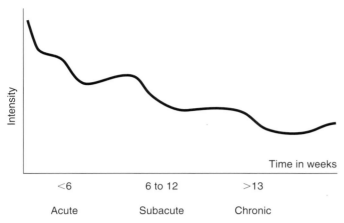

Figure 16.1 A representation of pain duration. These time periods relate to low-back pain.

clinical relevance is for the application of wet ice which is useful in the acute stage of injury but not of much benefit after about 3 days postinjury (Ebrall et al 1992).

Presentations such as low-back pain may be differentiated between being a chronic injury or a sudden-onset injury, in which case there may be acute tissue damage amenable to ice treatment in the first 3 days, and it is appropriate to consider that those tissues shift to a subacute phase after that time. The syndrome of low-back pain rarely arises from one simple tissue injury and is more likely to be due to a variety of complex processes recurring over time. This is the reason why a clinical presentation such as low-back pain can be considered acute within a 6-week window, subacute up to 13 weeks, and then chronic. Further, early intervention in patients with low-back pain seems to prevent progression to chronicity (Ebrall 1992c, 1993).

Intensity

Pain has an intensity which may be quantified on a visual analog scale (VAS), as discussed in Chapter 7. In terms of taking the history, the three most useful words to describe the intensity of the pain experience as both perceived and demonstrated by the patient are mild, moderate, and severe (Box 16.3).

The selection of these descriptors includes a judgment by the practitioner of the patient's pain response which in turn reflects his or her expressed experience of a negative kinesthetic event. For example, the patient may report the pain as severe, yet still be able to walk unaided in and out of the clinic and perhaps may even continue performing activities of daily living (ADL). A patient with pain that is truly severe is unlikely to be physically able to behave in that manner.

The majority of patients attending for manual healthcare will describe their pain as mild or moderate and reserve the term "severe" as a descriptor of the pain at its onset, especially if the onset was traumatic. These terms are therefore of little use as outcomes measurements and the VAS is the preferred tool. However, the terms are useful in the context of understanding the patient's pain experience and for guiding subsequent examination of the patient.

Box 16.3 Measures of the intensity of pain

Objective
Measurements on pain scales or other instruments
The amount of time taken off work
Restrictions in the activities of daily living (ADL)

Subjective
Does the patient rate the pain as mild, moderate, or severe?

Abstract
How is the patient expressing his or her embodiment of the pain experience? (consider tough macho male and stoic female)
What is the nature of the psychosociocultural context (is there evidence of secondary gain?)
Are there other complaints and relationships which may modulate intensity? (the patient does not understand any relationships between pains, so this must be specifically explored by the practitioner)

- Is there any referred pain? If so, is it more nerve root or from trigger point?
- Is there evidence of underlying visceral pain?
- Is there any altered function or sensory change?
- Are there any other problems which may not seem related?

A patient with mild pain should be able to perform the tasks of clinical assessment with minimal, if any, limitation. The tasks may need to be modified for patients who report moderate pain as some degree of restriction and limitation of movement will be present. Patients need to be warned that some of the tests may reproduce and temporarily worsen the pain experience and that they may even briefly experience severe pain again, especially with clinical presentations of disk herniation.

Frequency

The pain experience may be constant from its onset, or it may be recurrent. Constant pain should be explored to determine whether it is worsening, easing, or remaining about the same. Recurrent pain is explored to determine its frequency in terms of being daily, several days a week, weekly, several weeks a month, or monthly. Pains which come and go throughout the day can be considered intermittent, whilst the remainder are recurrent when the same signs and symptoms are present.

The patient may have experienced the same or similar pain on a previous occasion. If the interval is greater than several months, then the pain may be considered familiar. If the intervals are shorter, than the pain is recurrent. Questions about the frequency of pain are given in Box 16.4.

Location

The descriptors presented above must be anchored in the patient record to a well-described location. For example, the phrase "low-back pain" may be useful to convey an impression of a complex problem but it does little to describe the pain experience. Anatomical levels and areas should be documented to identify clearly the area to which the descriptors apply.

Mechanical dysfunction commonly produces referred pain and these patterns must also be described in association with duration, intensity, and frequency. The clinical implication is that the pain history will rarely be one simple statement; it may

---

Box 16.4 Questions about the frequency of pain

- Is this the first time for this pain?
- Is the pain constant and always there?
  - If "no", then how does the pain vary during the day?
  - How does the pain vary during the week?
- Is the pain related to you doing any specific activity?
- Are there times when you have no pain at all? (This may point to a functional overlay. Most mechanical pain is episodic)
- Is this pain a familiar pain to you?
- Has there been a previous occurrence of this pain? (Familiar pain is less of a concern than a new pain. Look for cycles and recurrences and any temporal aspect which may be causative)
- What treatment did you have previously for this pain? (It is even better when a familiar pain is reported to respond to a particular intervention or type of adjustment)

Box 16.5 Eight key prompts for the case history

The first four prompts act as review questions for the case history. The second four screen the patient for indications of problems which may be relevant to the presentation and which are responsive to early, cost-effective intervention:

1. Please summarize any past illnesses or admissions to hospital.
2. Please summarize any past accidents or trauma.
3. Is there any other health problem bothering you at the moment?
4. Were you born with any health problem?
5. Have you noticed any unusual lumps or swellings?
6. Have you noticed any recent changes in a mole or freckle?
7. Have you had any unexplained weight loss?
8. Have you noticed any abnormal bleeding from any body part?

---

require several statements to document adequately the experiences of the patient in more than one location.

INSTRUMENTATION

Pain is an emotional experience and the instruments which attempt to capture and explore this experience are complex. They make useful outcomes measures to quantify the patient's progress, and in some cases may also provide an important measurement at the initial interaction. Their use is a decision of the practitioner with consideration of the overall patient presentation.

There are certain types of clinical practice when pain and functionality instruments are completed as a matter of course at the entry of the patient to the clinic. These include rehabilitation clinics and those who accept work-injured patients under insurance and/or compensation schemes. An underlying principle is that, when a third party is involved in the payment of services for a particular patient, a greater obligation exists to demonstrate evidence-based progress of the patient. A range of outcomes measurements are available for a variety of purposes (Yeomans 2000).

EIGHT SUMMARY QUESTIONS

No matter how thorough the case history, there is often something the patient does not think of at the time. It is useful to have a short set of questions which review broad areas of the history (Box 16.5) as a prompt for completeness.

These questions are effective near the end of the oral history and act as a reminder to the patient for completeness. The last four questions are especially powerful by acting as a quick screen for underlying problems which the patient may be ignoring, yet which usually respond well to early intervention.

PREHISTORY FORMS

In some cases the practitioner may require patients to complete their own past history and review of systems forms in the belief that it will save time during the face-to-face encounter. Forms of this nature may be useful for gathering information from the patient in a manner which minimally inconveniences the practitioner; however it is a false economy. Also, there is no

guarantee that patients understand the questions or the terminology and therefore their responses cannot be taken as an accurate representation of their condition.

There are two further principles of clinical record keeping which apply to this matter. The first is that information should not be collected simply for the sake of attempting to appear complete. Information hidden away in a file is useless; moreover it can be dangerous to the patient and the practitioner in that it may be in the record, but not considered.

The second principle is that the practitioner is responsible for all of the information in the patient file. This is not suggesting that only the practitioner can add material; rather it is stating the obvious, that the practitioner must be aware of the contents of the clinical record. The extension of this principle is that the practitioner is responsible for what appears on plain radiographs and other images which the practitioner is trained to interpret, and must not rely solely on the radiologist's report.

In the same manner, the practitioner is responsible for knowing whatever the patient may write on a prehistory form and its interpretation, then interpolation, where necessary, with other data. Hence any prehistory form completed by the patient must be thoroughly reviewed by the practitioner in the presence of the patient so that he or she may clarify the responses to ensure the practitioner has complete disclosure. Given that the practitioner must spend this time with the patient, they may elect to complete the form themselves in a face-to-face conversation, using the form as a prompt to direct the discussion.

CONCLUSION

The case history and the pain history form the patient history, which is an integral component of the clinical record. A number of possible diagnoses may be included or excluded on the basis of a thorough history alone. Eliciting an effective history is a complex sociological process which benefits from a structured approach to ensure it is comprehensive and relevant. The history drives the examination of the patient and is a vital element of the working diagnosis which in turn generates the management plan.

Perhaps the most important attributes of the practitioner are to know which questions to ask, how to ask them, and how to listen to the answers.

17

The process of diagnosis

KEY CONCEPTS

The purpose of the diagnosis is to assist in determining the level and type of care to be provided to the patient. It is the link between the source data and the management plan and is the evidence that a clinical decision-making process has been undertaken to determine the nature of the clinical problem.

The three themes in diagnostic decision making are pattern recognition, probability reasoning, and causal thinking. These themes are linked within the strategy of the hypothetico-deductive clinical decision-making process.

The diagnosis may be disease-centered or patient-centered. A strong characteristic of manual healthcare is its tendency to be patient-centered and this is complemented by the patient-centered diagnosis which explores the significance of the disorder to the patient and its effect on family, relationships, sexuality, work, income, attitudes, and spirituality.

There are multiple levels of diagnosis. These start with the possible diagnosis which literally means the patient may have any one or more of any clinical conditions; these are narrowed through the history and clinical assessment to several probable diagnoses, from which one or two are taken forward to form the working diagnosis.

The working diagnosis is a series of statements which identify the temporal dimension of the presentation and the demographics of the patient and describe the clinical entity in terms of its causation where known, its associations, modifiers, and effects on the patient, culminating in the specific cause to be addressed.

The working diagnosis is tested by the management plan and both are continuously informed by a feedback loop from each subsequent treatment interlude which allows either or both to be amended to improve the quality of care to the patient.

When the working diagnosis responds favorably to the management plan it becomes the presumed diagnosis. The highest level in the hierarchy is a confirmed diagnosis but as this needs quantitative evidence it is not often achieved in the practice of manual healthcare.

INTRODUCTION

A diagnosis is the determination of the nature of a disease, injury, or congenital defect (Stedman's Medical Dictionary 2000). The essential purpose of a diagnosis is to differentiate one disorder from another. The differentiation of disorders by diagnosis effectively identifies the problem or problems for which treatment will be selected and delivered. A difficulty arises when some disorders are generalized and non-specific as they can be difficult to differentiate into one diagnostic term or category.

The diagnosis becomes the driver of the management plan and its therapeutic intervention. It encapsulates the entire purpose of generating source data through the process of assessment subsequent to the patient presentation. It is a statement or series of statements synthesized within the process of the practitioner gathering the source data and interpreting it within the context of his or her own clinical acumen (Fig. 17.1).

The process of synthesizing the diagnostic statement represents the applied clinical decision-making technique of the practitioner. Three themes in diagnostic decision making have been described by Jamison (1999). These are:

• Pattern recognition – where the practitioner identifies and compares the patient's presentation with a known disease picture. This is a form of inductive reasoning (Higgs & Jones 1995) and, while the recognition of patterns of presenting signs and symptoms is a powerful component of clinical practice, it has weaknesses for diagnosis. The first weakness is that it is dependent on the variety of patterns set for recall by the practitioner. The second is that minor variations in the pattern may derail the process. Third, the practitioner must maintain

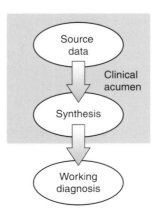

Figure 17.1 Generating the diagnosis. The working diagnosis results from the process of synthesis with the source data and the clinical acumen of the practitioner.

awareness for problems which may masquerade as a particular pattern (Murtagh 1994). If pattern recognition alone was an effective and safe approach to differential diagnosis, then practitioners would be replaced by computers.

• Probability reasoning – where the most probable conditions given the patient's presentation are considered. This theme is important in manual healthcare for the reason that many musculoskeletal problems have mechanical causation and predictable effects. Probability reasoning is enhanced by pattern recognition and informed by the history and examination, and represents a stage in the diagnostic hierarchy where probable diagnoses are ruled out by clinical findings (Fig. 17.2).

• Causal thinking – where an effort is made to identify the factors responsible for the condition. This includes the mechanism of injury (history) for musculoskeletal conditions, as well as findings from the assessment. Its weakness is the degree of clinical uncertainty of associating particular findings, such as degenerative change about the spinal motion unit (SMU), with specific painful presentations. A reliance on simple cause-and-effect relationships opens the practitioner to missing serious disorders (Murtagh 1994).

No single theme of clinical decision making is effective on its own and the typical practitioner applies a range of strategies to move between the observations contained within the source data and the diagnostic possibilities. Strategies include the exhaustion method (Lopes 1993), which is a common practice of the student and the novice practitioner. It gathers and assesses every conceivable element in the hope that by exhausting every possibility something will be left which is clinically relevant. It is a cumbersome and inefficient approach confounded by the overwhelming number of findings it generates.

A second strategy is the multiple branching method of algorithms which advance through a predetermined sequence of steps to advance towards a diagnosis (Lopes 1993). Algorithms are useful to provide a checklist for completeness (Souza 2001); however, the wealth of clinical information available from a patient may be constrained by a rigid checklist (Gatterman 1990 p. 88). A second weakness of algorithms is the need to identify the presenting condition in order to select an appropriate algorithm. This simply means that the process of diagnosis has already begun without the algorithm.

A third and common strategy is the hypothetico-deductive reasoning approach. This integrates the three themes and recognizes the multiple thought processes which occur in clinical decision making. The practitioner moves from a set of observations to a generalization by inductive reasoning. The generalizations form a belief of what may be happening with the patient which becomes a hypothesis tested by deductive reasoning. This allows the practitioner to move from a generalization to a conclusion in relation to specific data (Higgs & Jones 1995). This spiral of hypothetico-deductive reasoning represents the process of synthesis which both directs and links the source data to the working diagnosis (Fig. 17.1).

THE PURPOSE OF THE DIAGNOSIS

The generation of a diagnosis is the evidence that a clinical decision-making process has been undertaken to determine the

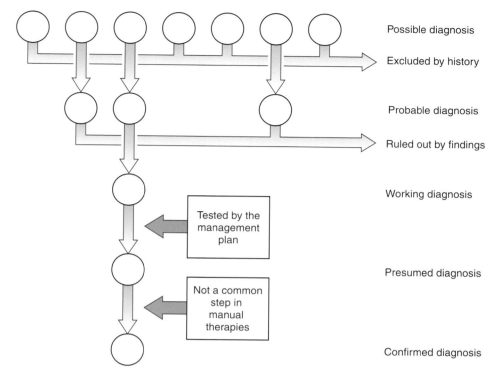

Figure 17.2 The diagnostic hierarchy. The step between the presumed and confirmed diagnosis requires autopsy and is more applicable to known pathological disease processes than functional change secondary to spinal dysfunction.

nature of the clinical problem. The diagnosis assists greatly in determining the level and type of care to be provided to the patient and is the link between the source data and the management plan.

The processes of contextualization and socioculturalization (Fig. 15.2) allow the synthesis of the working diagnosis. Contextualization represents the main patient history, which will be extensive on the initial visit. The resultant working diagnosis takes into account the presenting demeanor of the patient, the case and pain histories, family history, and the physical examination findings, review of body systems, and any other information which could have a direct bearing on the patient's health status at that moment in time. This material represents the source data.

Socioculturalization integrates the biopsychosocial issues, including the expectations of the patient, environmental issues which may affect recovery, and issues of health maintenance and preventive care. It allows the working diagnosis to be translated into a management plan which includes specification of the nature of the intervention as well as the frequency and duration of care.

The management plan thus tests the working diagnosis and must always retain ample opportunity for new data to inform and modify the ongoing treatment. These data are drawn from each subsequent treatment interlude (Fig. 17.3) and are informed by the progress notes and response to therapy. If the working diagnosis continues to be validated then the management plan continues; however, if the outcomes are not as positive

as expected then that information is fed back into the synthesis process where the practitioner must review, reflect, and reconsider.

In manual healthcare the diagnosis is subject to change. This is part of the process of identifying and applying therapeutic intervention and it is expected that a patient with a specific acute or subacute musculoskeletal complaint which can be encapsulated within a diagnostic statement will have that complaint resolved through appropriate treatment. Ergo, the diagnosis changes as the problem changes and resolves. The process is not so predictable with chronic musculoskeletal disorders and it is not unusual for a patient to carry a complex diagnostic grouping such as low-back pain for a considerable period of time.

The use of the feedback loop (Fig. 17.3) therefore does not imply a negative outcome ☹. It may also reflect no change ☺ or a positive improvement ☺. These are powerful arguments against cookbook scheduling: the patient may demonstrate dramatic improvement within a shorter time than predicted and thus the frequency and duration of care must be reduced to avoid overservicing; on the other hand, the patient may demonstrate signs and symptoms which demand review. These may be associated with the therapeutic intervention or they may be unrelated and secondary to an external event such as a motor vehicle accident. At the very least such an external event would warrant a review of the management plan, if not independent assessment and treatment for its effects in addition to the original problem.

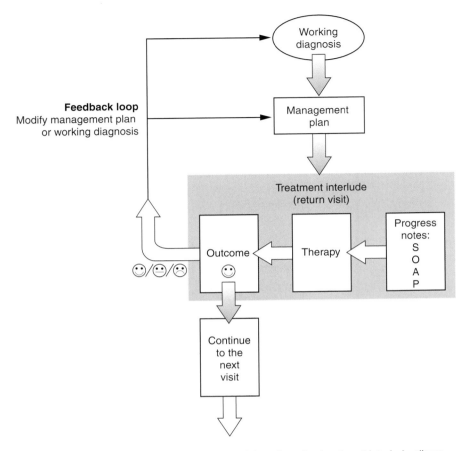

Figure 17.3 The living diagnosis. The feedback loop from the treatment interlude allows modification of the working diagnosis or management plan to improve the quality of care.

TYPES OF DIAGNOSIS

The diagnosis may be disease-centered or patient-centered (Murtagh 1994). A disease-centered diagnosis is typically short, to the point of being a label, and allows the prescription of drugs or intervention such as surgery. Once a patient has been labeled with a diagnosis it tends to stick and patients may never move beyond the labeled reinforcement that they have "asthma" or "cancer" or "a bulging disk".

A patient-centered diagnosis explores the significance of the disorder to the patient and its effect on family, relationships, sexuality, work, income, attitudes, and spirituality (Murtagh 1994). This type of diagnosis is significantly more comprehensive and inclusive than a disease-centered label.

A strong characteristic of manual healthcare is its tendency to be patient-centered (Gatterman 1995b). The patient-centered diagnosis is therefore the appropriate type of diagnosis for use in this type of practice. The entire process of establishing the clinical record and eliciting the patient history as described in this text is patient-centered. This approach is time-consuming in the first instance but more rewarding over time through its inclusion of the patient in the healing process.

The diagnosis should aim to bring all the clinical elements together, including those which underscore the patient-centered aspects, including the biopsychosocial dimensions, into a series of statements which form the diagnostic statement.

The practitioner must exercise care with the terms selected for use within the diagnostic statements. For example, "subluxation" is neither a diagnosis nor a label; it is a technical term for two surfaces of a joint which are slightly removed from their correct anatomical alignment. The term "subluxation complex" is a diagnostic label which needs explanation through the identification of its many dimensions and the evidence for them which may be found in the patient. Conversely, "posterior joint dysfunction" is not a diagnosis, it is one possible mechanism for a presumed component of a larger clinical entity.

LEVELS OF DIAGNOSIS

The diagnosis assumes different status at different points of the clinical interaction, and while there will usually be one diagnosis which informs the management plan, it will have multiple diagnostic elements and will be reached after the exclusion of diagnostic options (Fig. 17.2). Finally, depending on the response of the patient, the practitioner will have some idea of whether the diagnosis was what it was presumed to be.

Possible diagnosis

The moment a patient enters the clinical environment, any diagnosis is possible. In fact, a fundamental principle of primary care practice is that patients have the right to present with whatever condition or conditions they please. Fortunately, the majority of patients selecting manual healthcare as an option do so in the belief that their condition will be amenable to such treatment. However, while there is a degree of patient self-selection, the possible diagnoses which could explain the presenting complaint must be considered.

The possible diagnoses include what Murtagh (1994) calls the "serious disorders which must not be missed". These include severe infections such as meningoencephalitis, septicemia, epiglottitis, and infective endocarditis. There are also coronary diseases, including myocardial infarct, unstable angina, and arrhythmias, which may generate pain patterns which mimic musculoskeletal pain. The manual physician must also consider neoplasia, especially metastatic spread to or from the spine, cauda equina syndrome, and vertebrobasilar insufficiency as possible confounders or diagnoses.

Generally these possible diagnoses may be excluded by the history but those which remain become probable diagnoses and must be excluded by examination or diagnostic testing. This reflects the clinical decision-making process whereby the possible diagnoses include a range of options which advance to the second level of the diagnostic hierarchy where they are either ruled in or ruled out by specific testing and assessment. Clinical findings are equally as powerful to rule out a condition in their absence as they are to suggest its inclusion by their presence.

The "not-to-be-missed" conditions are compounded by a number of conditions which may masquerade as a musculoskeletal problem. Generally a suspicion that there may be a masquerade arises after a trial of conservative manual care is implemented with no response. Yet again this is a powerful reason why each treatment interlude must review the patient's progress.

Probable diagnosis

Each general presentation in manual healthcare has a group of probable diagnoses of musculoskeletal relevance as well as those which must not be missed and those which may masquerade to confuse the issue. There is no substitute for a thorough history, physical examination, and spinal assessment of the patient for sorting through the probabilities.

The probable diagnoses are those from the list of possible diagnoses which are not excluded by the history in the first instance, and then by further testing in the second. In the case of a patient presenting with generalized low-back pain with stiffness and radiating pain into one leg to about the knee, five probable diagnoses of a musculoskeletal nature are suggested in addition to those of a more sinister nature. The probable musculoskeletal diagnoses are:

- lumbar disk protrusion with nerve root involvement
- facet syndrome (posterior joint dysfunction)
- subluxation complex within the lumbar spine and/or pelvis
- sacroiliac joint syndrome
- a myofascial pain syndrome of low-back and pelvic musculature.

The practitioner should first act to exclude the non-musculoskeletal diagnoses and, where this is not possible, retain them as a fall-back consideration should the patient be

non-responsive to treatment delivered for the eventual working diagnosis. The practitioner then acts to exclude the probable musculoskeletal diagnoses until there is sufficient evidence to include one or two, or at times, three. Given that musculoskeletal disorders frequently coexist and appear as layers over each other, it is difficult at times to be so exclusionary that only one option remains. The working diagnosis will take this into account.

The exclusion of probable diagnoses by clinical assessment is a process which leads to the inclusion of the most probable diagnosis which then becomes the working diagnosis. If the assessment fails to provide convincing evidence of spinal dysfunction or other biomechanical dysfunction, with specific findings which satisfactorily explain the pain and nature of the presenting complaint, then there is little, if any, evidence for a diagnosis suitable to manual healthcare and the patient should be referred for medical assessment.

Working diagnosis

The working diagnosis is a descriptive statement or series of statements which integrate the believed cause of the presentation with the many clinical elements which are manifested in various forms. The truthfulness of the working diagnosis reflects the comprehensiveness of the assessment yet can only remain a best guess of what is happening to the patient.

The fact that the working diagnosis is usually a "best guess" is not really a problem as long as the process of reaching this point is exhaustive and documented. On the other hand, if a guess is made within seconds of the patient entering the clinic then there is reason for suspicion.

The musculoskeletal diagnosis in general, and a diagnosis of subluxation complex in particular, can really only be best guesses at this point of the evolution of manual healthcare. There is, of course, a clear distinction between that range of musculoskeletal presentations which reflect clear and defined injury with well-established clinical signs and symptoms and known findings from diagnostic imaging. These presentations include cruciate ligament tears and other similar injuries which are beyond dispute.

On the other hand, spinal dysfunction remains largely a "black box" and it is the manual physicians who have pursued this elusive entity to a point where it has a certain substance through clinical findings. Spinal dysfunction is largely a neurophysiological disorder manifested through functional changes as opposed to physical pathological changes. The working diagnosis of somatic lesion or subluxation complex is one which must be tested by the application of specific therapies.

A positive response of the patient can be taken as suggesting the working diagnosis had validity only when all other probable diagnoses were excluded. This is almost an impossible expectation, which is why the end-point in most manual healthcare is a presumed diagnosis.

Presumed diagnosis

Manipulation and adjustment of the spine are diagnostic as well as therapeutic. A positive response to treatment can be seen as evidence that the problem intended to be treated by the treatment was most likely present and that the treatment adequately corrected the problem. This is a fairly bold presumption, which is why the working diagnosis can only become a presumed diagnosis.

Manual physicians cannot be criticized for working at the level of presumed diagnoses as this is a common trait of all health disciplines and a lot of medical practice is conducted at this level. If patients have high blood pressure which responds to one of a number of drug regimes then they are presumed to have hypertension. Moreover, this diagnostic label usually includes the term "idiopathic," which means "of unknown cause" (Stedman's Medical Dictionary 2000).

Definitive diagnosis

Disorders and diseases which result in pathological changes can be evidenced on autopsy and represent the group of presumptive diagnoses which become definitive. The majority of spinal lesions are functional and their effects non-pathological in the sense that they do not result in known organic change. These conditions are not evidenced at autopsy, although there may be a range of objective findings such as disk herniation and hypertrophy of the facet joints, neither of which are pathognomonic indicators of subluxation complex.

It must be remembered that objective, biomechanical change about the SMU may have no causal relationship at all with the patient's pain and dysfunction. Such is the nature of spinal dysfunction in general and the subluxation complex in particular: if there were pathological changes demonstrable at autopsy then it is likely that the manual disciplines would have been well subsumed into mainstream medicine.

The very fact that the majority of lesions diagnosed and treated by manual physicians can only remain a presumed diagnosis at best is the reason why manual healthcare is an art as well as a science.

WRITING THE DIAGNOSIS

The content and structure of the working diagnosis are complex and must integrate all elements of the assessment process. Given that it is also patient-centered, the diagnosis must reflect those elements associated with patient-centered care.

The diagnosis must be written in the clinical record and should follow a structure which logically incorporates the various clinical and patient-centered elements. The result is a descriptive diagnosis which is typically a series of linked statements which integrate the clinical findings with their causation and subsequent effect on the patient.

The descriptive diagnosis may become a complex entity in itself, but it should always include a diagnostic label to provide an overview of what is believed to be happening, and conclude with a defined problem which encapsulates the evidence-based essence of the preceding statements and becomes the key driver of the management plan. The components of the descriptive diagnosis are explored below.

Temporal dimension

It is beneficial for the descriptive, working diagnosis to commence with words which anchor the presentation in time.

Appropriate terms include acute, subacute, chronic, recurrent, and familiar. The intent is to direct the management plan better as well as convey a mental picture of how the patient is experiencing the problem.

The temporal dimension may be supplemented by a demographic statement to set the scene for the diagnostic statements which follow. Examples include:

- "A 35-year-old female primary school teacher with recurrent …"
- "A 45-year-old female motor mechanic with acute …"
- "A 55-year-old male motor mechanic with chronic …"
- "An 18-year-old male apprentice motor mechanic with acute …"

No matter the subtlety of the changes in the above four opening statements, they each convey a very different impression to the experienced practitioner.

The clinical entity

The clinical entity is a broad diagnostic label which serves to position patients and their presentation within a context which is clearly appropriate to the provision of manual healthcare. It encapsulates the patient's perception of the problem which thus links the patient into the diagnostic statement. Examples of clinical entities include low-back pain, neck pain and headache, shoulder and arm pain, and mid thoracic pain and discomfort.

The entity envelopes the contextualization of the patient and in itself points to the various issues of socioculturalization which become an integrated aspect of the clinical interaction. For example, low-back pain is often attended by sexual dysfunction, and recurrent headaches may stimulate thoughts of suicide. This component of the descriptive diagnosis must be carefully considered as it may tend to categorize the patient unfairly if the subsequent information fails to explore the presentation adequately.

Using the opening statements from above, the following clinical entities can be added to demonstrate how a powerful mental picture may be generated by careful use of appropriate words:

- "A 35-year-old female primary school teacher with recurrent neck pain and headaches …"
- "A 45-year-old female motor mechanic with acute low-back pain and leg pain …"
- "A 55-year-old male motor mechanic with chronic mid thoracic pain and discomfort …"
- "An 18-year-old male apprentice motor mechanic with acute left-sided low-back pain …"

These four stems will be used to illustrate how the different elements of the diagnostic statement may be integrated. They are examples only and every patient must be individually assessed to identify the most relevant findings for inclusion within the diagnostic statement. The working diagnosis is thus highly variable in its content and comprehensiveness.

Causation

Causation is the mechanism of injury or disorder. The inclusion of causation within the diagnostic statement helps differentiate

Type 1 care (Box 15.1) from other levels:

A 45-year-old female motor mechanic with acute low-back pain and leg pain secondary to strain/sprain injury while lifting and turning with a heavy load from an engine bay ...

An 18-year-old male apprentice motor mechanic with acute left-sided low-back pain following a fall on the left buttock ...

The causation is either unclear or not known in Type 2 care:

A 35-year-old female primary school teacher with recurrent neck pain and headaches of unknown origin ...

The essence of Type 3 care is that, in the absence of care, familiar signs and symptoms return to the patient. The inclusion of this information in the diagnostic statement empowers the statement as a driver for ongoing maintenance care:

A 55-year-old male motor mechanic with chronic mid thoracic pain and discomfort which is known to be relieved by spinal manipulation ...

Causation is not a consideration in Type 4 (preventive) care as the presentation of the patient is more likely to be driven by a desire to improve health as opposed to the need to relieve pain.

Associations

The identification of associated findings is the essence of the working diagnosis. The quality of the diagnostic statements is only as good as the quality of the evidence it presents to drive the management plan. Manual healthcare physicians are able to identify and categorize the clinical signs, symptoms, and findings, especially in as much as they implicate certain levels of the spine as being the object of treatment.

The associated findings are the evidence for the spinal dysfunction and can be ordered as the elements of the functional spinal lesion. The benefits of including associations within the working diagnosis are that certain associated findings may form a clear clinical picture of a particular problem. They also identify findings which may be used as outcomes measures.

Kinematic change

A plain-language description is needed of any altered movement patterns within the SMU or related joints:

A 35-year-old female primary school teacher with recurrent neck pain and headaches of unknown origin associated with restricted intersegmental movement in the upper cervical spine ...

The kinematic change need only be described in broad terms at this stage as the working diagnosis will conclude with the specific problems to be addressed, such as "subluxation of the left atlanto-occipital joint listed as left posterior-superior occiput". Further, not all levels of kinematic change will be identified for treatment; some will be considered compensations and others incidental findings.

Connective tissue change

Findings of connective tissue change are important to direct the specific therapeutic intervention.

A 45-year-old female motor mechanic with acute low-back pain and leg pain secondary to strain/sprain injury while lifting and turning with a heavy load from an engine bay associated with edema and inflammation about the right iliolumbar ligament ...

Note that there is no inclusion of kinematic change at this time. An acute strain/sprain injury of the lumbosacral spine may preclude a valid assessment of kinematic change until the swelling has eased and the region can be assessed for intersegmental movement. The point is that the diagnostic statement is not meant to be the all-encompassing life story of the patient. Rather, it includes the findings which are apparent and relevant at a particular time. Hence it becomes living in the sense it is frequently modified by feedback from subsequent assessment (Fig. 17.3).

Muscle change

Muscle changes are included when they appear to be associated with the presenting complaint.

An 18-year-old male apprentice motor mechanic with acute left-sided low-back pain following a fall on the left buttock associated with movement restriction of L5 on S1, tenderness over the left sacroiliac joint and about the left gluteus medius and minimus, and weakness of the left gastrocnemius ...

Muscle change includes alterations to tonicity and the presence of tenderness, as well as gradings of strength and function and any finding of trigger points.

Neural change

The scheme of neural change (Fig. 7.1) allows for a wide variety of potential findings. These will range between objective, subjective, and abstract depending on the patient presentation. With the examples used in this chapter, the "35-year-old female primary school teacher with recurrent neck pain and headaches of unknown origin associated with restricted intersegmental movement in the upper cervical spine" could have an emphasis on subjective and abstract dimensions as opposed to motor, reflex, or sensory changes.

On the other hand, motor, sensory, and reflex changes, along with pain, are commonly associated with a traumatic onset:

An 18-year-old male apprentice motor mechanic with acute left-sided low-back pain following a fall on the left buttock associated with movement restriction of L5 on S1, tenderness over the left sacroiliac joint and about the left gluteus medius and minimus, and weakness of the left gastrocnemius demonstrated by decreased ability to plantar flex the left foot. The deep tendon reflex at the knee is absent on the left and 2+ right and at the ankle it is absent left and 2+ right. Radiating pain into the left leg to below the knee is found on supine straight leg raise at 30° ...

Vascular change

Vascular changes may range from the simple presence of bruising to the complexities of chronic regional pain syndrome. The principle of constructing the working diagnosis remains: if a finding is identified and considered relevant to the presentation, it is included:

An 18-year-old male apprentice motor mechanic with acute left-sided low-back pain following a fall on the left buttock associated with movement restriction of L5 on S1, tenderness over the left sacroiliac joint and about the left gluteus medius and minimus, and weakness of the left gastrocnemius demonstrated by decreased ability to plantar flex the left foot. The deep tendon reflex at the knee is absent on the left and 2+ right and at the ankle it is absent left and 2+ right. Radiating pain into the left leg to below the knee is found on supine straight leg raise at 30°. Mild bruising is noted over the left posterolateral buttock and hip region…

The inclusion of specific findings in this statement has now determined the preferred outcomes measurements, namely improvements in the supine straight-leg raise, return of muscle strength to the gastrocnemius, return of bilaterally equal reflexes, and the resolution of tenderness about the left sacroiliac joint and gluteals. For these improvements to be considered an outcome of treatment they would need to be demonstrated as occurring more quickly than resolution by natural history.

The correction of movement restriction at L5–S1 is also a valid outcome measure, although some may argue differently. In the clinical environment the determination of movement restriction is associated with a complex set of findings in each degree of movement, usually accompanied by pain and tenderness (Ch. 4). The finding of such changes at a spinal level, and their resolution as perceived by the treating practitioner, is the essence and purpose of manual healthcare.

Modifiers

The inclusion of modifiers in the sense of factors or actions which ease or worsen the presentation, or findings which may affect the healing process such as degenerative joint disease, or modify the treatment options such as osteoporosis, can be included. They add value by helping the working diagnosis to point to a preferred treatment plan.

Effect

The working diagnosis may also include a statement of the effect on the patient of this particular problem. The effect may be quantitative in that it has resulted in time off work or has affected other activities of daily living, or qualitative in that it

may be impacting on the biopsychosocial dimensions of the patient's existence, or both. For example, chronic low-back pain is commonly associated with time off work, sexual dysfunction, and depression.

Suggestive of

The statements culminate in the specific cause or working diagnosis to address. It is stated as an impression of what the findings most likely indicate:

An 18-year-old male apprentice motor mechanic with acute left-sided low-back pain following a fall on the left buttock associated with movement restriction of L5 on S1, tenderness over the left sacroiliac joint and about the left gluteus medius and minimus, and weakness of the left gastrocnemius demonstrated by decreased ability to plantar flex the left foot. The deep tendon reflex at the knee is absent on the left and 2+ right and at the ankle it is absent left and 2+ right. Radiating pain into the left leg to below the knee is found on supine straight-leg raise at 30°. Mild bruising is noted over the left posterolateral buttock and hip region and the patient is unable to work at this time. These findings are suggestive of left posterolateral protrusion of the L5–S1 disk with posttraumatic subluxation complex of the L5–S1 SMU.

As the management plan progresses, the working diagnosis can be revisited to incorporate the responses to treatment and any required amendments to the diagnosis. The entire diagnostic statements do not need to be reproduced in this process, rather they can be referred to as "the original working diagnosis was amended to reflect …".

CONCLUSION

The whole purpose of assessing the patient in general and the spine in particular is to identify areas of dysfunction associated with the complaints of the patient with a view to informing the most appropriate management plan for those problems. The goal is the restoration of optimal health for the individual patient.

The working diagnosis therefore becomes a mini-narrative which is descriptive of the problem and its effects on the patient. As such, it is a powerful patient-centered documentation of the clinical encounter. The more complete the diagnostic statements, the more justifiable the treatment, and justifiable treatment naturally leads to valid outcomes measurements which feed back to inform the healing journey further.

References

ACA Council on Technic 1988a Chiropractic terminology [report]. Journal of the American Chiropractic Association 25 (9): 68–70

ACA Council on Technic 1988b Chiropractic terminology [report]. Journal of the American Chiropractic Association 25 (10): 46–57

Adams M A, Hutton W C 1980 The effect of posture on the role of the apophyseal joints in resisting intervertebral compressive force. Journal of Bone and Joint Surgery – British 62-B: 358–362

Adams M A, Hutton W C 1982 Prolapsed intervertebral disc: a hyperflexion injury. Spine 7: 184–191

Adams M A, Dolan P, Hutton W C, Porter R W 1990 Diurnal changes in spinal mechanics and their clinical significance. Journal of Bone and Joint Surgery – British 72 (2): 2166–2270

Adams M A, McNally D S, Dolan P 1996 "Stress" distributions inside vertebral discs. The effects of age and degeneration. Journal of Bone and Joint Surgery – British 78 (6): 965–972

Adams M A, Freeman B J, Morrison H P et al 2000 Mechanical initiation of intervertebral disc degeneration. Spine 25: 1625–1636

Adams M A, Bogduk N, Burton K, Dolan P 2002 The biomechanics of back pain. Churchill Livingstone, Edinburgh, UK

Ader R, Cohen N, Felten D 1995 Psychoneuroimmunology: interactions between the nervous system and the immune system. Lancet 345 (8942): 99–103

Aker P D, Lopes A A, Yong-Hing K, Cassidy J D 1989 Cervical calcification in children: a case report. Journal of the Canadian Chiropractic Association 33: 191–194

Akhaddar A, Mansouri A, Zrara I et al 2002 Thoracic spinal cord compression by ligamentum flavum ossifications. Joint, Bone, Spine: Revue du Rhumatisme 69 (3): 319–323

Albarran J W, Durham B, Chappel G et al 2000 Are manual gestures, verbal descriptors and pain radiation as reported by patients reliable indicators of myocardial infarction? Preliminary findings and implications. Intensive and Critical Care Nursing 16 (2): 98–110

Al-Hadidi M T, Badran D H, Al-Hadidi A M, Abu-Ghaida J H 2001 Magnetic resonance imaging of normal lumbar intervertebral discs. Saudi Medical Journal 22 (11): 1013–1018

Alix M E, Bates D K 1999 A proposed etiology of cervicogenic headache: the neurophysiologic basis and anatomic relationship between the dura mater and the rectus capitis posterior muscle. Journal of Manipulative and Physiological Therapeutics 22: 534–539

AMA Council on Scientific Affairs Report 1987 Thermography in neurological and musculoskeletal conditions. Thermology 2: 600–607

Amonoo-Kuofi H S, El-Badawi M G Y 1997 Ligaments related to the intervertebral canal and foramen. In: Giles L G F, Singer K P (eds) Clinical anatomy and management of low back pain. Butterworth Heinemann, Oxford, UK

Amonoo-Kuofi H S, El-Badawi M G, Fatani J A 1988 Ligaments associated with lumbar intervertebral foramina. 1, L1 to L4. Journal of Anatomy 56: 177–183

Andersson E A, Oddsson L I, Grundstrom H et al 1996 EMG activities of the quadratus lumborum and erector spinae muscles during flexion-relaxation and other motor tasks. Clinical Biomechanics 11 (7): 392–400

Aprill C, Bogduk N 1992 High-intensity zone: a diagnostic sign of painful lumbar disc on magnetic resonance imaging. British Journal of Radiology 65 (773): 361–369

Arafat Q W, Jackowski A, Chavda S V, West R J 1993 Case report: ossification of the thoracic ligamenta flava in a Caucasian: a rare cause of myelopathy. British Journal of Radiology 66 (729): 1193–1196

Arai E, Matsumoto M, Takaiwa H, Maruo S 1985 Biomechanical behaviour of the posterior elements of the lumbar spine under loading – a study of stress analysis by means of three dimensional photoelastic experiments. Nippon Seikeigeka Gakkai Zasshi 59 (8): 853–863

Ariyoshi M, Nagata K, Sonoda K et al 1999 Spondylolysis at three sites in the same lumbar vertebra. International Journal of Sports Medicine 20 (1): 56–57

Association of Chiropractic Colleges 1996. Position paper #1. Journal of Manipulative and Physiological Therapeutics 19: 634–647

Atasoy C, Fitoz S, Karan B et al 2002 A rare cause of cervical spinal stenosis: posterior arch hypoplasia in a bipartite atlas. Neuroradiology 44 (3): 253–255

Axelsson P, Johnsson R, Stromqvist B 2000 Is there increased intervertebral mobility in isthmic adult spondylolisthesis? A matched comparative study using roentgen stereophotogrammetry. Spine 25: 1701–1703

Bagatur A E, Zorer G, Centel T 2001 Natural history of paediatric intervertebral disc calcification. Archives of Orthopaedic Trauma Surgery 121 (10): 601–603

Bakkum B W, Mestan M 1994 The effects of the transforaminal ligaments on the sizes of T11 to L5 human intervertebral foramina. Journal of Manipulative and Physiological Therapeutics 17: 517–522

Baldry P E 2001 Myofascial pain and fibromyalgia syndromes, p. 354. Churchill Livingstone, Edinburgh, UK

Banzai Y, Aoki T 2001 Muscle sympathetic nerve activity in patients with lumbar spinal canal stenosis. Journal of the Nippon Medical School 68 (5): 376–383

Barbaix E, Girardin M D, Hoppner J P et al 1996 Anterior sacrodural attachments – Trolard's ligaments revisited. Manual Therapy 2: 88–91

Barbaix E, Lapierre M, Van Roy P, Clarijs J P 2000 The sternoclavicular joint: variants of the discus articularis. Clinical Biomechanics 15 (S1): S3–S7

Barker P J, Briggs C A 1999 Attachments of the posterior layer of lumbar fascia. Spine 24: 1757–1764

Baron R, Maier C 1996 Reflex sympathetic dystrophy: skin blood flow, sympathetic vasoconstrictor reflexes and pain before and after surgical sympathectomy. Pain 67 (2–3): 317–326

Barthes X, Walter B, Zeller R, Dubousset J F 1999 Biomechanical behaviour in vitro of the spine and lumbosacral junction. Surgical and Radiologic Anatomy 21 (6): 377–381

Barton P M 1991 Piriformis syndrome: a rational approach to management. Pain 47 (3): 345–352

Bartsch T, Goadsby P J 2002 Stimulation of the greater occipital nerve induces increased excitability of dural afferent input. Brain 125 (7): 1496–1509

Bartsch T, Janig W, Habler H J 2000 Reflex patterns in preganglionic sympathetic neurons projecting to the superior cervical ganglion in the rat. Autonomic Neuroscience 83 (1–2): 66–74

Batson O V 1940 The function of the vertebral veins and their role in the spread of metastases. Annals of Surgery 112: 138–149. Also published as a classic article (1995). The function of the vertebral veins and their role in the spread of metastases. Clinical Orthopedics (312): 4–9

Beal M C 1989 Viscerosomatic reflexes. In: Patterson M M, Howell J N (eds) The central connection: somatovisceral/viscerosomatic interaction, pp. 19–29. University Classics Ltd, Athens, OH

Beatty R A 1994 The piriformis muscle syndrome: a simple diagnostic manoeuvre. Neurosurgery 34 (3): 512–514. Discussion 514. Comment 34 (3): 545

Bednar D A, Orr F W, Simon G T 1995 Observations on the pathomorphology of the thoracolumbar fascia in chronic mechanical back pain. A microscopic study. Spine 20: 1161–1164

Behrsin J F, Briggs C A 1988 Ligaments of the lumbar spine: a review. Surgical Radiologic Anatomy 10: 211–219

Bendtsen L, Norregaard J, Jensen R, Olesen J 1997 Evidence of qualitatively altered nociception in patients with fibromyalgia. Arthritis and Rheumatism 40: 98–102. Comment 40: 2275–2277

BenEliyahu D J 1989 Thermography in the diagnosis of sympathetic maintained pain. American Journal of Chiropractic Medicine 2: 55–60

BenEliyahu D J 1992. Infrared thermal imaging of the vertebral subluxation complex. International Review of Chiropractic Jan/Feb: 14–17

Bennett R M 1999 Emerging concepts in the neurobiology of chronic pain: evidence of abnormal sensory processing in fibromyalgia. Mayo Clinic Proceedings 74 (4): 385–398

Bergmann T F, Peterson D H, Lawrence D L 1993 Chiropractic technique. Churchill Livingstone, New York, NY

Berman B M, Swyers J P 1999 Complementary medicine treatments for fibromyalgia syndrome. Baillière's best practice and research. Clinical Rheumatology 13 (3): 487–492

Berthelot J M, Delecrin J, Maugars Y et al 1996 A potentially underrecognised and treatable cause of chronic back pain: entrapment neuropathy of the cluneal nerves. Journal of Rheumatology 23 (10): 2179–2181

Berthoud H R, Neuhuber W L 2000 Functional and chemical anatomy of the afferent vagal system. Autonomic Neuroscience 20 (1–3): 1–17

Bharihoke V, Gupta M 1986 Muscular attachments along the medial border of the scapula. Surgical and Radiologic Anatomy 8 (1): 71–73

Biedermann H 1992 Kinematic imbalances due to suboccipital strain in newborns. Journal of Manual Medicine 6: 151–156

Bilkey W J 1992 Involvement of fascia in mechanical pain syndromes. Journal of Manual Medicine 6: 157–160

Birklein F, Schmelz M, Schifter S, Weber M 2001 The important role of neuropeptides in complex regional pain syndrome. Neurology 57(12): 2179–2184. Comment 57 (12): 2161–2162

Bland J H 1991 Cervical and thoracic pain. Current Opinion in Rheumatology 3: 218–225

Blix E, Sviggum O, Koss K S, Oian P 2003 Inter-observer variation in assessment of 845 labour admission tests: comparison between midwives and obstetricians in the clinical setting and two experts. BJOG: an international journal of obstetrics and gynaecology 110 (1): 1–5

Blume H G 2000 Cervicogenic headaches: radiofrequency neurotomy and the cervical disc and fusion. Clinical and Experimental Rheumatology 18 (S19): S53–S58

Bogduk N 1991 The lumbar disc and low back pain. Neurosurgical Clinics of North America 2 (4): 791–806

Bogduk N, Marsland A 1988 The cervical zygapophyseal joints as a source of neck pain. Spine 13: 610–617

Bogduk N, Mercer S 2000 Biomechanics of the cervical spine. I: Normal kinematics. A review paper. Clinical Biomechanics 15: 633–648

Bogduk N, Modic M T 1996 Lumbar discography. Spine 21: 402–404

Bogduk N, Twomey L T 1987 Clinical anatomy of the lumbar spine. Churchill Livingstone, Melbourne, NSW

Bogduk N, Johnson G, Spalding D 1998 The morphology and biomechanics of latissimus dorsi. Clinical Biomechanics 13 (6): 377–385

Bogduk N, Wilson A S, Tynan W 1982 The human lumbar dorsal rami. Journal of Anatomy 134 (Pt 2): 383–397

Bolton P S 1998 The somatosensory system of the neck and its effects on the central nervous system. Journal of Manipulative and Physiological Therapeutics 21: 553–563

Bolton P S 2000 Reflex effects of vertebral subluxations: the peripheral nervous system. An update. Journal of Manipulative and Physiological Therapeutics 23: 101–103. Comment 23: 512–513

Bolton S P 2002 Words as weapons in the politics of power: a commentary of words, phrases, language and jargon. Chiropractic Journal of Australia 32: 135–138

Bolton P S, Kerman I A, Woodring S F, Yates B J 1998 Influences of neck afferents on sympathetic and respiratory nerve activity. Brain Research Bulletin 47 (5): 413–419

Bone C M, Hsieh G H 2000 The risk of carcinogenesis from radiographs to pediatric orthopaedic patients. Journal of Pediatric Orthopedics 20 (2): 251–254

Borenstein D G, O'Mara J W Jr, Boden S D et al 2001 The value of magnetic resonance imaging of the lumbar spine to predict low back pain in asymptomatic subjects: a seven-year follow-up study. Journal of Bone and Joint Surgery – American 83-A: 1306–1311

Bornke C, Schmid G, Szymanski S, Schols L 2002 Vertebral body infarction indicating midthoracic spinal stroke. Spinal Cord 40 (5): 244–247

Bough B, Thakore J, Davies M, Dowling F 1990 Degeneration of the lumbar facet joints. Journal of Bone and Joint Surgery – British 72-B (2): 275–276

Bowers L J 1994 The "slippery slope": boundary issues for the chiropractic physician. Topics in Clinical Chiropractic 1 (3): 1–8

Bowers L J 2000 Intimate strangers: issues of touch. Topics in Clinical Chiropractic 7 (3): 11–18

Boyd-Clark L C, Briggs C A, Galea M P 2001 Comparative histochemical composition of muscle fibres in a pre- and postvertebral muscle of the cervical spine. Journal of Anatomy 199 (Pt 6): 709–716

Boyd-Clark L C, Briggs C A, Galea M P 2002 Muscle spindle distribution, morphology, and density in longus colli and multifidus muscles of the cervical spine. Spine 27: 694–701

Boyle J J W, Singer K P, Milne N 1998 Pattern of intervertebral disc degeneration in the cervicothoracic junctional region. Manual Therapy 3 (2): 72–77

Boyle J J, Milne N, Singer K P 2002 Influence of age on cervicothoracic spinal curvature: an ex vivo radiographic survey. Clinical Biomechanics (Bristol, Avon) 17 (5): 361–367

Brand N E, Gizoni C M 1982 Moire contourography and infrared thermography: ranges resulting from chiropractic adjustments. Journal of Manipulative and Physiological Therapeutics 5: 113–116

Brelsford K L, Uematsu S 1985 Thermographic presentation of cutaneous sensory and vasomotor activity in the injured peripheral nerve. Journal of Neurosurgery 62: 711–715

Brier S R 1999 Primary care orthopedics. Mosby, St Louis, MO

Briggs C A, Chandraraj S 1995 Variations in the lumbosacral ligament and associated changes in the lumbosacral region resulting in compression of the fifth dorsal root ganglion and spinal nerve. Clinical Anatomy 8 (5): 339–346. Comment: 1996; 9 (4): 278–279

Brightbill T C, Pile N, Eichelberger R P, Whitman M Jr 1994 Normal magnetic resonance imaging and abnormal discography in lumbar disc disruption. Spine 19: 1075–1077. Comment: 1995; 20: 120

Browning J E 2001 Pelvic pain and pelvic organ dysfunction. In: Masarsky C, Todres-Masarsky M (eds) Somatovisceral aspects of chiropractic, pp. 109–135. Churchill Livingstone, New York, NY

Brumagne S, Lysens R, Swinnen S, Verschueren S 1999 Effect of paraspinal muscle vibration on position sense of the lumbosacral spine. Spine 24: 1328–1331

Brumagne S, Cordo P, Lysens R et al 2000 The role of paraspinal muscle spindles in lumbosacral position sense in individuals with and without low back pain. Spine 25: 989–994

Bucciero A, Vizioli L, Cerillo A 1998a Soft cervical disc herniation: an analysis of 187 cases. Journal of Neurosurgical Science 42 (3): 125–130

Bucciero A, Carangelo B, Cerillo A et al 1998b Myeloradicular damage in traumatic cervical disc herniation. Journal of Neurosurgical Science 42 (4): 203–211

Bucknill A T, Coward K, Plumpton C et al 2002 Nerve fibres in lumbar spine structures and injured spinal roots express the sensory neuron-specific sodium channels SNS/PN3 and NaN/SNS2. Spine 27: 135–140

Buckwalter J A, Woo S L Y, Goldberg V M et al 1993 Current concepts review: soft-tissue aging and musculoskeletal function. Journal of Bone and Joint Surgery – American 75-A (10): 1533–1548

Budgell B S 1999 Spinal manipulative therapy and visceral disorders. Chiropractic Journal of Australia 29: 123–128

Budgell B S 2000 Reflex effects of subluxation: the autonomic nervous system. Journal of Manipulative and Physiological Therapeutics 23: 104–106

Budgell B, Hirano F 2001 Innocuous mechanical stimulation of the neck and alterations in heart-rate variability in healthy young adults. Autonomic Neuroscience: Basic and Clinical 91 (1–2): 96–99

Budgell B, Suzuki A 2000 Inhibition of gastric motility by noxious chemical stimulation of interspinous tissues in the rat. Journal of the Autonomic Nervous System 80: 162–168

Budgell B, Sata A, Suzuki A, Uchida S 1997 Responses of adrenal function to stimulation of lumbar and thoracic interspinous tissues in the rat. Neuroscience Research 28 (1): 33–40

Budgell B S, Hotta H, Sato A 1998 Reflex responses of bladder motility after stimulation of interspinous tissues in the anesthetized rat. Journal of Manipulative and Physiological Therapeutics 21: 593–599

Buirski G, Silberstein M 1993 The symptomatic lumbar disc in patients with low back pain. Magnetic resonance imaging appearances in both a symptomatic and control population. Spine 18: 1801–1811

Buna M, Coghlan W, deGruchy M et al 1984 Ponticles of the atlas: a review and clinical perspective. Journal of Manipulative and Physiological Therapeutics 7: 261–266

Burke J G, Watson R W, McCormack D et al 2002 Intervertebral discs which cause low back pain secrete high levels of proinflammatory mediators. Journal of Bone and Joint Surgery – British 84 (2): 196–201

Burns L 1937 Certain remote effects of upper cervical lesions. Journal of the American Osteopathic Association 37: 55–58

Buttermann G R, Kahmann R D, Lewis J L, Bradford D S 1991 An experimental method for measuring forces on the spinal facet joint: description and application of the method. Journal of Biomechanical Engineering 113 (4): 375–386

Byfield D 1996 Chiropractic manipulative skills. Butterworth Heinemann, Oxford, UK

Cabre P, Pascal-Moussellard H, Kaidomar S et al 2001 Six cases of cervical ligamentum flavum calcification in Blacks in the French West Indies. Joint, Bone, Spine: Revue du Rhumatisme 68 (2): 158–165

Cai C Y, Palmer C A, Paramore C G 2001 Exuberant transverse ligament degeneration causing high cervical myelopathy. Journal of Spinal Disorders 14 (1): 84–88

Camacho A, Villarejo A, de Aragón A M et al 2001 Spontaneous carotid and vertebral artery dissection in children. Pediatric Neurology 25: 250–253

Carragee E J, Paragioudakis S J, Khurana S 2000 Lumbar high-intensity zone and discography in subjects without low back problems [2000 Volvo Award winner in clinical studies]. Spine 25: 2987–2992

Carrick F R 1997 Changes in brain function after manipulation of the cervical spine. Journal of Manipulative and Physiological Therapeutics 20: 529–245

Caruso W, Leisman G 2000 A force/displacement analysis of muscle testing. Perception and Motor Skills 91 (2): 683–692

Caruso W, Leisman G 2001 The clinical utility of force/displacement analysis of muscle testing in applied kinesiology. International Journal of Neuroscience 106: 147–157

Cassidy J D, Kirkaldy-Willis W H, Thiel H W 1992 Manipulation. In: Kirkaldy-Willis W H, Burton C V (eds) Managing low back pain, 3rd edn, pp. 283–296 Churchill Livingstone, New York, NY

Cattley P, Tuchin P J 1999 Chiropractic management of migraine without aura. Australian Chiropractic and Osteopathy 8 (3): 85–90

Cavanaugh J M, Ozaktay A C, Yamashita T, King A I 1996 Lumbar facet pain: biomechanics, neuroanatomy and neurophysiology. Journal of Biomechanics 29 (9): 1117–1129

Cavanaugh J M, Ozaktay A C, Yamashita T et al 1997 Mechanisms of low back pain: a neurophysiologic and neuroanatomic study. Clinical Orthopaedics Feb (335): 166–180

Chaitow L 1999 Cranial manipulation theory and practice Churchill Livingstone, Edinburgh, UK

Chaitow L 2000 The muscle designation debate: the experts respond. Journal of Bodywork and Movement Therapies 4 (4): 225–227

Chaitow L, DeLany J W 2000 Clinical application of neuromuscular techniques, vol. 1. The upper body. Churchill Livingstone, Edinburgh, UK

Chaitow L, DeLany J W 2002 Clinical application of neuromuscular techniques, vol. 2. The lower body. Churchill Livingstone, Edinburgh, UK

Chance M A, Peters R E 2001 A subluxation is a subluxation is a subluxation [editorial] Chiropractic Journal of Australia 31 (4): 121

Chandraraj S, Briggs C A, Opeskin K 1998 Disc herniation in the young and end-plate vascularity. Clinical Anatomy 11 (3): 171–176

Chang H P, Liao C H, Yang Y H et al 2001 Correlation of cervical vertebra maturation with hand-wrist maturation in children. Kaohsiung Journal of Medical Science 17 (1): 29–35

Chapman-Smith D 2001 Safety and effectiveness of cervical manipulation, vol. 15, pp. 1–8. The Chiropractic Report, Toronto, ON

Chapman-Smith D 2003 Manipulation as safe as normal neck movements, vol. 17, pp. 1–8. The Chiropractic Report, Toronto, ON

Chen T Y 2000 The clinical presentation of uppermost cervical disc protrusion. Spine 25: 439–442

Chen R, Cohen L G, Hallett M 2002 Nervous system reorganisation following injury. Neuroscience 111 (4): 761–773

Cheng C K, Chen H H, Kuo H H et al 1998 A three-dimensional mathematical model for predicting spinal joint force distribution during manual liftings. Clinical Biomechanics 13 (1, S1): S59–S64

Christensen H W, Vach W, Vach K et al 2002 Palpation of the upper thoracic spine: an observer reliability study. Journal of Manipulative and Physiological Therapeutics 25 (5): 285–292. Erratum 25 (6): 425

Christiansen J, Gerow G 1990 Thermography. Seminars in chiropractic, a quarterly series. Williams & Wilkins, Baltimore, MD

Christiansen J, Mueller J 1990 History of thermography. In: Christiansen J, Gerow G (eds) Thermography. Seminars in chiropractic, a quarterly series, pp. 3–10. Williams & Wilkins, Baltimore, MD

Chun J Y, Dillon W P, Berger M S 2002 Symptomatic enlarged cervical anterior epidural venous plexus in a patient with Marfan syndrome. American Journal of Neuroradiology 23 (4): 622–624

Cinotti G, De Santis F, Nofroni I, Postacchini F 2002 Stenosis of lumbar intervertebral foramen Spine 27: 223–229

Clark W C, Janal M N, Hoben E K, Carroll J D 2001 How separate are the sensory, emotional, and motivational dimensions of pain? A multidimensional scaling analysis. Somatosensory and Motor Research 18 (1): 31–39

Clark B C, Manini T M, Mayer J M et al 2002 Electromyographic activity of the lumbar and hip extensors during dynamic trunk extension exercise. Archives of Physical Medicine and Rehabilitation 83 (11): 1547–1552

Clausen J D, Goel V K, Traynelis C, Scifert J 1997 Uncinate processes and Luschka joints influence the biomechanics of the cervical spine: quantification using a finite element model of the C5–C6 segment. Journal of Orthopaedic Research 15: 342–347

Cole W V 1947 The effects of the atlas lesions. Journal of the American Osteopathic Association 47: 150–152

Conwell T D 1990 Thermography in the diagnosis of myofascial pain syndromes and localising trigger points. DC Tracts 2: 207–220

Conwell T D 1991a Infrared thermographic imaging, magnetic resonance imaging, CT scan, and myelography in low back pain. DC Tracts 3: 14–19

Conwell T D 1991b Thermography in the diagnosis of radiculopathies. DC Tracts 3: 20–26

Cooke P M, Lutz G E 2000 Internal disc disruption and axial back pain in the athlete. Physical Medicine and Rehabilitation Clinic of North America 11 (4): 837–865

Cooke E D, Pilcher M F 1973 Thermography in the diagnosis of deep vein thrombosis. British Medical Journal 2: 523–526

Cooke E D, Harris J, Fleming C F et al 1995 Correlation of pain with temperature and blood-flow changes in the lower limb following chemical lumbar sympathectomy in reflex sympathetic dystrophy. A case report. International Angiology. A Journal of the International Union of Angiology 14 (3): 226–228

Coppes M H, Marani E, Thomeer R T W N, Groen G J 1997 Innervation of "painful" lumbar discs. Spine 22: 2342–2349

Côté P 1999 Editorial. Screening for stroke: let's show some maturity. Journal of the Canadian Chiropractic Association 43: 72–74

Côté P, Kreitz B G, Cassidy J D, Thiel H 1996 The validity of the extension-rotation test as a clinical screening procedure before neck manipulation: a secondary analysis. Journal of Manipulative and Physiological Therapeutics 19: 159–164

Côté P, Kreitz B G, Cassidy J D et al 1998 A study of the diagnostic accuracy and reliability of the Scoliometer and Adam's forward bend test. Spine 23: 796–802; Discussion 803; Comment 1999; 24: 307–308; 2411–2412

Coughlin P 2001 Manual therapies. In: Micozzi M S (ed.) Fundamentals of complementary and alternative medicine, pp. 100–127. Churchill Livingstone, New York, NY

Coulter I D 1991 An institutional philosophy of chiropractic. Chiropractic Journal of Australia 21: 136–141

Coulter I D 1999 Chiropractic – a philosophy for alternative health care. Butterworth Heinemann, Oxford, UK

Coulter I D 2000 The roles of philosophy and belief systems in complementary and alternative health care. In: Papers distributed to delegates, conference on Philosophy in Chiropractic Education. World Federation of Chiropractic, Toronto, ON

Cox J M 1999 Low back pain. Mechanisms, diagnosis and treatment, 6th edn. Williams & Wilkins, Baltimore, MD

Cramer G D, Darby S A 1995 Basic and clinical anatomy of the spine, spinal cord, and ANS. Mosby, St Louis, MO

Cramer G D, Tuck N R, Knudsen J T et al 2000 Effects of side-posture positioning and side-posture adjusting on the lumbar zygapophyseal joints as evaluated by magnetic resonance imaging: a before and after study with randomization. Journal of Manipulative and Physiological Therapeutics 23: 380–394

Cramer G D, Skogsbergh D R, Bakkum B W et al 2002 Evaluation of transforaminal ligaments by magnetic resonance imaging. Journal of Manipulative and Physiological Therapeutics 25: 199–208

Cyriax J H, Cyriax P J 1996 Cyriax's illustrated manual of orthopaedic medicine, 2nd edn. Butterworth Heinemann, Oxford, UK

Dabbs V, Lauretti W J 1995 A risk assessment of cervical manipulation vs. NSAIDs for the treatment of neck pain. Journal of Manipulative and Physiological Therapeutics 18: 530–536. Comment 1996; 19: 220–221

Daffner S D, Vaccaro A R 2002 Managing disorders of the cervicothoracic junction. American Journal of Orthopedics 31 (6): 323–327

Dai L, Cheng P, Tu K et al 1992 The stress distribution of the lumbar spine and disc degeneration. Chinese Medical Science Journal 7 (3): 166–168

Dankiw W 1990 Medical thermography. Australian Institute of Health: Health care and technology series no. 4. Australian Government Publication Service, Canberra, Australia

Davey N J, Lisle R M, Loxton-Edwards B et al 2002 Activation of back muscles during voluntary abduction of the contralateral arm in humans. Spine 27: 1355–1360

Davis M J, Hill M A 1999 Signalling mechanisms underlying the vascular myogenic response. Physiological Reviews 79 (2): 287–423

Dean N A, Mitchell B S 2002 Anatomic relation between the nuchal ligament (ligamentum nuchae) and the spinal dura mater in the craniocervical region. Clinical Anatomy 15 (3): 182–185

Debiais F, Bataille B, Debiais P et al 2000 Femoral neuropathy secondary to ossification of the ligamentum flavum. Journal of Rheumatology 27 (5): 1313–1314

Degenhardt B F, Kuchera M I 1996 Update on the osteopathic medical concepts and the lymphatic system. Journal of the American Osteopathic Association 96 (2): 97–100

de la Calle-Reviriego J L 2000 Complex regional pain syndrome: the need for multidisciplinary approach. Revista de Neurologia 30 (6): 555–561

Delp S L, Hess W E, Hungerford D S, Jones L C 1999 Variation of rotation moment arms with hip flexion. Journal of Biomechanics 32 (5): 493–501

Demondion X, Delfaut E M, Drizenko A et al 2000 Radio-anatomic demonstration of the vertebral lumbar venous plexuses: an MRI experimental study. Surgical and Radiologic Anatomy 22 (3–4): 151–156

DeToledo J C, David N J 2001 Innervation of the sternocleidomastoid and trapezius muscles by the accessory nucleus. Journal of Neuroophthalmology 21: 214–216

DeToledo J C, Dow R 1998 Sternomastoid function during hemispheric suppression by Amytal: insights into the inputs to the spinal accessory nerve nucleus. Movement Disorders 13: 809–812

Devillè W L J M, van der Windt D A W M, Džafergić A et al 2000 The test of Lasègue. Spine 25: 1140–1147

Diakow P R P 1988 Thermographic imaging of myofascial trigger points. Journal of Manipulative and Physiological Therapeutics 11: 114–117

Diakow P R P, Ouellet S, Lee S, Blackmore E J 1988 Correlation of thermography with spinal dysfunction: preliminary results. Journal of the Canadian Chiropractic Association 32: 77–80

Dick B, Eccleston C, Crombez G 2002 Attentional functioning in fibromyalgia, rheumatoid arthritis, and musculoskeletal pain patient. Arthritis and Rheumatology 47 (6): 639–644

Dietz V 2002 Do human bipeds use quadrupedal coordination? Trends in Neurosciences 5 (9): 462–476

Diop M, Parratte B, Tatu L et al 2002 Anatomical basis of superior gluteal nerve entrapment syndrome in the suprapiriformis foramen. Surgical Radiologic Anatomy 24 (3–4): 155–159

Di Sebastiano P, Fink T, di Mola F F et al 1999 Neuroimmune appendicitis. Lancet 354 (9177): 461–466. Comment: 354 (9190): 1648

Dishman J D, Bulbulian R 2000 Spinal reflex attenuation associated with spinal manipulation. Spine 25: 2519–2525

Dishman J D, Ball K A, Burke J 2002 Central motor excitability changes after spinal manipulation: a transcranial magnetic stimulation study. Journal of Manipulative and Physiological Therapeutics 25: 1–9

Dittrick K, Allmendinger N, Wolpert L et al 2002 Calcified abdominal aortic aneurysm in a 12 year old boy. Journal of Pediatric Surgery 37 (9): E24

Dolan P, Adams M A 2001 Recent advances in lumbar spinal mechanics and their significance for modelling. Clinical Biomechanics 16 (S1): S8–S16

Donaldson C C S, Nelson D V, Schulz R 1998 Disinhibition in the gamma motoneuron circuitry: a neglected mechanism for understanding myofascial pain syndromes? Applied Psychophysiology Biofeedback 23: 43–57

DonTigny R L 1997 Mechanics and treatment of the sacroiliac joint. In: Vleeming A, Mooney V, Dorman T et al (eds) Movement, stability and low back pain, pp. 461–476. Churchill Livingstone, Edinburgh, UK

Dorman T 1997 Pelvic mechanics and prolotherapy. In: Vleeming A, Mooney V, Dorman T et al (eds) Movements, stability and low back pain, pp. 501–522. Churchill Livingstone, Edinburgh, UK

Dreher J C, Grafman J 2002 The roles of the cerebellum and basal ganglia in timing and error prediction. European Journal of Neuroscience 16: 1609–1619

Dreyfuss P, Michaelsen M, Fletcher D 1994 Atlanto-occipital and lateral atlantoaxial joint pain patterns. Spine 19: 1125–1131

Dudley W N 1987 Thermography: tracking nerve traps. American Chiropractic Association Journal of Chiropractic 21: 63–65

Dulhunty J 1987 Basic mechanics of the vertebral subluxation. Journal of the Australian Chiropractors' Association 1: 49–52

Dulhunty J A 1996 A mathematical basis for defining vertebral subluxations and their correction. Chiropractic Journal of Australia 26: 130–138

Dulhunty J A 1997 Anthropometrical and mechanical considerations in determining normal parameters for the sagittal lumbar spine [review of the literature]. Journal of Manipulative and Physiological Therapeutics 20: 90–102

Dumas J L, Sainte Rose M, Dreyfus P et al 1993 Rotation of the cervical spinal column: a computed tomography in vivo study. Surgical and Radiologic Anatomy 15 (4): 333–339

Dunlop R B, Adams M A, Hutton W C 1984 Disc space narrowing and the lumbar facet joints. Journal of Bone and Joint Surgery – British 66 (5): 706–710

Dunn G 1989 Design and analysis of reliability studies, pp. 1–58. Oxford University Press, Oxford, UK

Duval-Beaupere G 1992 Rib hump and supine angle as prognostic factors for mild scoliosis. Spine 17: 103–107

Dvořák J 1998 Epidemiology, physical examination, and neurodiagnostics. Spine 23: 2663–2672

Dvořák J, Dvořák V 1984 Manual medicine, diagnostics, Thième Stratton, New York, NY

Dvořák J, Dvořák V 1990 Manual medicine, diagnostics, 2nd edn. Thième Medical, New York, NY

Ebrall P S 1989 Meralgia paraesthetica. A historical perspective. Journal of the Australian Chiropractors' Association 19: 137–141

Ebrall P S 1990 Meralgia paraesthetica part 2: a clinical update. Journal of the Australian Chiropractors' Association 20: 15–16

Ebrall P S 1992a A descriptive report of the case-mix within Australian Chiropractic practice. Chiropractic Journal of Australia 23: 92–97

Ebrall P S 1992b A determination of the applied laboratory error of the Metrecom computer assisted goniometer. Journal of Chiropractic Technique (4): 46–51

Ebrall P S 1992c Mechanical low back pain: a comparison of medical and chiropractic management in Victoria. Chiropractic Journal of Australia 22: 47–53

Ebrall P S 1993 Residual disability from delayed manipulative treatment for mechanical low back pain: a case review. Chiropractic Journal of Australia 23: 54–58

Ebrall P S 1994 Some anthropometric dimensions of male adolescents with idiopathic low back pain. Journal of Manipulative and Physiological Therapeutics 17: 296–301

Ebrall P S 2001a Guest editorial. Philosophy in chiropractic education: the importance of globalisation as opposed to Americanisation. Chiropractic Journal of Australia 31: 1–7

Ebrall P S 2001b A survey of sets of principles of chiropractic. Chiropractic Journal of Australia 31: 58–69

Ebrall P S 2001c Commentary: The nature of the principles of chiropractic. Chiropractic Journal of Australia 31: 98–106

Ebrall P S, Bales G, Frost B 1992 An improved clinical protocol for ankle cryotherapy. Journal of Manual Medicine 6: 161–165

Ebrall P S, Ellis W B 2000 Transient syncope in chiropractic practice: a case series. Chiropractic Journal of Australia 30: 82–91

Ebrall P S, Molyneux T P 1993 Rotary subluxation of the atlas: an exploration of the diagnostic potential of the CT scan. Chiropractic Journal of Australia 23: 42–47

Ebrall P S, Alevaki H, Cust S L, Roberts N J 1993 Preliminary report: evidence of temporal variation in the values of three sagittal spinal angles. In: Minter W (ed.) Proceedings of the National Conference, Chiropractors' Association Australia, p. 81. Chiropractors' Association of Australia, Sydney, NSW

Ebrall P S, Hobson P, Iggo A, Farrant G 1994a A description of the thermal characteristics of spinal regions identified as having differential temperature by contact thermocouple measurement (the Nervo Scope). Chiropractic Journal of Australia 24: 139–146

Ebrall P S, Hobson P, Iggo A, Farrant G 1994b Preliminary communication: the thermal characteristics of spinal regions identified as having differential temperature by contact thermocouple measurement (the Nervo Scope). In: Minter W (ed.) Proceedings of the National Conference, Chiropractors' Association Australia, pp. 12–13. Chiropractors' Association of Australia, Sydney

Editorial 1945 National Chiropractic Journal (United States) 15 (1): 6

Edwards W T, Ordway N R, Zheng Y et al 2001 Peak stresses observed in the posterior lateral anulus. Spine 2001 (16): 1753–1759

Eingorn A M, Muhs G J 1999 Rationale for assessing the effects of manipulative therapy on autonomic tone by analysis of heart rate variability. Journal of Manipulative and Physiological Therapeutics 22: 161–162

Ellis W B, Ebrall P S 1991 The resolution of chronic inversion and plantar flexion of the foot: a pediatric case study. Journal of Chiropractic Technique 3: 55–59

Ellis W V, Morris J M, Swartz A A 1989 Screening thermography of chronic back pain patients with negative neuromusculoskeletal findings. Thermology 3: 125–126

Erwin W M, Jackson P C, Homonko D A 2000 Innervation of the human costovertebral joint: implications for clinical back pain syndromes. Journal of Manipulative and Physiological Therapeutics 23: 395–403

Escolar D M, Henricson E K, Mayhew J et al 2001 Clinical evaluator reliability for quantitative and manual muscle testing measures of strength in children. Muscle and Nerve 24: 787–793

Evans R C 2001 Illustrated orthopedic physical assessment, 2nd edn. Mosby, St Louis, MO

Faridi T J 1995 Spinal manipulation and visceral diseases. Sdi Systems, Dallas, TX

Faye L J 1986 Spinal motion palpation and clinical considerations of the lumbar spine and pelvis [lecture notes]. Motion Palpation Institute, Huntington Beach

Feipel V, Rondelet B, Le Pallec J P, Rooze M 1999 Normal global motion of the cervical spine: an electrogoniometric study. Clinical Biomechanics 14: 462–470. Comment 2001; 16 (5): 455–458

Ferezy J S 1989 Chiropractic management of meralgia paresthetica: a case report. Journal of Chiropractic Technique 1 (2): 52–56

Fernandez E, Towery S 1996 A parsimonious set of verbal descriptors of pain sensation derived from the McGill pain questionnaire. Pain 66: 31–37. Erratum: 68: 437

Field D 2001 Anatomy palpation and surface markings, 3rd edn. Butterworth-Heinemann, Oxford, UK

Fine E J, Ionita C C, Lohr L 2002 The history of the development of the cerebellar examination. Seminars in Neurology 22 (4): 375–384

Firth J N 1948 A text-book on chiropractic diagnosis, 5th edn. Self-published, James N Firth, Indianapolis, IN

Fishman L M, Dombi G W, Michaelsen C et al 2002a Piriformis syndrome: diagnosis, treatment, and outcome – a 10-year study. Archives of Physical Medicine and Rehabilitation 83 (3): 295–301

Fishman L M, Anderson C, Rosner B 2002b Botox and physical therapy in the treatment of piriformis syndrome. American Journal of Physical Medicine and Rehabilitation 81 (12): 936–942

Fitzcharles M A, Costa D D, Pohhia R 2003 A study of standard care in fibromyalgia syndrome: a favourable outcome. Journal of Rheumatology 30 (1): 154–159

Fligg D B 1986 The anterior thoracic adjustment. Journal of the Canadian Chiropractic Association 30: 211–213

Foreman S M, Croft A C 2002 Whiplash injuries, 3rd edn. Lippincott Williams & Wilkins, Philadelphia, PA

Forrester K, Griffiths D 2001 Essentials of law for health professionals. Harcourt, Sydney, NSW

Forster A L 1920 Principles and practice of chiropractic, 2nd edn. National Publishing, Chicago, IL

Franz B, Altidis P, Altidis B, Collis-Brown G 1999 The cervicogenic otoocular syndrome: a suspected forerunner of Ménière's disease. International Tinnitus Journal 5 (2): 125–130

Freeman R, Komaroff A L 1997 Does the chronic fatigue syndrome involve the autonomic nervous system? American Journal of Medicine 104 (4): 357–364

Freeman M D, Fox D, Richards T 1990 The superior intracapsular ligament of the sacroiliac joint: presumptive evidence for confirmation of Illi's ligament. Journal of Manipulative and Physiological Therapeutics 13: 384–390

Freeman L W, Lyn W, Lawlis G F 2001 Mosby's complementary and alternative medicine. A research-based approach. Mosby, St Louis, MO

Freemont A J, Peacock T E, Goupille P et al 1997 Nerve ingrowth into diseased intervertebral disc in chronic back pain. Lancet 350: 178–181

Freemont A J, Watkins A, Le Maitre C et al 2002a Nerve growth factor expression and innervation of the painful intervertebral disc. Journal of Pathology 197 (3): 286–292

Freemont A J, Jeziorska M, Hoyland J A et al 2002b. Mast cells in the pathogenesis of chronic back pain: a hypothesis. Journal of Pathology 197 (3): 281–285

Frobin W, Brinckmann P, Biggemann M et al 1997 Precision measurement of disc height, vertebral height and sagittal plane displacement from lateral radiographic views of the lumbar spine. Clinical Biomechanics 12 (S1): S1–S63

Frobin W, Leivseth G, Biggemann M, Brinckmann P 2002 Sagittal plane segmental motion of the cervical spine. A new precision measurement protocol and normal motion data of healthy adults. Clinical Biomechanics 17 (1): 21–31

Fujimoto T, Budgell B, Uchida S et al 1999 Arterial tonometry in the measurement of the effects of innocuous mechanical stimulation of the neck on heart rate and blood pressure. Journal of the Autonomic Nervous System 75 (2–3): 109–115

Fukuda K, Kawakami G 2001 Proper use of MR imaging for evaluation of low back pain (radiologist's view). Seminars in Musculoskeletal Radiology 5 (2): 133–136

Fuller G 1999 Neurological examination made easy, 2nd edn. Churchill Livingstone, Edinburgh, UK

Gamber R G, Shores J H, Russo D P et al 2002 Osteopathic manipulative treatment in conjunction with medication relieves pain associated with fibromyalgia syndrome: results of a randomized clinical pilot project. Journal of the American Osteopathic Association 102 (6): 321–325

Gashev A A 2002 Physiologic aspects of lymphatic contractile function: current perspectives. Annals of the New York Academy of Sciences 979: 178–187

Gashev A A, Zawieja D C 2001 Physiology of human lymphatic contractility: a historical perspective. Lymphology 34 (3): 124–134

Gatterman M I 1990 Chiropractic management of spine related disorders. Williams & Wilkins, Baltimore, MD

Gatterman M I 1992 The vertebral subluxation syndrome: is a rose by any other name less thorny? Journal of the Canadian Chiropractic Association 36 (2): 102–104

Gatterman M I 1995a Advances in subluxation terminology and usage. In: Lawrence D J (ed.) Advances in chiropractic, vol. 2., pp. 461–469. Mosby, St Louis, MO

Gatterman M I 1995b A patient centered paradigm: a model for chiropractic education and research. Journal of Alternative and Complementary Medicine 1: 415–432

Gatterman M I 1995c Foundations of chiropractic, subluxation. Mosby, St Louis, MO

Gatterman M I 1997 Teaching chiropractic principles through patient centered outcomes. Journal of the Canadian Chiropractic Association 41 (1): 27–35

Gatterman M I, Hansen D T 1994 Development of chiropractic nomenclature through consensus. Journal of Manipulative and Physiological Therapeutics. 17 (5): 302–309

Gerlach R, Zimmermann M, Kellermann S et al 2001 Intervertebral disc calcification in childhood – a case report and review of the literature. Acta Neurochirurgica 143 (1): 89–93

Gibbons P, Tehan P 2000 Manipulation of the spine, thorax and pelvis. Churchill Livingstone, Edinburgh, UK

Gibbs R W Jr 2003 Embodied experience and linguistic meaning. Brain and Language 84: 1–15

Giles L G F 1992 The pathophysiology of zygapophyseal joints. In: Haldeman S (ed.) Principles and practice of chiropractic, 2nd edn, pp. 197–210. Appleton & Lange, Norwalk, CT

Giles L G F, Singer K P 1997 Clinical anatomy and management of low back pain. Butterworth Heinemann, Oxford, UK

Giles L G F, Singer K P 1998 Clinical anatomy and management of cervical spine pain. Butterworth Heinemann, Oxford, UK

Giles L G F, Singer K P 2000 Clinical anatomy and management of thoracic spine pain. Butterworth Heinemann, Oxford, UK

Gillet H 1972 Gillet talks about Illi. Journal of the Australian Chiropractors' Association 6 (2): 16–18

Gillet H 1973 A definition of the subluxation. Journal of the Australian Chiropractors' Association 7 (4): 8, 17

Gillet J J, Gaucher-Peslherbe P L 1996 New light on motion palpation [commentary]. Journal of Manipulative and Physiological Therapeutics 19 (1): 52–59

Goh S, Price R I, Leedman P J, Singer K P 1999 The relative influence of vertebral body and intervertebral disc shape on thoracic kyphosis. Clinical Biomechanics 14 (7): 439–448

Goldman A B, Ghelman B, Doherty J 1990 Posterior limbus vertebrae: a cause of radiating back pain in adolescents and young adults. Skeletal Radiology 19: 501–507

Goldstein D S, Robertson D, Esler M et al 2002 Dysautonomias: clinical disorders of the autonomic nervous system. Annals of Internal Medicine 137 (9): 753–763

Golub B S, Silverman B 1969 Transforaminal ligaments of the lumbar spine. Journal of Bone and Joint Surgery – American 51 (5): 947–956

Goodheart G 1965 Applied kinesiology manual. Privately published, Detroit, MI

Gore D R 2001 Roentgenographic findings in the cervical spine in asymptomatic persons: a ten-year follow-up. Spine 26: 2463–2466

Gracely R H, Petzke F, Wolf J M, Clauw D J 2002 Functional magnetic resonance imaging evidence of augmented pain processing in fibromyalgia. Arthritis and Rheumatism 46 (5): 1333–1343

Granata K P, Wilson S E 2001 Trunk posture and spinal stability. Clinical Biomechanics 16 (8): 650–659

Green J, Coyle M, Becker C, Reilly A 1986 Abnormal thermographic findings in asymptomatic volunteers. Thermology 2: 13–15

Greenman P E 1990 Clinical aspects of sacroiliac function in walking. Journal of Manual Medicine 5: 125–130

Greenstein G M 1997 Clinical assessment of neuromusculoskeletal disorders. Mosby, St Louis, MO

Grice A S 1979 Radiographic, biomechanical and clinical factors in lumbar lateral flexion. Part I. Journal of Manipulative and Physiological Therapeutics 2 (1): 26–34

Gu Y, Hasegawa T, Yamamoto Y et al 2001 The combined effects of MRI and X-rays in ICR mouse embryos during organogenesis. Journal of Radiation Research (Tokyo) 42 (3): 262–272

Gudavalli M R, Triano J J 1999 An analytical model of lumbar motion segment in flexion. Journal of Manipulative and Physiological Therapeutics 22: 201–208

Guiot B H, Khoo L T, Fessler R G 2002 A minimally invasive technique for decompression of the lumbar spine. Spine 27: 432–438

Haas M 1990a The physics of spinal manipulation. Part I. The myth of $F = ma$. Journal of Manipulative and Physiological Therapeutics 13: 204–206

Haas M 1990b The physics of spinal manipulation. Part II. A theoretical consideration of the adjustive force. Journal of Manipulative and Physiological Therapeutics 13: 253–256

Haas M 1990c The physics of spinal manipulation. Part III. Some characteristics of adjusting that facilitate joint distraction. Journal of Manipulative and Physiological Therapeutics 13: 305–308

Haas M 1990d The physics of spinal manipulation. Part IV. A theoretical consideration of the physician impact force and energy requirements needed to produce synovial joint cavitation. Journal of Manipulative and Physiological Therapeutics 13: 378–383

Haas M, Nyiendo J, Peterson C et al 1992 Lumbar motion trends and correlations with low back pain. Part I. A roentgenological evaluation of coupled lumbar motion in lateral bending. Journal of Manipulative and Physiological Therapeutics 15: 145–158

Haas M, Raphael R, Panzer D, Peterson D 1995 Reliability of manual end play palpation of the thoracic spine. Journal of Chiropractic Technique 7: 120–124

Hack G D, Koritzer R T, Robinson W L et al 1995 Anatomic relation between the rectus capitis posterior minor muscle and the dura mater. Spine 20: 2484–2486

Hagg O, Wallner A 1990 Facet joint asymmetry and protrusion of the intervertebral disc. Spine 15 (5): 356–359.

Haijiao W, Koti M, Smith F W, Wardlaw D 2001 Diagnosis of lumbosacral nerve root anomalies by magnetic resonance imaging. Journal of Spinal Disorders 14 (2): 143–149

Halbert J, Crotty M, Cameron I D 2002 Evidence for the optimal management of acute and chronic phantom pain: a systematic review. Clinical Journal of Pain 18 (2): 84–92

Haldeman S, Kohlbeck F J, McGregor M 1999 Risk factors and precipitating neck movements causing vertebrobasilar artery dissection after cervical trauma and spinal manipulation. Spine 24: 785–794

Haldeman S, Carey P, Townsend M, Papadopoulos C 2001 Arterial dissections following cervical manipulation: the chiropractic experience. Canadian Medical Association Journal 165 (7): 905–906

Haldeman S, Kohlbeck F J, McGregor M 2002a Unpredictability of cerebrovascular ischemia associated with cervical spine manipulation therapy. Spine 27: 49–55

Haldeman S, Kohlbeck F J, McGregor M 2002b Stroke, cerebral artery dissection, and cervical spine manipulation therapy. Journal of Neurology 249 (8): 1098–1104

Hall E J 1994 Radiobiology for the radiologist, 4th edn. J B Lippincott, Philadelphia, PA

Hankey G J, Khangure M S 1988 Cervical myelopathy due to calcification of the ligamentum flavum. Australian and New Zealand Journal of Surgery 58 (3): 247–249

Hannecke V, Mayoux-Benhamou M A, Michel P et al 2001 Fetal development and postnatal maturation of the longus colli muscle. Morphologie 85 (269): 13–17

Hanson P, Sonesson B 1994 The anatomy of the iliolumbar ligament. Archives of Physical Medicine and Rehabilitation 75 (11): 1245–1246

Hanson P, Magnusson S P, Sorenson H, Simonsen E B 1998 Differences in the iliolumbar ligament and the transverse process of the L5 vertebra in young white and black people. Acta Anatomica 163 (4): 218–223

Härkäpää K, Järvikoski A, Mellin G et al 1991 Health locus of control beliefs and psychological distress as predictors for treatment outcome in low back pain patients: results of a 3-month follow-up of a controlled intervention study. Pain 46: 35–41

Harrington J Jr, Sungarian A, Rogg J et al 2001 The relation between vertebral endplate shape and lumbar disc herniations. Spine 26: 2133–2138

Harris A J 1999 Cortical origin of pathological pain. Lancet 354: 1464–1466; Comment 355: 318–319

Harris R I, MacNab I 1954 Structural changes in the lumbar intervertebral discs: their relationship to low back pain and sciatica. Journal of Bone and Joint Surgery – British 36-B: 304–322

Harrison E 1820 Remarks upon the different appearances of the back, breast and ribs, in persons affected with spinal diseases: and on the effects of spinal distortion on the sanguineous circulation. London Medical Physicians' Journal 14: 365–378

Harrison E 1827 Pathological impractical observations on spinal diseases. Thomas & George Underwood, London, UK

Harrison D D, Troyanovich S, Harrison D E et al 1996a A normal sagittal spine configuration: a desirable clinical outcome. Journal of Manipulative and Physiological Therapeutics 19: 398–405

Harrison D D, Colloca C J, Troyanovich S J, Harrison D E 1996b Torque: an appraisal of misuse of terminology in chiropractic literature and technique. Journal of Manipulative and Physiological Therapeutics 19: 454–462

Harrison D D, Janik T J, Harrison G R et al 1996c Chiropractic biophysics technique: a linear algebra approach to posture in chiropractic. Journal of Manipulative and Physiological Therapeutics 19: 525–535

Harrison D E, Harrison D D, Troyanovich S J 1997 The sacroiliac joint: a review of anatomy and biomechanics with clinical implications. Journal of Manipulative and Physiological Therapeutics 20: 607–617

Harrison D E, Harrison D D, Troyanovich S J, Harmon S 2000 It's time to accept the evidence for a normal spinal position. Journal of Manipulative and Physiological Therapeutics 23: 623–644

Harrison D E, Cailliet R, Harrison D D et al 2002a A new 3-point bending traction method for restoring cervical lordosis and cervical manipulation: a nonrandomized clinical controlled trial. Archives of Physical Medicine and Rehabilitation 83 (4): 447–453

Harrison D E, Cailliet R, Harrison D D, Janik T J 2002b How do anterior/posterior translations of the thoracic cage affect the sagittal lumbar spine, pelvic tilt, and thoracic kyphosis? European Spine Journal 11 (3): 287–293

Harrison D E, Harrison D D, Haas J W 2002c CBP structural rehabilitation of the cervical spine. Harrison Chiropractic Biophysics Seminars, Evanston, Wyoming

Hasan W, Smith P G 2000 Nerve growth factor expression in parasympathetic neurons: regulation by sympathetic innervation. European Journal of Neuroscience 12 (12): 4391–4397

Hasan M, Shukla S, Siddiqui M S, Singh D 2001 Posterolateral tunnels and ponticuli in human atlas vertebrae. Journal of Anatomy 199 (pt 3): 339–343

Hasegawa T, Mikawa Y, Watanabe R, An H S 1996 Morphometric analysis of the lumbosacral nerve roots and dorsal root ganglia by magnetic resonance imaging. Spine 21: 1005–1009

Hassel B, Farman A G 1995 Skeletal maturation evaluation using cervical vertebrae. American Journal of Orthodontic Dentofacial Orthopedics 107 (1): 58–66

Hauri P P 1975 Biofeedback and self-control of physiological functions: clinical applications. International Journal of Psychiatry Medicine 6 (1–2): 255–265

Hayashi T, Hirose Y, Sagoh M, Murakami H 1998 Ossification of transverse ligament of the atlas associated with atlantoaxial dislocation – case report. Neurologia Medico-chirurgica (Tokyo) 38 (7): 425–428

Haynes M J 1996 Doppler studies comparing the effects of cervical rotation and lateral flexion on vertebral artery blood flow. Journal of Manipulative and Physiological Therapeutics 19: 378–384

Haynes M J 2000 Vertebral arteries and neck rotation: Doppler velocimeter and duplex results compared. Ultrasound in Medicine and Biology 26 (1): 57–62

Haynes M J 2002 Vertebral arteries and cervical movement: Doppler ultrasound velocimetry for screening before manipulation. Journal of Manipulative and Physiological Therapeutics 25: 556–567

Haynes M J, Milne N 2001 Color duplex sonographic findings in human vertebral arteries during cervical rotation. Journal of Clinical Ultrasound 29 (1): 14–24

Haynes M J, Hart R, McGeachie J 2000 Vertebral arteries and neck rotation: Doppler velocimeter interexaminer reliability. Ultrasound Medical Biology 26 (8): 1363–1367

Haynes M J, Cala L A, Melsom A et al 2002 Vertebral arteries and cervical rotation: modelling and magnetic resonance angiography studies. Journal of Manipulative and Physiological Therapeutics 25: 370–383

He X, Oyadiji S O 2001 Application of coefficient of variation in reliability-based mechanical design and manufacture. Journal of Materials Processing Technology 119 (1–3): 374–378

Heggeness M H, Doherty B J 1998 Morphologic study of lumbar vertebral osteophytes. Southern Medical Journal 91 (2): 187–189

Herbst R W 1968 Gonstead chiropractic science and art. Sci-Chi Publications, Mt Horeb, WI

Herrick R T 1990 Thermography. Neurology 40: 1146

Herzog W 1998 Torque: misuse of a misused term [commentary]. Journal of Manipulative and Physiological Therapeutics 21: 57–59

Herzog W 2000 Clinical biomechanics of spinal manipulation. Churchill Livingstone, New York, NY

Hestback L, Leboeuf-Yde 2000 Are chiropractic tests for the lumbo-pelvic spine reliable and valid? A systematic critical literature review. Journal of Manipulative and Physiological Therapeutics 23: 258–275

Heylings D J 1978 Supraspinous and interspinous ligaments of the human lumbar spine. Journal of Anatomy 123: 127–131

Hides J A, Richardson C A, Jull G A 1996 Multifidus muscle recovery is not automatic after resolution of acute, first-episode low back pain. Spine 21: 2763–2769

Higgs J, Jones M 1995 Clinical reasoning in the health professions. Butterworth Heinemann, Oxford, UK

Hildebrandt R W 1977 Chiropractic spinography, a manual of technology and interpretation. Hilmark Publications, Des Plaines, IL

Hill M A, Zou H, Potocnik S J, Meininger G A, Davis M J 2001 Invited review: arteriolar smooth muscle mechanotransduction: Ca(2+) signalling pathways underlying myogenic reactivity. Journal of Applied Physiology 91 (2): 973–983

Hoffman R M, Daniel L K, Deyo R A 1991 Diagnostic accuracy and clinical utility of thermography for lumbar radiculopathy – a meta analysis. Spine 16: 623–628

Holm S, Indahl A, Solomonow M 2002 Sensorimotor control of the spine. Journal of electromyography and Kinesiology 12 (3): 219–234

Homewood A E 1981 The neurodynamics of the vertebral subluxation, 3rd edn. Parker Chiropractic Research Foundation, Fort Worth, TX

Honda H 1983 [Histopathological study of aging of the posterior portion of the human cervical vertebral bodies and discs – with special reference to the early ossification of the posterior longitudinal ligament.] Nippon Seikeigeka Gakkai Zasshi 57 (12): 1881–1893

Hongo M, Abe E, Shimada Y 1999 Surface strain distribution on thoracic and lumbar vertebrae under axial compression. Spine 24 (12): 1197–1202

Hoppenfeld S 1976 Physical examination of the spine and extremities. Appleton-Century-Crofts, Norwalk, CT

Hoppenfeld S 1997 Orthopaedic neurology. A diagnostic guide to neurologic levels. Lippincott Williams & Wilkins, Philadelphia, PA

Howarth D, Burstal R, Hayes C et al 1999. Autonomic regulation of lymphatic flow in the lower extremity demonstrated on lymphoscintigraphy in patients with reflex sympathetic dystrophy. Clinical Nuclear Medicine 24 (6): 383–387

Howe J W 1975 The role of X-ray findings in structural diagnosis. In: Goldstein M (ed.) The research status of spinal manipulative therapy, pp. 239–247. US Department of Health, Education, and Welfare, Bethesda, MD

Hsueh T C, Yu S, Kuan T S, Hong C Z 1998 Association of active myofascial trigger points and cervical disc lesions. Journal of the Formosan Medical Association 97 (3): 174–180

Hubbard J E 1990 Neuromuscular thermography: an analysis of criticisms. Thermology 3: 160–165

Hukuda S, Kojima Y 2002 Sex discrepancy in the canal/body ratio of the cervical spine implicating the prevalence of cervical myelopathy in men. Spine 27: 250–253

Humzah M D, Soames R W 1988 Human intervertebral disc: structure and function. Anatomical Record 220 (4): 337–356

Hurwitz E L, Aker P D, Adams A H et al 1996 Manipulation and mobilization of the cervical spine. A systematic review of the literature. Spine 21: 1746–1759. Discussion 1759–1760. Comment 22: 1676–1677

Hutton W C, Elmer W A, Bryce L M et al 2001 Do the intervertebral disc cells respond to different levels of hydrostatic pressure? Clinical Biomechanics 16 (9): 728–734

Ibatullin I A, Zaitseva R L, Chudnovskii N A, Chudnovskaia M N 1987 Structure and histo-topography of meniscoid structures of the atlanto-occipital and atlantoaxial joints. Arkhiv Anatomii Gistologii i Embriologii 92 (1): 30–38

Igarashi Y, Budgell B S 2000 Case study: response of arrhythmia to spinal manipulation: monitoring by ECG with analysis of heart-rate variability. Chiropractic Journal of Australia 30: 92–95

Inan N, Ceyhan A, Inan L et al 2001 C2/C3 nerve blocks and greater occipital nerve block in cervicogenic headache treatment. Functional Neurology 16 (3): 239–243

Indahl A, Kaigle A M, Reikeras O et al 1997 Interaction between the porcine lumbar intervertebral disc, zygapophyseal joints, and paraspinal muscles. Spine 22: 2834–2840

Indahl A, Kaigle A M, Reikeras O, Holm S 1999 Sacroiliac joint involvement in activation of the porcine spinal and gluteal musculature. Journal of Spinal Disorders 12 (4): 325–330

Inufusa A, An H, Lim T et al 1996 Anatomic changes of the spinal canal and intervertebral foramen associated with flexion-extension movement. Spine 21: 2412–2420

Ishida Y, Ohmori K, Inoue H, Suzuki K 1999 Delayed vertebral slip and adjacent disc degeneration with an isthmic defect of the fifth lumbar vertebra. Journal of Bone and Joint Surgery – British 81 (2): 240–244

Ito M, Incorvaia K M, Yu S F et al 1998 Predictive signs of discogenic lumbar pain on magnetic resonance imaging with discography correlation. Spine 23: 1252–1258. Discussion: 1259–1260

Ito T, Takano Y, Yuasa N 2001 Types of lumbar herniated disc and clinical course. Spine 26: 648–651

Ito H, Kanno I, Shimosegawa E et al 2002 Hemodynamic changes during neural deactivation in human brain: a positron emission tomography study of crossed cerebellar diaschisis. Annals of Nuclear Medicine 16 (4): 249–254

Ivancic J J, Bryce D, Bolton P S 1993 Use of prevocational tests by clinicians to predict vulnerability of patients to vertebrobasilar insufficiency. Chiropractic Journal of Australia 23: 59–63

Iwamura Y, Onari K, Kondo S et al 2001 Cervical intradural disc herniation. Spine 26: 698–702

Jackson R P 1992 The facet syndrome: myth or reality? Clinical Orthopedics and Related Research 279 (June): 110–121

Jackson M, Solomonow M, Zhou B et al 2001 Multifidus EMG and tension-relaxation recovery after prolonged static lumbar flexion. Spine 26: 715–723

Jacob S W, Francone C A, Lossow W J 1992 Structure and function in man, 5th edn. W B Saunders, Philadelphia, PA

Jacobs W B, Perrin R G 2001 Evaluation and treatment of spinal metastases: an overview. Neurosurgical Focus 11 (6): 1–11

Jacobsen S, Danneskiold-Samsoe B, Lund B (eds) 1993 Musculoskeletal pain, myofascial pain syndrome, and the fibromyalgia syndrome. Proceedings from the 2nd World Congress on myofascial pain and fibromyalgia. Consensus document on fibromyalgia: the Copenhagen declaration, pp. 295–312. Haworth Press, Binghamton, NY

Jamison J R 1991 Preventative chiropractic and the chiropractic management of visceral conditions: is the cost to chiropractic acceptance justified by the benefit to health care? Chiropractic Journal of Australia 21: 95–101

Jamison J R 1996 Psychoneuroendoimmunology: the biological basis of the placebo phenomenon? Journal of Manipulative and Physiological Therapeutics 19: 484–487

Jamison J R 1998 Mind–body medicine: the evolving science of chiropractic care. Journal of Chiropractic Humanities 8: 8–15

Jamison J R 1999 Differential diagnosis for primary practice. Churchill Livingstone, Edinburgh, UK

Jamison J R 2001 Maintaining health in primary care. Guidelines for wellness in the 21st century. Churchill Livingstone, Edinburgh, UK

Jamison J R, McEwen A P, Thomas S J 1992 Chiropractic adjustment in the management of visceral conditions: a critical appraisal. Journal of Manipulative and Physiological Therapeutics 15: 171–180

Jamison R N, Gracely R H, Raymond S A et al 2002 Comparative study of electronic vs. paper VAS ratings: a randomised, crossover trial using healthy volunteers. Pain 99: 341–347

Janda V 1991 Muscle spasm – a proposed procedure for differential diagnosis. Journal of Manual Medicine 6: 136–139

Janse J 1948a The vertebral subluxation. National Chiropractic Journal 18 (10): 9–11, 66, 67

Janse J 1948b The vertebral subluxation (2). National Chiropractic Journal 18 (11): 17–18, 66

Janse J 1948c The vertebral subluxation (3). National Chiropractic Journal 18 (12): 18–21

Janse J 1976 Principles and practice of chiropractic. An anthology. National College of Chiropractic, Lombard

Jaovisidha S, Ryu K N, De Maeseneer M et al 1996 Ventral sacroiliac ligament. anatomic and pathologic considerations. Investigative Radiology 31 (8): 532–541

Jayson M L V 1983 Compression stresses in the posterior elements and pathologic consequences. Spine 6 (3): 338–339

Jende A, Peterson C K 1997 Validity of static palpation as an indicator of atlas transverse process asymmetry. European Journal of Chiropractic 45: 35–42

Jenis L G, An H S 2000 Spine update. Lumbar foraminal stenosis. Spine 25: 389–394

Jenkins D B 1998 Hollinshead's functional anatomy of the back and limbs, 7th edn. W B Saunders, Philadelphia, PA

Jinkins J R 2002 Lumbosacral interspinous ligament rupture associated with acute intrinsic muscle degeneration. European Radiology 12: 2370–2376

Johansson H, Sojka P 1991 Pathophysiological mechanisms involved in genesis and spread of muscular tension in occupational muscle pain and in chronic musculoskeletal pain syndromes: a hypothesis. Medical Hypotheses 35: 196–203

Johnson G M, Zhang M 2002 Regional differences within the human supraspinous and interspinous ligaments: a sheet plastination study. European Spine Journal 11 (4): 382–388

Johnson G M, Zhang M, Jones G 2000 The fine connective tissue architecture of the human ligamentum nuchae. Spine 25: 5–9

Johnston M G, Hayashi A, Elias R 1986 Quantitative approaches to the study of lymphatic contractile in vitro and in vivo: potential role of this dynamic "lymph pump" in the re-expansion of the vascular space following haemorrhage. Lymphology 19 (2): 45–54

Jutkowitz J 1997 A normal sagittal spine configuration: a desirable clinical outcome [letter]. Journal of Manipulative and Physiological Therapeutics 20: 288–290

Jutkowitz J 1998 A normal sagittal spine configuration: a desirable clinical outcome [letter]. Journal of Manipulative and Physiological Therapeutics 21: 60–61

Kadel R E, Godbey W D 1983 Meralgia paresthetica: a study of incidence in one chiropractic clinic. Journal of Manipulative and Physiological Therapeutics 6: 76–77

Kadel R E, Godbey W D, Davis B P 1982 Conservative and chiropractic treatment of meralgia paresthetica: review and case report. Journal of Manipulative and Physiological Therapeutics 5: 73–78

Kahn J L, Sick H, Koritke J G 1992 The posterior intervertebral spaces of the craniovertebral joint. Acta Anatomica 144: 65–70

Kambin P, Nixon J E, Chait A, Schaffer J L 1988 Annular protrusion: pathophysiology and roentgenographic appearance. Spine 13: 671–675

Kang Y M, Wheeler J D, Pickar J G 2001 Stimulation of chemosensitive afferents from multifidus muscles does not sensitize multifidus muscle spindles to vertebral loads in the lumbar spine of the cat. Spine 26: 1528–1536

Kang Y M, Choi W S, Pickar J G 2002 Electrophysiologic evidence for an intersegmental reflex pathway between lumbar paraspinal tissues. Spine 27: E56–E63

Kankaanpaa M, Laaksonen D, Taimela S et al 1998 Age, sex, and body mass index as determinants of back and hip extensor fatigue in the isometric Sorensen back endurance test. Archives of Physical Medicine and Rehabilitation 79 (9): 1069–1075

Kapandji I A 1974 The physiology of the joints, vol. 3. The trunk and the vertebral column. Churchill Livingstone, Edinburgh, UK

Kazemi M 1999 Adolescent lumbar disc herniation in a tae kwon do martial artist: a case report. Journal of the Canadian Chiropractic Association 43 (4): 236–242

Keating J C 1992a The evolution of Palmer's metaphors and hypotheses. Philosophical Constructs for the Chiropractic Profession 2 (1): 9–19

Keating J C 1992b Toward a philosophy of the science of chiropractic. Stockton Foundation for Chiropractic Research, Stockton, CA

Keating I, Lubke C, Powell V et al 2001 Mid-thoracic tenderness: a comparison of pressure pair threshold between spinal regions, in asymptomatic subjects. Manual Medicine 6 (1): 34–39

Keats T E, Smith T H 1988 An atlas of normal developmental roentgen anatomy, 2nd edn. Year Book Medical Publishers, Chicago, IL

Kellgren J H 1977 The anatomical source of back pain. Rheumatology and Rehabilitation 16 (3): 3–12

Kieler H, Cnattingius S, Haglund B et al 2001 Sinistrality – a side-effect of prenatal sonography: a comparative study of young men. Epidemiology 12 (6): 618–623

Kierner A C, Zelenka I, Burian M 2001 How do the cervical plexus and the spinal accessory nerve contribute to the innervation of the trapezius muscle? Archives of Otolaryngology and Head and Neck Surgery 127: 1230–1232

Kikuchi S, Hasue M, Nishiyama K, Ito T 1984 Anatomic and clinical studies of radicular symptoms. Spine 9: 23–30

Kikuchi S, Hasue M, Nishiyama K, Ito T 1986 Anatomic features of the furcal nerve and its clinical significance. Spine 11: 1002–1007

Kirici Y, Ozan H 1999 Double gluteus maximus muscle with associated variations in the gluteal region. Surgical and Radiologic Anatomy 21 (6): 397–400. Comment: 2000; 22 (1): 3

Kirkaldy-Willis W H 1992a Orthopedics: past, present, and future. In: Kirkaldy-Willis W H, Burton C V (eds) Managing low back pain, 3rd edn., pp. 397–402. Churchill Livingstone, New York, NY

Kirkaldy-Willis W H 1992b The three phases of the spectrum of degenerative disease. In: Kirkaldy-Willis W H, Burton C V (eds) Managing low back pain, 3rd edn, pp. 105–119. Churchill Livingstone, New York, NY

Kirkaldy-Willis W H 1992c Pathology and pathogenesis of low back pain. In: Kirkaldy-Willis W H, Burton C V (eds) Managing low back pain, 3rd edn, pp. 49–79. Churchill Livingstone, New York, NY

Kirkaldy-Willis W H, Hill R J 1979 A more precise diagnosis for low back pain. Spine 4: 102–109

Kirkaldy-Willis W H, Burton C V, Cassidy J D 1992 The site and nature of the lesion. In: Kirkaldy-Willis W H, Burton C V (eds) Managing low back pain, 3rd edn, pp. 121–148. Churchill Livingstone, New York, NY

Kissling R O, Jacob H A 1996 The mobility of the sacroiliac joint in healthy subjects. Bulletin of Hospital Joint Disease 54 (3): 158–164

Kissling R O, Jacob H A C 1997 The mobility of sacroiliac joints in healthy subjects. In: Vleeming A, Mooney V, Dorman T et al (eds) Movement, stability and low back pain, pp. 177–185. Churchill Livingstone, Edinburgh, UK

Kleihues H, Albrecht S, Noack W 2001 Topographic relations between the neural and ligamentous structures of the lumbosacral junction: in-vitro investigation. European Spine Journal. 10 (2): 124–132

Knutson G A 1999 Dysafferentation: a novel term to describe the neuropathological effects of joint complex dysfunction. A look at likely mechanisms of symptom generation [letter]. Journal of Manipulative and Physiological Therapeutics 22: 491–494

Kobrossi T, Steiman I 1986 Reflex sympathetic dystrophy of the upper extremity: a new diagnostic approach using flexi-therm liquid crystal contact thermography. Journal of the Canadian Chiropractic Association 30: 29–32

Koch L E, Biedermann H, Saternus K-S 1998 High cervical stress and apnoea. Forensic Science International 97: 1–9

Koch L E, Koch H, Graumann-Brunt S et al 2002 Heart rate changes in response to mild mechanical irritation of the high cervical spinal cord region in infants. Forensic Science International 128: 168–176

Kojima K, Maeda T, Arai R, Shichikawa K 1990 Nerve supply to the posterior longitudinal ligament and the intervertebral disc of the rat vertebral column as studied by acetylcholinesterase histochemistry. 1. Distribution in the lumbar region. Journal of Anatomy 169: 237–246

Korr I M 1975 Proprioceptors and somatic dysfunction. Journal of the American Osteopathic Association 74: 638–650

Koumantakis G A, Wistanley J, Oldham J A 2002 Thoracolumbar proprioception in individuals with and without low back pain: intratester reliability, clinical applicability, and validity. Journal of Orthopaedic and Sports Physical Therapy 32 (7): 327–335

Krakenes J, Kaale B R, Rorvik J, Gilhus N E 2001 MRI assessment of normal ligamentous structures in the craniovertebral junction. Neuroradiology 42 (12): 1089–1097

Krespi Y, Gurol M E, Coban O et al 2002 Vertebral artery dissection presenting with isolated neck pain. Journal of Neuroimaging 12 (2): 179–182

Kucukkeles N, Acar A, Biren S, Arun T 1999 Comparisons between cervical vertebrae and hand–wrist maturation for the assessment of skeletal maturity. Journal of Clinical Pediatric Dentistry 24 (1): 47–52

Kulkarni V, Chandy M J, Babu K S 2001 Quantitative study of muscle spindles in suboccipital muscles of human foetuses. Neurology India 49 (4): 355–359

Kumaresan S, Yoganandan N, Pintar F A et al 2001 Journal of Orthopedic Research 19 (5): 977–984

Kurunlahti M, Kerttula L, Jauhiainen J et al 2001 Correlation of diffusion in lumbar intervertebral discs with occlusion of lumbar arteries: a study in adult volunteers. Radiology 221: 779–786

Ladenheim C J, Sherman R P, Sportelli L 2001 Professional chiropractic practice: ethics, business and risk management. PracticeMakers Products, Palmerton, PA

Lam K S, Carlin D, Mulholland R C 2000 Lumbar disc high-intensity zone: the value and significance of provocative discography and the determination of the discogenic pain source. European Spine Journal 9 (1): 36–41

Lantz C A 1989 The vertebral subluxation complex. ICA International Review of Chiropractic Sep/Oct: 37–61

Lantz C A 1995a The vertebral subluxation complex. In: Gatterman M I (ed.) Foundations of chiropractic, subluxation, pp. 149–174. Mosby, St Louis, MO

Lantz C A 1995b A review of the evolution of chiropractic concepts of subluxation. Topics in Clinical Chiropractic 2 (2): 1–10

Large R, Butler M, James F, Peters J 1990 A systems model of chronic musculoskeletal pain. Australian and New Zealand Journal of Psychiatry 24: 529–536

Lawrence D J (ed.) 2000 Year book of chiropractic 2000, p. xiii. Mosby, St Louis, MO

Lebkowski W J, Dzieciol J 2002 Degenerated lumbar intervertebral disc. A morphological study. Polish Journal of Pathology 53 (2): 83–86

Leclaire R, Esdaile J M, Jequier J C et al 1996 Diagnostic accuracy of technologies used in low back pain assessment. Thermography, triaxial dynamometry, spinoscopy, and clinical examination. Spine 21: 1325–1330

Lederman E 1997 Fundamentals of manual therapy. Physiology, neurology and psychology. Churchill Livingstone, Edinburgh, UK

Lee D 1997 Treatment of pelvis instability. In: Vleeming A, Mooney V, Dorman T et al (eds) Movement, stability and low back pain, pp. 445–459. Churchill Livingstone, Edinburgh

Lee D 2000 The pelvic girdle, 2nd edn. Churchill Livingstone, Edinburgh, UK

Lee H M, Kim H S, Kim D J et al 2000 Reliability of magnetic resonance imaging in detecting posterior ligament complex injury in thoracolumbar spinal fractures. Spine 25: 2079–2084

Lehman G J, McGill S M 2001 Spinal manipulation causes variable spine kinematic and trunk muscle electromyographic responses. Clinical Biomechanics 16: 293–299

Leinonen V, Kankaanpää M, Airaksinen O, Hänninen O 2000 Back and hip extensor activities during trunk flexion/extension: effects of low back pain and rehabilitation. Archives of Physical Medicine and Rehabilitation 81 (1): 32–37

Leinonen V, Kankaanpää M, Luukkonen M et al 2001 Disc herniation-related back pain impairs feed-forward control of paraspinal muscles. Spine 26: E367–E372

Leonardi M, Simonetti L, Agati R 2002 Neuroradiology of spine degenerative diseases. Best Practice in Research and Clinical Rheumatology 16 (1): 59–87

Leong J C, Luk K D, Chow D H, Woo C W 1987 The biomechanical functions of the iliolumbar ligament in maintaining stability of the lumbosacral junction. Spine 12: 669–674

Lestini W F, Wiesel S W 1989 The pathogenesis of cervical spondylosis. Clinical Orthopaedics and Related Research 239: 69–93

Lewit K, Rosina A 1999 Why yet another diagnostic sign of sacroiliac movement restriction? Journal of Manipulative and Physiological Therapeutics 22: 154–160

Licht P B, Christensen H W, Hojgaard P, Marving J 1998 Vertebral artery flow and spinal manipulation: a randomised, controlled and observer-blinded study. Journal of Manipulative and Physiological Therapeutics 21: 141–144. Erratum 21: inside back cover

Licht P B, Christensen H W, Svendensen P, Hoilund-Carise P F 1999 Vertebral artery flow and cervical manipulation: an experimental study. Journal of Manipulative and Physiological Therapeutics 22: 431–435

Licht P B, Christensen H W, Hoilund-Carise P F 2000 Is there a role for premanipulative testing before cervical manipulation? Journal of Manipulative and Physiological Therapeutics 23: 175–179

Liebenson C (ed.) 1996 Rehabilitation of the spine. Williams & Wilkins, Baltimore, MD

Lin Y H, Chen C S, Cheng C K et al 2001 Geometric parameters of the *in vivo* tissues at the lumbosacral joint of young Asian male adults. Spine. 26: 2362–2367

Lopes M A 1993 Spinal examination. In: Plaugher G (ed.) Textbook of clinical chiropractic. A specific biomechanical approach, pp. 73–111. Williams & Wilkins, Baltimore, MD

Lowe T G 1990 Current concepts review: Scheuermann disease. Journal of Bone and Joint Surgery – American 72-A (6): 940–945

Lu J, Ebraheim N A, Huntoon M et al 1998 Anatomic considerations of superior cluneal nerve at posterior iliac crest region. Clinical Orthopedics (347): 224–228

Luk K D, Ho H C, Leong J C 1986 The iliolumbar ligament. A study of its anatomy, development and clinical significance. Journal of Bone and Joint Surgery – British 68 (2): 197–200

Lumley J S P 2002 Surface anatomy, 3rd edn. Churchill Livingstone, Edinburgh, UK

Lund T, Nydegger T, Schlenzka D, Oxland T R 2002 Three-dimensional motion patterns during active bending in patients with chronic low back pain. Spine 27: 1865–1874

Luo Z P, Butterman G R, Lewis J L 1996 Determination of spinal facet joint loads from extra articular strains – a theoretical validation. Journal of Biomechanics 29 (6): 785–790

Luoma K, Riihimäki H, Luukkonen R et al 2000 Low back pain in relation to lumbar disc degeneration. Spine 25: 487–492

Luoma K, Vehmas T, Riihimäki H, Raininko R 2001 Disc height and signal intensity of the nucleus pulposus on magnetic resonance imaging as indicators of lumbar disc degeneration. Spine 26: 680–686

Macklin J 1993 Pathways to better health. Issue paper 7. March. National Health Strategy Secretariat, Department of Health, Housing and Community Services, Canberra, Australia

MacLean J G B, Tucker J K, Latham J B 1990 Radiographic appearances in lumbar disc prolapse. Journal of Bone and Joint Surgery – British 72-B: 917–920

Maezawa Y, Baba H, Uchida K et al 2001 Ligamentum flavum hematoma in the thoracic spine. Clinical Imaging 25 (4): 265–267

Mak K H, Mak K L, Gwi-Mak E 2002 Ossification of the ligamentum flavum in the cervicothoracic junction: case report on ossification found on both sides of the lamina. Spine 27: E11–E14

Maigne R 1996 Diagnosis and treatment of pain of vertebral origin, Williams & Wilkins, Baltimore, MD

Maigne J Y, Maigne R 1991 Trigger point of the posterior iliac crest: a painful iliolumbar ligament insertion or cutaneous dorsal ramus pain? An anatomic study. Archives of Physical Medicine and Rehabilitation 72 (10): 734–737

Maigne J Y, Maigne R, Guerin-Surville H 1991 The lumbar mamillo-accessory foramen: a study of 203 lumbosacral spines. Surgical Radiologic Anatomy 13: 29–32

Maitland G D, Banks K, English K, Hengeveld E (eds) 2001 Maitland's vertebral manipulation, 6th edn. Butterworth Heinemann, Oxford, UK

Mannion A F 1999 Fibre type characteristics and function of the human paraspinal muscles: normal values and changes in association with low back pain. Journal of Electromyography and Kinesiology 9: 363–377

Marino E A 1997 A pilot study using the first cervical vertebra as an indicator of race. Journal of Forensic Science 42: 1114–1118

Marques A P, Rhoden L, de Oliveira J et al 2001 Pain evaluation of patients with fibromyalgia, osteoarthritis, and low back pain. Revista do Hospital das Clinicas 56 (1): 5–10

Marshall G L, Little J W 2002 Deep tendon reflexes: a study of quantitative methods. Spinal Cord Medicine 25 (2): 94–99

Masarsky C S, Todres-Masarsky M 2001 Introduction: somatovisceral considerations in the science of tone. In: Masarsky C S, Todres-Masarsky M (eds) Somatovisceral aspects of chiropractic – an evidence-based approach, pp. 1–5. Churchill Livingstone, New York, NY

Mathiak K, Hertrich I, Grodd W, Ackermann H 2002 Cerebellum and speech perception: a functional magnetic resonance imaging study. Journal of Cognitive Neuroscience 14 (6): 902–912

Mayer H M 2001 Discogenic low back pain and degenerative lumbar spinal stenosis – how appropriate is surgical treatment? Schmerz 15 (6): 484–491

Mayoux-Benhamou M A, Revel M, Vallee C et al 1994 Longus colli has a postural function on cervical curvature. Surgical and Radiologic Anatomy 16 (4): 367–371

Mayoux-Benhamou M A, Revel M, Vallee C 1997 Selective electromyography of dorsal neck muscles in humans. Experimental Brain Research 113 (2): 353–360

McArdle W D, Katch F I, Katch V L 1999 Sports and exercise nutrition. Lippincott/Williams & Wilkins, Philadelphia, PA

McCarthy P W 2001 Rumours and proven facts on the effects of manipulation: the role of neuroplasticity in understanding the physiological basis for chiropractic. European Journal of Chiropractic 46: 87–88

McCrory P 2001 "The piriformis syndrome" – myth or reality? British Journal of Sports Medicine 35 (4): 209–210

McCrory D C, Penzien D B, Hasselblad V, Gray R N 2001 Evidence report: behavioural and physical treatments for tension-type and cervicogenic headaches. Foundation for Chiropractic Education and Research, Des Moines, I

McKenzie R A 1990 The cervical and thoracic spine. Mechanical diagnosis and treatment. Spinal Publications (NZ) Ltd, Waikanae

McLeod J G, Tuck R R 1987 Disorders of the autonomic nervous system: part 1. Pathophysiology and clinical features. Annals of Neurology 21 (5): 419–430

McPartland J M, Brodeur R R, Hallgren R C 1997 Chronic neck pain, standing balance, and suboccipital muscle atrophy – a pilot study. Journal of Manipulative and Physiological Therapeutics 20: 24–29

Melzack R 1975 The McGill pain questionnaire: major properties and scoring methods. Pain 1: 277–279

Melzack R 1982 Pain measurement and assessment. Raven Press, New York, NY

Mense S 1991 Physiology of nociception in muscles. Journal of Manual Medicine 6: 24–33

Mercer S R, Jull G A 1996 Morphology of the cervical intervertebral disc: implications for McKenzie's model of the disc derangement syndrome. Journal of Manual Medicine 2: 76–81

Meyers S, Cros D, Sherry B, Vermeire P 1989 Liquid crystal thermography: quantitative studies in abnormalities of carpal tunnel syndrome. Neurology 39: 1465–1469

Micozzi M C 2001 Fundamentals of complementary and alternative medicine, 2nd edn. Churchill Livingstone, New York, NY

Middleton F A, Strick P L 1994 Anatomical evidence for cerebellar and basal ganglia involvement in higher cognitive function. Science 266 (5184): 458–461

Middleton F A, Strick P L 2000 Basal ganglia and cerebellar loops: motor and cognitive circuits. Brain Research, Brain Research Reviews 31 (2–3): 236–250

Milette P C, Fontaine S, Lepanto L et al 1999 Differentiating lumbar disc protrusions, disc bulges, and discs with normal contour but abnormal signal intensity. Magnetic resonance imaging with discographic correlations. Spine 24 (1): 44–53

Miller J A A, Haderspeck K A, Schultz A B 1983 Posterior element loads in lumbar motion segments. Spine 8 (3): 331–337

Mimura M, Moriya H, Watanabe T et al 1989 Three-dimensional motion analysis of the cervical spine with special reference to the axial rotation. Spine 14: 1135–1139

Mintz A C, Albano A, Reisdorff E J et al 1990 Stress fracture of the first rib from serratus anterior tension: an unusual mechanism of injury. Annals of Emergency Medicine 19: 411–414

Mitchell B S, Humphreys B K, O'Sullivan E 1998 Attachments of the ligamentum nuchae to cervical posterior spinal dura and the lateral part of the occipital bone. Journal of Manipulative and Physiological Therapeutics 21: 145–148

Mooney V, Robertson J 1976 The facet syndrome. Clinical Orthopaedics and Related Research 115: 149–156

Moore K L 1980 Clinically oriented anatomy. Williams & Wilkins, Baltimore, MD

Mootz R D 1995 Theoretic models of chiropractic subluxation. In: Gatterman M I (ed.) Foundations of chiropractic, subluxation, pp. 175–189 Mosby, St Louis, MO

Mootz R D, Talmage D M 1999 Evaluation of midback pain. Clinical assessment strategies for the thoracic area. Topics in Clinical Chiropractic 6 (3): 1–19

Moran R W, Gibbons P 2001 Intraexaminer and interexaminer reliability for palpation of the cranial rhythmic impulse at the head and sacrum. Journal of Manipulative and Physiological Therapeutics 24: 183–190

Morgan L 1997 A normal sagittal spine configuration: a desirable clinical outcome [letter]. Journal of Manipulative and Physiological Therapeutics 20: 130–131

Morgan L G 1998 Psychoneuroimmunology, the placebo effect and chiropractic [commentary]. Journal of Manipulative and Physiological Therapeutics 21 (7): 484–491

Morley S, Pallin V 1995 Scaling the affective domain of pain: a study of the dimensionality of verbal descriptors. Pain 62: 39–49

Morrison M L, McCluggage W G, Price G J et al 2002 Expert system support using a Bayesian belief network for the classification of endometrial hyperplasia. Journal of Pathology 197 (3): 402–414

Moser E A, Harbaugh R E, Cromwell L, Nordgren R E 1993 Os odontoideum and posterior circulation stroke in childhood. Journal of the Neuromusculoskeletal System 1: 170–173

Murphy D R 2000 The muscle designation debate: the experts respond. Journal of Bodywork and Movement Therapies 4 (4): 229–232

Murtagh J 1994 General practice. McGraw-Hill, Sydney, NSW

Murtagh J E, Kenna C J 1997 Back pain and spinal manipulation, 2nd edn. Butterworth Heinemann, Oxford, UK

Naderi S, Mertol T 2002 Simultaneous cervical and lumbar surgery for combined symptomatic cervical and lumbar spinal stenosis. Journal of Spinal Disorders and Techniques 15 (3): 229–232

Nansel D, Szlazak M 1995 Somatic dysfunction and the phenomenon of visceral disease simulation: a probable explanation for the apparent effectiveness of somatic therapy in patients presumed to be suffering from true visceral disease. Journal of Manipulative and Physiological Therapeutics 18: 379–397

National Better Health Secretariat 1991 The role of primary health care in health promotion in Australia. Department of Community Services and Health, Canberra, Australia

Neidre A, MacNab I 1983 Anomalies of the lumbosacral nerve roots. Spine 8: 294–299

Neumann M, Friedl S, Meining A et al 2002 A score card for upper GI endoscopy: evaluation of intraobserver variability in examiners with various levels of experience. Zeitschrift fur Gastroenterologie 40 (10): 857–862

Newcomer K, Laskowski E R, Yu B et al 2000a Repositioning error in low back pain. Spine 25: 245–256

Newcomer K, Laskowski E R, Yu B et al 2000b Differences in repositioning error among patients with low back pain compared with control subjects. Spine 25: 2488–2493

Newman R I, Seres J L, Miller E B 1984 Liquid crystal thermography in the evaluation of chronic back pain. Pain 20: 293–305

Nguyen D K, Botez M I 1998 Diaschisis and neurobehaviour. Canadian Journal of Neurological Sciences 25 (1): 5–12

Nikolajsen L, Staehelin Jensen T 2000 Phantom limb pain. Current Review of Pain 4 (2): 166–170

Nitta H, Tajima T, Sugiyama H, Moriyama A 1993 Study on dermatomes by means of selective lumbar spinal block. Spine 18: 1782–1786

Norman R, Wells P, Neumann P et al 1998 A comparison of peak vs. cumulative physical work exposure risk factors for the reporting of low back pain in the automotive industry. Clinical Biomechanics 13: 561–573

Nygaard Ø P, Mellgren I 1998 The function of sensory nerve fibres in lumbar radiculopathy. Spine 23: 348–352

Nystrom B, Weber H, Amundsen T 2001 Microsurgical decompression within laminectomy in lumbar spinal stenosis. Ups Journal of Medical Science 1–6 (2): 123–131

Oguz H, Akkus S, Tarhan S et al 2002 Measurement of spinal canal diameters in young subjects with lumbosacral transitional vertebra. European Spine Journal 11 (2): 115–118

Ohman J C 1986 The first rib of hominoids. American Journal of Physical Anthropology 70 (2): 209–229

Okuda S, Myoui A, Nakase T et al 2001 Ossification of the ligamentum flavum associated with osteoblastoma: a report of three cases. Skeletal Radiology 30 (7): 402–406

Olszewski W L 2002 Contractility patterns of normal and pathologically changed human lymphatics. Annals of the New York Academy of Sciences 979: 52–63

O'Malley J N 1997 How real is the subluxation? Journal of Manipulative and Physiological Therapeutics 20: 482–487

Otani K, Konno S, Kikuchi S 2001 Lumbosacral transitional vertebrae and nerve-root symptoms. Journal of Bone and Joint Surgery – British 83: 1137–1140

Otte A, Ettlin T M, Nitzsche E U et al 1997 PET and SPECT in whiplash syndrome: a new approach to a forgotten brain? Journal of Neurology, Neurosurgery and Psychiatry 63 (3): 368–372

Owens C 1937 An endocrine interpretation of Chapman's reflexes, 2nd edn, pp. 1–2. Chattanooga Printing and Engraving, Chattanooga, TN

Owens E F 1997 A normal sagittal spine configuration: a desirable clinical outcome [letter]. Journal of Manipulative and Physiological Therapeutics 20: 133–134

Paajanen H, Alanen A, Erkintalo M et al 1989 Disc degeneration in Scheuermann disease. Skeletal Radiology 18: 523–526

Pal G P, Routal R V, Saggu S K 2001 The orientation of the articular facets of the zygapophyseal joints at the cervical and upper thoracic region. Journal of Anatomy 98 (pt 4): 431–441

Palmer B J 1966 Our masterpiece, vol. XXXIX. Palmer College of Chiropractic, Davenport, LA

Palmer D D 1910 The science, art and philosophy of chiropractic. Portland Publishing House, Portland, OR

Panattoni G L, Todros T 1989 Fetal motor activity and spine development. Panminerva Medicine 31 (4): 183–186

Panegyres P K, Moore N, Gibson R et al 1993 Thoracic outlet syndromes and magnetic resonance imaging. Brain 116 (pt 4): 823–841

Panjabi M M, White A A 2001 Biomechanics in the musculoskeletal system. Churchill Livingstone, New York, NY

Panjabi M, Yamamoto I, Oxland T, Crisco J 1989 How does posture affect coupling in the lumbar spine? Spine 14 (9): 1002–1011

Panjabi M M, Crisco J J, Vasavada A et al 2001 Mechanical properties of the human cervical spine as shown by three-dimensional load-displacement curves. Spine 26: 2692–2700

Panzer D M, Fechtel S G, Gatterman M I 1990 Postural complex. In: Gatterman M I (ed.) Chiropractic management of spine related disorders, pp. 256–284. Williams & Wilkins, Baltimore, MD

Parekh H C, Gurusinghe N T, Perera S S, Prabhu S S 1993 Ossification of the ligamentum flavum in a Caucasian: case report. British Journal of Neurosurgery 7 (6): 687–690

Park J B, Chang H, Kim K W, Park S J 2001a A comparison between far lateral and posterolateral lumbar disc protrusions. Spine 26: 677–679

Park J B, Kim K W, Han C W, Chang H 2001b Expression of Fas receptor on disc cells in herniated lumbar disc tissue. Spine 26: 142–146

Patriquin D A 1992 Viscerosomatic reflexes In: Patterson M M, Howell J N (eds) The central connection: somatovisceral/ viscerosomatic interaction. Proceedings of the 1989 American Academy of Osteopathy International Symposium, pp. 4–18. University Classics, Athens, OH

Pelz D M, Fox A J 1990 Radiologic investigation (of the cervical disc and degenerative disease). Current Orthopaedics 4: 9–14

Penning L 2000 Psoas muscle and lumbar spine stability: a concept uniting existing controversies. Critical review and hypothesis. European Spine Journal 9 (6): 577–585

Penning L, Wilmink J T 1987 Rotation of the cervical spine: a CT study in normal subjects. Spine 12: 732–738

Peters D (ed.) 2001 Understanding the placebo effect in complementary medicine. Theory, practice and research. Churchill Livingstone, Edinburgh, UK

Peterson D H, Bergmann T F 2002 Chiropractic technique: principles and procedures. 2nd edn. Mosby, St Louis, MO

Petty N J, Moore A P 2001 Neuromuscular examination and assessment, 2nd edn. Churchill Livingstone, Edinburgh, UK

Pfirrmann C W, Binkert C A, Zanetti M et al 2000 Functional MR imaging of the craniocervical junction. Correlation with alar ligaments and occipito-atlantoaxial joint morphology: a study in 50 asymptomatic subjects. Schweizerische Medizinische Wochenschrift. 130 (18): 645–651. Data from this paper have also been published by the authors in Radiology 2001; 218: 133–137

Phillips R B 1992 Plain film radiology in chiropractic. Journal of Manipulative and Physiological Therapeutics 15 (1): 47–50

Pickar J G, Kang Y-M 2001 Short-lasting stretch of lumbar paraspinal muscle decreases muscle spindle sensitivity to subsequent muscle stretch. Journal of the Neuromusculoskeletal System 9: 88–96

Pietrzykowski J, Chmielowski K, Shrzynski S, Krzysztof Podgorski J 1997 Diaschisis phenomenon. Crossed cerebellar diaschisis. Neurologia I Neurochirurgia Polska 31 (6): 1207–1215

Piovesan E J, Kowacs P A, Tatsui C E et al 2001 Referred pain after painful stimulation of the greater occipital nerve in humans: evidence of convergence of cervical afferences on trigeminal nuclei. Cephalgia 21 (2): 107–109

Plaugher G 1993 Textbook of clinical chiropractic. A specific biomechanical approach. Williams & Wilkins, Baltimore, MD

Pletain S 1997 Motion palpation of the pelvis. In: Lawrence D J (ed.) Advances in chiropractic, vol. 4, pp. 69–101. Mosby Year Book, St Louis, MO

Pletain S 2001 Approaches to motion palpation: detecting primary and secondary fixations in the cervical spine. European Journal of Chiropractic 46: 67–68

Pochaczevsky R, Wexler C E, Meyers P H et al 1982 Liquid crystal thermography of the spine and extremities: its value in the diagnosis of spinal root syndromes. Journal of Neurosurgery 56: 386–395

Pool-Goudzwaard A L, Kleinrensink G J, Snijders C J et al 2001 The sacroiliac part of the iliolumbar ligament. Journal of Anatomy 199 (pt. 4): 457–463

Pope M H, Aleksiev A, Panagiotacopulos N D et al 2000 Evaluation of low back muscle surface EMG signals using wavelets. Clinical Biomechanics 15 (8): 567–573

Potocnik S J, Hill M A 2001 Pharmacological evidence for capacitative Ca(2+) entry in cannulated and pressurized skeletal muscle arterioles. British Journal of Pharmacology 134 (2): 247–256

Prabhakar S, Bhatia R, Khandelwai N et al 2001 Vertebral artery dissection due to indirect neck trauma: an underrecognised entity. Neurology India 49: 384–390

Prassopoulos P K, Faflia C P, Voloudaki A E, Gourtsoyiannis N C 1999 Sacroiliac joints: anatomical variants on CT. Journal of Computer Assisted Tomography 23 (2): 323–327

Prentice W E 2001 Impaired muscle performance: regaining muscular strength and endurance. In: Prentice W E, Voight M I (eds) Techniques in musculoskeletal rehabilitation, pp. 59–72. McGraw-Hill, New York, NY

Price C J, Warburton E A, Moore C J et al 2001 Dynamic diaschisis: anatomically remote and context-sensitive human brain lesions. Journal of Cognitive Neurosciences 13 (4): 419–429

Putzke J D, Richards J S, Hicken B L et al 2002 Pain classification following spinal cord injury: the utility of verbal descriptors. Spinal Cord 40: 118–127

Qiu M L (ed.) 1993 Chinese acupuncture and moxibustion. Churchill Livingstone, New York, NY

Quint U, Wilke H J, Shirazi-Adl A et al 1998 Importance of the intersegmental trunk muscles for the stability of the lumbar spine. Spine 23: 1937–1945

Radebold A, Cholewicki J, Polzhofer G K, Greene H S 2001 Impaired postural control of the lumbar spine is associated with delayed muscle response times in patients with chronic idiopathic low back pain. Spine 26: 724–730

Rahlmann J F 1987 Mechanisms of intervertebral joint dysfunction: a literature review. Journal of Manipulative and Physiological Therapeutics 10: 177–187

Raskin M M, Martinez-Lopez M, Sheldon J J 1976 Lumbar thermography in discogenic disease. Radiology 119: 149–152

Rebain R, Baxter G D, McDonough S 2002 A systematic review of the passive straight leg raising test as a diagnostic aid for low back pain (1989–2000). Spine 27: E388–E395

Refshauge K M 1994 Rotation: a valid premanipulative dizziness test? Does it predict safe manipulation? Journal of Manipulative and Physiological Therapeutics 17: 15–19. Comment 17: 413–414

Refshauge K M, Parry S, Shirley D et al 2002 Professional responsibility in relation to cervical spine manipulation. Australian Journal of Physiotherapy 48 (3): 171–179

Remier P A 1957 Modern X-ray practice and chiropractic spinography, 3rd edn. Palmer School of Chiropractic, Davenport, LA

Rend M T 2002 The "piriformis syndrome" – myth or reality [comment]. British Journal of Sports Medicine 36 (1): 76

Rho R H, Brewer R P, Lamer T J, Wilson P R 2002 Complex regional pain syndrome. Mayo Clinical Proceedings 77 (2): 174–180. Comment 77 (7): 733–734. Discussion 734

Richardson C 2000 The muscle designation debate: the experts respond. Journal of Bodywork and Movement Therapies 4 (4): 235–236

Ricketson R, Simmons J W, Hauser B O 1996 The prolapsed intervertebral disc. The high-intensity zone with discography correlation. Spine 21: 2758–2762. Comment: 1997, 22: 1538

Risk Management Seminar 2002 The Chiropractors' Association of Australia (Victoria), Guild Insurance, The Chiropractic Registration Board of Victoria, Melbourne, NSW

Ritchie W G M, Soulen R L, Lapayowker M S 1979 Thermographic diagnosis of deep vein thrombosis. Radiology 131: 341–344

Rivett D A, Sharples K J, Milburn P D 1999 Effect of premanipulative tests on vertebral artery and internal carotid artery blood flow: a pilot study. Journal of Manipulative and Physiological Therapeutics 22: 368–375

Rivierez M, Vally P 2001 Ossification of ligamentum flavum unmasked by acute paraplegia. Neurochirurgie 47 (6): 572–575

Rodgers W B, Coran D L, Kharrazi F D et al 1997 Increasing lordosis of the occipitocervical junction after arthrodesis in young children: the occipitocervical crankshaft phenomenon. Journal of Pediatric Orthopedics 17 (6): 762–765

Rodrigue T, Hardy R W 2001 Diagnosis and treatment of piriformis syndrome. Neurosurgical Clinics of North America 12 (2): 311–319

Rogawski K M 1990 The rhomboideus capitis in man – correctly named rare muscular variation. Okajimas Folia Anatomica Japonica 67 (2–3): 161–163

Ross J K, Bereznick D E, McGill S M 1999 Atlas-axis facet asymmetry, implications in manual palpation. Spine 24: 1203–1209

Rossi P, Cardinali P, Serrao M et al 2001 Magnetic resonance imaging findings in piriformis syndrome: a case report. Archives of Physical Medicine and Rehabilitation 82 (4): 519–521

Rothwell D M, Bondy S J, Williams J I 2001 Chiropractic manipulation and stroke. A population-based case-control study. Stroke 32: 1054–1060

Rousseaux M, Steinling M 1999 Remote regional cerebral blood flow consequences of focused infarcts of the medulla, pons and cerebellum. Journal of Nuclear Medicine 40 (5): 721–729

Routal R V, Pal G P 2000 Location of the spinal nucleus of the accessory nerve in the human spinal cord. Journal of Anatomy 196: 263–268

Routal R V, Pal G P 2000 Location of the spinal nucleus of the accessory nerve in the human spinal cord. Journal of Anatomy 196 (pt 2): 263–268

Rubinstein S M, Haldeman S 2001 Cervical manipulation in a patient with a history or traumatically induced dissection of the internal carotid artery: a case report and review of the literature on recurrent dissection. Journal of Manipulative and Physiological Therapeutics 24: 520–525

Rucco V, Basadonna P T, Gasparini D 1996 Anatomy of the iliolumbar ligament: a review of its anatomy and a magnetic resonance study. American Journal of Physical Medicine and Rehabilitation 75 (6): 451–455

Rygh L J, Tjolsen A, Hole K, Svendsen F 2002 Cellular memory in spinal nociceptive circuitry. Scandinavian Journal of Psychology 43 (2): 153–159

Saadeh F A 1988 A bifid piriformis muscle with dual insertion. Gegenbaurs Morphologisches Jahrbuch 134 (2): 185–187

Sackett D 2002 Testimony at Lewis Inquest, Coroner's Court, Toronto, ON, November 20

Saeed A B, Shuaib A, Al-Sulaiti G, Emery D 2000 Vertebral artery dissection: warning symptoms, clinical features and prognosis in 26 patients. Canadian Journal of Neurological Sciences 27 (4): 292–296

Sakamoto H, Akita K, Sato T 1996 An anatomical analysis of the relationships between the intercostal nerves and the thoracic and abdominal muscles in man. Ramification of the intercostal nerves. Acta Anatomica 156 (2): 132–142

Sakamoto N, Yamashita T, Takebayashi T et al 2001 An electrophysiologic study of mechanoreceptors in the sacroiliac joint and adjacent tissues. Spine 26: E468–E471

Sanchez-Chavez J J 1999 The penumbra area. Revista de Neurologia 28 (8): 810–816

Sandoz R 1976 Some physical mechanisms and effects of spinal adjustments. Annals of the Swiss Chiropractors' Association 6: 91–141

Sandoz R 1989 Some critical reflections on subluxations and adjustments. Annals of the Swiss Chiropractors' Association 9: 7–29

Santiago F R, Milena G L, Herrera R O et al 2001 Morphometry of the lower lumbar vertebrae in patients with and without low back pain. European Spine Journal 10 (3): 228–233

Sasaki H, Iton T, Takei H, Hayashi M 2000 Os odontoideum with cerebellar infarction: a case report. Spine 25: 1178–1181

Sato A 1992 The reflex effects of spinal somatic nerve stimulation on visceral function. Journal of Manipulative and Physiological Therapeutics 15: 57–61

Sato A, Swenson R S 1984 Sympathetic nervous system responses to mechanical stress of the spinal column in rats. Journal of Manipulative and Physiological Therapeutics 7: 141–147

Schafer R C 1983 Clinical biomechanics, musculoskeletal actions and reactions. Williams & Wilkins, Baltimore, MD

Schellhas K P, Pollei S R, Gundry C R, Heithoff K B 1996 Lumbar disc high-intensity zone. Correlation of magnetic resonance imaging and discography. Spine 21: 79–86

Schmorl G, Junghans H 1971 The human spine is health and disease. E F Beseman (translation), p. 158. Grune & Stratton, New York, NY

Schneider M J 1999 Principles of manual myofascial therapy. Self-published, Pittsburgh

Schneider M J, Brady D M 2001 Fibromyalgia syndrome: a new paradigm for differential diagnosis and treatment [commentary]. Journal of Manipulative and Physiological Therapeutics 24: 529–541

Schultz G D, Bassano J M 1997 Is radiography appropriate for detecting subluxations? Topics in Clinical Chiropractic 4 (1): 1–8

Schwarzer A C, Aprill C N, Derby R et al 1995 The prevalence and clinical features of internal disc disruption in patients with chronic low back pain. Spine 20: 1878–1883. Comment 15: 776–777

Schwenkreis P, Witscher K, Janssen F et al 2001 Assessment of reorganisation in the sensorimotor cortex after upper limb amputations. Clinical Neurophysiology 112 (4): 627–635

Seaman D R, Cleveland III C 1999 Spinal pain syndromes: nociception, neuropathic, and psychologic mechanisms. Journal of Manipulative and Physiological Therapeutics 22: 458–472

Seaman D R, Winterstein J F 1998 Dysafferentation: a novel term to describe the neuropathophysiological effects of joint complex dysfunction. A look at likely mechanisms of symptom generation. Journal of Manipulative and Physiological Therapeutics 21: 267–280

Seidel H M, Bell J W, Dains J E, Benedict G W 1999 Mosby's guide to physical examination. Mosby, St Louis, MO

Seitsalo S, Österman K, Hyvärinen H et al 1990 Severe spondylolisthesis in children and adolescents. Journal of Bone and Joint Surgery – British. 72-B (2): 258–265

Shao Z, Rompe G, Schiltenwolf M 2002 Radiographic changes in the lumbar intervertebral discs and lumbar vertebrae with age. Spine 27: 263–268

Shibata Y, Shirai Y, Miyamoto M 2002 The aging process in the sacroiliac joint: helical computed tomography analysis. Journal of Orthopedic Science 7 (1): 12–18

Shiokawa K, Hanakita J, Suwa H et al 2001 Clinical analysis and prognostic study of ossified ligamentum flavum of the thoracic spine. Journal of Neurosurgery 94 (2 suppl): 221–226

Shirazi-Adl A, Parnianpour M 1999 Effect of changes in lordosis on mechanics of the lumbar spine–lumbar curvatures in lifting. Journal of Spinal Disorders 12 (5): 436–447

Sihvonen T, Lindgren K A, Airaksinen O, Manninen H 1997 Movement disturbances of the lumbar spine and abnormal back muscle electromyographic findings in recurrent low back pain. Spine 22: 289–295

Silver J K, Leadbetter W B 1998 Piriformis syndrome: assessment of current practice and literature review. Orthopedics 21 (10): 1133–1135

Silver I, Li B, Szalai J, Johnston M 1999 Relationship between intracranial pressure and cervical lymphatic pressure and flow rates in sheep. American Journal of Physiology 277 (6 Pt 2): R1712–R1717

Simons D G 1991 Muscle pain syndromes. Journal of Manual Medicine 6: 3–23

Simons D G, Travell J G, Simons L S 1999 Travell & Simons' myofascial pain and dysfunction, the trigger point manual, vol. 1. Upper half of body. 2nd edn. Williams & Wilkins, Baltimore, MD

Singer K P 1989 Thoracolumbar mortice joint: radiological and histological observations. Clinical Biomechanics 4: 137–143

Singer K P, Day R E, Breidahl P D 1989 In vivo axial rotation at the thoracolumbar junction: an investigation using low dose CT in healthy male volunteers. Clinical Biomechanics 4: 145–150

Singer K P, Giles L G F, Day R E 1990 Intra-articular synovial folds of thoracolumbar junction zygapophyseal joints. Anatomical Record 226: 147–152

Siracusano S, Sau G, Aiello I et al 1994 The skin response in evaluation of the sympathetic chains after retroperitoneal lymphadenectomy, preliminary report. Scandinavian Journal of Urology and Nephrology 28 (4): 405–407

Sjolander P, Johansson H, Djupsjobacka M 2002 Spinal and supraspinal effects of activity in ligament afferents. Journal of Electromyography and Kinesiology 12 (3): 167–176

Slosberg M 1988 Effects of altered afferent articular input on sensation, proprioception, muscle tone and sympathetic reflex responses. Journal of Manipulative and Physiological Therapeutics 11: 400–408

Smart L J, Smith D L 2001 Postural dynamics: clinical and empirical implications. Journal of Manipulative and Physiological Therapeutics 24: 340–349

Smith O G, Langworthy S M, Paxson M C 1906 Modernized chiropractic. Lawrence Press, Cedar Rapids, IO

Smith B M, Hurwitz E L, Solsberg D et al 1998 Interobserver reliability of detecting lumbar intervertebral disc high-intensity zone on magnetic resonance imaging and association of high-intensity zone with pain and annular disruption. Spine 23 (19): 2074–2080

Snijders C J, Vleeming A, Stoeckart R et al 1997 Biomechanics of the interface between spine and pelvis in different postures. In: Vleeming A, Mooney V, Dorman T et al (eds) Movement, stability and low back pain, pp. 103–113. Churchill Livingstone, Edinburgh, UK

So Y T, Olney R K, Aminoff M J 1989a Evaluation of thermography in the diagnosis of selected entrapment neuropathies. Neurology 39: 1–5

So Y T, Aminoff M J, Olney R K 1989b The role of thermography in the evaluation of lumbosacral radiculopathy. Neurology 39: 1154–1158

Solinger A B 1996a Equations of motion for the "flopping doctor" model of spinal manipulative therapy. Journal of Manipulative and Physiological Therapeutics 19: 26–31

Solinger A B 1996b The physics of spinal manipulation: a critical review of four articles by Haas [commentary]. Journal of Manipulative and Physiological Therapeutics 19: 141–145

Solinger A B 1996c Oscillations of the vertebrae in spinal manipulative therapy. Journal of Manipulative and Physiological Therapeutics 19: 238–243

Solinger A B 2000 Theory of small vertebral motions: an analytical model compared to data. Clinical Biomechanics 14: 87–94

Solomonow M, Zhou B H, Harris M et al 1998 The ligamento-muscular stabilizing system of the spine. Spine 23: 2552–2562

Solomonow M, Eversull E, Zhou B H et al 2001 Neuromuscular neutral zones associated with viscoelastic hysteresis during cyclic lumbar flexion. Spine 26: E314–E324

Southall J P C (ed.) 1962 Helmholtz's treatise on physiological optics. Translated from the 3rd German edn. Dover Publications, New York, NY

Souza T A 1994 Decision making with scoliosis management. Topics in Clinical Chiropractic (3): 39–54

Souza T A 2001 Differential diagnosis and management for the chiropractor, 2nd edn. Aspen, Gaithersburg

Speldewinde G C, Bashford G M, Davidson I R 2001 Diagnostic cervical zygapophyseal joint blocks for chronic cervical pain. Medical Journal of Australia 174 (4): 174–176

Standaert C J, Herring S A 2000 Spondylolysis: a critical review. British Journal of Sports Medicine 34 (6): 415–422

Standaert C J, Herring S A, Halpern B, King O 2000 Spondylolysis. Physical Medicine Rehabilitation Clinic of North America 11 (4): 785–803

Stanford M R, Gras L, Wade A, Gilbert R E 2002 Reliability of expert interpretation of retinal photographs and the diagnosis of toxoplasma retinochoroiditis. British Journal of Ophthalmology 86 (6): 636–639

Stedman's Medical Dictionary, 27th edn 2000 Lippincott/Williams & Wilkins, Baltimore, MD

Stengel R F, Ghigliazza R, Kulkarni N, Laplace O 2002 Optimal control of innate immune response. Optimal Control Applications and Methods 23: 91–104. Also published as Stengel R F, Ghigliazza R, Kulkarni N 2002 Optimal enhancement of immune response. Bioinformatics 18 (9): 1227–1235

Stephens D, Gorman F 1997 The association between visual incompetence and spinal derangement: an instructive case history. Journal of Manipulative and Physiological Therapeutics 20: 343–350

Stephenson R W 1948 Chiropractic textbook. Palmer School of Chiropractic, Davenport, LA

Stern J T Jr, Jungers W L 1990 The capitular joint of the first rib in primates: a re-evaluation of the proposed link to locomotion. American Journal of Physical Anthropology 82 (4): 431–439

Stevinson C, Ernst E 2002 Risks associated with spinal manipulation. American Journal of Medicine 112 (7): 566–571

Stewart J M 2000 Autonomic nervous system dysfunction in adolescents with postural orthostatic tachycardia syndrome and chronic fatigue syndrome is characterized by attenuated vagal baroreflex and potentiated sympathetic vasomotion. Pediatric Research 48 (2): 218–226

Stewart R 1972 The reality of organisations. Pan Books, London, UK

Stillwagon G, Stillwagon K L, Stillwagon B S, Dalesio D L 1992 Chiropractic thermography. International Review of Chiropractic Jan/Feb: 8–13

Stroman P W, Krause V, Malisza K L et al 2002 Functional magnetic resonance imaging of the human cervical spinal cord with stimulation of different sensory dermatomes. Magnetic Resonance Imaging 20 (1): 1–6

Stubbs D M 1992 The arcuate foramen. Variability in distribution related to race and sex. Spine 17: 1502–1504

Sturesson B 1997 Movement of the sacroiliac joint: a fresh look. In: Vleeming A, Mooney V, Dorman T et al (eds) Movement, stability and low back pain, pp. 171–176. Churchill Livingstone, Edinburgh, UK

Suseki K, Takahashi Y, Takahashi K et al 1997 Innervation of the lumbar facet joints, origins and functions. Spine 22: 477–485

Sviatova G S, Abil'dinova G Zh, Berezina G M 2001 Frequency, dynamics, and structures of congenital malformations in populations under long-term exposure to ionizing radiation [article in Russian]. Genetika 37 (12): 1696–1704

Swärd L, Hellstrom M, Jacobsson B, Peterson L 1990 Back pain and radiologic changes in the thoraco-lumbar spine of athletes. Spine 15: 124–129

Swinkels A, Dolan P 1998 Regional assessment of joint position sense in the spine. Spine 23: 590–597

Swinkels A, Dolan P, Saal J S 2000 Spinal position sense is independent of the magnitude of movement. Spine 25: 98–104, discussion 105

Symons B P, Leonard T, Herzog W 2002 Internal forces sustained by the vertebral artery during spinal manipulative therapy. Journal of Manipulative and Physiological Therapeutics 25: 504–510

Szuba A, Rockson S G 1997 Lymphodema: anatomy, physiology and pathogenesis. Vascular Medicine 2 (4): 321–326

Taimela S, Kankaanpää M, Luoto S 1999 The effect of lumbar fatigue on the ability to sense a change in lumbar position. Spine 24: 1322–1327

Takasita M, Matsumoto H, Uchinou S et al 2000 Atlantoaxial subluxation associated with ossification of posterior longitudinal ligament of the cervical spine. Spine 25: 2133–2136

Tambe A, Monk J, Calthorpe D 2002 "Spinolith": case report of a loose body in the spinal canal. Spine 27: E248–E249

Tamura T 1989 Cranial symptoms after cervical injury. Journal of Bone and Joint Surgery – British 71-B; 2: 283–287

Tan S H, Teo E C, Chua H C 2002 Quantitative three-dimensional anatomy of lumbar vertebrae in Singaporean Asians. European Spine Journal 11 (2): 152–158

Taylor J A M, Resnick D 2000 Skeletal imaging atlas of the spine and extremities, W B Saunders, Philadelphia, PA

Terrett A G J T 1987 The search for the subluxation: an investigation of medical literature to 1985. Journal of Chiropractic History 7 (1): 29–33

Terret A G J 1995a The cerebral dysfunction theory. In: Gatterman M I (ed.) Foundations of chiropractic, subluxation, pp. 340–352. Mosby, St Louis, MO

Terrett A G J 1995b Misuse of the literature by medical authors in discussing spinal manipulative therapy injury [review]. Journal of Manipulative and Physiological Therapeutics 18: 203–210

Terrett A G J T 2002 Did the SMT practitioner cause the arterial injury? Chiropractic Journal of Australia 32: 99–110

Terrett A G J, Terrett R G 2002 Referred posterior thoracic pain of cervical posterior rami origin: a cause of much misdirected treatment. Chiropractic Journal of Australia 32: 42–51

Thunberg J, Hellstrom F, Sjolander P et al 2001 Influences of the fusimotor-muscle spindle system from chemosensitive nerve endings in cervical facet joints in the cat: possible implications for whiplash induced disorders. Pain 91: 15–22

Todres-Masarsky M, Masarsky C, Anrig C A et al 2001 Somatovisceral involvement in the pediatric patient. In Masarsky C, Todres-Masarsky M (eds) Somatovisceral aspects of chiropractic, pp. 203–211. Churchill Livingstone, New York, NY

Tokuhashi Y, Matsuzaki H, Uematsu Y, Oda H 2001 Symptoms of thoracolumbar junction disc herniation. Spine 26: E512–E518

Topinard P 1877 Des anomalies de nombre de la colonne vertebrale chez l'homme. Revue d'Anthropologie 6: 577–649

Toppenberg K S, Hill D A, Miller D P 1999 Safety of radiographic imaging during pregnancy. American Family Physician 59 (7): 1813–1818, 1820

Triano J J 2001a Biomechanics of spinal manipulative therapy. Spine Journal 1 (2): 122–130

Triano J J 2001b The functional spinal lesion: an evidence-based model of subluxation. Topics in Clinical Chiropractic 8 (1): 16–28

Trott P H, Pearcy M J, Ruston S A et al 1996 Three-dimensional analysis of active cervical motion: the effect of age and gender. Clinical Biomechanics 11 (4): 201–206

Troyanovich S J 1997 Anthropometrical and mechanical considerations in determining normal parameters for the sagittal lumbar spine [letter]. Journal of Manipulative and Physiological Therapeutics 20: 420–422

Turk Z, Ratkolb O 1987 Mobilization of the cervical spine in chronic headaches. Manual Medicine 3: 15–17

Ugarriza L F, Cabezudo J M, Porras L F, Rodriguez-Sanchez J A 2001 Cord compression secondary to cervical disc herniation associated with calcification of the ligamentum flavum: case report. Neurosurgery 48 (3): 673–676

Uhtoff H K 1993 Prenatal development of the iliolumbar ligament. Journal of Bone and Joint Surgery – British 75 (1): 93–95

Urban M R, Fairbank J C, Etherington P J, Loh L et al 2001 Electrochemical measurement of transport into scoliotic intervertebral discs in vivo using nitrous oxide as a tracer. Spine 26: 984–990

van der Schans C P, Geertzen J H, Schoppen T, Dijkstra P U 2002 Phantom pain and health-related quality of life in lower limb amputees. Journal of Pain and Symptom Management 24 (4): 429–436

Vanharanta H, Sachs B L, Spivey M et al 1988 A comparison of CT/discography, pain response and radiographic disc height. Spine 13: 321–324

van Oostenbrugge R J, Herpers M J, de Kruijk J R 1999 Spinal cord compression caused by unusual location and extension of ossified ligamenta flava in a Caucasian male. A case report and literature review. Spine 24: 486–488

Van Roy P, Caboor D, De Boelpaep S et al 1997 Left–right asymmetries and other common anatomical variants of the first cervical vertebra. Manual Therapy 2 (1): 24–36

Vasavada A N, Li S, Delp S L 1998 Influence of muscle morphometry and moment arms on the moment-generating capacity of the human neck muscles. Spine 23: 412–422

Vautravers P, Maigne J Y 2000 Cervical spine manipulation and the precautionary principle. Joint, Bone and Spine 67 (4): 272–272

Vernon L F, Cala B M 1992 High-level disc herniations: are they more prevalent that originally thought? Journal of Manual Medicine 6: 205–207

Vilensky J A, Baltes M, Weikel L et al 2001 Serratus posterior muscles: anatomy, clinical relevance, and function. Clinical Anatomy 14 (4): 237–241

Visscher C M, de Boer W, Naeije M 1998 The relationship between posture and curature of the cervical spine. Journal of Manipulative and Physiological Therapeutics 21 (6): 388–391

Vlasuk S L 1991 The role of thermography in the evaluation of lumbosacral radiculopathy. DC Tracts 3: 8–13

Vleeming A, Pool-Goudzwaard A L, Stoeckart R et al 1995 The posterior layer of the thoracolumbar fascia: its function in load transfer from spine to legs. Spine 20: 753–758

Vleeming A, Pool-Goudzwaard A L, Hammudoghlu D et al 1996 The function of the long dorsal sacroiliac ligament: its implication for understanding low back pain. Spine 21: 556–562

Vleeming A, Mooney V, Dorman T et al (eds) 1997a Movement, stability and low back pain. Churchill Livingstone, Edinburgh, UK

Vleeming A, Snijders C, Stoeckart R, Mens J M A 1997b The role of the sacroiliac joints in coupling between spine, pelvis, legs and arms. In: Vleeming A, Mooney V, Dorman T et al (eds) Movement, stability and low back pain, pp. 53–71. Churchill Livingstone, Edinburgh, UK

Vleeming A, de Vries H J, Mens J M, van Wingerden J P 2002 Possible role of the long dorsal sacroiliac ligament in women with peripartum pelvic pain. Acta Obstetricia et Gynecologica Scandinavica 81 (5): 430–436

Vogt L, Banzer W 1997 Dynamic testing of the motor stereotype in prone hip extension from neutral position. Clinical Biomechanics 2 (2): 22–127

von der Weid P Y 2001 Review article: lymphatic vessel pumping and inflammation – the role of spontaneous constrictions and underlying electrical pacemaker potentials. Alimentary Pharmacology Therapeutics 15 (8): 1115–1129

Waddell G 1998 The back pain revolution. Churchill Livingstone, Edinburgh, UK

Walker B F 1998 Most common methods used in combination to detect spinal subluxation. Australian Chiropractic and Osteopathy 7 (1): 109–111

Walter S D 1984 Measuring the reliability of clinical data: the case for using three observers. Revue d'Epidemiologie et de Santé Publique 32: 206–211

Walther D S 1981 Applied Kinesiology. vol. 1 Basic procedures and muscle testing. Systems DC, Pueblo, CO

Wang H A, Davis M J, Rajanayagam M A et al 1999 Myogenic reactivity of rat epineural arterioles potential role in local vasoregulatory events. American Journal of Physiology 2767 (1 Pt 2): H144–H151

Wang J C, Nuccion S L, Feighan J E et al 2001 Growth and development of the pediatric spine documented radiographically. Journal of Bone and Joint Surgery – American 83-A: 1212–1218

Wang M, Dumas G A 1998 Mechanical behaviour of the female sacroiliac joint and influence of the anterior and posterior sacroiliac ligaments under sagittal loads. Clinical Biomechanics 13 (4–5): 293–299

Wardwell W I 1992 Chiropractic – history and evolution of a new profession. Mosby, St Louis, MO

Watson P J, Booker C K, Main C J, Chen C A N 1997 Surface electromyography in the identification of chronic low back pain patients: the development of the flexion relaxation ratio. Clinical Biomechanics 12 (3): 165–171

Wedge J H, Tchang S 1992 Differential diagnosis of low back pain. In: Kirkaldy-Willis W H, Burton C V (eds) Managing low back pain, 3rd edn, pp. 225–241. Churchill Livingstone, New York, NY

Westcott D J 2000 Sex variation in the second cervical vertebra. Journal of Forensic Science 45 (2): 462–466

Whatmore G B, Kohi D R 1968 Dysponesis: a neurophysiologic factor in functional disorders. Behavioural Science 13 (2): 102–124

White A A, Panjabi M M 1978 Clinical biomechanics of the spine. J B Lippincott, Philadelphia, PA

White A A, Panjabi M M 1990 Clinical biomechanics of the spine, 2nd edn. J B Lippincott, Philadelphia, PA

Wight S, Osborne N, Breen A C 1999 Incidence of ponticulus posterior of the atlas in migraine and cervicogenic headache. Journal of Manipulative and Physiological Therapeutics 22: 15–20

Wilke A, Wolf U, Lageard P, Griss P 2000 Thoracic disc herniation: a diagnostic challenge. Manual Therapy 5 (3): 181–184

Wilkinson I M S 1993 Essential neurology, 2nd edn. Blackwell Scientific Publications, Oxford, UK

Willems J M, Jull G A, Ng J K-F 1996 An *in vivo* study of the primary and coupled rotations of the thoracic spine. Clinical Biomechanics 11: 311–316

Williams M, Solomonow M, Zhou B H et al 2000 Multifidus spasms elicited by prolonged lumbar flexion. Spine 25: 2916–2924

Williams P L, Warwick R (eds) 1980 Gray's anatomy, 36th edn. Churchill Livingstone, Edinburgh, UK

Wiltse L L 2000 Anatomy of the extradural compartments of the lumbar spinal canal. Peridural membrane and circumneural sheath. Radiology Clinics of North America 38 (6): 1177–1206

Wiltse L L, Fonesca A S, Amster J et al 1993 Relationship of the dura, Hofmann's ligaments, Batson's plexus, and a fibrovascular membrane lying on the posterior surface of the vertebral bodies and attaching to the deep layer of the posterior longitudinal ligament. An anatomical, radiologic, and clinical study. Spine 18: 1030–1043

Wolfe F, Smythe H, Yunus M et al 1990 The American College of Rheumatology 1990 criteria for the classification of fibromyalgia. Arthritis and Rheumatism 33 (2): 160–172

Wurdinger S, Humbsch K, Reichenbach J R et al 2002 MRI of the pelvic ring joints postpartum: normal and pathological findings. Journal of Magnetic Resonance Imaging 15 (3): 324–329

Wurster R D 1992 Cardiac autonomic control – interaction of somatic and visceral afferents. In: Patterson M M, Howell J N (eds) The central connection: somatovisceral/viscerosomatic interaction. Proceedings of the 1989 American Academy of Osteopathy International Symposium, pp. 266–273. University Classics, Athens OH

Xiong L, Zeng Q Y, Jinkins J R 2001 CT and MRI characteristics of ossification of the ligamenta flava in the thoracic spine. European Radiology 11: 1798–1802

Yahia L H, Rhalmi S, Newman N, Isler M 1992 Sensory innervation of human thoracolumbar fascia. An immunohistochemical study. Acta Orthopaedica Scandinavica 63 (2): 195–197

Yahia L H, Pigeon P, DesRosiers E A 1993 Viscoelastic properties of the human lumbodorsal fascia. Journal of Biomedical Engineering 15 (5): 425–429

Yamamoto A, Nishiura I, Handa H, Kondo A 2001 Ganglion cyst in the ligamentum flavum of the cervical spine causing myelopathy: report of two cases. Surgical Neurology 56 (6): 390–395

Yamashita T, Cavanaugh J M, El-Bohy A A, King A L 1990 Mechanosensitive afferent units in the lumbar facet joint.

Journal of Bone and Joint Surgery – American 72-A (6): 865–870

Yamashita T, Cavanaugh J M, Ozaktay A C et al 1993 Effect of substance P on mechanosensitive units of tissues around and in the lumbar facet joint. Journal of Orthopedic Research 11 (2): 205–214

Yamashita T, Minaki Y, Ozaktay A C et al 1996 A morphological study of the fibrous capsule of the human lumbar facet joint. Spine 21: 538–543

Yeomans S G 2000 The clinical application of outcomes measurement. Appleton & Lange, Stamford, CT

Yingling V R, McGill S M 1999 Anterior shear of spinal motion segments. Spine 24 (18): 1882–1889

Yochum T R, Rowe L J 1996 Essentials of skeletal radiology, 2nd edn, Williams & Wilkins, Baltimore, MD

Yoshii S, Ikeda K, Murakami H 2001 Myxomatous degeneration of the ligamentum flavum of the lumbar spine. Spinal Cord 39 (9): 488–491

Yoshimura N, Dennison E, Wilman C et al 2000 Epidemiology of chronic disc degeneration and osteoarthritis of the lumbar spine in Britain and Japan: a comparative study. Journal of Rheumatology 27 (2): 429–433

Yoshio M, Murakami G, Sato T et al 2002 The function of the psoas major muscle: passive kinetics and morphological studies using donated cadavers. Journal of Orthopaedic Science 7 (2): 199–207

Yrjama M, Tervonen O, Vanharanta H 1996 Ultrasonic imaging of lumbar discs combined with vibration pain provocation compared with discography in the diagnosis of internal anular fissures of the lumbar spine. Spine 21: 5771–5775

Yu H, Hou S, Wu W 1998 The relationship of facet orientation to intervertebral disc protrusion and lateral recess stenosis in lower lumbar spine. Zonghua Wai Ke Za Zhi 36 (3): 176–178

Yunus M B, Inanici F 2001 Clinical characteristics and biopathophysiological mechanisms of fibromyalgia syndrome. In: Baldry P E (ed.) Myofascial pain and fibromyalgia syndromes. A clinical guide to diagnosis and management, pp. 351–377. Churchill Livingstone, Edinburgh, UK

Zachman Z J, Bolles S, Bergmann T F 1989 Understanding the anterior thoracic adjustment (a concept of a sectional subluxation). Journal of Chiropractic Technique Jan/Feb: 30–33

Zapletai J, Hekster R E, Straver J S et al 1995 Association of transverse ligament calcification with anterior atlanto-odontoid osteoarthritis: CT findings. Neuroradiology 37 (8): 667–669

Zawieja D C 1996 Lymphatic microcirculation. Microcirculation 3 (2): 241–243

Zedka M, Prochazka A, Knight B et al 1999 Voluntary and reflex control of human back muscles during induced pain. Journal of Physiology 520 (2): 591–604

Zhang Y, Yu L, Li T K 2002 Clinical anatomy of the fibrous capsule of human lumbar facet joint. Di Yi Jun Yi Da Xue Xue Bao 22 (7): 600–601

Zheng N, Watson L G, Yong-Hing K 1997 Biomechanical modelling of the human sacroiliac joint. Medical Biology and Engineering Computing 35 (3): 77–82

Zhou S H, McCarthy I D, McGregor A H et al 2000 Geometric dimensions of the lower lumbar vertebrae – analysis of data from digitised CT images. European Spine Journal 9 (3): 242–248

Zink G, Lawson W 1979 An osteopathic structural examination and functional interpretation of the soma. Osteopathic Annals 12 (7): 433–440

Zorn M 2002 Implementation of an X-ray radiation protective equipment inspection program. Health Physics 82 (2 suppl): S51–S53

Index

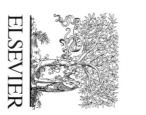
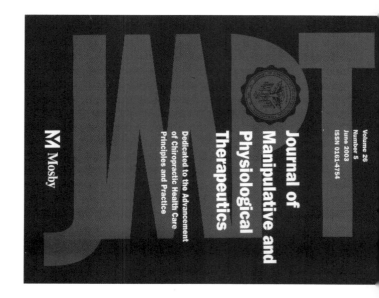